NEW
CHOICES
in
NATURAL
HEALING

NEW CHOICES
in
NATURAL HEALING

Over 1,800 of the Best
Self-Help Remedies
from the World of
Alternative Medicine

Edited by Bill Gottlieb, Editor-in-Chief,
PREVENTION Magazine Health Books

with Susan G. Berg, Senior Copy Editor,
and Patricia Fisher, Senior Managing Editor,
PREVENTION Magazine Health Books

Written by Doug Dollemore, Mark Giuliucci, Jennifer Haigh,
Sid Kirchheimer and Jean Callahan

Rodale Press, Inc.
Emmaus, Pennsylvania

Library of Congress Cataloging-in-Publication Data

    New choices in natural healing : over 1,800 of the best self-help remedies from the world of alternative medicine / edited by Bill Gottlieb, with Susan G. Berg and Patricia Fisher : written by Doug Dollemore... [et al.].
      p.   cm.
    Includes index.
    ISBN 0–87596–257–2   hardcover
    ISBN 0–87596–364–1   paperback
    1. Self-care, Health. 2. Alternative medicine. 3. Medicine, Popular. I. Gottlieb, Bill. II. Dollemore, Doug.
    RA776.95.N48   1995
615.5—dc20   95–15907

Distributed in the book trade by St. Martin's Press

    14   16   18   20   19   17   15   13   hardcover

      4   6   8   10   9   7   5   3   paperback

—— OUR PURPOSE ——

"We inspire and enable people to improve their lives and the world around them."

NOTICE TO OUR READERS

CONTENTS

PART II

NATURAL REMEDIES FOR 160 HEALTH PROBLEMS

CONTENTS

CONTENTS

CONTENTS

ILLUSTRATIONS

PART III

RESOURCES FOR NATURAL HEALING

EDITOR'S INTRODUCTION

You Asked Us for Choices—And Here They Are!

By Bill Gottlieb
Editor-in-Chief
Prevention Magazine Health Books

Dear Reader:

A couple of years ago, the editors at *Prevention* Magazine Health Books met with 20 of you in a "focus group"—an event arranged by companies to find out what their customers like and dislike about their products and what their customers want for the future.

You wanted choices.

You didn't want to be limited to just one kind of doctor—a medical doctor. You wanted to be able to sample from the new field of "alternative medicine," with its broad range of practitioners.

You didn't want to be limited to just one kind of treatment—the medical treatment of a drug or an operation. You wanted to explore the world of natural healing, because you thought those methods might be safer and more effective.

(In fact, you told us that a lot of the medical care you used didn't work and that it sometimes created even more health problems than you started with.)

But you wanted more than a new kind of doctor and a new kind of treatment. You wanted the option to solve your health problems at home.

You were fed up with the arrogance of medical doctors who thought they knew everything and would hardly give you the time of day. Sure, you wanted to go to a doctor for medical problems that were beyond self-care—but you wanted a way to minimize your contact. You wanted, whenever possible, to take care of yourself.

We listened carefully.

We thought about what you said.

And we created a unique and practical book that we hope gives you exactly what you want: *New Choices in Natural Healing: Over 1,800 of the Best Self-Help Remedies from the World of Alternative Medicine.*

Unique, because never before has there been such a large compilation of remedies from such a wide variety of alternative approaches. For every one of the 160 health problems in this book, you'll find one or more *natural choices*: the vitamin, the herb, the acupressure point, the yoga pose, the food, the mental image (to name just a few of the techniques) that can make you feel better.

Practical, because all of the remedies in this book are from health professionals who have used them with their patients and clients and have proved their effectiveness.

You asked us for choices—and we hope this book allows you to make the best choice of all: the choice for better health.

Bill Gottlieb

PART I

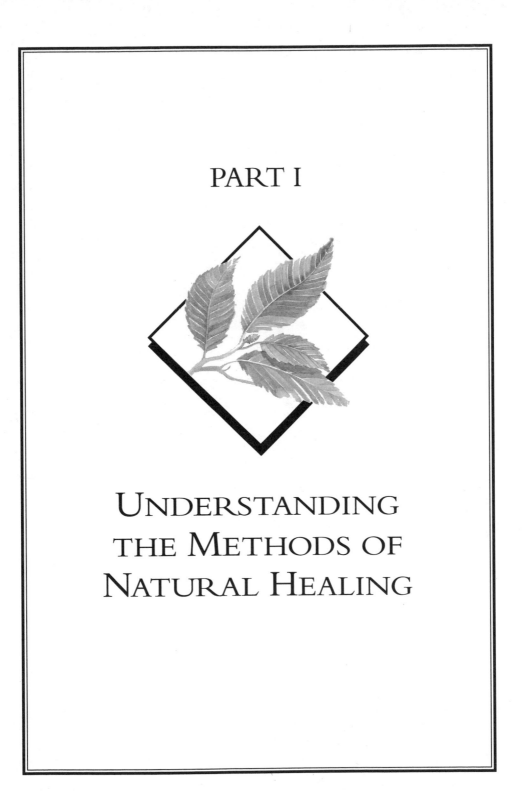

UNDERSTANDING
THE METHODS OF
NATURAL HEALING

THE MOST NATURAL OF REMEDIES

For These, What's Old Is New

From pacemakers to birth control pills, from kidney transplants to artificial hearts, America has an international reputation for making medical breakthroughs.

But even as revolutionary medical techniques continue to make the headlines, another, quieter health revolution is happening in homes across the country. As conventional medicine becomes ever more complicated and costly, a growing number of people are turning to natural healing—simple, traditional, decidedly low-tech methods of preventing illness and solving everyday health problems.

Consider:

- In 1990, Americans made an estimated 425 million visits to alternative health practitioners—more than they made to primary care physicians.
- In 1992, the National Institutes of Health in Bethesda, Maryland, established the Office of Alternative Medicine, which devotes more than $3 million a year to exploring unconventional healing techniques such as meditation, massage, vitamin therapy and herbal therapy.
- In 1993, Americans spent an estimated $1.5 billion on herbal remedies, including teas and supplements. While that's a lot less than the $13.3 billion spent on over-the-counter drugs, it's more than ten times the amount we spend on over-the-counter sleeping pills from grocery stores and drugstores.

MORE FAMILIAR THAN YOU THINK

What's going on here? What do homeopaths and nutritionists, massage therapists and Ayurvedic practitioners have to offer a society that boasts the most advanced medical technology in the world? Why are people flocking to health food stores, with their lotions and potions, and what keeps them going back for more?

"There has been a real shift in the way people think about their health," says Andrew Weil, M.D., a teacher of alternative medicine at the University of Arizona College of Medicine in Tuscon, founding director of the university's Center for Integrative Medicine and a physician emphasizing natural and preventive medicine. "At the same time, they're realizing that conventional medicine is expensive and sometimes dangerous—and not always effective."

While the term *alternative medicine* may conjure up some pretty exotic images, many of these therapies are more familiar than you think. If you've ever massaged your temples to ease a headache, applied an ice pack to a sprained ankle or listened to your car radio to de-stress during a traffic jam, you've already practiced some simple natural healing techniques.

Most of us know we can bolster our diets with vitamin supplements or drink prune juice to avoid constipation. What we may not realize is that these are time-tested therapies and they're usually cheaper, safer and better for what ails us than painkillers, laxatives or after-work cocktails.

Until a few years ago, herbal teas, those age-old remedies for everything from insomnia to morning sickness, were sold mainly in health food stores. Today, you'll find seemingly endless varieties stacked next to the java and hot chocolate in your local supermarket. And a cosmetics company, Origins, uses aromatherapy oils in its Sensory Therapy line, which includes peppermint, wintergreen, cinnamon, licorice and patchouli among its ingredients.

Even mainstream doctors have begun to recommend natural, drugless therapies to treat both everyday complaints and serious illnesses. Dietary modification, for instance, has become the weapon of choice against a number of diseases that would have been treated mainly with prescription drugs a generation ago. "We know that many conditions are caused by the wrong diet and can be reversed by the right diet," says Neal Barnard, M.D., president of the Physicians Committee for Responsible Medicine in Washington, D.C., and author of *Food for Life* and other books on the healing aspects of food. "Heart disease, cancer, weight problems, arthritis, diabetes, high blood pressure—they can all be treated to some degree with foods."

Yoga, once dismissed as a hobby for hippies and double-jointed contortionists, has also been rediscovered. Actress/fitness guru Jane Fonda released a yoga workout video, and yogic breathing and relaxation techniques get a full chapter in the best-selling *Dr. Dean Ornish's Program for Reversing Heart Disease*.

The wide appeal of the Ornish program, which includes relaxation, meditation and emotional sharing in support groups as well as exercise and dietary changes, suggests that many people are ready for a more holistic approach to health.

"Western thought has always regarded the mind and body as separate entities," says Dennis Gersten, M.D., publisher of *Atlantis*, a bi-monthly imagery newsletter, and a San Diego psychiatrist whose therapies include techniques such as guided imagery, nutritional counseling and meditation as well as medication. If needed, Dr. Gersten will refer patients for treatment with a homeopath, an acupuncturist, a chiropractor, an Ayurvedic practitioner or an orthopedic surgeon. "A holistic approach means recognizing that the mind and the spirit have a direct, powerful effect on how the body functions," he says.

NATURAL HEALING THROUGH THE AGES

While natural therapies have been described as the wave of the future, they're actually much older than Western treatments such as surgeries and antibiotics. Experts estimate that herbal remedies and Ayurveda, the traditional medicine of India, have been around for 5,000 years. Ancient Egyptians used fragrant oils in what may have been an early version of aromatherapy, and hydrotherapy was practiced in ancient Greece and Rome. And homeopathy, one of the newest techniques, is more than 200 years old.

Homeopathy, in fact, was as big as allopathy, the type of medicine practiced by conventional doctors, in the early nineteenth century, according to David Edelberg, M.D., an internist and medical director of the American Holistic Center/Chicago, one of the largest alternative treatment facilities in the country. He says that "there were dozens of 'eclectic' medical colleges in the nineteenth century, which taught an approach to medicine that ultimately became naturopathy," a type of medicine still practiced today that uses a number of alternative techniques, including homeopathy, acupuncture, massage, hydrotherapy, nutritional counseling and herbal and vitamin therapies.

It wasn't until the early twentieth century, the golden age of drug development, that Americans developed the attitude that good health was found in the medicine chest. "Technological medicine made some incredible advances in the first half of the century," says Dr. Weil. In light of lifesaving discoveries such as penicillin and the Salk polio vaccine, it seemed only reasonable to assume that scientists would one day develop similar "wonder drugs" to wipe out cancer, heart disease and other dread diseases.

"It wasn't long, though, before people realized that technology creates as many problems as it solves," says Dr. Weil.

A prime example is the widespread use of antibiotics, which has given rise to strains of bacteria that are highly resistant to most drugs in the conventional arsenal, says Sheila Quinn, association manager of the American Association of Naturopathic Physicians, a Seattle-based organization that provides information on naturopathic medicine and referrals to naturopathic physicians. While antibiotics have saved millions of lives, they haven't really solved problems such as tuberculosis, which is turning up in new forms that don't respond to conventional therapies, Dr. Edelberg says.

THE MOST NATURAL OF REMEDIES

"The naturopaths are really on to something," says Dr. Edelberg. For example, instead of prescribing an antibiotic to wipe out an infection, a naturopathic physician might prescribe a combination of natural remedies to attack the infection but then will also try to determine which factors in the patient's daily life—such as stress, poor nutrition or inadequate exercise—made him susceptible to the illness in the first place. Natural healers may use a combination of juices, vitamin and mineral supplements, dietary changes and other therapies to build up the immune system, the body's natural defense against infection. And as the immune system becomes stronger, antibacterial and antiviral herbs and homeopathic preparations can be used to zero in on the infection.

COMPLEMENTARY MEDICINE

That's not to say that alternative treatment should be a substitute for conventional medicine. Most alternative health practitioners believe that the best care involves considering all options, including conventional medicine. "Good holistic doctors recognize that regular medicine really is best in certain areas, especially emergency situations," says Dr. Gersten. "Using an inhaler during an attack can save the life of someone with asthma. What it can't do is improve the condition in the long term. That's where other treatments come in."

One area where alternative treatment is particularly helpful is the managing of stress, which has been implicated in a wide range of conditions, from allergies and skin problems to gastrointestinal disorders and heart disease. Meditation, sound therapy and touch therapies such as massage and reflexology offer simple, practical techniques to keep stress at bay.

In the United Kingdom, where natural techniques are better known and more widely used than in the United States, they're called complementary therapies, which both conventional physicians and alternative practitioners seem to like. "In some ways it's a better name," says Dr. Edelberg. "It illustrates the proper place of these therapies: side by side with conventional medical treatment."

And while some in the medical community have been slow to accept unconventional treatments, there are a number of indications that these attitudes are changing. "Physicians are intellectually curious," says Dr. Edelberg. "We've had M.D.'s call and visit from all over the country, and many have wanted to rotate here to spend a few days talking to the practitioners."

This willingness to consider alternative therapies is also beginning to spread to the health insurance industry. A few large carriers have started to experiment with covering alternative treatments. A pilot program at Mutual of Omaha, for instance, covers the Dean Ornish cardiac rehabilitation program, and Blue Cross of Washington has a policy that covers naturopathy and homeopathy. But no carrier has made a greater commitment to natural healing than the American Western Life Insurance Company of Foster City, California. The company's Wellness plan covers naturopathic treatments, including Ayurveda, homeopathy, nutritional counseling, massage and physical therapy.

"We were looking for a cost containment mechanism, not a new philosophy," says Lisa WolfKlain, an American Western vice-president who oversees the Wellness plan. But in researching ways to cut health care costs, American Western discovered naturopathy. Today, the company maintains a full-time Wellness Line, staffed by trained naturopathic doctors who answer clients' health care questions.

Premiums for the Wellness plan are about 20 percent lower than for the company's traditional plans, says WolfKlain, "because we believe very strongly that if people do take care of themselves, if they take preventive measures, it's going to save us all a lot of money in the long run."

While the Wellness plan has more than 2,000 subscribers, it's offered in only five western states. For more information on coverage for alternative treatments, contact your insurance company.

THE BACK-TO-NATURE MOVEMENT

Interest in natural healing has been increasing since the 1960s, says Dr. Edelberg. "It was a combination of the anti-establishment tenor of the 1960s and President Nixon's 1974 visit to China, which led to a loosening of immigration laws for people coming from the East," says Dr. Edelberg. "In this country, you had a very curious, open-minded group of young people who were already interested in natural living. Suddenly, there were thousands of Asians immigrating with their own culture and medical background. Americans were very interested, particularly in California."

But while the back-to-nature movement may have started out as a West Coast phenomenon, people across the country are exploring natural therapies in record numbers, says Gene BeHage, vice-president of marketing for General Nutrition Center (GNC), a nationwide chain of health food stores. GNC is the largest specialty retailer of herbs, health foods and vitamin and mineral supplements in the nation. The Pittsburgh-based company has 1,900 stores across the country, up from 800 ten years ago.

MEDICINE FOR A NEW CENTURY

Why the recent surge in interest? Rising health care costs may be a factor, says BeHage. "People are taking more control of their destinies as far as health is concerned," he says. "They have to, because with the cost of health care, they can't afford not to."

At the same time, more and more Americans have been affected by newly discovered chronic degenerative diseases such as AIDS and chronic fatigue syndrome, conditions that Western medicine can't cure. "Conventional medicine doesn't do all that well with chronic illnesses, which are definitely on the increase," notes Dr. Edelberg. Many patients with chronic fatigue, arthritis or irritable bowel syndrome either aren't helped by medication, he says, or experience such severe side effects that they stop treatment altogether.

"Conventional doctors often tell patients to learn to live with these problems, but for a 32-year-old woman with irritable bowel who doesn't want to live with diarrhea and stomach cramps for the next half-century, that's just not acceptable," says Dr. Edelberg. "People are willing to try unconventional treatments because they want to get well."

Many patients are also attracted to the alternative practitioner's emphasis on treating the whole person—mind, body and spirit. Ayurvedic practitioners treat patients according to mind/body type, believing that true healing depends on balancing physical, mental and emotional influences. Flower remedy/essence therapy is chosen to even out emotional imbalances, which, therapists believe, are at the root of most physical problems. And holistic physicians such as Dr. Edelberg use intensive counseling to help patients find out whether aspects of their daily lives, such as job stress, marital problems, diet or sleeping habits, might be behind their symptoms.

In this age of managed care and impersonal group practices, patients find this individualized approach particularly appealing, says Dr. Gersten.

"It's definitely a reaction to how depersonalized allopathic medicine has become," says Dr. Gersten. "It wasn't always this way. The family doctor of a century ago was really a holistic doctor. He knew three generations of the family, and he knew that the mother's diabetes got worse when the teenager acted up. He saw the big picture. That's something conventional medicine has definitely lost."

TAKE CONTROL OF YOUR HEALTH

Finally, whether they're changing their diets or relaxing with meditation, patients who take the natural approach report feeling more in charge of their health.

This is one of the principal goals of natural healing, says WolfKlain. "The whole idea is to break the cycle of dependency, to get people well and keep them out of the doctor's office when it's not necessary. Many people go to the

HOW TO USE THIS BOOK

The book you're holding is a potent natural medicine—a concentrated collection of hundreds of ways for you to feel better. And like any potent medicine, you need some simple instructions on how to "take" it so that it's maximally effective. You need to know how to use this book.

Obviously, when using this book you'll probably turn first to Part II, "Natural Remedies for 160 Health Problems," to find remedies for the health problem that's bothering you (or someone you care about).

You can use any of those remedies right away, of course. But you'll notice that almost all of the individual remedies refer you to a chapter in Part I of this book, "Understanding the Methods of Natural Healing." You may want to read that chapter *before* you use the remedy. So for example, if you have arthritis and you've decided to try the Ayurvedic remedy for the disease, you may want to read the Ayurveda chapter first. If you've decided to try juicing, you may want to read the juice therapy chapter first. If you've decided to try a homeopathic remedy, you may want to read the homeopathy chapter first. (You get the idea.) You don't have to read these chapters first—in fact, you don't have to read them at all—but reading them may make you a more informed (and perhaps more successful) user of the natural remedies in this book.

(Of course, feel free to read *all* of these chapters before you use the remedies in *New Choices in Natural Healing*. Each chapter is a fascinating guide to a particular "country" in the varied world of alternative healing.)

The remedy may also ask you to turn to a page in the illustration section in Part II. Some of the remedies involve exercises that we've illustrated, and we've put all of these illustrations together in one part of the book for your reading convenience.

Finally, you may want more information about the alternative methods discussed in this book. Or certain remedies that the book suggests may not be readily available, and you may have to order them through the mail. For this, please turn to Part III, "Resources for Natural Healing." You will find a complete listing of organizations, sources of mail-order products and books for each of the 16 natural healing methods that are covered in this book.

And here's a final "instruction" for using *New Choices in Natural Healing*: Use it in good health!

doctor with a victim mentality: 'Here, I'm a body, take care of me.' Instead, we want them to ask how they can take care of themselves."

Alternative practitioners admit that this approach isn't for everyone. "There are plenty of people who think 'I don't want to change my life. I don't want to hear that my job is giving me a coronary. Just give me a pill for it,' " says Dr. Edelberg. "We send these patients back to conventional physicians, who will probably do just that."

"Changing behavior is hard," says Quinn. "Alternative practitioners are better at helping people change behavior because that's what their training emphasizes and because they spend more time getting to know the patient—body, mind and spirit."

ACUPRESSURE

Let Your Fingers Do the Healing

Y ou've probably heard of acupuncture, or seen a photo of someone receiving the treatment—looking a bit like a human pincushion, with dozens of little needles sticking out of his body.

But how much do you know about acu*pressure*?

With acupressure, you use finger or hand pressure instead of needles. But its goal is the same as acupuncture's: to stimulate what Chinese medical practitioners call chi—the body's most basic healing energy.

Acupressure is the older, original technique, a Chinese home remedy that gave rise to the more "technological" approach of acupuncture. (In much the same way, the herb willow bark was the predecessor of aspirin.)

Many American physicians and health professionals say that both of these techniques are powerful methods for pain relief and disease treatment.

"But acupressure can be even more powerful than acupuncture for relieving everyday aches, pains and stress," says Michael Reed Gach, Ph.D., director of the Acupressure Institute in Berkeley, California, and author of *Acupressure's Potent Points*. Those common complaints include headaches, backaches, sinus pain, neck pain, eyestrain and menstrual cramps, he says. Acupressure can also reduce the pain of ulcers, help heal sports injuries, relieve insomnia and alleviate constipation and other digestive problems.

Another advantage of pressure over puncture is that you can do it yourself—all you need are your hands, a little knowledge and some time. It's also cheap—free, in fact, once you've learned the basics. And it's simple and safe. If you use common sense, the only thing you can do wrong is be a little too vigorous.

Ready to let your fingers do the healing? Well, before you use the acupressure remedies in this book, you might enjoy reading a bit more about the theory and practice of the technique itself. Think of the rest of this chapter as a tour of an exotic foreign country—your body, as understood by Chinese medicine and as healed by acupressure.

THE INSTINCT OF HEALING

"Acupressure is as old as instinct," says Dr. Gach. "When your head hurts, you rub your temples. When your stomach aches, you bend over and hold the place where it hurts."

11

THE MANY FLAVORS OF ACUPRESSURE

Ice cream is one food, but it has lots of flavors. It's the same with acupressure. It's one technique with a lot of varieties. Here are your choices.

Do-in. This system of stretches, breathing, exercises and acupressure techniques is great for beginners. You can use do-in every day as a kind of acupressure workout.

Acu-yoga. This method uses yoga postures for the purpose of pressing many acupressure points with your whole body instead of with just your hands. It's meant for use at home. The yoga stretches are particularly helpful when you want to work on your back and other hard-to-reach places. (For more on yoga, see page 150.)

Jin Shin Jyutsu. This is a Japanese form of self-help acupressure that involves gentle touching or cradling of the body rather than massagelike movements. The goal of Jin Shin Jyutsu is to harmonize body, mind and spirit by touching 26 "safety energy locks" found along energy pathways in the body. Sessions can include a series of touches or can be as simple as the holding of one finger.

Shiatsu. This technique, also from Japan, involves rhythmic pressing of acupressure points for short periods, from three to ten seconds. The thumbs are used whenever possible, because they can exert firmer pressure than the fingers. Shiatsu, which means "finger pressure" in Japanese, tends to be more vigorous than acupressure.

Zen shiatsu. Zen is a form of Buddhism that originated in Japan, and it often involves strenuous practices such as hours of meditation a day. Zen shiatsu is also strenuous, adding yogalike stretches to help open the meridians. Health professionals who practice this technique also apply heavy pressure, using their full body weight when they press the points. This isn't an at-home technique.

Barefoot shiatsu. No, this isn't a massage you receive with your shoes off. You use your feet to rub and press the points. Practitioners say this method delivers more pressure.

Some of these acupressure therapies are do-it-yourself; some require a qualified professional. But if you choose to visit a health professional who practices acupressure, make sure he is properly certified or licensed. (Look for a degree such as C.A.T., which indicates that the practitioner is adequately trained.) And ideally, just as when you go to a dentist or a doctor for the first time, it's always best to have a recommendation from a friend or relative who has used the practitioner's services. Refer to the resource list on page 631 for organizations that will help you locate an acupressurist.

Acupressure

"These are ancient peasant remedies," says Betsy Ruth Dayton, founder of High Touch Network, a professional organization in Friday Harbor, Washington, whose members practice acupressure. "Women used these techniques when their kids were sick. Neighbors gave each other treatments. They were gifts anybody could afford to give."

These basic human impulses—to touch, to heal—were combined in China with the principles of traditional Chinese medicine, which has as its original text the nearly 4,000-year-old *Yellow Emperor's Classic of Internal Medicine*. In that text, and over the next two millennia, Chinese doctors discovered a system of channels and points on the body that, if correctly touched or stimulated, would relieve pain and speed healing.

The traditional Chinese doctors said these channels, called meridians, were the invisible wires that conducted the body's chi, or energy. If these channels were disturbed—if the energy flowing through them was too slow or too fast, too turbulent or too static—the body's chi was said to be imbalanced. The goal of traditional Chinese medicine was to restore chi to a state of balance, and acupressure (along with diet, herbs, deep breathing, gentle exercises and other methods) was one of its techniques.

"If a person is totally healthy—mentally, emotionally and physically—energy will flow through the body freely, like electricity is conducted through circuits," says Dayton. "But none of us is totally healthy. We all experience disease, injury and emotional trauma. And there are environmental assaults, too, such as air pollution and noise. You can use acupressure to rebalance or unblock the energy that flows through your body, so your body can begin to heal itself."

And you can use acupressure not only to ease your aches and pains but also to prevent the development of illnesses, says Subhuti Dharmananda, director of the Institute for Traditional Medicine in Portland, Oregon.

You can also use acupressure to feel better mentally and spiritually, Dayton says.

How to Be a Block Buster

If a block in your body is physical, such as a swollen ankle, you can use acupressure to tone muscles and improve circulation in the injured area. As you gently press acupressure points on the ankle, the muscle tension lessens as the muscle fibers relax and lengthen, and blood flows more freely to the injury. The swelling goes down, and the pain goes away.

Pressing on the points can also free an emotional block by releasing the accumulated tension you hold in your body, says Dayton. In this book, you'll find points on your back, near your shoulder blades, that can relieve sadness and depression and points on your wrists and in the center of your forehead that can quell anxiety, according to Ayurveda experts.

Even spiritual blocks, such as difficulty meditating, can be relieved with acupressure. Lightly holding a point at the center of your forehead just above the bridge of your nose for one minute with your eyes closed is a wonderful way to help you enter a meditative state, says Dr. Gach. And he says that pressing two points underneath the base of the skull called the Gates of Consciousness not only helps relieve headaches but also makes you more receptive to spiritual wisdom.

Those are only a few of the dozens of acupressure points. Where are the rest?

Well, imagine that your body is a big city, the meridians are the subway lines and the points are the subway stops. In acupressure, there are 14 main subway lines, with 365 stops. But don't worry about getting lost. You'll find simplified maps of the most important self-care points beginning on page 564.

We don't want you to feel like an out-of-towner, however. So here's a little bit more about meridians and points.

GO WITH THE FLOW

First, there are 12 major meridians, each of which is connected to a specific organ, such as the stomach or spleen. Six of these meridians—lung, heart, pericardium, liver, spleen and kidney—flow up the front of the body. Six others—small intestine, large intestine, bladder, stomach, gallbladder and triple warmer—run down the back. (Don't worry if you've never heard of your triple warmer organ; you don't have one. The Chinese system identifies some connections in the energy system that don't fit the conceptual framework of Western medicine.)

There is another set of meridians, called the eight extraordinary channels, that run through the body in routes not directly related to the major organs. Acupressure points are located on two of these meridians. One, called the governing channel, links the spinal column, brain and nervous system and runs from the tailbone at the base of the spine up the back and over the top of the head to the center of the upper lip. The other, called the conception channel, is linked to the digestive and reproductive systems and flows from the head to the perineum (the space between the anus and the genitals).

In this book, the names of the meridians have been abbreviated. Each acupressure point is identified by the abbreviation of its meridian and a specific number. (In Chinese medicine, the points have poetic names such as Sea of Tranquillity, Wind of Heaven and Welcoming Perfume.) So LI 4, for example, means point 4 on the large intestine meridian, while St 36 is point 36 on the stomach meridian. (For a list of these abbreviations, see "Shorthand for the Meridians.")

SHORTHAND FOR THE MERIDIANS

In this book, the names of the 14 major meridians, or energy channels, have been abbreviated. Here they are.

ABBREVIATION	MERIDIAN	ABBREVIATION	MERIDIAN
B	Bladder	Lu	Lung
CV	Conception vessel (channel)	Lv	Liver
		P	Pericardium
GB	Gallbladder	SI	Small intestine
GV	Governing vessel (channel)	Sp	Spleen
H	Heart	St	Stomach
K	Kidney	TW	Triple warmer
LI	Large intestine		

You'll find that the acupressure remedies usually combine points near the area of pain or tension with points that seem to have no obvious connection to the immediate problem. Chinese medicine calls the nearby points local points and the faraway points trigger points. Trigger points work because the meridian pathways connect the points.

APPLYING PRESSURE THAT'S JUST RIGHT

How do you turn your fingers and hands into healing instruments? It's easy, but you'll need some basic guidelines: how hard to press, how long, when to knead, when to maintain a constant, light pressure and when to rub. Dr. Gach says you always need to use both common sense and your intuition for what kind of touch you need to apply.

But the basic acupressure technique is: Use firm pressure. To apply the pressure, you can use your thumbs, fingers, palms or knuckles, depending on what is easiest and most comfortable for you. (When you're applying pressure with one finger, the middle finger is usually the best choice, since it's the longest and strongest.)

The general guideline, according to Dr. Gach, is that pressure should be firm enough to "hurt good." In other words, the sensation should fall somewhere between pain and pleasure. Don't be a masochist; the point of acupressure isn't to cause pain. But don't be a wimp, either; if you're too gentle, you won't do yourself any good.

Most acupressure points occur in symmetrical pairs—that is, one point is on the left side of your body, and the other is in the same location on the right side of your body. Both points in a pair should be pressed simultaneously, when possible. So if you're working the Lu 1 points on your chest, for example, you should use your thumbs to press the points on both sides of your chest at the same time. Some pairs of points—such as the LI 4 points, which are located in the webbing between the thumb and index finger of each hand—can't be stimulated this way, so you need to work first one point, then the other. "Working both sides balances your body and increases the effectiveness of acupressure," says Dr. Gach.

To relax an area or relieve pain, first press the points gently for 30 seconds. Increase the pressure until it's quite firm, holding it for one to three minutes. Then release slowly and gently, again taking about 30 seconds to gradually come off the points.

When you're working on acupressure points in a large muscle group, such as the muscles in your shoulders or calves, kneading is often an excellent warm-up before using acupressure. Use your thumbs and fingers and the heels of your hands to knead the points as well as the areas around them, just like you would knead dough to make bread. But always be gentle. You don't want to injure yourself.

Quick tapping with the fingertips stimulates muscles that are located just under the surface of the skin. Work gently on acupressure points on sensitive parts of the body, such as the face and abdomen, and on areas where there is very little cushioning between skin and bone, such as the top of the head, recommends Cindy Banker, co-founder of the New England Shiatsu Center in Boston and education director for the American Oriental Bodywork Therapy Association.

If you're using acupressure to work on a chronic health problem or to relieve muscle tension, be persistent and consistent. Acute conditions such as a flare-up of back pain or shoulder tension may require acupressure two or three times a day. Even after you've obtained relief, weekly pressure point stimulation can help prevent recurrences.

Brisk rubbing in general, and especially on the acupressure points, helps in-

THE FIVE-MINUTE ACUPRESSURE WORKOUT

You exercise a few times a week to keep your muscles and circulatory system in shape. But how do you keep your energy system in shape? How do you keep your chi flowing? With an acupressure workout, of course.

Like a regular workout, this routine is best done at least three days a week, but if you can do it every day, or even twice a day, that's great. And it doesn't take long—just five minutes. It was adapted from the book *Acupressure's Potent Points* by Michael Reed Gach, Ph.D., director of the Acupressure Institute in Berkeley, California. The acupressure points described in this workout can be found in the illustrations beginning on page 564.

Begin your workout by sitting in a chair in a comfortable position with your spine straight. Then:

- Find the Sea of Vitality points (B 23 and B 47) on your lower back. Place the backs of your hands along both sides of the spine. Rub briskly up and down for one minute, feeling a warmth from the friction.
- Place your middle and index fingers under one side of the base of the skull, using the thumb of the same hand on the other side to gently press the Gates of Consciousness points (GB 20) at the base of your skull. With the middle finger of your other hand, gently press the Third Eye point (GV 24.5) for a couple of minutes before slowly releasing all points. Tilt your head back comfortably, close your eyes and take three long, slow, deep breaths.
- Now keep breathing deeply as you do a quick mental survey of your body to locate tension. Let the tension stream out of your body with each exhalation until you feel your body release any tightness. Continue breathing deeply for a minute or two; with each inhalation, imagine healing energy flowing into your body.
- Hold the Sea of Energy point (CV 6), three finger-widths below your navel on your lower abdomen. Sit straight with your shoulders relaxed. Close your eyes, press this point firmly and breathe deeply for one minute.

crease blood flow. You can use that technique to warm up your body if you're feeling cold, Dr. Gach says. This technique can be especially beneficial for the bedridden or for older people with sluggish circulation.

For an energizing acupressure workout, try applying pressure to a series of points for short periods of time—say, five to ten seconds each.

You don't have to be an expert to use your hands as healing tools either on yourself or on others. A hug or a pat on the back can be shared with family and friends; so can acupressure.

"We live in a touch-deprived culture," says Banker. "I think this is one of the reasons why we have so much domestic violence and so much depression among the aged. I've done treatment on elderly people who haven't been touched in a caring or meaningful way in 30 years. You'd be amazed at how quickly the pulse decreases and how the body relaxes just a few minutes into the treatment."

AROMATHERAPY

The Power of 'Scentual' Medicine

I t's good for you."
  Tell this to anyone who's about to brave the dentist's chair or the doctor's examination table, and he'll expect nothing short of pain and suffering.

Tell this to anyone who's about to try aromatherapy, and odds are he won't expect a lavender-scented bath or a cup of tea that tastes like peppermint candy. But these fragrant, pleasurable treatments are typical of aromatherapy, a system of caring for the body with botanical oils such as rose, lemon, lavender and peppermint. Whether they're added to a bath or massaged into the skin, inhaled directly or diffused to scent an entire room, these natural, aromatic oils have been used for nearly a thousand years to relieve pain, care for the skin, alleviate tension and fatigue and invigorate the entire body.

AROMATHERAPY THROUGH THE AGES

While no one called it aromatherapy until the late 1920s, aromatic plants have played an important role in maintaining health for several thousand years. "Ancient Egypt was a very fragrant civilization," says John Steele, an aromatic consultant in Los Angeles. "They infused fragrant oils for massage, bathing and medicine, burned incense in religious ceremonies and used aromatic cedar oil to embalm their dead."

But it wasn't until the eleventh century A.D. that European healers began working with essential oils, potent, highly volatile liquids extracted from plants through distilling or squeezing. The most concentrated, therapeutic form of the plant, an essential oil isn't greasy, like mineral oil. It is more like water in texture, evaporates quickly and penetrates the skin easily.

Essential oils were introduced to Europe by crusaders returning from the East. Valued for their antiseptic properties, these oils were burned in homes and public buildings during the bubonic plague in hopes of stopping the disease from spreading. Legend has it that glove makers, who used essential oils in their craft, enjoyed special protection from the plague.

Eclipsed by the development of synthetic drugs in the late 1800s and early 1900s, the tradition of healing with aromatics was revived in the 1920s and 1930s by René-Maurice Gattefossé, the French chemist who first coined the term *aromatherapy*.

But while aromatherapy has been popular in Europe for many years—essential oils are available in many French drugstores, and pharmacists are often trained in their uses—it wasn't until the late 1980s that Americans began to discover this fragrant medicine. "When I wrote my book *Herbs and Things* in 1969, my editors took 'aromatherapy' out of the index because nobody knew what the word meant," says San Francisco herbalist Jeanne Rose, chairperson of the National Association for Holistic Aromatherapy and author of *Aromatherapy: Applications and Inhalations*, a practical guide to using aromatherapy at home.

Twenty-five years later, "aromatherapy" still isn't a household word, but essential oils have been discovered by top-selling cosmetic companies such as Estée Lauder and the Body Shop, and aromatherapy creams and oils are showing up everywhere from department store cosmetics counters to the Home Shopping Network.

"People are feeling the need to take their health into their own hands," says Judith Jackson, a Greenwich, Connecticut, aromatherapist and author of *Scentual Touch: A Personal Guide to Aromatherapy*. "They're looking for ways to help themselves that are natural and without side effects. And if the treatment has an element of pleasure as well, so much the better."

THE SENSE OF SMELL

Essential oils work on the body on several different levels. The most obvious is by stimulating the powerful but little understood sense of smell.

In recent years, medical research has uncovered what aromatherapists have always known: that the odors we smell have a significant impact on the way we feel.

"Smells act directly on the brain, like a drug," says Alan Hirsch, M.D., a neurologist, a psychiatrist and director of the Smell and Taste Treatment and Research Center in Chicago.

In the course of treating patients who have lost the sense of smell, Dr. Hirsch has found that a life without fragrance seems to lead to a high incidence of psychiatric problems such as anxiety and depression.

And while most depressed, stressed-out people can smell just fine, Dr. Hirsch believes that their emotional states are also affected by the odors they are—or aren't—smelling.

Scientific research supports the notion that smelling particular odors has a direct effect on brain activity. "We know from brain wave frequency studies that smelling lavender increases alpha waves in the back of the head, which are associated with relaxation," says Dr. Hirsch. "An odor such as jasmine increases beta waves in the front of the head, which are associated with a more alert state."

And since most people can detect many different odors, the potential therapeutic uses of smell seem endless. Experts say that inhaling essential oils can benefit many conditions linked to nervous tension, including headaches, insomnia and anxiety. Inhalations are also used to treat respiratory complaints such as colds, allergies and bronchitis.

Experiencing the mood–altering power of scent can be as simple as adding several drops of essential oil to your bath or placing a couple of drops of essential oil on a scent ring, which sits on a warm lightbulb. A longer-lasting way to scent a room is with an aroma lamp, a porcelain or clay pot in which essential oils are mixed with water and heated over a candle, or an electric aromatic diffuser, which reduces essential oils to a fine spray and disperses the scent throughout the room. These are sold in some health food stores and through mail order (refer to the resource list on page 633).

MORE THAN MEETS THE NOSE

But fragrance isn't the only way that essential oils work on the body. " 'Aromatherapy' is actually a very bad name," says Galina Lisin, a European-trained aromatherapist and president of Herba-Aromatica in Hayward, California. "Essential oils have never been used in perfumes. They're medicines, and inhalation is only one of many ways they can be used."

Essential oils are also effective when used topically. "Unlike mineral oils, which just hang around on the skin, essential oils are made up of very small mol-

SOME WORDS OF CAUTION

When used wisely, essential oils are less likely to cause side effects than most over-the-counter drugs. But experts still advise using caution. In general, people with fair or freckled skin are more likely to experience skin irritation from essential oils, says Los Angeles aromatic consultant John Steele. He advises all first-time users to perform a simple skin test to avoid allergic reactions: Place a drop of the oil on a cotton swab and apply it to the inside of the wrist or to the inner elbow. Cover with a bandage and don't wash the area for 24 hours. If no itching or redness occurs, the oil should be safe for external use.

Pregnant women should take particular care in using essential oils. The essential oils calamus, mugwort, pennyroyal, sage and wintergreen can induce miscarriage when taken internally, but even inhalation and topical application are strongly discouraged. Basil, hyssop, myrrh, marjoram and thyme can also cause adverse reactions and should be avoided as well.

Tea tree oil is safe to use by the drop, but should never be ingested. Amounts as small as one teaspoon can be fatal if swallowed.

ecules that actually penetrate through the skin into the blood system," says Steele.

Topical application is used to treat a wide range of skin problems, and essences are popular ingredients in skin care products and other cosmetics. Mild essential oils such as lavender can even be applied full strength, or "neat," to treat cuts, burns, headaches and other simple first-aid conditions.

"For the layperson, there aren't many essential oils I would recommend using neat on the skin," says Steele. "Even a trained aromatherapist can't always predict who will have an allergic reaction to an essential oil, so using them diluted provides an extra measure of safety." While an essential oil diluted in a carrier oil is less quickly absorbed into the skin, many experts prefer this method because it guards against skin irritation. "A rule of thumb is that more is not always better with essential oils," adds Steele.

Another topical use of essential oils is aromatherapy massage. When added to traditional massage oils such as almond, olive and sesame, essential oils enhance the benefits of massage, relieving stress, improving circulation and creating a feeling of well-being.

While European medical doctors also administer essential oils orally, in suppositories and even transdermally (as in a patch on the skin), experts recommend consulting a medically trained aromatherapist before taking any oils internally. Steele also advises that you learn about essential oils before using them, since some aren't recommended for certain conditions. (For more information on using essential oils safely, see "Some Words of Caution" on page 21.)

USING AROMATHERAPY

To explore the healing power of aromatherapy, begin in your local health food store. Essential oils vary widely in price and quality: A ½-ounce vial of lavender oil, for example, can set you back as little as $7 or as much as $15, depending upon its purity and where it's produced. The most popular home care oils retail at $5 to $16 per five-milliliter bottle, says Steele, but because essential oils are highly concentrated, a small quantity can last for months with normal use. (If you have trouble finding essential oils in your area, try one of the mail-order companies that specialize in aromatherapy supplies. Refer to the resource list on page 633.)

Experimenting with aromatherapy shouldn't cost a fortune. By investing in a few versatile, inexpensive essential oils, you can try many of the remedies in this book and explore basic aromatherapy massage. (See "Essential Oils for Beginners.")

Because many applications involve blending essential oils with other ingredients, you'll also need a few glass or hard plastic bottles to store the mixtures in.

ESSENTIAL OILS FOR BEGINNERS

Don't be put off by the confusing array of essential oils available from dealers. You can begin to explore the benefits of aromatherapy at home with only a handful of inexpensive oils, says Los Angeles aromatherapist Michael Scholes of Aromatherapy Seminars, an organization that trains professionals and others in the use of essential oils. Scholes recommends the following six oils for their safety, versatility and value.

Citrus oils. Great for dispelling a somber mood, citrus oils work well in a diffuser and create a bright, uplifting atmosphere, says Scholes. Lemon, lime, orange and grapefruit oils can be had for $3 to $5 for five milliliters, says Los Angeles aromatic consultant John Steele, while mandarin goes for about $5 to $6.

Floral oils. They're the best for stress relief, according to Scholes. "Aesthetically, most people find florals the most appealing." He suggests adding florals to unscented lotions and bath oils or mixing them with carrier oils for a soothing massage. While rare, precious floral oils such as rose and jasmine can be pricey—a tiny, ⅓-ounce bottle of rose oil imported from Turkey can cost over $175, for instance—the same quantity of geranium, which smells very much like rose, costs only $10.

Lavender. "If there is one oil no home should be without, it's lavender," says Scholes. An excellent first-aid oil, lavender soothes cuts, bruises and insect bites and can also be added to your usual bath oil for a relaxing, stress-relieving soak. Average price: $5 to $6.50 for a five-milliliter bottle.

Peppermint. This is a great mental stimulant, says Scholes, who recommends adding a drop to an unscented facial lotion and applying the lotion under the nose or behind the ears. Peppermint can also help your stomach: Add a drop, mixed with a teaspoon of honey, to a cup of herbal tea to ease intestinal discomfort, suggests Scholes. (Honey is added to help quickly disperse the essential oil within the water.) Average price: $5 for five milliliters.

Rosemary. An invigorating oil for low-energy days, it works well in an aroma lamp or a diffuser, says Scholes. "You can also inhale right from the bottle," he adds. Average price: $3 to $4 for five milliliters.

Tea tree. A versatile antiseptic and very gentle to the skin; Scholes suggests applying a single drop directly to the skin to speed the healing of cuts and pimples. Average price: $5 for five milliliters.

And since light can damage essential oils, experts recommend using tinted glass bottles and storing them in a cool, dark place. Stores that sell essential oils often sell bottles as well, as do many mail-order houses.

Finally, whether you are serious about learning aromatherapy or just enjoy discovering new fragrances, experts say a home diffuser is a great investment. "A year ago, you couldn't buy a good diffuser for under $150," says Rose. "But the market is getting more competitive every year, and diffusers are now in the price range of the average American." Rose herself uses a $40 electric diffuser from the Maryland mail-order company Phybiosis. (See the resource list on page 633.) "The diffuser is a must for respiratory treatments," says Rose, who suffers from asthma. "And it makes a great alarm clock! I run mine on a timer, so I can wake up to whatever scent I like."

AYURVEDA

5,000 Years Old—And Still Going Strong

What do Santa Claus, Dan Rather and Diana Ross have in common? Each typifies one of the three doshas, which are Ayurveda's guide to human nature and health. Santa Claus, a jolly, generous, round-bellied soul, is a good example of the earthy kapha dosha. Hard-driving journalist Dan Rather makes his living asking piercing questions, a perfect profession for the incisive pitta dosha. And with her creative gifts and exotic demeanor, Diana Ross is the epitome of the vata dosha's airy exuberance.

To understand doshas, the cornerstone of Ayurvedic diagnosis and treatment, think first of the more familiar Western body types: ectomorph (light and slim), endomorph (heavy and soft) and mesomorph (husky and muscular). The definitions of the doshas begin with similar physical descriptions, then add layers of information about emotional tendencies, intellectual styles and spiritual inclinations, creating a detailed portrait of each type of individual.

Learning about your dosha is like getting a medical exam and a psychological test at the same time. When you understand your dosha, say Ayurvedic practitioners, you can make diet and lifestyle changes that will help you live a healthier, longer and happier life—and maybe even achieve spiritual illumination.

"The most important thing to know about Ayurveda is that it treats the whole person, not just the person's health problems," says Robert E. Svoboda, B.A.M.S., an American who graduated from the Tilak Ayurveda Mahavidyalaya, an Ayurvedic school in Pune, India, and who now works with the Ayurvedic Institute, a training center in Albuquerque, New Mexico. "It isn't just about clearing up symptoms or even curing disease. It's also about restructuring the content of a person's consciousness so that he can be aware of the essential nature and meaning of life."

Ayurveda experts trace the beginning of this unique approach to physical health, mental clarity and spiritual fulfillment to the sages of ancient India, the rishis. They say the rishis discovered the principles of Ayurveda while in deep meditation. The principles were then codified in the Vedas (which means "knowledge"), the essential religious texts of Hinduism, which scholars say are more than 5,000 years old. There are the Rig Veda, the Sama Veda, the Yajur Veda and the Atharva Veda, which is the origin of Ayurveda.

Imagine one of the books of the Old Testament being a treatise on every practical detail of achieving physical, mental and emotional balance in order to

HOW TO MAKE GHEE

Many Ayurvedic home remedies use ghee, or clarified butter, as a primary ingredient. The following recipe is from Vasant Lad, B.A.M.S., M.A.Sc., director of the Ayurvedic Institute in Albuquerque, New Mexico, a native of India and one of the few classically trained Ayurvedic practitioners teaching in the United States. The mixture produces enough to last for several weeks. Store in a tightly closed container on the kitchen shelf. Ghee does not need refrigeration, and according to Ayurvedic practitioners, the cooking process burns off the cholesterol.

- Melt two pounds of unsalted butter in a heavy saucepan over medium heat.
- As soon as the butter begins to boil and foam, reduce the heat to a simmer. Keep the melted butter at a steady simmer until it is golden in color and no foam remains on top.
- Stir occasionally after the whitish curds sink to the bottom. When these curds turn light tan, the ghee is ready.
- Cool the mixture and strain it into a sterile quart jar. Discard the curds from the bottom, as they are almost pure cholesterol.

perfect the individual's relationship with the Divine Power, and you'll have a sense of the breadth and depth of Ayurveda.

DYING MACHINE OR LIVING LIGHT?

What's the difference between the Ayurvedic approach to health and the typical approach found in America and other countries of the Western world? According to proponents of Ayurveda, their discipline sees the body as a material expression of divine intelligence, while Western medicine sees the body as a kind of machine with parts. The arteries to the heart are clogged? Take some arteries out of the leg and attach them to the heart. Or replace the heart with a new one. Or put a part-specific substance, a drug, in the machine to keep the machine running in spite of its being broken. But no matter how the machine is fixed, it eventually wears out and stops.

Philosophically, the ideas at the foundation of Western medicine are called deterministic and materialistic, and they're based on nineteenth-century Newtonian physics, which said that reality is composed of pieces of matter that bounce into each other like balls on a billiard table.

But the physics of the twentieth century—the physics of Einstein known as quantum physics—paints a very different picture of reality. You know its central formula: $E = mc^2$. What this formula means is that all matter is nothing but a dense version of energy or light. And this energy or light is an eternal substance that never dies but that constantly changes into many forms. Surprisingly, this is the same point of view of those sages from India who discovered Ayurveda. But, say twentieth-century Ayurveda experts, these sages went one step further. They also said that this energy or light is alive and intelligent—in fact, that it is the Divine Life Force and Creative Intelligence. And then they went a final step: They said that the Divine Life Force and Creative Intelligence are also the essential nature of the individual—and that realizing this essential nature is the purpose of life.

Realizing the essential nature of reality allows one to make any change in the forms of reality, such as increasing the health of the body or the emotional and mental well-being of the mind, says Deepak Chopra, M.D., author of the best-sellers *Quantum Healing* and *Ageless Body, Timeless Mind* and many other books on Ayurveda.

"Because the intelligence of the universe and the intelligence of the self are the same, the new physics turns out to be a great support for (the idea) . . . that reality can be changed once you reach the level of the self," says Dr. Chopra in *Creating Health*, another of his books on Ayurveda. "The universe and the human organism are united at the level of intelligence."

One of those changes, for example, is the ability to prolong life—to make it more like energy or light, more immortal and less mortal. "I've seen yogis in India who have lived to be 300 and 400 years old," says Vasant Lad, B.A.M.S., M.A.Sc., director of the Ayurvedic Institute, a native of India and one of the few classically trained Ayurvedic practitioners teaching in the United States. (Dr. Lad's B.A.M.S. degree from the prestigious University of Pune in India is equivalent to an M.D. in the United States. In India, a classically trained Ayurvedic practitioner spends five years in medical school and then a year or more in internship, which is equivalent to a Western residency.)

Aging is "a mistake of the intellect," says Dr. Chopra in his book *Perfect Health*. "This mistake consists of identifying oneself solely with the physical body."

DOSHAS AND INDIVIDUAL CONSTITUTION

One of the core ideas of Ayurveda is that the fundamental energy of life expresses itself through the three doshas we discussed earlier—vata, pitta and kapha. (For a description of each one, see "All about Vata, Pitta and Kapha" on page 28.) Every person has a different mixture of doshas; usually, one dosha is predominant, and another is secondary. According to Ayurveda, your doshas
(continued on page 30)

ALL ABOUT VATA, PITTA AND KAPHA

To understand Ayurveda, it's essential to know something about each of the doshas. Once you understand this system, guessing whether someone is a vata, pitta or kapha is irresistible. And fun.

The following descriptions of the three doshas are from Vasant Lad, B.A.M.S., M.A.Sc., director of the Ayurvedic Institute in Albuquerque, New Mexico, a native of India and one of the few classically trained Ayurvedic practitioners teaching in the United States. They'll help acquaint you with the characteristics of vata, pitta and kapha. To pinpoint your own dosha, take the test in "What's Your Dosha?" on page 33.

VATA

Vata people are creative, quick-witted and resourceful. Associated with the elements of space and air, vatas are active and alert and enjoy being on the move. Like the wind, vata people are light, cool, clear, exuberant and expansive. Vatas can be quite soft-hearted and romantic. They are seldom very good at managing money. Physiologically, vata people tend to be thin, with curly hair, dry skin and prominent bones. Thrown off balance, they can be nervous and fearful.

With an overabundance of vata, people get spacey, irresponsible, ungrounded, out of touch with life's earthier aspects. Vata energy is based in the colon, and vatas are prone to conditions such as flatulence, tics and twitches, aching joints, dry skin and hair, nerve disorders, constipation and anxiety. Vata energy is strongest during the fall season.

Maintaining a routine is crucial to vata's good health. Vata people are particularly sensitive to sugar, alcohol and drugs and should use these substances sparingly, if at all. Cold foods aren't the best choice for vatas, especially during the fall and winter. If you're a vata, you're advised to stay away from ice cream and other cold sweets. Choose warming foods and spices, and limit your intake of raw foods. You can eat some salads and raw vegetables in summer, preferably at lunchtime, when digestive fire, which Ayurveda calls agni, is strongest. Vatas thrive in warm, coastal climates.

PITTA

Pitta people are fiery, determined, strong-willed and passionate. They are tough-minded, clearheaded, enthusiastic and ambitious and can be quite successful. Pittas work well under pressure and can be courageous in emergencies. Out of balance, the pitta temper can be scary, however. Un-balanced pittas fly off the handle, scream and lash out, criticize and judge. Or they seethe in private and develop ulcers. The pitta dosha combines the elements of fire and water. Think of diving into the ocean on a hot summer's day at the beach. That's pitta intensity.

Anyone with red hair and freckles is probably pitta. Blondes are fre-quently pitta, too, as are those with prematurely gray hair. But pittas can also have dark hair. Of all of the doshas, pittas most easily maintain weight proportionate to height because of their strong metabolisms. Pitta is based in the small intestine, and pittas tend to have efficient di-gestive systems. (A little pitta energy is essential for everyone, since any-thing that enters the body, from food to new ideas to new experiences, must be digested.)

Pittas can be fad followers, moving quickly from one passion to the next. They often are very good at making money but not so good at ac-cumulating wealth. Pittas like to spend money as fast as they make it.

Summer is pitta season, and problems such as sunburn and poison ivy typify pitta's tendency to develop skin rashes and outbreaks. Pittas are also prone to burning sensations such as ulcers, to fevers and to inflammations and irritations such as conjunctivitis, colitis and sore throats. At meno-pause, pitta women may have the most trouble with hot flashes.

The optimal pitta diet emphasizes cooling foods such as cottage cheese, mint tea, oatmeal, basmati rice and sweet-tasting fruits. Pittas often love to eat hot, spicy foods but should do so only rarely, because spicy foods aggravate pitta's natural fire.

While vatas may skip meals because they simply forget to eat, pittas al-ways know when it's time for dinner. Everyone needs to eat regularly, but pittas are most adamant about doing so. The best place for pittas to live is in cool climates where seasons visibly change. New England, for instance, is prime pitta territory.

KAPHA

Kaphas are sensuous, strong, calm, soft-spoken and forgiving. They tend to have well-developed bodies with big but not prominent bones. Hair is plentiful, usually dark and wavy or curly. Kaphas frequently have oily complexions and large, soulful eyes. Of all of the doshas, kaphas have

(continued)

ALL ABOUT VATA, PITTA AND KAPHA—Continued

the most trouble keeping their weight proportionate. Vatas worry and fidget themselves skinny. Pittas burn off the pounds with their fiery energy. But sweet, self-satisfied kaphas can turn into couch potatoes who kick back and pack on the pounds.

At their best, kaphas are wise, relaxed, tolerant and loyal. Connected to the elements of earth and water, kaphas are usually well-grounded, fluid and able to accept changes. Down-to-earth and good-humored, they can make wonderful friends and excellent hosts. But when their energy goes out of whack, kaphas become greedy, possessive and selfish. While their tendency to live in the present is advantageous to their spiritual development, their deep, abiding attachments to people and things can be obstacles on the spiritual path.

Kapha energy dominates in winter and early spring, and some of the diseases kaphas are most vulnerable to are associated with those seasons. Kaphas can be more susceptible to colds and flus, sinusitis and headaches. Kaphas frequently suffer seasonal allergies. Their metabolisms can be sluggish, making them feel tired, gain weight easily and retain water.

The good news for kaphas is that if they eat sensibly and exercise regularly, their natural strength and endurance give them an advantage for living long, healthy lives. A good kapha diet emphasizes pungent, bitter and astringent foods. Kaphas can safely use plenty of spices but are advised to stay away from sweet foods and follow a low-fat diet.

From the financial perspective, kaphas are the most likely to build up wealth. They're good at making money and at saving it. Kaphas thrive in the desert or in mountainous regions, as long as the weather is moderate to warm. New Mexico is a great place for kaphas to live.

are determined at the moment of conception, when the vata, pitta and kapha from your parents' bodies unite to create your constitution, which Ayurveda calls prakruti. Of course, the constitution you were born with is affected by day-to-day factors such as your work, the people you spend time with and the foods you eat. That daily constitution is called vikruti. The way to have a healthy vikruti is to keep your doshas balanced, so no single one of them becomes too active or too inactive.

There are many Ayurvedic remedies in this book. But Ayurveda says that one of the main ways to keep your doshas balanced is through diet. Vatas, for instance, fare best on a diet that includes what in Ayurveda are considered "sweet" foods such as rice, breads and pasta, "sour" foods such as yogurt, grapefruit and aged cheese and salty foods such as . . . well, anything salty. Pittas need to eat sweet foods as well as "bitter" foods such as leafy greens and "astringent" foods such as beans and peas. Kaphas, say Ayurveda, feel best when they emphasize bitter, astringent and "pungent" foods, which means anything hot and spicy such as jalapeño peppers and dry mustard.

If you don't eat according to your dosha, says Ayurveda, you create imbalances. Kaphas who eat lots of sweet foods may develop diabetes. Pittas who eat too many spicy foods may develop heartburn. Vatas eating astringent foods may develop gas, constipation or insomnia.

But Ayurveda says there are many signs and symptoms of an imbalanced state of the doshas. When vata is out of balance, for instance, it may lead to dry skin, joint pain, constipation, insomnia, fear, anxiety and insecurity. An aggravated kapha can produce a cold, congestion, a cough, poor appetite, water retention, greed and possessiveness. Too much pitta can cause heartburn, nausea, diarrhea, hives, rash, anger, hate and envy.

HOW TO FIND AN AYURVEDIC PRACTITIONER

In the United States, there are very few properly trained Ayurvedic practitioners, says Dr. Lad. But there has been growing interest in both the philosophy of Ayurveda and in the practical details of Ayurvedic self-care. Dr. Lad says that Westerners are attracted to the integration of body, mind and spirit that Ayurveda teaches, to the peace its meditative practices offer and to the elegant mystery of its ancient wisdom.

In America, interest in Ayurveda has also been sparked by the work of Dr. Chopra, who has popularized Ayurvedic teachings through his books, television appearances, audiotapes and seminars.

There are, however, no licensing procedure and no accrediting board for Ayurvedic practitioners in the United States. Courses in Ayurveda are offered at various centers here and in Canada and Europe, but in the United States, graduates can only consult with clients, not practice medicine.

If you're interested in exploring Ayurvedic therapies, choose a practitioner who combines Western medical training with Ayurvedic training or coordinate Ayurvedic consultations with your regular M.D., suggests Scott Gerson, M.D., an internist in New York City who has studied Ayurveda in India and is an Ayurvedic consultant.

"Modern Western medicine works best when surgery or some other acute intervention is necessary," says Dr. Gerson. "Ayurveda may serve better for the treatment of some chronic conditions and as preventive medicine."

That's because Ayurveda treats the causes of health problems, not the symptoms. Dr. Lad says that Westerners who try Ayurveda are usually pleased with the attention that this health care system pays to what mainstream doctors might consider to be insignificant minor symptoms or psychosomatic complaints, such as flatulence or sensitivity to cold foods.

Ayurveda can provide simple, effective treatment for chronic problems such as dizziness, fatigue, digestive complaints and tension headaches—problems that tend to frustrate Western medicine.

THE DAILY ROUTINE OF AYURVEDA

If you're not in the care of an Ayurvedic practitioner but would like to try out Ayurveda's health care philosophy, you can begin with some simple lifestyle changes that are part of the optimal Ayurvedic routine.

- Rise early—by 6:00 A.M., if possible.
- Meditate for at least 20 minutes once or twice each day.
- Keep your diet simple. A vegetarian or modified vegetarian diet is best. Make lunch the major meal of the day and eat a light dinner early in the evening, preferably between 5:00 and 6:00.
- Take short walks after meals to aid digestion.
- Get to bed early—ideally, by 10:00 P.M.

Ayurvedic treatments are usually simple, involving lifestyle changes that can be made at once or gradually. One of the hardest things for Westerners when they first try Ayurveda is "the necessity to take personal responsibility for changing a lifestyle that causes disease," says Dr. Svoboda.

Eating foods because they are good for you rather than because they taste good is one such adjustment, he says. Rising early and going to bed early is another, as is learning to meditate.

"People spend so much time on crutch activities," Dr. Svoboda says, "doing things that help them avoid their feelings." He says Ayurveda urges you to face your feelings, to look at your life and make constructive changes, so you may journey farther along the road to optimal physical, emotional and spiritual health.

WHAT'S YOUR DOSHA?

This test, from *A Woman's Best Medicine: Health, Happiness and Long Life through Ayurveda* by Nancy Lonsdorf, M.D., Veronica Butler, M.D., and Melanie Brown, Ph.D., will help you learn your dosha. Try taking it twice: once with general traits in mind to determine your prakruti, and again, thinking about how you feel right now, for a reading of your vikruti.

Evaluate your constitutional traits as you've observed them throughout your lifetime, using the following rating system and putting a number in each blank.

0 = Doesn't describe me at all
1 = Describes me a little
2 = Describes me quite well
3 = Describes me almost perfectly

	VATA	PITTA	KAPHA
1. My hair texture tends to be	__ Dry, curly, wavy, shiny	__ Straight, fine	__ Thick, full of body
2. My hair color is	__ Medium or light brown	__ Blond or reddish tone, early gray	__ Dark brown, black
3. My skin tends to be	__ On the dry side	__ Delicate, sensitive	__ Oily, smooth
4. My complexion (when compared with others of my race) is	__ Darker	__ More reddish, freckled	__ Lighter
5. Compared with others of my height, I have	__ Smaller bones	__ Average-size bones	__ Larger bones
6. My weight is	__ Thin; I don't gain easily	__ Average	__ Heavy; I gain easily

(continued)

WHAT'S YOUR DOSHA?—Continued

	VATA	PITTA	KAPHA
7. My energy level	___ Tends to fluctuate, to come in waves	___ Is moderate or high; I can push myself too hard	___ Is steady
8. Regarding temperature, I	___ Dislike cold, am comfortable in the heat	___ Dislike heat, perspire easily, thrive in winter	___ Dislike damp cold, tolerate extremes well
9. My typical hunger level	___ Can vary from excessive to no interest in food	___ Is intense; I need regular meals	___ Is usually low but can be emotionally driven
10. I prefer my food/drink	___ Warm, moist, oily	___ Cold	___ Warm, dry
11. I generally eat	___ Quickly	___ Moderately fast	___ Slowly
12. My sleep is most often	___ Interrupted, light	___ Sound, moderate	___ Deep, long; I am slow to waken
13. My dreams often include	___ Flying, looking down at the ground, mountains, chase scenes	___ Fire, waterfalls, battles, fights	___ Oceans, clouds, romance
14. My resting pulse rate (in beats per minute) is			
FOR WOMEN	___ 80–100	___ 70–80	___ 60–70
FOR MEN	___ 70–90	___ 60–70	___ 50–60

	VATA	PITTA	KAPHA
15. My sexual interest is	__ Strong when romantically involved, low to moderate otherwise	__ Moderate to strong	__ Slow to awaken but sustained, generally strong
16. I am most sensitive to	__ Noise	__ Bright light	__ Strong odors
17. My emotional moods	__ Change easily; I'm very responsive	__ Are intense; I'm quick-tempered	__ Are even; I'm slow to anger
18. My general reaction to stress is	__ Anxious, fearful	__ Irritated	__ Mostly calm
19. With regard to money, I	__ Am easy and impulsive	__ Am careful, but I spend	__ Tend to save, accumulate
20. My way of learning is	__ To learn quickly, enjoy more than one thing at a time; I can lose focus	__ To focus sharply, discriminate, finish what I start	__ To take my time, tend to be methodical
21. I learn new material best by	__ Listening to a speaker	__ Reading or using visual aids	__ Associating it with another memory
22. My memory is	__ Best in the short term	__ Good overall	__ Best in the long term
23. My way of speaking is	__ Quick, often imaginative or excessive	__ Clear, precise, detailed, well-organized	__ Soothing, rich with moments of silence

(continued)

WHAT'S YOUR DOSHA?—CONTINUED

	VATA	PITTA	KAPHA
24. If there was one trait to best describe me, it would be	__ Vivacious	__ Determined	__ Easygoing
25. Regarding my relationships, I	__ Easily adapt to different kinds of people	__ Often choose friends on the basis of their values	__ Am slow to make new friends but am forever loyal
26. My family and friends might prefer me to be more	__ Settled	__ Tolerant	__ Enthusiastic
27. This evaluation made me feel	__ Indecisive	__ Annoyed	__ Sleepy
	VATA	PITTA	KAPHA
TOTALS	____	____	____

ASSESSING YOUR SCORE

If one column total is 15 or more points higher than the other two column totals, this is clearly your dominant constitutional type—vata, pitta or kapha. If two of the column totals are 0 to 15 points apart, you are a dual-dosha constitutional type—vata-pitta (or pitta-vata), pitta-kapha (or kapha-pitta) or vata-kapha (or kapha-vata). And if all three column totals are within 0 to 10 points of each other, you are a tri-dosha constitutional type.

FLOWER REMEDY/ ESSENCE THERAPY

Power for Mind and Body

When a friend is sick, recovering from surgery or grieving the loss of a loved one, our first response is to send flowers. Whether because of their vibrant colors or their lovely fragrances, flowers seem to have a therapeutic effect when we're fighting illness, fatigue or flagging spirits.

But for some alternative practitioners, flower power goes way beyond stimulating the senses. For anyone who practices flower remedy/essence therapy, a system of natural medicine that uses remedies distilled from blooming plants and trees, flowers are nature's gentle tools for treating and preventing disease.

Healing with flowers isn't a new idea. Early societies, from those in ancient Egypt and Rome to many Native American tribes, used flowering plants for medicinal purposes.

The modern tradition of healing with flowers began with Edward Bach, an English physician. In the early 1930s, Dr. Bach discovered that many of his patients displayed various emotional and psychological difficulties before the onset of physical disease. (He also noted that those same responses, such as fear, anger, jealousy and anxiety, would *complicate* physical disorders, making them more difficult to treat.) Concerned about the side effects of drugs, Dr. Bach searched in nature for a solution to the problem of *emotional* healing, eventually discovering 38 flowering plants and trees that alleviated a wide range of emotional and psychological difficulties. Today, these 38 "flower remedies" are used worldwide.

"The main reason for the failure of modern medicine is that it is dealing with results and not causes," Dr. Bach wrote in 1931. True healing, he believed, involves treating the cause of the suffering—emotional and mental imbalances.

For Dr. Bach, who died in 1936, finding the right remedy to correct a particular emotional or mental imbalance was a combination of intuition and clinical research. For several days before discovering a new remedy, Dr. Bach would often experience the emotional symptoms the remedy was to treat. By placing different flower petals in his hand or on his tongue and observing their effects, Dr. Bach believed he could tell which flower would be most able to stabilize a particular emotional or physical state.

CHOOSING THE ESSENCES

For modern men and women accustomed to Western medicine's emphasis on symptoms, the idea that emotions such as grief and jealousy could lead to acne, heartburn or worse takes some getting used to.

"Many people are uncomfortable with the idea that their attitudes and emotions create health problems, because it makes them feel as if their illnesses were their fault," says Lynda Hamner, M.D., an Ayurvedic practitioner in Leavenworth, Washington, who uses the 38 flower remedies. But she believes these attitudes are changing. "Now that studies have shown the connection between emotional stress and heart disease, people are beginning to recognize and respect the link between body and mind."

Flower remedies are not directly used to treat physical conditions, says herbalist Leslie J. Kaslof, author of *The Traditional Flower Remedies of Dr. Edward Bach*, but "physicians note that when emotional and psychological stress are stabilized, functional and other disorders, which have strong emotional and psychological components as their underlying causes, often resolve themselves or can be treated more easily."

"It's not enough to recognize your physical symptoms; you have to get to know yourself on a deeper level," says Patricia Kaminski, co-director of the Flower Essence Society, a Nevada City, California, organization that studies and promotes the therapeutic use of flower remedies/essences.

HOW DO THEY WORK?

Though the exact way in which the flower remedies/essences work is not yet understood, some researchers think the substances stimulate the brain to release neurochemicals that alter emotions such as fear, anger and anxiety. The result, they say, is a strengthening of the body's innate ability to heal itself.

As Kaslof points out, it's a theory that is as difficult to prove as it is to refute. "It may be some years before science is capable of measuring the kinds of subtle changes we're talking about," he says.

Flower remedy/essence therapy has developed an enthusiastic following, first in Europe and more recently in North America. The Flower Essence Society is in touch with more than 30,000 professionals and laypeople worldwide who use flower remedies/essences as a healing modality. They include naturopathic and holistic doctors who use the remedies/essences along with herbs, nutritional therapy and homeopathy, medical doctors and dentists who use them in tandem with conventional treatment and individuals interested in preventive medicine for themselves and their families.

A CAUTION FOR PREGNANT WOMEN

All flower remedy concentrates contain a very small amount of alcohol as a preservative, says Leslie Kaslof, an herbalist and author of *The Traditional Flower Remedies of Dr. Edward Bach*. But even though many experts say it's unlikely alcohol would be harmful in such a small dosage, Kaslof recommends that pregnant women consult a health professional before using a flower remedy.

Besides the 38 Bach remedies, some practitioners also use the essences of flower species native to California, many of them traditional Native American cures. These essences are distilled in a manner similar to the one Dr. Bach used and, like the Bach flowers, are prescribed according to the mental and emotional state of the patient.

USING THE REMEDIES/ESSENCES

Part II of this book recommends flower remedies/essences to treat over 40 conditions. The remedies/essences are available in some health food stores or may be ordered directly from the manufacturer (refer to the resource list on page 635). Sold in a highly concentrated form, they can be given in one-fourth of a glass of water and sipped at intervals—first thing in the morning, before meals and at bedtime—or diluted in a separate dosage bottle before using. Because only a few drops of the remedy or essence are needed, a 10.5-milliliter bottle (retail price: approximately $8 to $9) can last three to six months depending on use, according to Kaslof.

In cases where there seems to be more than one emotional issue at the root of a physical problem, two or more flower remedies/essences can be combined in one-fourth of a glass of water and sipped at intervals or diluted in a single dosage bottle. Experts advise using two to four drops of each remedy/essence.

But don't overdo it. Mixing several remedies/essences—say, six or more—may be confusing, because it's impossible to tell which substance is having an effect.

"In general, up to six remedies can be used in combinations," says Kaslof. "However, when more are indicated, I often suggest reducing the number by having people deal with the most pressing emotional issues first and using one remedy at a time whenever possible."

WHAT TO EXPECT

For those accustomed to the quick action of prescription drugs and over-the-counter medicines, using flower remedies/essences takes patience. Kaslof estimates that most people see results in 1 to 12 weeks, depending on each person's sensitivity and type of emotional difficulty. He also cautions that for those conditions or symptoms requiring medical attention, or if symptoms persist, a qualified health professional should be consulted.

"The remedies aren't quick fixes," he emphasizes. "For example, if you have trouble sleeping one night, a sleeping pill can put you out in a matter of minutes—but there's no guarantee that you won't have the same problem again the next night. If you take the right flower remedy when indicated, you're addressing the underlying cause of your problem. It may take a few weeks, but your chances for a long-term solution are much better."

The action of the remedy/essence is quite subtle. "You might not be sure the remedy is working until you discover one day that your attitude toward and relationship to prior difficulties have changed," says Kaslof.

This gentle action makes flower remedies/essences ideal for home use. Unlike many pharmaceutical drugs, the flower remedies/essences aren't habit forming; they can be taken for as long as needed, until the individual feels his emotional issues have been resolved. The flower remedies/essences have a self-diminishing effect. As the individual moves closer to resolving conflicts, the need for and the effectiveness of the remedy/essence diminish.

DR. BACH'S STRESS-RELIEVING FORMULA

In addition to the 38 remedies and the North American essences, many flower therapists use the emergency stress relief formula, a blend of five remedies developed by Dr. Bach for use in everyday stress and emergency situations. Legend has it that Dr. Bach discovered the formula while treating a shipwrecked sailor, who had washed up on the beach near his laboratory in Cromer, England. After being treated with a blend of three remedies—Rockrose, Clematis and Impatiens—the sailor regained consciousness and later recovered.

The modern version of this formula, which also contains the remedies Cherry Plum and Star-of-Bethlehem, has been used for everything from stage fright to insect bites, from temper tantrums to labor pains. Marketed under brand names such as Calming Essence, Rescue Remedy and Five-Flower Formula, this blend is said to have a calming, balancing effect on people and even on animals in distress.

"The formula is not a substitute for medical attention. In emergencies and other circumstances requiring medical attention, one should seek the help of a qualified health professional," says Kaslof. "The remedy can be of great assistance in stabilizing emotional stress in a crisis, which may help ease physical symptoms." Practitioners use the formula to help treat conditions as acute as an angina attack or as benign as Monday morning lethargy.

The emergency formula can be particularly helpful for patients grieving over a divorce or the death of a loved one, according to Eve Campanelli, Ph.D., a holistic family practitioner in Beverly Hills, California. And Cincinnati dentist William Westendorf, D.D.S., has used it for the past ten years to soothe tense, fearful patients. "People experience a lot of anxiety when they go to see the dentist," says Dr. Westendorf. "I use the formula in conjunction with the usual anesthesia, and my patients—especially the children—are noticeably more relaxed."

The emergency formula may be used as often as needed in a crisis situation; some of Dr. Campanelli's patients use it every half-hour. It is taken directly from the bottle by placing four drops under the tongue. Some manufacturers also produce it in cream form, to be applied topically to injuries including, but not limited to, sprains, muscle aches, minor burns and cuts, bruises, insect bites and even tension headaches.

FOOD THERAPY

Beating Disease with Eating

No doubt there were those who thought Hippocrates was behind the times back in 400 B.C., when the so-called father of modern medicine said "Let food be your medicine and medicine be your food." And more than a few probably considered lightbulb-inventing visionary Thomas Edison to be a tad dim for his claim that "the doctor of the future will give no medicines but will interest his patients in the care of the human frame, in diet and in the causes of disease."

Heck, even you snickered when that wisest voice of all, Mom's, boasted of the curative powers of homemade chicken soup or nagged you to eat more vegetables.

So who's laughing now?

Not the statisticians. After all, the numbers they report are some frightening food for thought: Four of the ten leading causes of death in the United States—heart disease, cancer, stroke and diabetes—are linked to the way we eat. Diet also is increasingly being implicated as the cause of or a contributing factor to scores of other ailments, from acne to arthritis, from hair loss to hearing loss, from premenstrual syndrome to postnasal drip.

The experts aren't laughing, either. "What's really tragic about this is that we were so busy learning how to fix broken arms, deliver babies and do all of those 'doctor' things in medical school that we considered nutrition to be boring," says Michael A. Klaper, M.D., a nutritional medicine specialist in Pompano Beach, Florida, and director of the Institute of Nutritional Education and Research, an organization based in Manhattan Beach, California, that teaches doctors about nutrition and its relationship to disease. "But after we get into practice, we spend most of the day treating people with diseases that have huge nutritional components that have long been essentially ignored. I frequently get calls from doctors across the country saying that their patients are asking questions about nutrition and its role in their conditions and they don't know what to tell them."

Now, after decades of depending on drugs and high-tech surgery, more Americans are finally heeding the words of Hippocrates, Edison and dear ol' Mom—straight-faced, we might add—and realizing what has been known since the beginning of time: Food is strong medicine.

FOOD THERAPY

THE DOWNSIDE OF PROGRESS

This change in attitude didn't come overnight. In fact, it took nearly 100 years. Up until the turn of the century, food therapy was widely practiced as a way of healing the sick and keeping the healthy well. Archaeological findings in Mesopotamia believed to be 5,000 years old showed that the ancient Sumerians, Assyrians, Akkadians and Babylonians all used foods, herbs and spices as medicine. Ancient Egyptians treated asthma with figs, grapes and even beer and touted garlic for curing infection and other conditions—a practice we continue today. Celery has been used since 200 B.C. in Asian folk medicine to lower blood pressure. And through the generations, the much-ballyhooed claim by sailors that lime juice could protect against scurvy on long voyages proved to be anything but a fish story.

Until the twentieth century, food therapy was commonly practiced in the United States. Before that, we were primarily a nation of small farms. "People largely ate what they grew," says Dr. Klaper, and what they grew were fruits, vegetables and grains—"whole" foods high in nutrients and fiber and low in fat. And since they didn't have today's antibiotics and other medications, their gardens also served as their medicine chests, and their kitchens acted as pharmacies.

But then came the industrial revolution and, with it, a new way of eating and a new attitude toward food. "When Henry Ford started turning power tractors off the assembly line in 1905, the American diet started to change—and as a result, so did the health of Americans," says Dr. Klaper. "Suddenly, the farmer who did three acres a day behind a team of horses could plow 50 acres with a tractor. Prairies erupted with mountains of corn, soybeans and oats to be fed to millions of cattle, pigs and chickens, and so meat became a plentiful staple in the diet instead of a special-occasion dish."

The American diet went from low-fat, high-fiber and plant-based to one that centered around high-fat, low-fiber animal sources. "This contributed to many of the diseases we're seeing today, such as heart disease and cancer," adds Dr. Klaper. "People rarely got cancer back then. Heart disease is a twentieth-century disease; the first heart attack was described in the *Journal of the American Medical Association* in 1908. In fact, if you look at a medical book from the 1860s, you won't find anything on coronary atherosclerosis (hardening of the arteries). If the condition existed, it was rare and generally unrecognized. Now it's one of our most prevalent conditions."

By the end of World War II, factories and processing plants had all but replaced the mom-and-pop farm, and our post-war prosperity found new healing heros. "People started relying on the so-called wonder drugs, such as antibiotics, and paid less attention to food as medicine," says registered pharmacist Earl Mindell, R.Ph., Ph.D., professor of nutrition at Pacific Western University in

Los Angeles and author of *Earl Mindell's Food as Medicine* and other books on nutrition. "About the same time, as television became more popular and was introduced in more people's homes, foods went from being whole and nutritious to being processed and refined and void of necessary nutrients. People started eating these quick-to-prepare meals quickly, in front of their television sets."

By the 1950s, food had lost its status as a healing agent and was regarded strictly as fuel for the body. Fast-food burger joints sprang up everywhere "to offer a quick fill-up of heavily processed, high-fat fare," says Dr. Mindell. "When patients asked physicians about nutrition or vitamins, their questions were often dismissed with 'As long as you're eating a well-balanced diet, you have nothing to worry about.' "

PROBLEMS ON THE PLATE

They were wrong. There was plenty to worry about, as we're learning today with our rates of disease. Our nation's diet is the single biggest contributor to heart disease, the top cause of death in the United States, according to Basil Rifkind, M.D., of the National Heart, Lung and Blood Institute in Bethesda, Maryland. And diet is believed to play a crucial role in approximately 30 percent of cancers. More and more, researchers are learning how the way we eat can influence our physical and emotional health, playing a leading role in scores of other diseases—everything from arthritis to wrinkles.

"When you're sitting down for meals, three times a day you are dosing yourself with huge quantities of things that will determine what's coursing through your arteries and blood vessels for the rest of the day," says Neal Barnard, M.D., president of the Physicians Committee for Responsible Medicine in Washington, D.C., and author of *Food for Life* and other books on the healing aspects of food. "Most people don't think of food as medication, but in reality, it's the single biggest medication we're exposed to."

And unfortunately, most of such "medicine" is ailing itself. Most foods in the American diet are no longer *whole*, a term used to describe a food in its most natural, unadulterated form—free of processing, preservatives and additives. Even most fresh fruits and vegetables, clearly the most nutritional foods in the American diet, are suspect: Only 1 percent of the U.S. produce is organic, grown without the use of cancer-causing pesticides and other dangerous chemicals.

When a food is processed or refined, it loses its nutritional punch. There are fewer vitamins and fiber, more fat and more sugar, says Elson Haas, M.D., director of the Preventive Medical Center of Marin in San Rafael, California, and author of *Staying Healthy with Nutrition*. And that spells trouble.

"The reason why so many of us are sick and stay sick is nutritional imbalance," he says. "And when you think of nutritional imbalance, there are two primary problems: congestion—too many of the wrong foods going in and not being processed and eliminated properly—and deficiency, from not getting enough vitamins, minerals, amino acids and essential fatty acids. Both of these problems interfere with the body being able to do the functions it needs to, so we get colds, dry skin and hair loss and feel fatigued."

Perhaps even more significant is the possible danger of many common food additives. Aspartame, the artificial sweetener sold as NutraSweet and Equal, can cause headaches and migraines, rashes, ringing ears, depression, insomnia and loss of motor control, according to a study by the Food and Drug Administration. Nitrates and nitrites, used as preservatives in meats and fish, form cancer-causing compounds. Other common additives, such as monosodium glutamate, butylated hydroxyanisole and brominated vegetable oil, can create an alphabet soup's worth of problems; they've been linked with heart palpitations, nausea, headaches and nerve damage.

"Within minutes after you eat, molecules of that food are in every cell of your body," says Dr. Klaper. "There they produce changes in every level, from pH changes in your blood to membrane changes in your muscles and nerve cells."

THE SKINNY ON FAT

Even additive-free foods can cause problems if they're high in fat, like much of what's in the typical American diet. Most of us have diets that are approximately 40 percent fat. Ideally, experts say, fat should comprise about 25 percent of total calories.

"Around every cell is a cell membrane that contains a little envelope of fat; this is needed so that cells can talk to each other," says Dr. Klaper. "One way these cells communicate is by throwing little pieces of these cell membranes back and forth at each other." So when you get an infection or catch a virus, or even get a splinter, your body is able to call on the inflammatory reaction and then turn it off again (when the splinter is removed, for example) because of this cell-to-cell membrane communication.

If this little envelope of fat becomes a big envelope, as it does in many Americans, cell communication becomes muddy. "Fat acts like an oil slick on cells, especially on the immune cells that help fight disease and other invaders," adds Dr. Barnard. "It keeps the cells from working well."

The only problem is, it's not always easy to detect the dangerous fat in your diet. "All people see are those three letters: F-A-T. But the reality is that all fats are not created equal," says Dr. Klaper. "There's a big difference between beef fat and flaxseed oil: One can clog your arteries, and the other has the opposite effect and can help lower cholesterol. Everybody needs about 30 grams of fat every day to build new cells and nerves as well as for other functions, including helping to heal certain health problems, so you might as well make it the right kind of fat."

TRANS-FORMING YOUR DIET

You probably already know that saturated fat, the kind abundant in animal sources such as meats, cheeses and whole dairy products, is nasty, clogging arteries and linked with scores of other health problems. And you may have heard that polyunsaturated and monounsaturated fats, found in vegetables, nuts and seeds, are the "healthy" kinds, playing a role in lowering cholesterol and reducing inflammation.

But reputations can sometimes be deceiving. Take trans-fatty acids, which are made from heart-healthy vegetable oils. Through a cooking process called hydrogenation, these healthy oils are made unhealthy, transformed into a spreadable consistency resembling butter that can raise cholesterol levels. Hundreds of food manufacturers use this process to give their products— including many labeled as "low-fat" or "cholesterol-free"—more texture and a richer, more appealing taste.

You'll know a product is hydrogenated by reading the label. If you see the words "partially hydrogenated vegetable oil," the food contains trans-fatty acids and should be avoided or eaten sparingly, especially if the oil is listed among the top four ingredients. Another tip: Labels that read "May contain one or more of the following" and then list partially hydrogenated cottonseed oil, soybean oil or other oils also indicate that the product has been chemically changed and contains trans-fatty acids.

While they may lack saturated fat, hydrogenated products such as margarine can be even more dangerous to your heart. Three studies have found that trans-fatty acids can raise cholesterol even higher than saturated fat, according to Alberto Ascherio, M.D., Dr.P.H., assistant professor of nutrition at the Harvard School of Public Health. And the damage isn't only to your arteries.

"When you eat foods containing these processed hydrogenated oils, it's like putting sugar in a gas tank—it messes up the combustion of your body," says Dr. Klaper. "The cell membrane is transformed from having this flexible, pliable curve that it gets from the 'right' fats such as polyunsaturates to becoming straight and rigid through hydrogenation. The trans-fatty acids are not incorporated into the new cell membrane, so cells can't divide properly. When they do divide, they can have unstable membranes that are prone to breaking, which might put you at increased risk for various diseases, including cancer."

THE BEEF ABOUT MEAT

To many people eating their way to better health, "beef" and "meat" have become a new breed of four-letter word. While no one argues that too much of this good-tasting stuff is bad for your health, you can have your steak and eat it, too—provided it's a cut relatively low in fat and cholesterol and you do not add fat in cooking and serving.

Among beef choices, select-grade eye of round is considered by some to be just that: A 3½-ounce serving has approximately four grams of fat, less than half of the amount in a 1-ounce serving of Cheddar cheese. It also contains 69 milligrams of cholesterol, among the lowest for meats, and it's a good source of zinc, iron and other nutrients. Tip round, bottom round and top sirloin are also relatively lean and high in these nutrients.

Turkey breast and chicken breast are poultry prizes—as long as you remove the skin. Turkey has less than 1 gram of fat and 83 milligrams of cholesterol; chicken has 3.6 grams of fat and 85 milligrams of cholesterol. Pork tenderloin is the top choice for the "other white meat," while leg shank is the leanest choice among lamb cuts.

GUT RESPONSE

Some say the center of your healing potential is your center—quite literally. "Most people aren't aware just how important intestinal health is to overall health," says Dr. Haas.

Literally dozens of health woes, including unexpected ones such as mood swings, acne and rashes, may result from problems formed in the gut: bacteria overgrowths, congestion in the intestines or other conditions caused by eating the wrong foods, according to Dr. Haas. And conversely, they can be treated with simple changes in the diet.

Dr. Haas recommends what he calls a detoxification diet (see "Detoxing Your Ills" on page 48), a three-week eating plan that he says purifies the body and helps rid it of scores of congestive problems. Unlike a fast, which avoids solid foods, Dr. Haas's plan includes plenty of solids: steamed vegetables, whole grains, fresh fruits and, after the initial three-week period, legumes, nuts and other whole foods. "It's a transition plan to help rid the body of toxins and rebalance abnormal yeasts, bacteria and parasites that cause diseases. It helps the body heal itself," says Dr. Haas. "The proper elimination of these toxins is essential to intestinal and overall health."

DETOXING YOUR ILLS

The way to heal many health problems is with a detoxification diet that cleanses the body and re-establishes the nutritional balance needed for optimum health, says Elson Haas, M.D., director of the Preventive Medical Center of Marin in San Rafael, California, and author of *Staying Healthy with Nutrition*. His diet should be practiced for only three weeks—it's not nutritionally balanced enough for longer periods. Do not undergo it if you are pregnant or suffer from deficiency problems marked by fatigue, coldness or heart weakness. Here's the detox diet.

BREAKFAST

Immediately upon arising, drink two glasses of water, one of them containing the juice of half of a lemon. Also have one to two servings of fresh fruit—apples, pears, bananas, grapes or citrus fruits such as oranges or grapefruit.

About 15 to 30 minutes later, have one to two cups of cooked oatmeal, brown rice, millet, amaranth or untoasted buckwheat. For flavoring, you can add two tablespoons of fruit juice, or use the Better Butter described below.

Better Butter Recipe

Stir ½ cup of canola oil (look for one labeled "cold-pressed") into a dish with ½ pound of butter, melted or at least softened, and refrigerate. Use about one teaspoon per meal for flavoring, and don't exceed three teaspoons a day.

Another advantage of this type of diet is that it's high in fiber, a crucial part of healing with food. "High-fiber foods fill you up, so you eat less," says Rosemary Newman, R.D., Ph.D., a registered dietitian and professor of foods and nutrition at Montana State University in Bozeman who has studied fiber and its relationship to cholesterol since the early 1980s.

That's important, since many of the health problems that affect us are the result of being overweight, a condition that afflicts more than 47 million American adults. But perhaps even more significant, says Dr. Newman, is that fiber helps prevent the absorption of fat and cholesterol from the intestinal tract.

There are two kinds of fiber, and they are found in varying degrees in different foods. Soluble fiber is abundant in beans, fruits and grains such as oats, barley and

LUNCH

Have a big bowl (up to four cups) of steamed vegetables—potatoes, yams, green beans, broccoli, kale, cauliflower, carrots, beets, asparagus, cabbage or others. Use a variety, including stems, roots and greens. Better Butter can also be used. Then refrigerate the water from the vegetables for later use.

Within two hours, slowly drink one to two cups of the water from the steamed vegetables, mixing each mouthful with saliva. You can add a little sea salt or kelp for flavoring.

DINNER

Same as lunch, with a variety of vegetables.

EVENING (AFTER DINNER)

No food at all, but you can have noncaffeinated herbal teas such as peppermint, chamomile or blends. No caffeinated beverages.

Throughout the day, feelings of hunger should be satisfied by drinking plenty of water and eating pieces of carrot or celery. If you are feeling very fatigued or if hunger persists, then you may add up to four ounces of protein, such as fish, organic chicken, lentils or garbanzo, mung or black beans. Optimally, this should be eaten midafternoon, around 3:00 or 4:00.

rye. Insoluble fiber is found in vegetables, cereals and grains such as wheat.

Soluble fiber forms a gel-like material that keeps dietary fat and cholesterol from getting to the interior wall of the intestines, where it is absorbed by the body, says Dr. Newman. So if you're having a fatty food such as steak, be sure to include a soluble-fiber food such as beans with it.

"My belief is that you should have most of your fiber with your fattiest meal of the day in order to have it work most effectively," she adds. "Since soluble fiber inhibits the absorption of dietary fat, it makes sense that it would be most effective when we're having most of that dietary fat."

Meanwhile, the insoluble fiber found in most vegetables doesn't gel, so it's less effective at preventing fat from being absorbed. But it still provides a very important benefit—keeping you "regular," so food and the toxins in it pass through the intestines faster. "Once again, this prevents congestion, one of the two reasons for the nutritional imbalance that causes so many health problems," says Dr. Haas.

MEALS THAT HEAL

Once you reduce the fat in your diet (including those tricky trans-fatty acids) and increase your fiber intake, you lower your risk of developing certain diseases—and you also help your body's ability to recover from them. "It has been well-established that the right diet can protect against certain diseases, such as cancer, heart disease, hypertension (high blood pressure), arthritis, diabetes and problems associated with obesity," says Dr. Barnard. "But these conditions can also be treated with food—namely, a low-fat diet."

Probably the most widely studied is cardiovascular disease, which kills two of every five Americans, according to American Heart Association statistics. There have been nearly a dozen major medical studies showing that you can

WHAT'S COOKING WITH YOUR NUTRIENTS

If you're slaving over a stove of vitamin-packed vittles, you may think you're really cooking—nutritionally speaking. But if you're really cooking 'em, you're not. Because many vitamins and minerals are inactivated by heat, the higher the temperature and the longer the cooking time, the more you may be depriving yourself of nutrients in food.

"The key to getting the most nutrients from whatever you're cooking is to not overcook it," says Barbara Klein, Ph.D., professor of foods and nutrition at the University of Illinois at Urbana-Champaign and associate scientific editor for the *Journal of Food Science*. "Go for the shortest cooking time possible with the least amount of water, whether you're cooking in or on a stove, microwaving or steaming." Of dry cooking methods, baking and roasting are probably the worst, because they take the longest; broiling and grilling also subject a food to high heat. Stir-frying is often recommended for the nutrient-wise, since it's among the quickest cooking methods.

Preparing foods for cooking should also take short order. "If you chop vegetables two hours before you eat them, then you'll get a lot of oxidation, which causes the destructive activity of vitamins," says Dr. Klein. "If you have a garden, pick your vegetables just minutes before you plan to prepare them."

actually reverse plaque in the arteries—a leading cause of heart attack—by adopting a diet that's low in saturated fat, says Neil Stone, M.D., associate professor of medicine at Northwestern University Medical School in Chicago and chairman of the American Heart Association's Nutrition Committee. In fact, he notes that in some cases, a low-fat diet alone may be as effective in reducing heart attack risk as going on a low-fat diet while also taking cholesterol-lowering medication.

Meats, whole dairy products, eggs and snack foods such as potato chips, crackers and cookies are the biggest sources of saturated fat in the American diet.

"With a low-fat diet, especially one free of animal food sources and those processed junk foods, you'll see all kinds of welcome changes," says Dr. Klaper. "Joints often stop hurting. Asthma frequently improves. Psoriasis can get much better or completely disappear. You start to see that there is a large group of diseases with an inflammatory component that is improved with diet."

And it's not just fat that causes problems. "We were raised with the mistaken notion that protein makes us big and strong, so we ate huge amounts of meat and drank large quantities of milk—and now we're seeing a dramatic increase in cancer, arthritis and other health problems," says Dr. Barnard. That's because many proteins can have as harmful an effect as animal fat upon the blood and cell membranes.

"In the past few years, there has been a lot of research finding that arthritis can be treated with diet. When patients go on a low-fat vegetarian diet and get away from dairy products, in many cases their arthritis will go into complete remission," says Dr. Barnard. "And while we've always used diet as the treatment of choice for Type II (non–insulin-dependent) diabetes, it appears as though Type I (insulin-dependent) diabetes is caused at least in part by exposure to dairy proteins during infancy."

CANCER PHYT-ERS

That is not to say you need to become a full-fledged vegetarian to prevent and treat disease (although some certainly advise it). But most experts do recommend that you eat more like one. The National Cancer Institute in Rockville, Maryland, has spent about $1 million a year on a media campaign aimed at getting people to eat more fruits and vegetables.

Why? Because most of these plant foods—fruits, vegetables and legumes—are nutrient-dense, meaning they're extremely low in fat while being high in fiber and key nutrients that help protect against and treat illness. But fruits and vegetables offer an additional nutritional payback.

"While you could get the nutrients you need from taking vitamin supplements, the advantage to getting them in fruits and vegetables is that you also

FOOD SENSITIVITY: HOW TO DISCOVER THE "HEALTHY" FOODS THAT CAN CAUSE DISEASE

Orange juice, whole-wheat toast and some low-fat yogurt with a banana on top. Sounds like a healthy breakfast, right?

Maybe not, according to David Edelberg, M.D., an internist and medical director of the American Holistic Center/Chicago. He says that millions of Americans are "sensitive" to these and other everyday foods—and that these sensitivities can cause or complicate all kinds of health problems, from acne and arthritis to sinus problems and just plain feeling run-down. "Many of the common problems treated in a primary care practice have a component of food sensitivity," he explains.

Fortunately, says Dr. Edelberg, there's a somewhat limited list of foods and ingredients that cause most sensitivities. They are: dairy products; egg products; citrus fruits; wheat products; bananas; kidney, lima and string beans; chemicals in processed foods; and any food that you "crave excessively" or that you eat more than three times a week.

To discover if you're sensitive to these foods or ingredients, you need to cut them out of your diet for one month. (It's worth the effort, says Dr. Edelberg, because you might find yourself feeling really good for the first time in years.)

If at the end of the month your health problem is just the same, then you're *not* sensitive to any foods, and you can go back to your normal diet. But if you're feeling better, you now need to discover *which* of the foods or ingredients that you eliminated is causing your problem.

To do that, you need to start eating the foods you eliminated, but only

get other micronutrients that you can't get in a pill—trace minerals and other compounds that are believed to play key roles in protecting against certain diseases and possibly even helping to heal them," says Barbara Klein, Ph.D., associate scientific editor for the *Journal of Food Science*.

Among these compounds are phytochemicals, which are natural chemicals found in all plants—but not in most vitamin supplements—that may protect the plants against their stresses, such as sunlight, disease and being eaten by animals. Researchers believe that the protection they offer isn't limited to plants.

"We're just getting to the tip of the iceberg regarding phytochemicals, but what we're learning is very exciting," according to Dr. Klein, who is also professor of foods and nutrition at the University of Illinois at Urbana-Champaign, where studies of phytochemicals in soy products are ongoing. "It one food group a week. So say you decide to start eating dairy the first week. If the symptoms return any time during that week—even as long as two to three days after eating a dairy product—congratulations, Sherlock Holmes! You've detected your food sensitivity. If they don't, start eating another food or food group the following week—say, egg products. And once again, be on the lookout for a return of your symptoms.

There's one catch: You might discover that you're sensitive to more than one food or food group—to citrus fruits *and* egg products (*and* those cream-filled doughnuts you pick up on the way to work every morning). So you need to reintroduce the foods and food groups one by one— which means that even if you discover during the first week that you're sensitive to something, you still need to introduce another food or food group during week two. And another during week three. (We agree: You may be in for a tedious month or two. But imagine being free of arthritis pain—one of the problems frequently complicated by food sensitivities— for the rest of your life.)

Okay, you've discovered that you're sensitive to citrus fruits. Now what do you do? Well, you don't have to give them up forever, but you shouldn't eat them for four to six months, says Dr. Edelberg. At that point, you can probably return to eating citrus fruits about twice a week, with at least three days between the two times you eat it. And, says Dr. Edelberg, if you discover you're sensitive to more than one food group, you shouldn't eat those groups on the same day.

appears that these micronutrients may be the real secret to staying healthy."

Most research indicates that these tongue-twisting phytochemicals protect against an array of cancers, particularly those that line the body's organs, in- cluding the lungs, bladder, cervix, colon, stomach, rectum, larynx and pan- creas, says Herbert F. Pierson, Ph.D., vice-president for research and development at Preventive Nutrition Consultants in Woodenville, Washington. Researchers at Johns Hopkins University School of Medicine in Baltimore have already concluded that one phytochemical found in broccoli, sul- foraphane, appears to help protect against breast cancer in animal studies. And another research team found that animals exposed to tobacco carcinogens were half as likely to develop lung cancer when fed a diet rich in watercress com- pared with those who didn't eat the vegetable.

These phytochemicals stop cancer in different ways. Have a piece of orange or some strawberries, and you'll consume flavonoids that prevent cancer-causing hormones from latching on to a cell, says Dr. Pierson. Have some green pepper or pineapple, and you'll get p-courmaric acid and chlorogenic acid, substances that stop cancer cells from forming. Have a slice of tomato, and you'll get up to several hundred different phytochemicals, most of which seem to play some role in stopping tumors before they form. To further reduce your risk of oxidation-caused cancers, experts recommend that you thoroughly wash and even peel all fruits and vegetables before eating them to minimize ingesting sprayed-on pesticides.

EATING FOR IMMUNITY

Another bonus offered by fruits and vegetables: They're among the best sources of nutrients needed for a strong immune system, your body's defense against disease. It's your immune system that helps prevent and fight colds and other viruses, infections and even diseases such as cancer.

"When a patient of mine comes in with pneumonia, I may give him antibiotics," says Dr. Klaper. "But then I say 'Why did he get pneumonia? What is he is doing to his immune system?' Healthy people don't get pneumonia. Problems with immunity are often related to the way someone eats."

That's why a good diet becomes even more important as you age, since immunity naturally tends to weaken as time passes. By your fifties and sixties, your infection-fighting cells don't function as well, placing you at greater risk for infection and cancer, says Ronald Watson, Ph.D., research professor and a nutrition and immunology specialist at the University of Arizona College of Medicine in Tucson.

But if you eat right, your immunity stays strong no matter what your age. And to most experts, that means a diet rich in the so-called antioxidant nutrients, vitamins and minerals that help protect against the damage caused by oxidation.

When a freshly cut apple turns brown, that's oxidation, the process of deterioration that occurs from exposure to oxygen. Our bodies need oxygen to stay alive, but too much of it causes severe damage to cells. And in today's society, where the air we breathe also contains cigarette smoke, car exhaust, background radiation and other dangerous pollutants and our drinking water has oxidizing chlorine, oxidation leads to premature aging and weakens immunity. Wrinkles, cataracts, arthritis and scores of other illnesses, including cancer and heart disease, are all thought to be caused in part by this oxidation process.

"When people talk about antioxidants, they are usually referring to vitamins C and E, beta-carotene and selenium," says Judith S. Stern, R.D., Sc.D., professor of nutrition and internal medicine at the University of California, Davis. "But what we're learning is that there are hundreds of other properties in foods that also have antioxidant qualities. Some of these are the phytochemicals. There are also other carotenoids like beta-carotene and other substances that we don't even know about."

WHAT SUPPLEMENTS DON'T HAVE

What experts do know is that some of these goodies—phytochemicals, carotenoids and some micronutrients—aren't in supplements. "The closer something is to its natural state, the better it is," says Dr. Haas. "And vitamins and minerals are in their natural state in foods, not in supplements."

"It's like taking a fiber supplement. It may be better than not having any fiber, but you're always better off eating high-fiber foods than taking a supplement," adds Dr. Stern. "Once you take the fiber out of a food, the fiber is dehydrated, it doesn't represent all of the types of fiber in foods, and it may not work the same way."

Another problem with supplements: Exposure to air and light has a detrimental effect, so each time you open the bottle, the pills get weaker.

"The funny thing is, people hear about studies that show vitamin C helps for this and beta-carotene protects against that, so they run to the store and buy a bottle of vitamin supplements, thinking it will help them," says Dr. Stern. "In reality, most of those studies are done with fruits and vegetables, so the benefit may be not only from that particular nutrient but from all of the other compounds in the food."

Among those compounds are other nutrients that also play key roles in boosting immunity, even though they don't get the publicity of the big-name anitoxidants. "You hear a lot about the antioxidant vitamins, but they're only part of the story," says Terry M. Phillips, Ph.D., D.Sc., director of the immuno-chemistry laboratory at George Washington University School of Medicine and Health Sciences in Washington, D.C. "There are other nutrients that may be just as important—or even more so—in keeping immunity strong." Among them: vitamin B_6, zinc, folate, magnesium and copper.

When you bite into a carrot, a mango or broccoli, you are getting a great source of antioxidant vitamins as well as some of these other key nutrients—and a host of other goodies, too, including fiber, "good" essential fatty acids and even protein and calcium.

"The bottom line is this," says Dr. Stern. "It may be easier to take vitamins. But if you're really, really concerned about your health, there is only one thing you must do: You have to eat right."

HERBAL THERAPY

Cures from Nature's Medicine Chest

If you've ever taken aspirin, you've taken a drug derived from an herb.

If you've ever taken one of those oral decongestants that don't make you drowsy, you've taken a drug derived from an herb.

"In the past, almost all medicines were herbs," says Varro E. Tyler, Ph.D., professor of pharmacognosy (the study of drugs from natural sources) at Purdue University in West Lafayette, Indiana. Like aspirin and those decongestants, many of today's medicines are synthetic forms of herbs. Aspirin's main ingredient is acetylsalicylic acid, which is isolated from the bark of a willow tree. Those oral decongestants contain pseudoephedrine, which is made from the ephedra plant. In fact, at least one-fourth of all of the drugs that doctors prescribe contain active ingredients derived or synthesized from plant medicines, says Norman R. Farnsworth, Ph.D., director of the Program for Collaborative Research in the College of Pharmacy at the University of Illinois at Chicago.

How did primitive man discover that plants had medicinal properties? The first "herbalists" probably watched the animals, noticing which plants the beasts grazed on when they weren't feeling well. They tried those plants themselves. They also discovered by trial and error which plants helped and which harmed. When someone felt better after eating certain flowers, others would try them. If someone broke out in a rash after chewing certain roots, everyone would stay away from them. Eventually, primitive people found plants that helped them sleep, plants that helped them stay awake, plants that cured stomachaches and plants that soothed sunburned skin.

THE HISTORY OF HERBS

Those primitive discoveries were eventually systematized in ancient Rome, Greece, Egypt and China. In ancient Egypt, for example, there was the Papyrus Ebers, a sort of hieroglyphic version of the *Physician's Desk Reference*. Its remedies included aloe vera for cuts and burns and mint to aid digestion—remedies that are still used today.

This tradition of herbal remedies continued for centuries, until the beginning of modern science and its knowledge of chemistry. At that point, scientists and doctors could isolate the active ingredient from an herb and produce a more potent, faster-acting medicine. In 1806, a German apprentice pharmacist isolated an active element of the opium plant, a chemical alkaloid that he called morphine. Scientists soon isolated other chemicals: the antimalarial quinine from *Cinchona orperuvian* bark, the antispasmodic atropine from belladonna leaves, the anesthetic cocaine from coca leaves and the heart drug digitoxin from purple foxglove leaves.

By the late nineteenth century, doctors were beginning to view herbal remedies as old-fashioned. And why not? Dosages of medicines were standardized in synthesized drugs but required guesswork when administered in herbs. But even as synthetic pharmaceuticals began to dominate medical practice, some practitioners continued to administer herbal remedies: homeopaths, osteopaths, chiropractors and hydrotherapists as well as the eclectics, a group of

GROWING YOUR OWN

Here's some good news: You don't need a green thumb to raise a crop of herbs.

"Herbs are incredibly adaptable," writes Steven Foster in his book *Herbal Renaissance: Growing, Using and Understanding Herbs in the Modern World.* "As a general rule, an herb garden requires much less attention than a vegetable garden."

Most herbs thrive in the sun, with six to eight hours of exposure being the ideal. Herbs generally need less water than flowers or vegetables do. In fact, many need to be watered only under drought conditions, says San Francisco herbalist Jeanne Rose, author of several herb books, including *Jeanne Rose's Modern Herbal.*

Foster suggests that gardeners start small. First, estimate how much time you'll want to spend gardening. (The bigger the garden, the more time it will need.) Consider the realities of the space you have to use: how much sun the garden will get, what the soil is like, which herbs will do best in your climate (the seed packet often tells you the type of soil and climate the herb will need).

For urban dwellers who lack plots to cultivate, Rose recommends a back porch or window box garden. A basic herb garden might include feverfew, peppermint, rosemary, chamomile and lavender, she says. Many herbs will thrive in pots, so you can bring the magic of the garden inside during the winter months. Remember these two things when growing herbs in pots: Water before the soil dries out or before the leaves yellow and fall off, and use a soil that is a bit alkaline and has good drainage.

THE SCIENTIFIC EVIDENCE ON HERBS

Clinical and laboratory studies of herbs have generated scientific evidence that herbs can effectively treat many diseases, says Varro E. Tyler, Ph.D., professor of pharmacognosy (the study of drugs from natural sources) at Purdue University in West Lafayette, Indiana.

The following herbs have been subject to the most scrutiny in European, Asian and North American studies. Dr. Tyler says that these nine herbs stand up to the highest clinical standards.

Chamomile. In the United States, chamomile is generally used as a tea, but Europeans use chamomile extracts, ointments and tinctures as well to treat a range of health problems, from indigestion to skin rashes. Chamomile tea, a gentle relaxant, makes an excellent bedtime drink. Scientific studies support chamomile's antispasmodic, anti-infective and anti-inflammatory uses.

Echinacea. Native American healers used this plant as a remedy for snakebites and skin wounds. Research shows that echinacea stimulates the immune system, helping the body defend itself against bacterial and viral infections.

Feverfew. In the 1980s, several British studies proclaimed feverfew's ability to reduce the severity and frequency of migraine headaches. Scientists believe that parthenolide, one of the active ingredients of feverfew, inhibits the release of serotonin and prostaglandin, hormones that may trigger migraines.

Garlic. Ancient Egyptians were serious garlic fans. They fed the odoriferous bulb to their slaves to keep them healthy. Now research shows that garlic can lower blood pressure and blood cholesterol levels and may even help heart attack survivors live longer. The National Cancer Institute in Rockville, Maryland, is studying garlic's tumor-fighting properties. On a more mundane level, garlic relieves gas and aids digestion.

Americans who combined European herbal traditions with the plant lore borrowed from Native American traditions.

With the discovery of penicillin in 1928, the age of miracle drugs began. The hormone cortisone was isolated in 1930. The antibiotics streptomycin and Aureomycin, a brand of chlortetracycline, were produced in 1943 and 1945, respectively. The drug industry became a multinational, mega-billion-dollar enterprise. But with more powerful drugs came more powerful problems—what doctors call side effects. (The most dramatic and ghastly were the birth defects created by thalidomide, a sleeping pill often used by pregnant

Ginkgo. Research shows that ginkgo is particularly useful for treating problems caused by decreased blood flow to the brain. Elderly people who suffer from memory loss caused by circulatory problems may find that mental clarity increases when they take ginkgo. Studies also suggest that by improving circulation throughout the body, ginkgo can help prevent blood clots and mood swings accompanied by anxiety and can relieve the symptoms of tinnitus (ringing in the ears), asthma, phlebitis (inflammation of a vein) and vertigo.

Lemon balm. Studies show that this herb works well to calm nerves and to protect the body from bacterial infection. Europeans use lemon balm to treat cold sores caused by the herpes simplex virus. Preliminary tests suggest a cream containing lemon balm extract helps herpes lesions heal faster and extends the period between outbreaks of herpes.

Milk thistle. Animal and human trials show that this herb is a promising supplemental treatment for liver conditions, including hepatitis and cirrhosis. Milk thistle contains a mixture of flavonoid derivatives called silymarin that works directly on liver cells.

Saint-John's-wort. Traditionally used as a muscle relaxant to relieve menstrual problems, as a mild tranquilizer and as a treatment for depression and insomnia, Saint-John's-wort now also shows promise as a treatment for nervousness and anxiety. Active compounds in the herb appear to function as MAO (monoamine oxidase) inhibitors. An excess of MAO is a possible cause of depression.

Valerian. Studies show that this herb is a safe, effective alternative to prescription sleeping pills and tranquilizers. Scientists aren't exactly sure how or why it works, but valerian seems to depress central nervous system activity.

women in the 1960s.) Yes, synthetic medicines were the norm, but many doctors (and patients) began to see a reason to use the gentler, more natural medicines that are herbs.

BACK TO NATURE—BACK TO HERBS

Why do people try herbal therapy? One reason, says Robert McCaleb, president of the Herb Research Foundation, a research and education organization in Boulder, Colorado, is that they're searching for self-care and disease prevention techniques in a time of soaring health care costs. "To people who are in good health, herbal remedies offer opportunities for staying well," McCaleb says.

Taking ginseng capsules, for instance, may help people stay mentally alert when they're coping with the stresses of working too hard, says Dr. Tyler. And drinking a cup of lemon balm tea, a natural relaxant, can relieve stress and calm you down, says naturopathic physician Mary Bove, L.M., N.D., director of the Brattleboro Naturopathic Clinic in Vermont.

Bruises, swelling, sprains, cuts, colds, fevers, minor burns and rashes respond well to herbal treatments, says Cynthia Mervis Watson, M.D., a physician who specializes in homeopathic and herbal therapies in her family practice in Santa Monica, California. There are also effective herbal therapies for women's reproductive problems, including premenstrual syndrome, infertility, irregular periods, menstrual cramps, menopausal symptoms and vaginal infections, she says.

Herbal remedies form a strong first line of defense against colds, flus and other infectious diseases. Unlike antibiotics, herbs can be used to treat both bacterial and viral infections, says Rosemary Gladstar, a Barre, Vermont, herbalist and author of several books about herbs, including *Herbal Healing for Women*.

Herbal therapy has another benefit as well. "For people who are taking potent prescription drugs with lots of side effects, herbs provide safer, gentler alternatives," McCaleb says. Valerian, for instance, is an effective, nonaddictive alternative to prescription sleeping pills, says Dr. Tyler. For motion sickness, ginger is a good alternative to antihistamines, which can cause drowsiness, and to the scopolamine patch, which can cause dry mouth. Ginger has no significant side effects, he says.

McCaleb says the herbs ginkgo and saw palmetto can alleviate some of the afflictions of old age. Studies show that taking ginkgo can help elderly people who suffer from memory loss and confusion and that saw palmetto is effective at treating the prostate problems that plague many older men.

And herbal remedies sometimes work when Western medical treatments fail. "They're great for treating urinary tract infections, digestive problems, menstrual cramps, coughs, colds, skin rashes, allergies, chronic fatigue—all kinds of immune system problems," says Dr. Watson.

When it comes to treating serious illnesses such as heart disease, cancer and autoimmune disorders, many medical doctors are prescribing herbal remedies to be used in conjunction with mainstream medical techniques, says Dr. Watson. Herbs such as ginger, peppermint, papaya and fennel can help reduce the nausea caused by chemotherapy, for instance. Irish moss can thin the blood, and hawthorn berry, rosemary and motherwort can improve circulation in people with heart disease. (When using herbs in the treatment of major health problems, you must consult with a health professional, Dr. Watson cautions.)

But whether using them for prevention, as home remedies or as helper substances for drugs, people are using a lot of herbs. In 1993, total sales of herbal remedies were estimated to be about $1.5 billion, says Mark Blumenthal, executive director of the American Botanical Council in Austin, Texas.

SHOPPING FOR HERBS

Choosing herbal remedies has always been somewhat of a puzzle, with most consumers not getting much help from label instructions about what to take, for what purpose and in what dosage. The reason for this is that the U.S. Food and Drug Administration (FDA) forbids manufacturers of herbal products from putting therapeutic information on the labels, says James Duke, Ph.D., an economic botanist and toxicology specialist retired from the U.S. Department of Agriculture. That's because herbs are considered to be nutritional supplements,

A ROAD MAP FOR SHOPPERS

When you walk into a health food store, you'll find that herbs are sold in a variety of forms. Teas are probably the most familiar, but here's a quick consumer's guide to other types.

Capsules and tablets. Swallowing tablets is probably the easiest way to take any medicine, but many herbalists prefer tinctures and teas because they believe that the active ingredients of the herbs are released more quickly and more efficiently in these forms.

Extracts and tinctures. Technically, extracts are stronger and more concentrated than tinctures. But today, these terms are generally used interchangeably. To make these, fresh herbs are soaked for days or weeks in alcohol with varying amounts of water. (Some concoctions are available using glycerin and water as a solvent.) The mixture is shaken regularly and then strained and rebottled for use. Extracts and tinctures are taken two or three times daily as a specified number of drops mixed in a little water.

Teas. One of the easiest ways to use herbs, fresh or dried, is to make a tea. When using the leaves or flowers of a plant, pour a cup of boiling water over one teaspoon of the loose herb and let it steep for roughly ten minutes, then strain out the loose herb. Pour cold water over roots, seeds, bark or tough leaves, bring to a boil and simmer for ten minutes, then strain. Sweeten to taste with honey, if you like.

Ointments and creams. These herbal products are prepared for external use. Use according to label directions.

not drugs. Of course, if an herb manufacturer wants to prove the therapeutic value of an herb, it's welcome to do so. But the FDA's medical testing process is so expensive that most herbal manufacturers can't afford it, says Dr. Duke—especially since the return, financially, is never as great with herbal remedies as with pharmaceuticals. "Who can afford to invest $231 million to prove that an herb such as feverfew, which you and I could grow in our backyards, can prevent migraines? How would manufacturers get their $231 million back?" he says.

Even though these remedies are not drugs, they are used for therapeutic purposes.

"It's important to remember that herbs are medicines," says Dr. Watson. "As

---

HAZARDOUS HERBS

Some people believe that all herbal products are safe. This is far from true. Although this is not a complete list of unsafe plants, those mentioned deserve special attention.

The following herbs are dangerous and should not be used as remedies.

PLANT	POTENTIAL DANGER
Borage	Harmful in large doses; may cause liver damage and cancer
Broom	Toxic; diuretic
Chaparral	May cause illness; banned in the United States
Coltsfoot	May cause cancer
Comfrey	May cause liver damage and cancer (but not through external use)
Foxglove	Potent heart toxin
Pennyroyal	The essential oil may cause convulsions in large doses; possibly harmful to pregnant women
Pokeweed	May cause respiratory paralysis and convulsions

with any medication, it's important to know how to take herbs, how frequently and in what dosage."

Many people are guided by magazines and books. It's also a good idea, says Gladstar, to ask for advice from health professionals, including M.D.'s and R.N.'s who have an interest in herbal therapy, naturopathic doctors (N.D.'s), who specialize in prescribing herbs, and herbalists, who are usually self-trained and often very knowledgeable. Be sure to ask them about side effects or possible interactions with other drugs that you might be taking. (For recommended books on herbs, refer to the resource list on 635.)

No matter what you do, however, you must be aware that just because it's nat-

PLANT	POTENTIAL DANGER
Rue	May make skin more susceptible to damage from sunlight
Sassafras	May cause cancer

The following herbs are potentially dangerous and should be used with caution.

PLANT	POTENTIAL DANGER
Aloe vera	The juice can be a powerful laxative when used internally (gels labeled for internal use do not have this effect)
Ephedra	Should not be used by people with heart conditions, high blood pressure, diabetes or thyroid disease
Juniper	Should not be used by women who are pregnant or people with kidney disease
Licorice	Exessive amounts may cause fluid retention and high blood pressure
Yohimbe	Side effects include nausea, vomiting, high blood pressure, palpitations, insomnia and tremors

ural doesn't mean it's always safe. Most herbal remedies are, but a few can be quite dangerous, especially when used in combination with prescription or over-the-counter drugs or when used by people with pre-existing health problems. (For a list of herbs with potentially harmful side effects, see "Hazardous Herbs" on page 62.)

Pokeweed, for instance, a plant that has been used to treat arthritis, can produce serious side effects such as respiratory paralysis and convulsions, says Dr. Duke.

Goldenseal, a powerful natural antibiotic, may help you fight colds, flus and other types of infection. When used long term for chronic infections, however, it should be taken only in cycles, such as two to three weeks on and two weeks off. Taken without a break in the cycle, it may cause you to get sicker rather than better, says Gladstar.

GIVING IT TIME

Herbs don't necessarily work quickly for chronic health problems. For some long-term conditions, you may need to take an herbal remedy for at least three months before you see results, says Gladstar.

"Most people who don't get results with herbs make the mistake of giving up too soon," Gladstar says. "They don't wait long enough, and they don't take enough of the herb for it to be effective."

Used wisely, in the context of a healthy lifestyle that includes a nutritious diet and regular exercise, herbal remedies may be just the boost your body needs to keep you feeling vital and to protect you from illnesses, Gladstar says.

Keep in mind that since herbal remedies are not standardized, it is wise to follow the manufacturer's label directions for each product that you buy. If a product does not have clear directions on the package, or if you have any problems or questions concerning the product, be sure to consult a reputable herbalist before using it. For a list of organizations that may help you locate an herbal therapy practitioner near you, refer to the resource list on page 635.

HOMEOPATHY

Small Doses Yield Big Results

After years of trying to fend off his hay fever with antihistamines, Richard D. Fischer was fed up.

"It was so bad that by the time I blew my nose and washed my hands, my nose would be dripping again. It was getting to the point that I could barely practice dentistry," says Dr. Fischer (D.D.S.), a dentist in Annandale, Virginia.

Then a patient told him about a homeopathic physician nearby who had helped many people cope with their allergies. Dr. Fischer was skeptical, but on his third visit to the homeopathic doctor, a remarkable thing happened.

"He gave me a remedy that literally popped my sinuses open. You could actually hear it happen. It shocked the daylights out of me. When I experienced for myself what a profound change homeopathy could make, I knew I had to learn more about it," says Dr. Fischer, president of the International Academy of Oral Medicine and Toxicology, a 500-member group of dentists, physicians and researchers that promotes the use of safe dental materials and procedures.

After 15 years of training from the National Center for Homeopathy, a non-profit educational service in Alexandria, Virginia, that conducts seminars for physicians and dentists, Dr. Fischer says he now uses homeopathy to treat everything from bad breath to toothaches.

"I find it surprising that more dentists and doctors aren't using homeopathy," Dr. Fischer says. "It provides so many benefits with so little risk to the patient . . . I can't imagine practicing dentistry without it."

WHAT IS IT?

Homeopathy, a form of medicine that relies on minute amounts of herbs, minerals and other substances to stimulate a person's natural defenses and help the body heal itself, often tames illnesses with a single dose of medicine and causes virtually no side effects, proponents say. Worldwide, homeopathy is commonly practiced in many countries, including India, Mexico and Russia. About four in every ten people in France and one in three people in England—including the British royal family—use homeopathy, according to the National Center for Homeopathy.

HOMEOPATHY

In the United States, however, homeopathy is less well known. It was introduced in this country in 1825, and by 1890, there were 14,000 homeopathic physicians, 22 homeopathic medical schools and more than 100 homeopathic hospitals nationwide. But less than 50 years later, homeopathy was virtually forgotten in the United States as reliance on Western medicine steadily grew and scientists developed antibiotics and other powerful drugs that seemed capable of eradicating any disease.

But homeopathy is experiencing a renaissance in this country. Since 1970, when there were fewer than 200 practitioners nationwide, there has been a surge of interest in the medical community. While their number is small compared with the number of Western practitioners, today there are at least 2,500 doctors, dentists, chiropractors and nurse-practitioners who regularly prescribe homeopathic remedies, according to the National Center for Homeopathy.

Each year, more than 2.5 million people seek homeopathic care. Retail sales of homeopathic remedies have increased about 25 percent a year since 1988 and now top $200 million annually. In comparison, Americans spent $290 million for over-the-counter antacids and $56 billion for prescription medicines in 1992. But that disparity is somewhat misleading, proponents say, since homeopathic remedies cost a fraction of most conventional drugs. A typical homeopathic remedy, containing 30 to 100 doses, costs from $3 to $5, says Chris Meletis, N.D., a naturopathic physician and medicinary director at the National College of Naturopathic Medicine in Portland, Oregon.

LIKE CURES LIKE

Homeopathy, which is derived from two Greek words, literally means "similar suffering." Although the concept dates back to at least the tenth century B.C., modern homeopathy is based on the observations of Samuel Hahnemann, an eighteenth-century German physician. Dr. Hahnemann considered the medical practices of the time barbaric, because patients were regularly bled, leeched and blistered to purge them of fluids believed to cause most illnesses.

Disillusioned, he quit medicine and became a translator of scientific texts, says Maesimund Panos, M.D., a homeopathic physician in Tipp City, Ohio, and co-author with Jane Heimlich of *Homeopathic Medicine at Home*. But Dr. Hahnemann continued to experiment on himself with various substances in hopes of finding a more humane way of healing people. He suspected that disease represented an imbalance in what he called the body's vital force (modern homeopaths believe he meant the immune system) and that only a small stimulus was needed to restore balance in the body's natural defenses.

But that hunch didn't fully bloom until he began experiments to discover why small doses of quinine, an extract from a Peruvian tree bark, cured malaria. To his surprise, Dr. Hahnemann found that large doses of the drug had unexpected effects. After taking massive doses of quinine for several days, he developed trembling, heart palpitations and other symptoms of malaria. As soon as he stopped taking the drug, his symptoms disappeared. From this experiment, Dr. Hahnemann developed his belief that "like is cured by like," also known as the as law of similars, which is the basis of homeopathy.

Dr. Hahnemann theorized that if large amounts of a substance such as quinine cause symptoms of illness in a healthy person, then small doses of that same substance should cure an ill person who has similar symptoms. So if you have a cold, for example, taking a small amount of a substance that in large doses would cause coldlike symptoms should cure your sniffles, according to Dr. Hahnemann's theory. But the remedy will work only if its pattern of induced symptoms matches the symptoms of the ill person.

Dr. Hahnemann and his early followers conducted more experiments, called provings, in which they gave large amounts of herbs, minerals and animal extracts to healthy people and recorded all of the symptoms they developed. Later, Dr. Hahnemann compiled these experiments into a book, *Materia Medica*, a reference guide first published in 1811 that helps practitioners match a patient's symptoms with a corresponding homeopathic remedy.

MAKING POISONS WORK FOR US

But Dr. Hahnemann had to overcome one major obstacle. Some of the substances he used, such as arsenic, mercury and belladonna (deadly nightshade), were extremely poisonous. So Dr. Hahnemann diluted the substances in water and alcohol until he believed he had safe doses that would trigger healing in the body without causing any harmful effects. In fact, Dr. Hahnemann theorized that as the doses got smaller, the remedy not only would become less toxic but would actually be more potent and effective as well.

Today, more than 1,200 substances are recognized as homeopathic remedies. These remedies are diluted so that 1 drop of a medicine is mixed with either 9 or 99 drops of a solution that is 87 percent alcohol and 13 percent distilled water, creating a dilution of 1 to 10 or 1 to 100, Dr. Meletis says. This mixture is vigorously shaken, then 1 drop of the mixture is diluted and shaken into another 9 or 99 drops of solution. After about 24 dilutions, there usually isn't one molecule of the original homeopathic medicine left in the solution, Dr. Meletis says. This process, however, often continues for 1,000 or more dilutions and shakings to increase the solution's potency, homeopaths say.

Homeopathic remedies are regulated by the Food and Drug Administration.

Available as pill, powder or liquid, these remedies are considered safe enough that 95 percent of them are sold over the counter in the United States in many health food stores, according to the National Center for Homeopathy. (When buying, remember that remedies that are labeled X have been diluted 1 to 10, while remedies labeled C, which are more potent, have been diluted 1 to 100. So a 3C remedy, for example, has been diluted three times at a ratio of 1 to 100 and is the equivalent of one drop of homeopathic remedy in one million drops of a solution of water and alcohol.)

"Even poisons have a purpose in this world if you use them right," says Deborah Gordon, M.D., a homeopathic physician in Ashland, Oregon. "The important thing to remember about the remedies is that we're using very small amounts that are diluted to the point that they're just a mirror of the substances."

In fact, a toxicology expert has calculated that swallowing 100 times the homeopathic dose of the poison strychnine would still be too diluted to harm even a very young child.

FIVE QUESTIONS YOU SHOULD ASK YOUR HOMEOPATH

Finding a good homeopathic practitioner is like pinning down your teenager's plans for Saturday night. It takes patience and persistence.

Some medical doctors (M.D.'s) and osteopathic doctors (D.O.'s) specialize in homeopathy. Another large group of homeopaths are naturopathic physicians (N.D.'s), doctors who are considered the general practitioners of alternative medicine. But homeopathy is also practiced by chiropractors, dentists, acupuncturists, nurse-practitioners and certified midwives.

So how do you find a reputable homeopath? To start, write the National Center for Homeopathy and ask for its information packet, which includes a list of homeopathic practitioners in your area (refer to the resource list on page 637).

Then before choosing one, ask each homeopath these questions to narrow your choice.

Where did you receive your homeopathic training? "The answer you don't want to hear is that they were trained in self-help study groups. Study groups are great, but you want your homeopathic care to come from a professional," says Maesimund Panos, M.D., a homeopathic physician in Tipp City, Ohio, and co-author with Jane Heimlich of *Homeopathic Medicine at Home.*

How long have you been practicing homeopathy? The longer they've been in practice, the more likely they are skilled and knowledgeable, Dr.

EMERGING SCIENTIFIC PROOF

Much of the support for homeopathy is anecdotal. But proponents say that most conventional medical studies of homeopathy are flawed because these studies attempt to measure the effectiveness of one homeopathic remedy in fighting one disease. Since homeopaths believe that individuals can have the same disease but different symptoms and therefore need different remedies, they claim any study requiring that every participant be given the same homeopathic remedy is bound to have inconclusive results.

"Homeopathic physicians have always been more involved with caring for their patients and haven't had the time or motivation to do these kinds of controlled studies," Dr. Panos says.

That is changing, however, as more homeopaths conduct research that proponents say is likely to prove that homeopathy does work. In a study of 478 people who had flu symptoms, French scientists found that 17 percent of

Panos says. Some homeopaths are board-certified, meaning that they have been practicing homeopathy for at least three years and have passed a comprehensive exam.

How much time do you spend with each patient? An initial office visit for treatment of a chronic ailment should take at least an hour, Dr. Panos says. It often takes that long for a homeopath to learn enough about you and your symptoms to select the right remedy for you. If the homeopath spends significantly less time than that on your initial visit, it may be a signal to see another homeopath.

What percentage of your practice is devoted to homeopathy? "If he uses it only 50 percent of the time, you might wonder about him," Dr. Panos says.

Do you treat patients with one remedy at a time, or do you use several homeopathic remedies at once? Although some homeopaths successfully treat patients with several remedies at a time, most good homeopaths prescribe only the one remedy that most closely matches all of a person's symptoms. They avoid prescribing one remedy to treat one disease and a second remedy to treat another, says Dana Ullman, author of *Discovering Homeopathy* and *Homeopathic Medicine for Children and Infants* and founder and president of the Foundation for Homeopathic Education and Research in Berkeley, California.

the people who received homeopathic treatment improved within 48 hours of beginning treatment compared with 10 percent of the individuals who took placebos, compounds that look like the real medicine but have no pharmacological effect. A group of 40 Nicaraguan children who received homeopathic treatment recovered from bouts of diarrhea an average of one day earlier than children who were given placebos, according to researchers at the University of Washington in Seattle.

In another study often cited by homeopaths, Scottish researchers gave homeopathic grass remedies to 56 people with hay fever. After five weeks, these people were less likely to have runny noses, irritated eyes and other symptoms of hay fever than a group that took placebos.

LET THE SPIRIT MOVE YOU

Although these studies suggest that homeopathy may be effective, no one really knows how it works. But part of the answer may have to do with the di-

HOMEOPATHIC FIRST AID: THE TEN ESSENTIAL REMEDIES

Your daughter limps home with a nasty bruise on her leg after taking a dive on her bicycle. So you search through your conventional first-aid kit for something to stop the swelling and ease her pain.

There are bandages, antiseptic cream and a few packages of aspirin. Pretty standard stuff. For something a little different, homeopaths suggest stocking your medicine cabinet with a few of their essential remedies.

"I think everyone in the United States should have a homeopathic first-aid kit and homeopathic first-aid book," says Jacquelyn Wilson, M.D., a homeopathic physician in San Diego. "You can use that kit as an initial treatment for almost any illness, even while you're waiting for an ambulance to arrive."

Homeopathic first-aid kits containing from 20 to 40 remedies are available in many health food stores. But you can also create your own kit. Here are 10 basic remedies that should be in every home, according to Maesimund Panos, M.D., a homeopathic physician in Tipp City, Ohio, and co-author with Jane Heimlich of *Homeopathic Medicine at Home*. Warning: For first-aid treatment, do not give a person doses higher than 30X or 30C without consulting a homeopath.

The plant, animal or mineral compound each remedy is derived from is listed in parentheses.

lutions and shakings mentioned earlier. Dr. Hahnemann believed that vigor-ously shaking the solution during each dilution releases a "spiritlike" essence that has the potential to heal the body.

Now some homeopaths think they know the science behind Dr. Hahne-mann's insight. The shakings, they believe, energize a solution with an elec-tromagnetic impression of the original homeopathic substance. This impression remains long after the molecules of the original substance have been diluted. It may be the distinct electromagnetic energy pattern of each remedy that seems to jolt the body's defenses into action against a specific ailment, Dr. Panos says.

Researchers at Hahnemann Medical College (now Hahnemann University School of Medicine) in Philadelphia, for example, examined 23 homeopathic remedies to determine nuclear magnetic resonance, a measure of the activity of small molecules. The researchers found that the homeopathic remedies had ac-tive subatomic particles—a sign that the remedies had been energized—while the subatomic particles in a group of placebo remedies were inactive.

- Aconite (monkshood) is a good remedy for the early stages of swelling or fever. A person who needs Aconite may feel fearful and restless and crave cold drinks.
- Apis (honeybee) soothes bee stings and other insect bites.
- Arnica (leopard's bane) relieves bruises and muscle soreness.
- Arsenicum (arsenic) is the most commonly needed remedy for upset stomach, vomiting, diarrhea and food poisoning.
- Belladonna (deadly nightshade) commonly helps people who have sore throats, coughs, headaches, earaches or fevers. The person who needs this remedy may appear flushed and feel hot and restless.
- Gelsemium (yellow jasmine) often relieves flus, head colds and tension headaches.
- Ipecacuanha (ipecac root) relieves nausea and can also halt a bad bloody nose or bleeding from any part of the body.
- Ledum (marsh tea) is a common remedy for puncture wounds, bites and stings and can also help eye injuries and ankle sprains.
- Nux vomica (poison nut) is a wonderful hangover remedy.
- Ruta (rue) helps heal sprains and sore bones. If Arnica doesn't relieve your bruised, lame feeling after a fall, try Ruta.

MAKING THE MOST OF YOUR REMEDY

Here are a few things you can do to enhance the effectiveness of a homeopathic remedy.

First, keep your remedy in a cool, dark place away from direct sunlight and temperatures higher than 100°F. Avoid exposing the remedy to strong odors such as perfumes or mothballs, which can decrease its effectiveness, says Dana Ullman, author of *Discovering Homeopathy* and *Homeopathic Medicine for Children and Infants* and founder and president of the Foundation for Homeopathic Education and Research in Berkeley, California.

Steer clear of coffee, because many remedies are adversely affected by the essential oils in coffee that give the beverage its flavor, says Maesimund Panos, M.D., a homeopathic physician in Tipp City, Ohio, and co-author with Jane Heimlich of *Homeopathic Medicine at Home*.

Avoid using lip balms, facial creams and other products containing camphor while taking a remedy, because on rare occasions, camphor can wipe out the remedy's effectiveness, Ullman says.

Don't use mint-flavored toothpastes or mouthwashes for at least an hour before and after you take a remedy, says Richard D. Fischer, D.D.S., a dentist and homeopath in Annandale, Virginia, and president of the International Academy of Oral Medicine and Toxicology. Like camphor, mint can be an antidote to a remedy. Homeopathic toothpastes that contain ingredients safe to use with remedies are available in many health food stores.

Avoid using electric blankets, because they may cause slight disturbances in the body's nervous system that can make it harder for a remedy to work, Ullman says. "It's a rare complication, but a few homeopaths have noticed that for some unknown reason, remedies are antidoted by electric blankets," he says.

Take no more than three doses of a remedy in a day unless directed by your homeopath, says Deborah Gordon, M.D., a homeopathic physician in Ashland, Oregon. Stop taking the remedy when you begin to feel better, because excessive doses of a homeopathic medicine can actually revive the symptoms you're trying to corral.

"The key is the shaking," says Kelvin Levitt, P.D., a registered pharmacist in Randallstown, Maryland, who has made and used homeopathic remedies for more than 17 years. "It releases pure healing energy into the solution, and when you take it, that's what causes the body to start healing."

HOW HOMEOPATHY CAN HELP YOU

Before you treat yourself or go to a homeopath, there a few other things you should know. First, homeopaths say they don't treat specific diseases. Instead, they treat the whole person based on all of his emotional and physical symptoms. So depending on their symptoms, a person who has a wart and a person who has a headache may be given the same remedy.

On the other hand, homeopaths also believe that two people with the same illness can have very different symptoms and need very different remedies.

It's unlikely, for instance, that your migraine and your boss's migraine will be very similar, Dr. Panos says. You might feel better with an ice pack on your head, but your boss might feel better with a warm cloth. You might feel awful when you move around, but his pain might be relieved if he gets up and walks around. You might get your migraines in the morning, but he might get them in the late afternoon.

"Nobody, from a homeopathic standpoint, is a textbook case, because we're all individuals," Dr. Panos says. "The main focus of homeopathy is to figure out what symptoms are present in each individual."

Unlike a medical doctor who might give you aspirin for your headache, a decongestant for your stuffy nose, lozenges for your sore throat and a tranquilizer to lessen your anxiety, a homeopath looks for a single remedy that helps all of your symptoms.

"When a person is ill, we're looking for the remedy that in the provings caused the symptoms most similar to the physical and emotional symptoms he displays," Dr. Panos says. "To get the best results, you need to find the one remedy that is most similar."

Often a homeopath will spend more than an hour with each new patient, trying to learn as much as possible about all of his symptoms, Dr. Panos says. A homeopath, for instance, might ask if you feel worse at a particular time of day, if you crave certain foods such as lemons or bacon or if you've developed any sudden anxieties such as a fear of water or dogs.

"Common symptoms are worth very little as a prescribing tool," Dr. Panos says. "Knowing that you have a cough really doesn't tell us much. But there are certain characteristics of a cough, such as whether it occurs when you enter a warm room or as you're going outside, that help us narrow down to the right remedy."

GIVE YOURSELF A HELPING HAND

Although it sounds complex, homeopaths say the basics are easy to learn and many people can develop enough homeopathic skills to treat most of their families' minor ailments at home.

HOMEOPATHY

"People who use homeopathy as primary home care or for first aid don't have to go to the doctor very often except for really serious problems," says Jacquelyn Wilson, M.D., a homeopathic physician in San Diego. "They can handle many problems at home and never have to go back to the doctor for a lot of stuff, such as earaches, colds, flus, rashes and sore throats."

Try the remedies suggested in this book, but if you're serious about using homeopathy more extensively, then practitioners suggest that you get at least 20 hours of instruction from a trained homeopath or join a self-help study group. The National Center for Homeopathy has a list of publications, classes and local study groups that can help you hone your skills (refer to the resource list on page 637).

If you're uncertain which remedy is best for your condition, many health food stores sell combination homeopathic remedies for minor ailments such as colds, flus, headaches and allergies. Since these combinations contain several homeopathic remedies commonly used to treat an ailment, proponents say there's a good chance that the one remedy you need will be contained in the mixture. The other remedies shouldn't have any effect.

But if your symptoms persist, no matter if you're taking a single or combination remedy, see a homeopath. He may recommend another homeopathic remedy or suggest conventional care such as antibiotics or surgery if you have a life-threatening infection or disease, a serious burn, internal bleeding, broken bones or another severe medical problem.

"There are some cases where it is better to have surgery or other treatment and then use homeopathy to help heal the body afterward," says Cynthia Mervis Watson, M.D., a family practice physician specializing in homeopathic and herbal therapies in Santa Monica, California.

HYDROTHERAPY

The Everyday Miracle of Water

H₂O. This little molecule is so commonplace that it's hard to think of it as a wonder drug. Yet in many cases of injury or accident, our first, instinctive response is to treat ourselves with water. Every time you soothe a sprained ankle with an ice pack or hold a burned finger under a stream of cold tap water, you're practicing a basic form of hydrotherapy, an ancient healing art that is safe and painless and requires nothing more exotic than what flows out of your bathroom faucet.

First used by Hippocrates in the fourth century B.C., hydrotherapy has been a part of the healing tradition of nearly every civilization from ancient Greece and Egypt to Rome, where virtually all medicine was practiced at the public baths.

Modern hydrotherapy originated in nineteenth-century Austria with the work of Vincent Priessnitz, considered the father of the hydrotherapy movement. When one of Priessnitz's patients, Robert Wesselhoeft, and his brother immigrated to the United States in the 1840s, hydrotherapy—or hydropathy, as it was then called—came with them.

In 1845, they founded the Brattleboro Infirmary in Vermont, modeled after Priessnitz's famous Gräfenberg spa in Austria. One of the earliest and most famous "water cure establishments," the infirmary attracted a distinguished clientele that included poet Henry Wadsworth Longfellow and novelist Harriet Beecher Stowe.

In the late nineteenth century, John Harvey Kellogg, brother of the cereal magnate and one of the most renowned physicians of his day, used water treatments at his famous Battle Creek, Michigan, sanitarium to manage pain and treat serious infections such as pneumonia. Around the same time, cold water sprays and rubs were common treatments for typhoid and pneumonia, and by the 1920s, U.S. veterans hospitals were using hydrotherapy to treat mental illness and general medical and surgical cases.

THOROUGHLY MODERN HYDROTHERAPY

Today, most Americans turn to the medicine chest instead of the bathroom faucet to alleviate colds, headaches and minor injuries, and doctors are far more likely to treat patients with pills than with poultices. But in many Euro-

pean countries, spending a week or two at a spa remains a popular way to re-
cuperate from a host of complaints, from simple stress and fatigue to backaches,
allergies and arthritis.

And here in the States, hydrotherapy is still practiced in places such as the
Uchee Pines Institute, a natural healing center in Seale, Alabama. Founded in
1970 by Agatha Thrash, M.D., a medical pathologist, and her husband, an internist, Uchee Pines helps patients rebuild their health with hydrotherapy, exercise, dietary changes and other simple remedies.

By the late 1960s, years of practicing pathology and internal medicine had
left the Thrashes disillusioned with conventional treatment. "It began to seem
to us that nobody ever really got well," recalls Dr. Thrash, who is co-director
of the institute. "The same patients just kept on coming back."

While teaching a class in anatomy and physiology at a local college, she became convinced that many diseases could be successfully treated by simple
physiological methods such as massage and hydrotherapy. "These remedies are
far less taxing to the body than drugs, which often cause insidious complications years after you stop taking them," she says.

HOW TO PERFORM AN ENEMA

A traditional water remedy for everything from constipation to migraine headaches, an enema cleanses the lower colon and can often
provide pain relief when other methods fail, says Agatha Thrash, M.D., a
medical pathologist and co-founder and co-director of Uchee Pines Institute, a natural healing center in Seale, Alabama. Enemas are also used in
conjunction with fasting to encourage the elimination of toxins released
during the fast.

To prepare an enema, fill an enema bag (available in most pharmacies)
with lukewarm water—from ½ to 1 quart for a child ten years of age or
older to no more than 2 quarts for an adult, suggests Dr. Thrash. Use one
pint for younger children. Never give children under ten years of age
more than one enema a day, since water can be absorbed and can cause
blood sodium to drop dangerously low (a condition known as hyponatremia). Take the enema while sitting on the toilet. First, lubricate the
anus and the end of the enema tubing with lotion or oil. Hold the bag
about three feet above you and insert the tubing into the anus about 1½
to 2 inches deep. Holding the tubing in place, slowly release the valve to
let the water enter the colon. Hold the solution in for several minutes,
then release into the toilet.

So if water therapies are both safe and effective, why do so many doctors appear to favor the pharmaceutical approach? One reason is that unlike drug therapies, which have mountains of scientific evidence to document their effectiveness, hydrotherapy hasn't been widely studied. "It's not easy to find funding for the study of something that is so widely available to everyone at minimal cost," says Irene Von Estorff, M.D., assistant professor of rehabilitation medicine at Cornell University Medical College in New York City. "But there is a tremendous need out there for sound research to provide specific guidelines for the best uses of hydrotherapy."

Hydrotherapy also requires "a certain amount of dedication on the part of the patient," says Dr. Thrash. "People are conditioned to believe that getting well should be as easy as swallowing a pill; they don't want to accept the idea that they have to eat well, exercise and devote time to treatment."

GULP YOUR WAY TO HEALTH

But there's at least one hydrotherapy treatment whose benefits are widely recognized. Doctors and patients alike know that drinking enough fresh, pure water is essential to our health and well-being.

This most basic form of hydrotherapy should be second nature to us—and it probably would be if we didn't keep coffee, cold beer and sugary cola on hand to quench our thirst. Though caffeinated and alcoholic beverages do contain water, both cause the body to excrete more water than it actually takes in. The result is a fluid deficit, which, over time, can lead to a variety of health problems, including dry skin, constipation and bladder infections.

These problems become more common in late adulthood, says Dr. Thrash, because our need for water actually increases with age. She recommends a minimum of 6 to 8 eight-ounce glasses of water a day for people under age 50, 8 to 10 eight-ounce glasses for those in their fifties and 10 to 12 eight-ounce glasses for active people 60 and over.

"As we age, our skin and mucous membranes become thinner and lose more water, and our kidneys function less efficiently, so our need for water increases," Dr. Thrash says. "Older people just don't feel thirst the way we did when we were younger, so we need to get in the habit of drinking water even if we're not thirsty."

Water is also valuable as a digestive aid, especially when it's combined with activated charcoal, a substance made from wood or bone that has been burned and then oxidized by steam or air. (The charcoal briquettes you use on the grill are treated with chemicals to make them light faster and aren't safe for therapeutic use.) Available in most health food stores and some pharmacies,

(continued on page 80)

HYDROTHERAPY AT HOME

Cheap and easy, these simple hydrotherapy treatments require no special equipment and are ideal for home use, say hydrotherapy experts. To find out which of these techniques can benefit a particular condition, turn to Part II of this book. Note that specifics such as water temperature and length of application can vary depending on the condition being treated. You can check water temperature with a regular oral thermometer.

- *Baths and showers* can be used to treat a number of health problems. Hot baths are used to ease joint pain, constipation and respiratory ailments. Cold baths relieve fever and combat fatigue, and herbal baths are popular for relaxation and skin care.
- *Neutral baths*, in which the body is immersed up to the neck in water slightly cooler than body temperature, are used to treat insomnia, emotional agitation and menopausal hot flashes. Soak for 20 minutes, adding water as needed to maintain the temperature of the bath.
- *Sitz baths* are used to treat pain and infection in the pelvic area. Sit in a tub or large basin filled with enough water that the pelvic area is submerged up to the navel. Soaking in a sitz bath for 1½ to 5 minutes at temperatures ranging from 40° to 85°F—or for longer periods at higher temperatures—relieves anal and vaginal irritation, hemorrhoids and anal fissures. Cold sitz baths can improve pelvic muscle tone in people with stress incontinence.
- *Contrast sitz baths*, using separate basins of hot and cold water, improve circulation in the pelvic area, speed the healing of vaginal and urinary tract infections, reduce pelvis pain and treat ovarian cysts. Begin with a three- to four-minute soak in hot water, followed by a 30- to 60-second cold soak. Repeat three to five times, ending with cold.
- *Foot baths* aren't just for tired, achy feet. Alternating hot and cold soaks is great for relieving swelling in the feet and legs. By diverting blood away from the affected areas, hot foot baths are used to relieve head and chest congestion and even menstrual cramps. Soak in comfortably hot water (about 110°F) for 10 to 30 minutes, adding water as needed to maintain the temperature of the foot bath. Finish by rinsing your feet with cold water. Alternating foot baths can also play an important role as a supplementary treatment for serious illnesses such as congestive heart failure.

- *Cold mitten friction rubs*, in which the skin is rubbed vigorously with a towel or mitten dipped in cold water, are used to increase circulation and fortify the immune system. A simple, invigorating way to banish fatigue, the cold mitten friction rub is also used to speed healing from bronchitis and pneumonia and may benefit those with chronic fatigue syndrome. After a hot bath, shower or sauna, dip a towel or washcloth into cold (50° to 60°F) water, curl one hand into a fist and wrap the cloth around it. Use your fist to rub your other arm in a vigorous circular motion, beginning with the fingers and finishing at the shoulder. Dip the cloth in the cold water again and repeat. The skin should be pink. Dry the arm with a towel using the same vigorous circular movement, then repeat the process on your other arm and on your legs, feet, chest and abdomen.
- *Steam inhalation* is used for respiratory conditions such as bronchitis and pneumonia, easing breathing by loosening mucus in the chest. Inhale the steam from a pot filled with boiling water. Take the pot off the stove and let it cool, so no active boiling is taking place (if the water is actively boiling, you can scald your face and respiratory tract). Hold your face about a foot away from the pot, and cover your head and shoulders with a towel to trap the steam. Continue for up to an hour, reheating the water as needed.
- *Hot compresses* applied to the chest are also helpful for respiratory problems. To prepare a large compress for the chest, fold a large bath towel lengthwise, twist it as if you were wringing it out and dip the center third into almost-boiling water. Pull the ends apart as hard as you can to remove most of the water, then lay the hot towel over a dry one on your chest. Leave it in place for about five minutes. Repeat this procedure every two hours. Smaller hot compresses are used for localized pain relief from muscle spasms and certain types of arthritis.
- *Cold compresses* can help relieve the pain of gout and minimize swelling from bruises and sprains. Experts suggest limiting cold applications to 20 minutes at a time to prevent damage to the skin.
- *Alternating hot and cold compresses* stimulates circulation to help heal sprains and joint and muscle injuries. Begin with three to four minutes of heat followed by 30 to 60 seconds of cold. Repeat three to five times, ending with cold.

(continued)

HYDROTHERAPY AT HOME—Continued

- *Heating compresses* are actually cold compresses that are covered with a layer of dry cloth. They are left in place until the body's heat warms them, usually for several hours or overnight. Used for sore throats, ear infections, chest colds, joint pain and digestive problems, the heating compress creates a soothing warmth in the affected area and attracts an influx of nutrient- and oxygen-rich blood to speed healing.
- The *body wrap*, or *wet sheet pack*, works on the same principle as the heating compress. The entire body is wrapped in a cold, wet sheet and covered with a wool blanket; the feet are kept warm with blankets or a hot foot bath. The pack is left in place until the body heat dries the sheet. The effect depends on the duration of the treatment. If removed after about 20 minutes, the body wrap can reduce a fever. Left in place a little longer and removed in the warm, or neutral, stage, it encourages sleep and relaxation. Applications up to three hours long induce profuse sweating, an effective detoxifying treatment for those with drinking problems as well as for those who smoke. (This treatment usually requires a second set of hands.)
- The *salt glow*, in which the body is rubbed vigorously with sea salts or Epsom salts, is an invigorating treatment for those with poor circulation. It's also recommended as preventive medicine and for those following a detoxification program. Starting with damp skin, take a handful of damp sea salts or Epsom salts and massage your skin vigorously until it turns slightly pink. Repeat on the arms, legs, back, shoulders and abdomen—and don't forget the hands and feet. It should take one to two pounds of salt to work your entire body. The salt glow may make you perspire and will help you sleep more soundly. Salt rubs should not be used if you have a skin rash or sensitive skin.

activated charcoal is known for its ability to adsorb many times its weight in liquids or gases.

"Nobody really knows how or why charcoal works, but it is truly a miracle," says Dr. Thrash, who keeps some in the medicine chest at all times for household emergencies from indigestion and toothaches to sore throats and food poisoning. Added to a glass of water, charcoal provides quick relief from most gastric discomfort; mixed with enough water to form a paste, it's great first aid for sprains and insect bites, says Dr. Thrash.

HYDROTHERAPY

SOME LIKE IT HOT, OR COLD

While other hydrotherapy treatments are a little more complicated than drinking a glass of water, most are easy to learn and require no special equipment, so they're perfect for home use.

How can a treatment as simple as a cold compress or a hot water bottle exert such a profound effect on the way we feel? The secret lies in stimulating the circulation of blood and lymphatic fluid, says Tori Hudson, N.D., a naturopathic physician and professor at the National College of Naturopathic Medicine in Portland, Oregon.

Hydrotherapists control the effect by adjusting the temperature of the water and the duration of the treatment. "Heat expands and cold contracts," says Dr. Hudson. "In general, hot water is relaxing and cold water is stimulating, although the effect also depends on how long a treatment lasts." As a rule, shorter treatments are more stimulating than longer ones.

Many hydrotherapists also use alternating hot and cold applications. These treatments, known as contrast therapies, have a powerful effect on circulation; they speed healing by delivering a greater supply of oxygen and nutrients in the blood to the injured area, according to Dr. Hudson.

Other water treatments work on the principle of derivation—that is, relieving pain and congestion by drawing blood away from a particular area of the body. To treat a sinus headache, for example, Dr. Hudson would apply cold compresses to the head and soak the feet in a hot bath to draw blood into the lower extremities, relieving the congestion in the head.

But hydrotherapy isn't just for localized conditions such as cramps and backaches. Water treatments are also used for illnesses that affect the entire system, such as chronic fatigue syndrome. In these cases, full-body applications, such as hot immersion baths, are used to strengthen the immune system, helping the body to heal itself. These treatments work by raising the body temperature from 98.6° to 102°F and sometimes higher. This process, called hyperthermia, increases the number of white blood cells in the bloodstream and improves their movement, making them more active against infection, according to Dr. Thrash. Hot treatments also draw more blood to the surface of the skin, where immune system cells are stationed. These cells fortify the blood with disease-fighting proteins, including interferon, interleukin-1 and interleukin-2.

While Dr. Thrash says the hot immersion bath is safe for healthy adults, those who are pregnant or who suffer from medical conditions such as diabetes and high blood pressure should get a doctor's advice before starting hyperthermia treatments.

TAKING CARE WITH HYDROTHERAPY

While hydrotherapy is generally quite safe, certain treatments are not recommended during pregnancy or for those with chronic health problems such as diabetes and heart disease. To avoid complications, take note of the following precautions.

- If you have diabetes, avoid hot applications to the feet or legs. "Instead of using a hot foot bath to treat a boil on the calf, a person with diabetes could apply a small hot compress, no bigger than a washcloth," says Agatha Thrash, M.D., a medical pathologist and co-founder and co-director of Uchee Pines Institute, a natural healing center in Seale, Alabama. Full-body heating treatments, such as body wraps, should also be avoided.
- Avoid cold applications if you've been diagnosed with Raynaud's disease.
- Hot immersion baths and long, hot saunas aren't recommended for those with diabetes or multiple sclerosis, women who are pregnant or anyone with abnormally high or low blood pressure.
- Don't take cold foot baths if you're prone to bladder or rectal irritation, warns Dr. Thrash. People who suffer from sciatica, pelvic inflammation or rheumatism in the toes or ankles should also avoid cold foot baths.
- Elderly people and young children may be exhausted by too much heat and should avoid long full-body hot treatments such as immersion baths and saunas.
- If you are pregnant or have heart disease, consult a doctor before taking a sauna.

FROM SAUNAS TO WHIRLPOOLS

While most hydrotherapy treatments are suitable for home use, a few require special equipment found in clinics or health clubs. One such treatment is the sauna, a sealed, wood-lined room heated by a special stove that treats the occupants to a dry-heat "bath."

Sauna baths are said to stimulate circulation, relieve arthritis pain and respiratory congestion and improve the elimination of waste products through the skin. They can also be deeply relaxing and a great way to melt away stress. Experts suggest spending no more than 15 to 20 minutes at a time in a sauna and wiping your face frequently with a cool cloth to avoid overheating.

HYDROTHERAPY

Another popular water treatment is the whirlpool bath, long used in clinics and hospitals to treat muscle and joint injuries, burns, frostbite and skin sores. Whirlpools have also found their way into health clubs and homes, where they're used to soothe sports injuries and promote relaxation.

A less familiar water treatment is colonic irrigation, in which the colon is flushed with large quantities of water to promote detoxification. Unlike an enema, which cleanses only the lower portion of the colon, a colonic purges the entire bowel, which is about five feet long. Colonics come highly recommended by many alternative practitioners, who believe that accumulated waste matter puts a strain on the immune system and can contribute to the development of degenerative diseases such as rheumatoid arthritis. Because colonic irrigation can be dangerous if performed improperly, it's essential to find a qualified practitioner. A physician, chiropractor, naturopath or gastrointestinal specialist can recommend a reliable technician.

IMAGERY

One Image Is Worth 1,000 Cures

You mowed your lawn, weeded your garden and pruned your rose-bushes, and now your back sizzles like a red–hot firecracker. You figure that you just overdid it and that the pain will soon subside. But hours later, your back is swollen and sore. Most people would take a couple of aspirin and put up their feet for the rest of the day. But not you.

Instead, you might close your eyes, take a few deep breaths and imagine that a block of ice is melting inside your neck and dripping down your back. Within minutes, the pain ebbs, and you're ready to dance the night away.

Far-fetched? Hardly, say a growing number of doctors, nurses and other advocates of imagery, who contend that the imagination is a potent healer that has long been overlooked by practitioners of Western medicine. They say imagery can relieve pain, speed healing and help the body subdue hundreds of ailments, including depression, impotence, allergies and asthma.

"The power of the mind to influence the body is quite remarkable. Although it isn't always curative, imagery can be helpful in 90 percent of the problems that people bring to the attention of their primary care physicians," says Martin L. Rossman, M.D., co-director of the Academy for Guided Imagery in Mill Valley, California, and author of *Healing Yourself: A Step-by-Step Program for Better Health through Imagery*.

EVERY PICTURE TELLS A STORY

"Imagery is the most fundamental language we have. Everything you do the mind processes through images," says Dennis Gersten, M.D., a San Diego psychiatrist and publisher of *Atlantis*, a bi-monthly imagery newsletter. "If you think about your childhood, you will probably remember images, not words. You ask anyone about his first memory of his parents, and it's not going to be a conversation."

Images aren't necessarily visual but can be sounds, tastes, smells or a combination of sensations. One person's imagery may be sparked by imagining a smell. For others, imagining that they're touching an object, such as a tree, will trigger vivid images, Dr. Gersten says. In fact, the more senses you can conjure, the more powerful an image will be.

Think, for example, of holding a fresh, juicy lemon in your hand. Perhaps you can feel its texture or see the vividness of its yellow skin. As you slice it open, you see the juice squirt out of it. The lemon's tart aroma is overwhelming. Finally, you stick it in your mouth, suck on it and taste the sour flavor as the juices roll over your tongue.

More than likely, your body reacted in some way to that image. For example, you may have begun to salivate.

"Imagery is the language that the mind uses to communicate with the body," Dr. Gersten says. "You can't really talk to a wart and say 'Hey, go away,' because that's not the language that the brain uses to communicate with the body. You need to imagine that wart and see it shrinking. Imagery is the biological connection between the mind and body."

Unfortunately, many of the images popping into our heads do more harm than good. In fact, the most common type of imagery is worry, says David Bresler, Ph.D., co-director of the Academy for Guided Imagery. Because when we worry, what we worry about exists only in our imaginations.

In just 30 seconds, for instance, a fragment of a song may zip through your head, which in turn sparks images of a good friend. That friend, unfortunately, just lost her job. Oops, that couldn't happen to you, right? Well, there is that important presentation on Tuesday. Suppose you don't make your sales quota this month? Your boss was a bit testy with you yesterday; does that mean something? In less than a minute, you've gone from a pleasant memory of a good friend to imagining yourself getting fired.

The average person has 10,000 thoughts or images like these careening through his mind each day, Dr. Gersten estimates. At least half of those thoughts are negative. Unharnessed, a steady dose of worry and other negative images can alter your physiology and make you more susceptible to a cornucopia of ailments, ranging from acne to arthritis, headaches to heart disease, ulcers to urinary tract infections, he says.

But if you can learn to direct and control the images in your head, you can help your body heal itself, Dr. Rossman says.

"The imagination is like a spirited, powerful horse. If it's untamed, it can be dangerous and run you over," Dr. Rossman says. "But if you learn to use your imagination in a way that is purposeful and directed, it can be a tremendously powerful vehicle to get you where you want to go, which in this case is better health."

A NEW LOOK AT AN OLD REMEDY

The belief that your imagination can help cure your ills isn't a new one. Imagery has been considered a healing tool in virtually all of the world's cultures and is an integral part of many religions. Navajo Indians, for example, practice an elaborate form of imagery that encourages a person to "see" himself as healthy. Ancient Egyptians and Greeks, including Aristotle and Hippocrates, the father of modern medicine, believed that images release spirits in the brain that arouse the heart and other parts of the body. They also thought that a strong image of a disease is enough to cause its symptoms.

Imagery continued to flourish during the Renaissance in the fifteenth and sixteenth centuries, when the Swiss physician Paracelsus wrote that "the power of the imagination is a great factor in medicine. It may produce disease . . . and it may cure them." As recently as the early 1600s, imagery was thought to have such a powerful influence on the body that it could even affect embryos in pregnant women.

But over the next 300 years, Western medicine discarded imagery as a healing tool as more and more doctors were indoctrinated with the teachings of René Descartes, a seventeenth-century French philosopher who believed the mind and body were separate and couldn't possibly have any influence on each other.

Although Sigmund Freud, Carl Jung and other European psychiatrists dabbled in treating patients with imagery, it was largely ignored in the United States until O. Carl Simonton, M.D., a radiation oncologist in Los Angeles, began using it in the early 1970s to help cancer patients. Dr. Simonton claimed that activity of the immune system could be boosted by visualizing strong white blood cells attacking weak cancer cells. Dr. Simonton tracked 159 patients, all with incurable cancer and all told that they had about a year to live. Using imagery as part of their treatment, 40 percent of those patients were still living four years later, and 22 percent of those went into full remission. In another 19 percent, the tumors shrank. Overall, people in the study who used imagery in conjunction with medical treatment lived twice as long as those who received medical care alone.

THE PROOF ISN'T AN ILLUSION

"There's definite evidence from Dr. Simonton and others that using imagery can dramatically enhance the quality of life and, in some cases, extend life," Dr. Gersten says.

People with cancer, for instance, who used imagery while receiving chemotherapy felt more relaxed, better prepared for their treatment and more positive about care than those who didn't use the technique, according to researchers at Ohio State University in Columbus.

Several studies suggest that imagery can also boost your immunity. Danish researchers, for example, found increased natural killer cell activity among ten

WHAT DO YOU SAY TO A NAKED LEPRECHAUN?

Your head feels as if it were being squeezed into a jelly jar. No doubt about it: You're having another killer headache. So you close your eyes and take a few deep breaths, and the next thing you know, you see a naked leprechaun twisting a rubber band around your head.

What do you do? Talk to him, suggests Dennis Gersten, M.D., a San Diego psychiatrist and publisher of *Atlantis*, a bi-monthly imagery newsletter.

"The leprechaun is a symbolic image of your symptoms. So if you talk to that image—ask him why he's there, what he wants from you—you might find out this leprechaun is very concerned about your well-being," Dr. Gersten says. "That's why he's twisting that band around your head. He's trying to get your attention so that he can tell you about some underlying stresses in your life that you may not be consciously aware of."

From there, you can begin to negotiate with the image about a solution to the problem, he says. You might, for instance, promise to stop skipping meals, to get an extra hour of sleep each night and to do an imagery exercise twice a day. In exchange, the leprechaun might agree to loosen the rubber band a notch or two. After several sessions with the leprechaun, he might even agree to take the rubber band off your head and go away.

Symbolic images can take many forms, says David Bresler, Ph.D., co-director of the Academy for Guided Imagery in Mill Valley, California. A symbolic image can be a shape, color, light or lightning bolt. "Imagery is very fanciful," he says. "People can fly through the air; rocks can talk."

But images can also be fairly literal. "Literal images are more anatomically correct than symbolic images," Dr. Gersten says. "You're imagining things the way you want them to be. If you have asthma, you might picture your airways as being open. If you have cancer, you might picture white blood cells chewing on the tumor. If you have a migraine, you might picture the blood vessels in your head being very smooth and relaxed and the blood cruising through without any problems."

Both types of imagery are useful, but which is best for you? "Your unconscious mind will tell you," Dr. Gersten says. "Listen to what your intuition is saying about it. If you feel more comfortable using a literal image, such as picturing the headache going away, do that. If you feel better asking your mind to create a symbolic image, do that. It's a matter of trusting your intuition, practicing and experimenting."

college students who imagined that their immune systems were becoming very effective. Natural killer cells are an important part of the immune system because they can recognize and destroy virus-infected cells, tumor cells and other invaders.

In another small study, researchers at Pennsylvania State University in University Park and Case Western Reserve University School of Medicine in Cleveland found that seven people who suffered from recurrent canker sores in their mouths significantly reduced the frequency of their outbreaks after they began visualizing that the sores were bathed in a soothing coating of white blood cells.

Imagery can also help alter menstrual cycles and relieve symptoms of premenstrual syndrome. In a preliminary study, researchers at Massachusetts General Hospital in Boston found that 12 of 15 women, ages 21 to 40, who used imagery for three months lengthened their monthly menstrual cycles by an average of nearly four days and slashed their perceived levels of premenstrual distress in half. They also reported fewer mood swings.

At the University of South Florida in Tampa, researchers asked 19 men and women, ages 56 to 75, who had chronic bronchitis and emphysema to rate their levels of anxiety, depression, fatigue and discomfort before and after they began using imagery. The researchers concluded that imagery significantly improved the overall quality of these people's lives.

Other studies have shown that imagery can lower blood pressure, slow heart rate and help treat insomnia, obesity and phobias, according to Anees Sheikh, Ph.D., professor of psychology at Marquette University in Milwaukee and editor of *Eastern and Western Approaches to Healing*.

IS IMAGERY VIRTUAL REALITY?

How imagery works its wonders in the body is still a mystery. Some evidence suggests, however, that the brain reacts the same way to an imagined sensation as to a real one.

"Imagery is like reality in the sense that if you look at activity in the brain when you're imagining something, it is strikingly similar to the activity that occurs when you're perceiving reality," Dr. Sheikh says.

Remember the lemon described earlier and how it probably caused you to secrete saliva in your mouth? Scientists know from PET (positron-emission tomography) scans, tests that show areas of brain activity, that imagery has similar effects on other parts of the body. Vividly imagining that you're swinging a tennis racket, for instance, can actually stimulate the muscles in your shoulders and arms.

Some researchers theorize that images are formed as a result of electrochemical reactions in the limbic system, a portion of the brain that processes emotions such as pleasure, pain, fright and anger. As these images arise in the limbic system, they are probably interpreted by the cerebral cortex, which is involved in higher brain functions such as reasoning and memory. Without the cerebral cortex, these images would probably be meaningless to us, Dr. Gersten speculates. The limbic system is also connected by nerves to the hypothalamus, a portion of the brain that regulates body temperature, heart rate, hunger, thirst, sleeping and sexual arousal, and to the pituitary gland, which oversees all of your hormones.

So after an image forms in the limbic system and is deciphered by the cerebral cortex, the hypothalamus and pituitary gland scramble into action, causing physiological reactions throughout the body.

If you imagine yourself waterskiing, for example, your brain triggers the release of nerve impulses, chemicals and hormones from the hypothalamus and pituitary gland that affect every one of your cells. In return, the cells can send signals back to the brain that make the experience seem more vivid and cause the mind to release more chemicals to sustain that image.

So for better or worse, nearly every image has an effect on your body.

"Let's say you're stuck in traffic and you're going to be late for an important meeting. What happens? You see all of those people impatiently waiting for you at the meeting. You're not in that situation yet. You don't even know if that's what they're doing. But you've created that image, and as a consequence, your heart rate goes up, your breathing becomes more shallow, your palms get sweaty, your hands get cold, and your muscles get tense. So that image is having a real physiological effect. You're producing adrenaline, which is going to keep your body unnecessarily on alert," says Barbara Dossey, R.N., director of Holistic Nursing Consultants in Santa Fe, New Mexico, and co-author of *Rituals of Healing: Using Imagery for Health and Wellness.*

On the other hand, if you could momentarily forget about the meeting and imagine a favorite scene, such as lying on a beach, climbing a mountain or playing with your child, that could spark the release of natural tranquilizers that would slow your breathing and heart rate, lower your anxiety and stimulate your immune system, Dossey says.

GETTING DOWN TO BASICS

So if you can learn to use the images in your mind instead of letting them flow over you like a wild, untamed river, they can have positive, long-term effects on your health and well-being, Dr. Gersten says.

Is it difficult to master? "Everybody thinks, everyone feels, and everyone has images," Dr. Gersten says. "It's just a matter of practice. Virtually everyone can successfully use imagery. It's a question of patience and persistence. It's just like

MAKING THE MOST OF YOUR IMAGES

Before you exercise, you stretch. Before you drive a car, you put on a seat belt. And before you can elicit an image, you need to be in the right frame of mind. Here's a simple step-by-step guide to help make imagery work for you.

Take a few moments to relax. Studies indicate that imagery works best when it is used in conjunction with a relaxation technique, says Dennis Gersten, M.D., a San Diego psychiatrist and publisher of *Atlantis*, a bimonthly imagery newsletter. "When your physical body is relaxed, you don't need to be in such conscious control of your mind, and you can give it the freedom to daydream," he says.

Loosen your clothing, take off your shoes, lie down or sit in a comfortable chair and, if you'd like, dim the lights. Close your eyes and take a few deep breaths. Picture yourself descending an imaginary staircase, suggests Martin L. Rossman, M.D., co-director of the Academy for Guided Imagery in Mill Valley, California, and author of *Healing Yourself: A Step-by-Step Program for Better Health through Imagery*. With each step, notice that you feel more and more relaxed.

As an alternative, you might want to try meditation or progressive relaxation, a series of muscle-flexing exercises that some people use to relieve tension. A person, for example, might begin by flexing and releasing the muscles in the hands, then progressively tensing and relaxing the muscles in the arms, neck, head, back, legs and feet.

When you feel relaxed, imagine a favorite scene. It could be a beach, a mountain slope or a particularly enjoyable moment with friends or family. Try to go into this scene each time you practice your imagery. "If you can create a special, safe place where nothing can hurt you and you feel secure, it will make you more receptive to other images," says Barbara L. Rees, R.N., Ph.D., an imagery expert and professor of nursing at the University of New Mexico College of Nursing in Albuquerque.

Once you feel comfortable in your favorite scene, gradually direct your mind toward the ailment you're concerned about. Use one of the images

learning to play the piano. You put in the time, you put in the discipline, you can play the piano. Practice with imagery will produce results just like learning to play a musical instrument."

How much time it will take before you begin to see results depends on the severity of your ailment, the vividness of your imagery and your own determination. A person who has a sprained ankle, for example, may get pain relief in suggested in Part II of this book, or allow your mind to create one of its own. Let the image become more vivid and in focus. Don't worry if it seems to fade in and out. "These images aren't like turning on a television set and the picture instantly being there," Dr. Rossman says. "They can fade away and come back over the course of several minutes."

If several images come to mind, choose one and stick with it for that session, Dr. Gersten says. If you jump from image to image, it will likely break your concentration and make it more difficult for the imagery to work for you, he says.

On the other hand, if no images come to mind, try focusing on a different sensation, suggests Gerald Epstein, M.D., a New York City psychiatrist and author of *Healing Visualizations*. For instance, imagine hearing fish frying in a skillet or smelling wildflowers in a meadow. If all else fails, think about how you feel at the moment. Angry? Frustrated? What color is that anger? What image is evoked? Use these feelings to forge images.

Each time you do this, imagine that your ailment is completely cured at the end of the session. "That creates an internal blueprint that your body can follow to help heal you," says Patricia Norris, Ph.D., a psychophysiological therapist at the Life Sciences Institute of Mind-Body Health in Topeka, Kansas.

At the end of your session, take a few more deep breaths and picture yourself reclimbing the imaginary staircase and gradually becoming aware of your surroundings. Open your eyes, stretch, smile and go on with your day, Dr. Rossman suggests.

If you wish, sketch a picture of the image you used. It may help you recall it for use during other sessions, Dr. Gersten says.

In the beginning, practice this imagery exercise for 15 to 20 minutes at least once a day. As you become more skilled, you will probably be able to do it at will for just a few moments at a time several times a day and still receive the benefits.

just one five-minute imagery session, while it may take weeks for a person who has severe burns to notice any significant pain reduction.

"For almost any chronic ailment, it's going to take a lot more time for imagery to work," Dr. Gersten says.

Most proponents suggest practicing your imagery for 15 to 20 minutes a day initially to ensure that you're learning to do it properly. But as you become more skilled and comfortable with the technique, you'll be able to do it for just a few minutes at a time as needed throughout the day, Dr. Gersten says. (For more information on how to use imagery successfully, see "Making the Most of Your Images" on page 90.)

To improve the quality of your images, become a keen observer of life, Dr. Sheikh advises. "Improving your observational skills is the most important thing you can do to make your images more vivid. If you've never really paid attention to what a rose looks like, smells like or feels like, your image of that rose is going be very vague and weak."

The best images are the ones that you conjure for yourself, because they have personal meaning and will help you learn more about yourself than any imagery that can be suggested to you, Dr. Gersten says.

"Imagery always represents a part of yourself," Dr. Bresler says. "It's very much like the old Rorschach ink blot test, but people are making their own ink blots or images."

The images suggested in Part II of this book will probably help you. But if they don't, don't give up. Instead, use these images as catalysts to help you create your own, Dr. Gersten recommends.

"These images will give you an idea about how to get started, but they may lead you to an image that is totally different, and that's okay," he says.

Juice Therapy

Putting the Squeeze on Good Health

Fruit and vegetable juices aren't new to the American diet. From hospital cafeterias to fast-food outlets to our own kitchens, breakfast isn't breakfast without orange juice. Juices now come in special packages designed for toddlers' tiny hands, and health-conscious adults swill the stuff all day long as a tasty alternative to soda.

But as more and more people are discovering, fruit and vegetable juices aren't just delicious. Alternative practitioners say these tasty nectars are natural tonics, offering a safe, inexpensive way to stimulate digestion, bolster the immune system and encourage the elimination of toxins. Fresh juices are also believed to be a potent weapon against disease; studies show that juices can speed the healing of infections and can even help cure stomach ulcers. And when used in conjunction with other natural techniques, such as herbs, homeopathy and nutritional therapy, fresh juices can create an optimal nutritional foundation to bolster the body's innate healing abilities.

While health-conscious Americans caught the juicing bug in the 1970s, juicing wasn't born yesterday. Juice therapy has long been a component of the 5,000-year-old tradition of Ayurveda, says John Peterson, M.D., an Ayurvedic practitioner in Muncie, Indiana.

In Ayurveda, a traditional system of medicine that originated in India, specific juices are used to fortify each body tissue, or *dhatues*. Ayurvedic practitioners believe that stress, emotional imbalance and poor digestion can block the body's normal absorption of nutrients, resulting in undernourishment and illness. By prescribing specific juices to strengthen the weak tissue, Dr. Peterson says he has had excellent results with conditions as varied as anemia, constipation and arthritis.

Juices are also used therapeutically by naturopathic physicians, who treat patients with some combination of natural healing methods such as homeopathy, herbs, vitamins, nutritional counseling and acupuncture. At the Northwest Naturopathic Clinic in Portland, Oregon, Steven Bailey, N.D., a naturopathic physician, uses a supervised juice fast with many patients, including those suffering from arthritis, cancer and AIDS. During the fast, Dr. Bailey's patients abstain from solid foods for several days, drawing their nourishment from large doses of fresh vegetable and fruit juices.

"Juice fasting enhances the body's natural healing capacity," explains Dr.

Bailey. "Juices provide optimal nutrition yet take very little energy to digest. And because you're not spending six hours trying to digest a fatty, high-protein meal, the body has more energy to devote to repairing itself."

The juice fast also helps identify food sensitivities, a major factor in immune system disorders such as arthritis, asthma and chronic fatigue syndrome, according to Dr. Bailey. By gradually re-introducing foods after the fast, many patients discover that their symptoms worsen when they eat certain foods. "Most of my patients don't realize they have food sensitivities until they start a juice fast, see an improvement in their symptoms and then get sick all over again once they go back to eating foods as common as corn, wheat and tomatoes," he says.

"Removing the allergen from the diet lifts a tremendous burden from the immune system, so it can fight disease more effectively."

While many have benefited from juice fasting, it isn't for everybody. A hidden medical condition such as diabetes or hypoglycemia can make fasting dangerous without careful medical supervision, so be sure to get a professional's advice before starting a fast.

For those whose active lifestyles make fasting impractical, a cleansing diet offers many of the same benefits as a juice fast, says naturopathic physician Robert Broadwell, N.D., director of the Institute for Alternative Medicine in Fountain Valley, California. For two to three days, Dr. Broadwell's patients stick to a diet of raw fruits and vegetables supplemented by plenty of fresh juices; diluted beet juice is particularly effective at stimulating the liver, says Dr. Broadwell. "This allows the body to eliminate stored toxins caused by a poor diet and sometimes by prolonged use of antibiotics."

A raw-foods diet featuring plenty of fresh juices is safe for virtually everyone, says Dr. Broadwell. He finds the cleansing diet especially helpful in treating chronic degenerative conditions such as heart disease and arthritis.

Drink Your Vegetables

Juices aren't used just to treat illness; they're also a safe, inexpensive form of preventive medicine. Studies show that a diet rich in fruits and vegetables decreases our risk of developing a number of chronic degenerative diseases, including cancer, diabetes and heart disease. But even with organizations such as the National Cancer Institute in Rockville, Maryland, and the American Cancer Society urging us to eat more fruits and vegetables, many people still aren't getting the message. One study found that fewer than 10 percent of Americans eat the recommended two fruits and three vegetables a day.

A few glasses of fresh juice each day is a great way to increase the nutrient density of our diets, says Cherie Calbom, M.S., a certified nutritionist in Kirkland, Washington, and co-author of *Juicing for Life*. "There aren't too many people who manage to eat a pound of raw carrots a day. But anyone can squeeze in an eight-ounce glass of juice."

That eight-ounce glass of carrot juice packs a nutritional wallop of important vitamins, with more than ten times the Recommended Dietary Allowance of vitamin A and as much vitamin C as two bananas.

What juices can't provide, though, is fiber—at least not the 20 to 35 grams that adults need each day. Our eight-ounce glass of carrot juice contains a meager 2 grams of fiber, compared with the 14 grams in the pound of carrots that it takes to make a cup of juice. Fiber is essential for healthy digestion and may even help prevent certain types of cancer. "Drinking juice isn't a substitute for eating high-fiber fruits, vegetables and whole grains," stresses Calbom.

"I encourage people to think of juices as a supplement to a healthy diet," she says. "If we followed a perfect diet, we'd be eating raw vegetables and drinking them. But considering that most Americans do neither, adding a few glasses of fresh juice each day can do a lot to improve the average person's diet."

HIGH-OCTANE NUTRITION

Fresh juices have more going for them than vitamins and minerals. A growing body of scientific research suggests that when it comes to the health benefits of fresh produce, vitamins and minerals may be just the tip of the iceberg.

"Fruits and vegetables have therapeutic properties that science is only beginning to understand," says Stephen Blauer, former director of the Hippocrates Health Institute, a naturopathic clinic in Boston, and author of *The Juicing Book*. "We know a lot about vitamins and minerals, but there are many other substances in fruits and vegetables that haven't been as well-studied."

Known collectively as the anutrients, these substances include pigments, which give plants their color, and enzymes, substances produced in the plant that help humans digest it.

Probably the best-known pigments are the carotenes, which are responsible for the vivid color of vegetables such as carrots, sweet potatoes and squash. Though scientists have identified more than 400 different carotenes, the one most people have heard about is beta-carotene, a nutritional heavy hitter that the body easily converts to vitamin A. Studies indicate that beta-carotene has potent anti-cancer properties and may actually reverse precancerous conditions such as oral leukoplakia, a pattern of abnormal cell growth that often leads to mouth cancer in people who chew tobacco. Additional studies indicate that other members of the carotene family may have similar cancer-fighting potential.

A second group of pigments with potential healing power is the flavonoids, found in vegetables, fruits and beverages such as tea. Flavonoids give fruits and flowers their vibrant hues. While American scientists have yet to study the flavonoids in detail, European researchers have begun to investigate the health benefits of these pigments. A five-year Dutch study of 805 elderly men found that those who regularly consumed fruits and vegetables high in flavonoids were less likely to die of heart disease than those whose intakes were lower, regardless of their intakes of other nutrients.

Raw fruits and vegetables are also rich in enzymes, substances produced in plant tissue that kick off the many chemical reactions necessary for human digestion. "Natural foods come 'packaged' with just the right enzymes to help us digest them," says Blauer. "But when you destroy those enzymes, as in the case of highly refined and processed foods, the body has to manufacture its own and ends up working very hard to break down foods. This isn't the way human digestion was designed to work."

WHY FRESH IS BEST

It's important to note that when these experts recommend juices, they're not talking about the prepackaged juices sold in supermarkets. "Processed juices bear very little resemblance to fresh juice, either nutritionally or aesthetically," says Blauer.

While fresh juices and prepackaged ones may start out equal, all store-bought juices are pasteurized, a process that involves heating the juice at very high temperatures to maximize shelf life. While pasteurization is necessary to prevent spoiling, it destroys many of the juice's fragile vitamins and enzymes, according to Blauer. While store-bought juices are better for you than cola, coffee or alcohol, they aren't considered to have much therapeutic value.

To reap the health benefits of juicing, you'll need to buy a home juicer, sold in most department and health food stores at prices ranging from $25 to $2,000. While this involves some initial expense, the growing popularity of juicing has brought a number of new manufacturers into the market, and prices are more competitive than ever. "A juicer is one of the best investments you can possibly make in your health," says Calbom. (To find out what to look for when buying a juicer, see "Choose Your Weapon.")

PICKING YOUR PRODUCE

Juice is only as healthful as the fruits and vegetables that go into it, so choosing the best-quality produce is very important. Most experts are big fans of organic produce, fruits and vegetables grown without the pesticides used in almost all mainstream agriculture. "We know so little about the long-term ef-

CHOOSE YOUR WEAPON

It takes a powerful machine to distill a hard, fibrous vegetable into a sweet, smooth cocktail. Because it can't separate the liquid from the pulp, your blender can only turn fruits and vegetables into mushy, unappealing paste. And while the old hand-squeezed method still works for citrus, it isn't much help with beets and carrots.

To do the job right, you'll need an electric juicer, sold in most department and health food stores. While juicers can be had for as little as $25 or as much as $2,000, the best values are in the $100 to $200 range, suggests Cherie Calbom, M.S., a certified nutritionist in Kirkland, Washington, and co-author of *Juicing for Life*, who says she has tried nearly every juicer on the market.

Juicers come in two basic models: the masticating type, which "chews" the fruit into a paste and then squeezes the paste through a screen, and the centrifugal type, which chops and spins the fruit in a rotating mesh basket, separating the juice from the pulp. Both kinds are fast and effective. Most machines sold in department stores are the centrifugal type; most health food stores sell both kinds.

Whichever model you choose, Calbom recommends one with at least 0.4 horsepower. It will cost more, she admits, but with proper care, it can last for 20 years or more. She prefers a machine that ejects the pulp out one side and pours the juice from the other. "If you're making a large quantity of juice, it saves you the trouble of stopping to empty the pulp collector," she says. On the other hand, if you're juicing for one or two, a pulp ejector probably isn't necessary, says Stephen Blauer, former director of the Hippocrates Health Institute, a naturopathic clinic in Boston, and author of *The Juicing Book*.

Above all, your juicer should be easy to clean; the fewer parts, the better. "It doesn't really matter how good the machine is if it's a hassle to clean, because you won't use it," says Calbom. Blauer uses a juicer that breaks down into four dishwasher-safe parts. "It's a real time-saver," he says.

fects of pesticides," notes Calbom. "For me, that's reason enough to avoid them." Buying organic also gives you more valuable nutrients for your money, says Dr. Bailey, since organic farmers generally take pains to protect the mineral content of their soil.

If you juice daily and find organic produce prohibitively expensive, you can still reduce your exposure to pesticides by choosing organic versions of just the

READY, SET, JUICE!

Once you've selected your produce, it's important to use it as quickly as possible. The following guidelines are suggested by Cherie Calbom, M.S., a certified nutritionist in Kirkland, Washington, and co-author of *Juicing for Life*.

- Scrub produce thoroughly with a vegetable brush before juicing. Soak nonorganic produce in a sinkful of tepid water with a drop of pure castile soap, available in most health food stores, adds Stephen Blauer, former director of the Hippocrates Health Institute, a naturopathic clinic in Boston, and author of *The Juicing Book*. (A drop of dishwashing liquid also does the job.)
- If a fruit or vegetable has been waxed, be sure to peel it before juicing. While the wax itself won't hurt you, it makes it virtually impossible to remove pesticide residues from the skin.
- Remove all seeds and pits. When you're not using a juicer made specifically for citrus fruits, be sure to peel them before juicing. The skins of oranges and grapefruits contain a toxic oil that's an active ingredient in some household cleaners, according to Calbom. Leave as much of the white, pithy part as possible, though, since it's loaded with vitamin C and flavonoids.
- Cut fruits and vegetables into small-enough pieces to fit easily through your juicer. Cut off and discard any parts that look bruised or damaged; they don't add any nutritional value and may affect the taste of your juice.
- Wash and juice any stems or greens that are still attached to the fruit or vegetable. Many, such as beet greens, are rich in valuable minerals. Two exceptions are carrot and rhubarb greens, which can be toxic.
- Certain fruits, such as bananas and avocados, contain very little water and can't be juiced. If you'd like to include them in a juice recipe, juice all the other, moister produce first, transfer the juice to a blender and process with the (peeled) banana or avocado.
- Imported fruits and vegetables should be avoided when possible because they contain more harmful pesticide residue than domestic produce. But if you must use it, be sure to peel it before juicing.
- For maximum benefit, serve juice immediately. Juices stored in the refrigerator lose their nutritional value very quickly.

fruits and vegetables you use most often and scrubbing supermarket produce to remove pesticide residues. Avoid imported produce when possible, though, since many pesticides that have been banned in the United States are still legal in other countries. If you must use imported produce, be sure to peel it before juicing.

Whenever possible, buy locally grown fruits and vegetables; they're usually both cheaper and fresher than those shipped in from other parts of the country. For variety, explore local farmers markets and roadside stands, and be on the lookout for pick-your-own farms, where you can roll up your sleeves and select your own peaches, peas, apples or strawberries.

For maximum benefit, drink your juice immediately after you make it; within a half-hour is best. Juices stored in the refrigerator lose their nutritional value rather quickly. As soon as a fruit or vegetable is processed in your juicer, the natural enzymes in the juice begin to break down the other nutrients. Because vegetables contain more enzymes than fruits, their nutrients are depleted faster. "Once vegetable juices start to thicken, all that's left are water, minerals and calories," says Dr. Bailey. (For more information on how to maximize the health benefits of juices, see "Ready, Set, Juice!")

MASSAGE

The Touch That Heals

Back in the days before aspirin, heating pads and whirlpools, humans treated their sore bodies the old-fashioned way: with massage. When a caveman twisted one of his Neanderthal knees, he rubbed it. When a Greek princess developed pain in her temples, she rubbed them. And when folks ate too much at one of those ancient Italian toga parties, they did what the Romans did: They rubbed their aching bellies.

In many ways, massage is the most natural of natural remedies. Touching your body where it hurts seems to be a basic instinct, like running from danger or eating when you're hungry. And experts say that massage, no matter how humble or low-tech it may seem, can be a powerful healer.

"It really makes you feel great, and it can be a great aid to healing," says Vincent Iuppo, N.D., a naturopathic physician, a massage therapist and director of the Morris Institute of Natural Therapeutics, a holistic health education center in Denville, New Jersey. "Massage is one of the best ways to help with blood circulation, sore joints, headaches and lots of other problems."

Massage has come a long way over the centuries. People around the world have developed special techniques, from the famous Swedish massage to the lesser-known but growing forms such as Hellerwork, Trager and craniosacral therapy. Many of these require years of training to master and can't be done on yourself. But experts say there are self-massage techniques that you can use to help with many common health concerns. You can rub away stress, headaches, restless legs, muscle cramps and more—all with techniques that require only practice, a warm, quiet spot and a little massage oil, which you can make from ingredients in your kitchen.

HOW SWEDE IT IS

Massage has been around for at least 5,000 years, Dr. Iuppo says. Artifacts show that the Chinese, Japanese, Greeks, Romans, Egyptians and just about every other culture practiced some form of body manipulation to ease pain and prevent or cure illness. In different languages, massage has been referred to as *toogi-toogi*, *anmo* and *nuad bo-rarn*.

In the nineteenth century, a Swede named Peter Hendrik Ling began to de-

100

velop what is now the most widely known and studied form of massage in the Western world: Swedish massage. Ling, a fencing master, incorporated gymnastics, movement and massage in a health care regimen that he called the Swedish Movement Cure. He was the first westerner in modern times to systematize massage, and he set up an academy in Sweden to teach his techniques. Ling's followers have refined his techniques into a series of maneuvers.

If you've ever been treated to a full Swedish massage, you know how relaxing it can be. But many massage experts believe that it offers other benefits as well, including:

- Reduced muscle tension
- Stimulated or soothed nervous system
- Enhanced skin condition
- Improved blood circulation
- Better digestion and intestinal function
- Increased mobility in joints
- Relief of chronic pain
- Reduced swelling and inflammation

A therapist trained in Swedish massage uses soothing, tapping and kneading strokes to work the entire body, relieving muscle tension and loosening sore joints. Swedish massage therapists use five basic strokes, which anyone can learn and use on themselves and others. They are:

- *Effleurage*, a French word that means "stroking." It's a warm-up technique that lets a person get used to the feel of the therapist's hands. The gliding stroke primarily improves circulation, says Elliot Greene, past president of the American Massage Therapy Association, the largest and oldest national professional association for massage therapists.
- *Petrissage*, a technique in which you lightly grab and lift muscles, pulling them away from the bones. You can then "knead" the muscles, rolling and squeezing them. Massage therapists believe this stroke helps relieve sore muscles by clearing away lactic acid, a by-product created by your muscles when they work extra hard. Petrissage may also increase circulation to muscle tissue.
- *Friction*, which involves using thumbs and fingertips to work deep circles into the thickest parts of muscles as well as around the joints. These circular motions may help break adhesions, knots of tissue that form when muscle fibers bind together. Greene says friction may also make soft tissue and joints more flexible.
- *Tapotement*, which includes all of the chopping, beating and tapping strokes in Swedish massage. These can be used for two purposes. A few

seconds of tapotement can invigorate your muscles, stimulating them and giving you a burst of energy. But if you use the technique for a longer period, it will begin to fatigue and thereby relax the muscle—a welcome result for muscles that are cramped, strained or in spasm.

• *Vibration*, whose strokes involve pressing fingers or flattened hands firmly on a muscle, then shaking the area rapidly for a few seconds. This may help stimulate your nervous system, experts say, and could boost circulation and improve the function of your glands.

For specific instructions on these techniques, see the illustrations beginning on page 570.

HANDS OFF!

When should you have a massage? Whenever you feel like it. "A Swedish massage every day would be absolutely terrific, provided you have the time and money to do it," says Vincent Iuppo, N.D., a naturopathic physician, a massage therapist and director of the Morris Institute of Natural Therapeutics, a holistic health education center in Denville, New Jersey. You should have a massage particularly if you are feeling stressed or fatigued or if you have muscle soreness, adds Elliot Greene, past president of the American Massage Therapy Association (AMTA).

Still, there are a few occasions when you should not get a massage. "In some instances, it may aggravate existing conditions," Dr. Iuppo says. If you have any of the problems below, the AMTA strongly urges you to check with a doctor before seeking a massage.

• Heart disease or high blood pressure. While massage may benefit these conditions, it's up to you and your doctor to decide the best course of action.
• Infections from a cut or injury. Don't massage any open wound.
• Bad sprains or strains. The AMTA suggests waiting 24 to 48 hours after a sprain or strain before having any massage done on the affected area. This gives the inflammation a chance to diminish before anyone starts to manipulate the area.
• Contagious skin conditions or diseases. Again, you could spread it to other body parts.
• Phlebitis or other circulatory problems. There is the possibility of a blood clot breaking free.

A TOUCH OF RELAXATION

Even though massage is older than any history book, since 1920 there has been relatively little scientific study of how it affects the body. Still, a revival in research has begun to unravel the mystery behind how massage works, says Tiffany Field, Ph.D., director of the Touch Research Institute at the University of Miami School of Medicine.

For one thing, massage may slow the body's release of the stress hormone cortisol, Dr. Field says. In a study of 52 hospitalized children, a daily 30-minute back massage seemed to inhibit the body's production of cortisol, and nurses also reported that the children were less anxious and slept longer. Dr. Field says that massage before bedtime also seems to lengthen the deepest phase of sleep, allowing your muscles and other body parts more time to regenerate.

In addition, massage may increase your body's production of another hormone, serotonin, which can improve your mood, boost your immune system and possibly ward off migraine headaches, Dr. Field says. And a study of 28 cancer patients showed that men who received a ten-minute back massage reported significant short-term pain relief immediately after their rubdowns.

DIFFERENT STROKES

Sweden is only one country, and Swedish massage is only one form of massage. According to Greene, some of the most common forms in the United States, such as deep tissue massage, sports massage and neuromuscular massage, are refinements of Swedish massage.

Deep tissue massage targets chronic tension in muscles that lie far below the surface of your body. You have five layers of muscle in your back, for instance, and while Swedish massage may help the first couple of layers, it won't do much directly for the muscle underneath. Deep muscle techniques usually involve slow strokes, direct pressure or friction movements that go across the grain of the muscles. Massage therapists will use their fingers, thumbs or occasionally even elbows to apply the needed pressure.

A therapist may use Swedish massage in combination with deep tissue or other forms of massage, Greene says. "I may do Swedish massage techniques until I find muscles that need deep tissue techniques," he says.

Sports massage is designed to help you train better, whether you're a world champion or a weekend warrior. The techniques are similar to those in Swedish and deep tissue massage, but Greene says sports massage has been adapted to meet the athlete's special needs. Pre-event massage can help warm up muscles and improve circulation before competition, but it can also energize or relax an athlete and help him focus on the competition. Post-event massage can push waste products out of the body and improve recovery. Sports massage can help athletes prevent or work through minor aches and pains accumulated during training and can allow them to train more effectively. Massage also helps athletes recover from injuries and aids in rehabilitation. The massage is faster-paced than Swedish or deep tissue massage, Greene says.

Neuromuscular massage is a form of deep tissue massage that is applied to individual muscles. It is used to increase blood flow, reduce pain and release pressure on nerves caused by injuries to muscles and other soft tissue. Neuromuscular massage helps release trigger points, intense knots of tense muscle that can also "refer" pain to other parts of the body. Relieving a tense trigger point in your back, for example, could help ease pain in your shoulder or reduce headaches.

There are many other, lesser-known techniques that differ from the Swedish massage tradition.

"There really is a whole world of techniques out there," says Dan Bienenfeld, a certified Hellerwork practitioner, a massage therapist and director of the Los Angeles Healing Arts Center, a holistic healing practice that offers massage and other natural health alternatives. "You can find all sorts of massage, from gentle touching to pressure points to pretty vigorous stuff. Each offers you something different, a different way to heal."

Some massage therapists call these techniques bodywork. Here's a sample of some of the major types and the benefits you might expect from each.

Rolfing seeks to re-educate your body about posture. When posture is poor, Bienenfeld says, it can be reflected in a number of health problems, such as backaches, headaches and joint pain. Rolfing seeks to realign and straighten your body by working the myofascia, the connective tissue that surrounds your muscles and helps hold your body together. The ten-session, head-to-toe Rolfing program used to be rather painful, but Bienenfeld says new techniques that employ a therapist's hands and elbows are quite tolerable and just as effective at improving your posture.

Hellerwork is an offshoot of Rolfing that adds both mental and movement re-education to the physical work. In a series of 11 sessions, you get instruction on how to break bad posture habits—and you also get a massage that focuses on returning your muscles and other tissue to their proper positions. The result can be dramatic. "Sometimes we can greatly increase the spaces in your joints to the point where you may grow three-fourths of an inch taller before you're done," Bienenfeld says.

Craniosacral therapy focuses on the skull and spinal column. Therapists use very gentle pressure—no more than the weight of a nickel—to massage the bones, membranes and fluids that support and bathe your skull and spinal column. The theory is that these manipulations will reduce tension and counteract any physical trauma you may have experienced to your head over the years. Craniosacral therapy can be effective with jaw problems such as temporomandibular joint disorder, experts say. Bienenfeld says that it can also seem spiritual, since "it can really send your head spinning with relaxation."

Aston-Patterning, another offshoot of Rolfing, was developed to teach people to maintain the improved alignment that they got through Rolfing. Aston-Patterning uses posture re-education and stresses physical fitness techniques.

Feldenkrais treats every body as an individual work of art, with different postures and different movement patterns. Practitioners seek to teach their clients ideal patterns of movement through slow, gentle, exercise-like sessions. It also includes a gentle massage that is designed to teach a person how to expand his range of motion. Bienenfeld says it's often useful for victims of stroke or accidents who have lost movement.

Trager uses gentle, rocking massage to help release the body's harmful "holding patterns." If you injured your left shoulder as a child, for example, you still may unconsciously carry it lower than your right shoulder, throwing your body off balance and robbing you of energy. Therapists employ very light, gentle shaking techniques that are unlike traditional Swedish-style massage. The idea is to make people more aware of their bodies, especially the way they move and hold themselves. Trager work can be uplifting, Bienenfeld says. For some reason, freeing people of physical holding patterns also seems to rid them of emotional stress that they associated with the prior injury, he explains.

While most massage types focus on rubbing, stroking and swirling techniques, others have an entirely different basis. Therapists who use techniques such as shiatsu and reflexology believe that you can unlock your body's healing energy by manipulating pressure points on your body. For more information on these techniques, see the chapters on acupressure (page 11) and reflexology (page 108).

DO-IT-YOURSELF RELIEF

Self-massage isn't always the perfect answer to your health concerns. It's tough to give yourself a decent back rub, after all—and you can't get perfect relaxation in one part of your body when you're flexing muscles in another to do the massage.

But if you're in a hurry, can't afford a massage therapist or don't have a partner to massage you, there are techniques that you can try on yourself. Most of them are Swedish massage methods that you adjust for self-care. You can easily massage cramped muscles in your legs or rub your shoulders for a little stress relief. For hard-to-reach places such as your back, you may be able to use

GETTING RUBBED RIGHT

Fifteen or 20 years ago, finding a legitimate massage therapist could prove a little risky—or downright risqué. There were places to get a massage, after all, and then there were adult entertainment places that operated under the guise of massage.

Fortunately, things have changed for the better, says Elliot Greene, past president of the American Massage Therapy Association (AMTA). These days, to find a reputable massage therapist all you need are a phone and a couple of minutes to ask questions.

Start by calling the AMTA. This nonprofit national body can provide you with a list of qualified massage therapists in your area, including those who specialize in techniques other than Swedish massage. Some of these other massage types also have national organizations that will send additional information on their methods and help you find a therapist in your area. The address for the AMTA is listed in the resource list on page 641.

Different states and localities have different licensing and registration practices. A licensed massage therapist in one city, county or other place may have to meet entirely different requirements than one in another jurisdiction. While 19 states require some form of licensing, the others don't require that therapists be licensed or otherwise regulated. The AMTA can give you details about your home state's regulations for massage therapists. So when you call a therapist, be sure to ask a few additional questions: How long have you been practicing? Are you nationally certified by the National Certification Board for Therapeutic Massage and Body Work? Do you belong to a professional organization such as the AMTA? Did you train at a school accredited by the AMTA Commission on Massage Training Accreditation/Approval? Ask your friends and colleagues for recommendations.

When you go for your appointment with a therapist, you should feel comfortable. It is your right not to do anything that makes you uneasy, Greene says. And if you don't like the personality or mannerisms of the therapist, find someone else with whom you are more comfortable.

Prices vary widely depending on the area and the experience of the therapist, Greene says, but for Swedish massage, you can expect to spend $25 and up for an hour-long massage.

tennis balls, rolling pins or other objects to help massage your muscles.

When you use self-massage, be sure to find a warm, quiet place, free of drafts and distractions. Take along a pillow and a blanket, so you can stay warm and comfortable. Many techniques call for using a lubricant, so your hands can glide over muscles smoothly and gently. You can buy massage creams, oils and scented lotions in many health food stores or other shops that sell beauty aids. If you want something handy, you can just use vegetable oil from your kitchen. Dr. Iuppo says the fatty acids in the oil will work into your skin, leaving it soft as a baby's bottom. "But if you're going to use vegetable oil, be sure to use a sheet that you don't mind getting rid of," he says, "because it will stain anything it touches."

If you're looking for a general massage to get you started, try a ten-minute foot massage from Elaine Stillerman, L.M.T., a massage therapist in New York City. "It can be stimulating or incredibly relaxing," says Stillerman. "Feet take a beating, no doubt about it. A general foot massage is powerful, soothing and relaxing."

Instructions and illustrations for this massage begin on page 572.

REFLEXOLOGY

You Can't Beat the Feet

We squeeze them into socks. We shove them into shoes. We stand, walk, climb, twist, turn, run and jump on them for hours at a time. No wonder our feet are begging for a gentle touch at the end of the day.

So why not indulge them a little? Nothing is more gloriously relaxing than a foot rub. And if you take time to learn a few special techniques, experts say you might even be able to help your health with a process called reflexology.

"Working with feet can be quite powerful," says Dwight Byers, a St. Petersburg, Florida, reflexologist and author of *Better Health with Foot Reflexology*. "Everyone knows how great a foot massage feels. And reflexology takes it a step further than that.

"I think that it can actually help the body cure itself."

Reflexologists believe that certain spots on your feet are directly linked to other body parts, including muscles, bones, organs and more. Working these spots helps the body relax, returning its natural balance and giving it a chance to heal.

"The idea is that pressure applied to the feet (and hands) promotes a beneficial response throughout the body, providing a break from stress," say Kevin and Barbara Kunz, reflexology researchers in Santa Fe, New Mexico, and authors of *Hand and Foot Reflexology*.

It's tough to match a one-on-one session with a reputable reflexologist. But experts say you can do lots of things by yourself, or with a partner, that may help relieve conditions ranging from insomnia to indigestion.

"We're still trying to figure out all of the hows and whys of reflexology," Byers says. "Yet the results are obvious. Reflexology can be a great contributor to overall health."

AMAZING FEETS

Human beings have been stroking sore feet from the day we first stood up and learned to walk. Egyptian tomb paintings from 2300 B.C. show people massaging each other's toes. Similar artifacts have been uncovered in China, India, Russia and other places around the globe.

But it wasn't until the early twentieth century that modern reflexology began to develop. An American doctor, William Fitzgerald, M.D., discovered that applying gentle pressure to one part of the body could relieve pain in other areas.

Eunice Ingham, an American massage therapist, took Fitzgerald's work further. She developed special massage techniques and created "maps" of the feet that showed which spots to touch to aid healing elsewhere on the body.

How does all of this work? Reflexologists say that relaxation is the key. Stress and tension are responsible for about 75 percent of all health problems, Byers says. And since each foot contains more than 7,000 nerves, experts believe it's a great spot to start the soothing.

"The relaxation I see in people is amazingly strong," says New York City–based reflexologist Laura Norman, author of *Feet First: A Guide to Foot Reflexology*. "Reflexology really reduces stress, which helps everything function better."

Reducing stress allows the body to return to its natural state of balance, called homeostasis, according to the Kunzes. And when your body is in balance, they say, it's better able to deal with diseases and other problems.

Reflexologists believe that your body is divided into ten "energy zones" that run from your head to your toes. To picture the zones, imagine a gingerbread man sliced lengthwise into ten pieces. Every tendon, ligament, organ, muscle, bone and brain cell is included in one of these zones—and every zone ends at the soles of your feet.

Your feet, then, are like mirrors that reflect the entire body. Spots on your feet, called reflex points or reflex areas, correspond to specific body parts. And reflexologists say that working these reflex areas with your thumbs or fingers can help relax those matching spots on the body.

You also have reflex points on your hands. You can use these if you have injuries to your feet or if want to do reflexology in your office or in a public place such as on a train or bus, where taking off your shoes and socks may be impractical. For Norman, however, feet are the most receptive to reflexology, because "they need more help than the hands." She says that toxins settle in the feet because of gravity and points out that feet are constricted in shoes all day. "Hands work out a lot of stress on their own," she says.

Just how your feet deliver their comforting messages remains a mystery. Many reflexologists believe that messages from the foot reflexes are somehow relayed to other parts of the body. If you touch the kidney reflex on your foot, for example, your body immediately sends a relaxing message to your kidney.

Others, like the Kunzes, believe that the nervous system plays a role. Touching spots on the feet may stimulate nerve impulses that travel to the brain, they say. The brain then relays the message to a body part.

REFLEXOLOGY

Reflexologists say they can often tell from your feet when something's out of whack in the rest of your body. Tender spots on the feet indicate that you may have a problem in the corresponding part of the body. While they don't diagnose illnesses or treat specific diseases, reflexologists say they can help by paying special attention to the sore spots.

"We're just giving the body a better chance of helping itself," says Kevin Kunz.

YOUR REFLEXOLOGY SESSION

There's more to reflexology than pulling off your socks and pulling on your toes.

"It's not just a foot massage," says St. Petersburg, Florida, reflexologist Dwight Byers, author of *Better Health with Foot Reflexology*. "It's a complex, thorough system. And you won't get the benefit if you just rub your feet all over."

Fortunately, you can pick up the basics pretty quickly. With a few thumb and finger techniques and a guide map, you can start working on your own feet, or your partner's, right away. These techniques also work for hand reflexology, where you touch reflex points on the hand instead of the foot.

The thumb walk is the most common technique. You use the outside edge of your thumb to take small "bites" of the hand or foot, applying gentle, steady pressure as you go. The finger walk is similar to thumb walking, except that you use the edge of your index finger to take the bites on the hand or foot. The hook and back up technique puts steady pressure on a single point. You place your thumb on the reflex point, then pull back slightly to "grab" the point. Rotation on a point also puts pressure on a single point and is better to use when you encounter a tender area. And the single finger grip lets you apply pressure to small points on your hand. You can also use a golf ball to apply pressure to reflex points on the hand, according to Kevin and Barbara Kunz, reflexology researchers in Santa Fe, New Mexico, and authors of *Hand and Foot Reflexology*.

You'll find instructions and illustrations for all of these techniques, as well as charts that list which techniques can be used for a specific reflex point, beginning on page 582.

The key to reflexology is pressure, say the Kunzes. Which technique you need depends not only on how large the area is but also on how

PREVENTION: THE SOLE OF REFLEXOLOGY

Whatever is behind reflexology, evidence is mounting that it does indeed work. Scientific research remains limited, but one study shows a possible link between reflexology and relief of premenstrual syndrome (PMS) in women.

The study, involving 35 California women who complained of PMS symptoms, showed that those women receiving true reflexology reported feeling

much pressure you need to "hurt good" in the area you are working.

The Kunzes suggest that you think of reflexology as exercise and make it part of your daily routine. You can work your hands or feet while you watch your favorite television program or while you are paying the bills. The Kunzes recommend 10 to 15 minutes daily, but even 5 minutes done every day can be beneficial. If you are using reflexology to deal with a specific problem, you can increase the total time of your session to up to 30 minutes to pay special attention to the areas of concern. If the problem is recurrent or chronic, you can add a longer session to your daily routine once or twice a week.

Start your session with a few minutes of relaxation techniques, such as pressing between the toes, across the soles and over the tops of the feet. On your hands, press between the fingers and cross the palms. Do anything you like that loosens up your hands and feet.

Then starting at the top of your left foot, work down the foot, applying pressure to the entire foot. Then work your foot a second time, applying pressure to tender spots and to the specific areas described in the remedies in Part II of the book. Press each area at least four or five times before moving on to the next area. You should also work adjoining points before moving on. Repeat on the right foot. Use the same general patterns for your hands: Start at the top and work down, work the areas of special concern a second time and then repeat on your other hand. Finish up with a few more minutes of relaxation.

Press until you "hurt good." If an area feels as though it's bruised or injured when you press it, you are pressing too hard. How hard you press will depend on the area you are working. For example, you would press more lightly on the bony area on the top of your hand than you would on the fleshy, callused sole of the foot. The amount of pressure depends on how sensitive your hands and feet are.

significantly better than those who didn't. To make the study as realistic as possible, half of the women received placebo reflexology sessions, where someone worked on parts of their ears, hands and feet that are not supposed to have any effect on PMS.

One of the study's co-authors calls the results "very promising." "I think you have to be impressed with these data," says Terry Oleson, Ph.D., chairman of the Department of Psychology and the Division of Behavioral Medicine at California Graduate Institute in Los Angeles.

Experts say reflexology works best when it's used for prevention. It helps keep your body running smoothly by improving blood circulation, clearing out impurities, balancing your system and giving you more energy, Norman says.

"It's a holistic approach," Norman says. "When you are relaxed all over and don't have to deal with stress so much, your immune system will be better able to deal with whatever comes its way."

That's why it's a good idea to make reflexology part of your routine instead of waiting until a problem flares up. "You can do some work on your own feet every day," Norman says. She suggests spending 20 to 30 minutes per day on your feet and toes, making sure you hit all of the major spots outlined in the illustrations beginning on page 596. Spend a little extra time on any reflex points that feel tender or sore. (See "Your Reflexology Session" on page 110 for more information on how to use this healing technique.)

Experts also recommend finding a trained reflexologist to give you a "tune-up session" about once a week. To locate a reputable reflexologist, you'll have to be a smart consumer, Kevin Kunz says. There's no central board that tests and certifies all reflexologists. But experts agree that a practitioner certified by any of the following groups has enough training to give you valuable service: the International Institute of Reflexology, the North American Association of Reflexology and Laura Norman and Associates, Reflexology Center.

You shouldn't automatically overlook other practitioners, however, says Kevin Kunz. "Try them out a couple of times. If you feel like you're getting some benefit, by all means stay with them. Some people have years of experience and do great work but have never received formal training or certification." Expect to pay from $15 to $65 for a half-hour session and from $30 to $100 for an hour.

There are now more than 25,000 certified reflexologists around the world and thousands more with practical experience. The number continues to grow, Byers says, as more and more people look for natural health remedies.

"Reflexology is the number one form of alternative care in Denmark, and it's very popular across Europe," he says. And if it's good enough for commoners, it's good enough for kings: Britain's royal family reportedly uses reflexology to help work the Windsor knots out of their stress-filled bodies.

RELAXATION AND MEDITATION

Take a Rest from Stress and Poor Health

Peace of mind heals.

That idea is as ancient as civilization itself—and as modern as the scientific evidence that is proving it's true.

"Relaxation and meditation can have a very powerful effect on the body," says Steven Fahrion, Ph.D., director of research at the Life Sciences Institute of Mind-Body Health in Topeka, Kansas. "It can help you cope with all kinds of stress-related problems, including migraines, peptic ulcers and anxiety. So I think that people who develop and retain peace of mind do experience mental and physical healing."

In fact, researchers have found that relaxation and meditation techniques can boost immunity, short-circuit anger, curb smoking and relieve insomnia, back pain, high blood pressure, motion sickness, impotence, premenstrual syndrome, menopause and irritable bowel syndrome. With professional care, these techniques can also help control diabetes, psoriasis, rheumatoid arthritis, panic attacks, phobias and depression.

"I think everyone can benefit from learning how to relax. Learning to neutralize the effects of stress is one of the most important aspects of preventive medicine," says Andrew Weil, M.D., teacher of alternative medicine at the University of Arizona College of Medicine in Tucson, founding director of the university's Center for Integrative Medicine and a physician emphasizing natural and preventive medicine.

SURVIVING THE RAT RACE

Relaxing or meditating probably isn't the first thing that pops into your mind when you're stuck in traffic, scrambling to meet a deadline or confronted by an angry spouse.

In those situations, your muscles tense, your breathing becomes shallow, your heart races, your blood vessels constrict, your blood pressure rises, you start to sweat, and your digestive tract cramps up. Unlike our primitive ancestors, we may not be able to "fight or flee"—the two most natural responses to

113

stress—when we're in a modern stressful situation, such as a traffic jam. So we remain chronically tense.

But calming yourself is what you should do, says Robert S. Eliot, M.D., director of the Institute of Stress Medicine in Jackson Hole, Wyoming, and author of *From Stress to Strength: How to Lighten Your Load and Save Your Life.* "If you can't fight and you can't flee, then you need to learn how to flow," he says.

That's because excessive amounts of stress can adversely affect almost every part of your body. Chronic stress, for example, can elevate blood pressure, total blood cholesterol and blood platelet counts, all of which can lead to atherosclerosis (hardening of the arteries) and heart attack. Stress has been linked to many other ailments ranging from the common cold to colon cancer. In fact, eight of ten people seen by primary care physicians have some stress-related symptoms. Overall, stress-related ailments cost American business and industry more than $100 billion annually in lost productivity and absenteeism, Dr. Eliot says.

"Consistently evoking the stress response with images of danger in the past or stress in the future is tantamount to setting off a false fire alarm in your body," says Neil Fiore, Ph.D., a psychologist in Berkeley, California, and author of *The Road Back to Health: Coping with the Emotional Aspects of Cancer.* "You're calling out the fire trucks when there really isn't anywhere for them to go."

POP YOUR MIND OUT OF GEAR

For many of us, dousing the fires sparked by stress means pushing hard on a long, fast run, sinking a 25-foot putt or climbing a mountain.

But while those activities can relieve stress, they can also generate competition and frustration, which can make it harder to relax.

"Sports and recreational activities give some people a legitimate outlet for the stress that they can't relieve on the job or at home," Dr. Fiore says. "But for other people, these pursuits raise their blood pressure and perpetuate the view that their lives are ongoing battles in a hostile, competitive world."

To help you really calm yourself, Dr. Fiore and other experts recommend that you let your mind slip into idle several times a day, so for at least a few minutes you're not regretting yesterday or fretting about tomorrow. Instead, you're focused on the present moment without feeling compelled to make judgments about your life.

"It's like being an actor in an emotional drama, who can step offstage, take a seat in the audience and watch another part of himself performing in the chase scene," Dr. Fiore says.

More importantly, these mental rest stops can evoke the relaxation response, a physiological state that has been shown to lessen feelings of stress and anxiety. The relaxation response reduces muscle tension, lowers heart rate, blood pres-

FIVE RELAXATION ENHANCERS

Relaxation and meditation techniques can do wonders for your mind and body, especially if you take time to make a few other changes in your life. Here's a look at five things you can do to enhance your sense of inner peace, according to Robert S. Eliot, M.D., director of the Institute of Stress Medicine in Jackson Hole, Wyoming, and author of *From Stress to Strength: How to Lighten Your Load and Save Your Life*.

Stomp out the smokes. Besides increasing your risk for heart disease and lung cancer, smoking triggers the release of stress hormones in the body. Quitting is the most important thing you can do to feel less stressed and more relaxed.

Curb the caffeine. Caffeine is a stimulant that can trigger the fight-or-flight response to stress, so avoid coffee, tea, cola, chocolate and other foods and beverages containing caffeine.

Calm down with carbs. Eating grains, vegetables and fruits loaded with complex carbohydrates, such as spaghetti, baked beans and apples, can trigger the release of hormones that will help relax you.

Work up a sweat. Regular exercise is a fundamental part of any relaxation program. It can lower anxiety, fend off depression and help increase a person's self-esteem. Try walking for 15 to 20 minutes a day.

Make time for a daily chuckle. Humor is a powerful ally in your quest for relaxation. A good laugh triggers the release of endorphins, chemicals in the brain that produce feelings of euphoria. It also suppresses the production of cortisol, a hormone released when you're under stress that indirectly raises blood pressure by causing your body to retain salt. So try to find humor in daily life.

sure, metabolism and breathing and sparks tranquil feelings, says Eileen Stuart, R.N., director of cardiovascular programs at the Mind–Body Medical Institute, a behavioral medicine clinic at Deaconess Hospital in Boston.

Although the relaxation response is often associated with a simple form of meditation described by Herbert Benson, M.D., president of the Mind–Body Medical Institute, it may easily be conjured by other relaxation and meditation techniques, Stuart says.

The relaxation response blunts the release of adrenaline, catecholamines and other stress hormones that trigger the fight–or–flight response, Stuart says. That's important, because an overdose of stress hormones can suppress the immune system and elevate blood cholesterol levels.

The relaxation response also performs another vital task.

"This type of deep relaxation is associated with healing in many different ways," Dr. Fahrion says. "When you get very deeply relaxed, for example, the body releases growth hormones that help repair and restore damaged tissue."

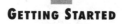

GETTING STARTED

Proponents say there are literally dozens of ways to produce the relaxation response. Some, such as meditation, are centuries old. Others, such as progressive relaxation and biofeedback, have been developed in the past 70 years.

"All of these techniques can work for you," Dr. Fiore says. "It's matter of discovering which ones you are most comfortable with."

In fact, the more techniques you know, the better off you may be, says Martha Davis, Ph.D., a psychologist at the Kaiser Permanente Medical Center in Santa Clara, California, and co-author of the *Relaxation and Stress Reduction Workbook*. "Using a combination of techniques, such as deep breathing followed by progressive relaxation, can increase the power of the relaxation effect. Each technique takes you down a notch and puts you into a deeper, longer-lasting state of relaxation," Dr. Davis says.

Before you begin, however, it's important to remember that these techniques won't prevent stress from occasionally disrupting your life.

"I don't think there is any way to eliminate stress," Dr. Weil says. "The challenge is to find ways to handle it better, so it doesn't damage your body."

Here's a glimpse at a few of the more common relaxation and meditation techniques that can help you cope with stress.

JUST TAKE A DEEP BREATH

Deep breathing is one of the simplest ways to relax, and it is an integral part of many of the other relaxation and meditation techniques.

"If I was to have one prescription for relaxation, it would be a breathing exercise," says Janet Messer, Ph.D., a psychologist in Eugene, Oregon. "When you slow down your breathing and focus your attention in your lower belly, it has really profound physiological and psychological effects."

Deep abdominal breathing relaxes tight chest muscles and opens up blood vessels, so your heart can pump more efficiently, Dr. Eliot says. It also helps you think clearly, so you can stay calmer in a stressful situation.

In addition, researchers at Wayne State University School of Medicine in Detroit found that menopausal women who practiced deep breathing had 50 percent fewer hot flashes than women who didn't.

"The wonderful thing about deep breathing is that it's always there," Dr.

Messer says. "You can do it on the subway, sitting at your desk or if the boss is starting to get on your nerves."

To do it, sit in a chair with your back straight, suggests Dr. Messer. Slowly breathe in and feel your lungs filling from the bottom to the top. Focus your attention in your belly; let it expand as you breathe. It should feel like your diaphragm, a muscular membrane separating your lungs from your abdomen, is being pulled down, as if it were attached to a string in your belly. Then slowly exhale, emptying your lungs from top to bottom. Feel your diaphragm relax into its natural position. Do this twice a day for five minutes.

To enhance the effect, Dr. Eliot suggests that as you inhale, think to yourself "Cool, clear mind," and as you exhale, "Calm, relaxed body."

MIND IF I MEDITATE?

Meditation isn't just for gurus anymore.

"Many people envision a meditator as someone who sits in a cave all day or as a wise man sitting on the mountaintop. But actually, a walker can do it as he strolls down the street, or a stockbroker can do it as he's reading stock quotes. So meditation isn't just sitting down and twisting yourself up like a pretzel," says Sundar Ramaswami, Ph.D., a clinical psychologist at F. S. Dubois Community Mental Health Center in Stamford, Connecticut, and a proponent and practitioner of meditation for more than 20 years.

Meditation is described by proponents as a type of intense inward concentration that allows you to focus on your senses, step back from your thoughts and feelings and perceive each moment as a unique event.

"I've always defined meditation as a form of mental martial arts. Normally, we're reactive to our thoughts; they attack us and we kick back. In meditation, we learn to sidestep out of the way. We learn how to keep ourselves centered so that we're no longer at the mercy of our own thoughts," says Joan Borysenko, Ph.D., a Boulder, Colorado, psychologist and author of *Minding the Body, Mending the Mind*.

Probably the best-known type of meditation is transcendental meditation (TM), an effortless technique introduced and taught by Maharishi Mahesh Yogi. During a seven-step course, practitioners of TM learn how to use a special, meaningless sound called a mantra.

But TM is just one of many meditation techniques. Generally, these techniques can be classified into two large categories.

Concentrative meditation uses a picture, a word (mantra), an object (such as a candle flame) or a sensation (such as breathing) to focus the mind, Dr. Ramaswami says. If your mind begins to drift, you refocus your attention on the object.

RELAXATION AND MEDITATION

TAPE YOUR WAY TO RELAXATION

You buy one of those fancy relaxation tapes, assuming that a calm voice and a bit of New Age music will help you find the inner tranquillity that has eluded you.

But you may be disappointed.

Commercially produced relaxation tapes have a couple of critical limitations, says Matthew McKay, Ph.D., clinical director of Haight Ashbury Psychological Services, a nonprofit counseling center in San Francisco, and co-author of *The Relaxation and Stress Reduction Workbook*. First, the tape may advocate a relaxation or meditation technique that isn't particularly effective for you. Second, you might not find the music soothing.

"There are tapes out on the market that claim to be relaxation tapes. But our studies show that if a person doesn't like the music, those tapes can actually increase anxiety," says Valerie Stratton, Ph.D., associate professor of psychology at Pennsylvania State University in Altoona. "The bottom line is if you want to relax, listen to something that is familiar and that you like rather than a preprogrammed relaxation tape."

Dr. McKay suggests that you try making your own relaxation tape. Creating your own tape allows you to combine relaxation techniques that work for you, and you can change the tape as your needs change. Using your own voice can also make your tape more personal and friendly.

"Using a tape frees you from trying to relax while giving yourself directions in your head. That can be difficult to do, even for people who have been using relaxation techniques for years," says Janet Messer, Ph.D., a psychologist in Eugene, Oregon.

Tape this chapter's instructions for the technique that works best for you, Dr. McKay suggests. Speak slowly and in a calm tone. Leave gaps in the tape to give yourself adequate time to follow the recorded instructions.

Experiment with dubbing your voice over background music if you want, but to simplify the process, Dr. McKay suggests recording the script without music. Then when you practice the relaxation technique, play the script on one tape deck, and if you wish, play music on a second deck or CD player. Finally, don't be discouraged if it takes several tries to get the instructions recorded at the right speed for you.

Mindfulness meditation is more complex. Instead of focusing on a single sensation or object, you allow thoughts, feelings and images to float through your mind.

"In mindfulness, you are a dispassionate observer," Dr. Ramaswami says.

"You note your thoughts, desires and sensations in the same way that a postal worker might notice stamps. You let these thoughts go in and out of your mind without expressing positive or negative feelings about them."

Some forms of meditation use a combination of concentrative and mindfulness techniques. In fact, you may already be practicing meditation without realizing it.

EVERYBODY'S DOING IT

"Everybody gets into a state of meditation several times a day without really calling it that," Dr. Borysenko says. "Just imagine a time when you were caught up in the moment. It could have been when you were digging in the garden, playing with a child or watching a sunset. For that moment, past and future faded away, and you were living in the present. That's a form of meditation."

Although it is often perceived as spiritually oriented, meditation can be used simply for relaxation and to improve your health, Dr. Borysenko says.

Studies have shown, for example, that meditation can reduce anxiety and soothe anger. Other studies have shown that it can reduce the severity of asthma, migraines and chronic pain.

Meditation can also help corral premenstrual syndrome, according to Harvard Medical School researchers. In a study of 46 women, the researchers found that meditation, twice daily for 15 to 20 minutes at a time, slashed premenstrual symptoms by 58 percent. That was double the improvement reported by women who read twice daily and nearly 3½ times better than women who merely kept track of their symptoms.

In a study at Maharishi International University in Fairfield, Iowa, of 29 men ages 18 to 32, researchers concluded that practicing TM twice a day can lower blood levels of cortisol, an important stress hormone that in excessive amounts can inhibit immunity, raise blood pressure and cause other damaging effects.

To try a simple mindfulness meditation, find a quiet spot and sit in a comfortable position. Take several slow, deep breaths. As you breathe out, ask yourself "Who am I?" Note the associations—"I'm a mother," "I'm a husband," "I'm a businessperson," "I'm tired," "I'm angry"—that pop into your head without judging them, Dr. Ramaswami says. If you think "I'm a homeowner," for example, and begin worrying about making the mortgage payment, refocus your mind on the question "Who am I?"

Dr. Ramaswami suggests practicing this meditation for 20 minutes twice a day at first. Then as you become more proficient and more aware of your body's sensations, you may find you can meditate less and still get the same effect. "This meditation will help you quickly get to the heart of your innermost thoughts," Dr. Ramaswami adds.

FEEL THE HEAT

Your mind speaks, your body listens.

That's the premise of autogenics, a technique that has much in common with yoga, imagery and meditation.

Autogenics, which means "self-generation," was developed in the 1930s by Johannes Schultz, M.D., a German neurologist and psychiatrist. Dr. Schultz— who compared the feelings generated by autogenics to taking a long, relaxing bath—wanted people to be able to generate deep relaxation in a versatile and practical way. In essence, the idea is to sit in a comfortable position and give your body a series of instructions such as "My hands are warm . . . my hands are heavy."

Proponents believe doing that stimulates blood flow and deep relaxation. Autogenics, for example, was found to be effective in reducing the number and severity of migraines and tension headaches in a study of 34 men and women at McMaster University in Hamilton, Ontario.

"An autogenic exercise is a good way for the average person to learn to speak to himself in a language that his body can cooperate with, without a lot of mumbo jumbo," Dr. Fiore says.

You need to find a quiet room, sit or lie in a comfortable position, close your eyes and take a few deep breaths, says Martin Shaffer, Ph.D., executive director of the Stress Management Institute in San Francisco and author of *Life after Stress.* As you exhale, repeat the following instructions to yourself.

"My hands and arms are warm and heavy" (five times).
"My feet and legs are warm and heavy" (five times).
"My abdomen is calm and comfortable" (five times).
"My breathing is deep and even" (ten times).
"My heartbeat is slightly calm and regular" (ten times).
"My forehead is cool" (five times).
"When I open my eyes, I will remain relaxed and refreshed" (three times).

Then take a moment to move your arms, hands, legs and feet around a bit. Rotate your head, open your eyes, and if you're lying down, sit up.

While doing this exercise, note what is happening to your body, but don't consciously try to analyze it. Avoid criticizing yourself if you have distracting thoughts. If your mind wanders, simply bring it back to your instructions as soon as possible.

Dr. Shaffer suggests doing two-minute sessions of this exercise ten times a day. Be patient, experts say, because in some cases, it may take weeks for autogenics to be effective.

RELAXATION AND MEDITATION

TUNE IN TO YOUR BODY'S SIGNALS

Biofeedback can help relieve a variety of conditions, including stuttering, muscle spasms, tooth grinding and epilepsy. Mental health professionals say it also works well in conjunction with other relaxation techniques.

In most cases, however, using biofeedback requires professional care. During traditional biofeedback, electrodes are attached to your body. These instruments monitor various body functions, such as temperature, muscle tension, brain wave activity and heart rate. Even a slight change in any one of these can be instantly detected by a biofeedback machine and transformed into a signal you can see or hear. With this enhanced feedback, you can learn how to regulate these bodily functions so that you feel more relaxed.

Although portable biofeedback devices are available, experts say you should still seek professional advice, since some guidance may be necessary to help you use these devices.

But there is at least one cheap and easy form of biofeedback that you can practice at home. It's called thermal biofeedback, and all it requires are a thermometer, your hands and about 15 minutes of your time, Dr. Fahrion says.

"Many people haven't heard of it, although it has been used in hospitals and clinics to treat stress-related disorders such as high blood pressure for more than 20 years," Dr. Fahrion says. "Most people can learn to do it in a single session."

Developed at the Menninger Clinic in Topeka, Kansas, thermal biofeedback is based on the premise that when a person is under stress, the body restricts blood flow to the extremities, such as the hands and feet, so they are colder than the rest of the body. But if you warm your hands, blood flow increases, stress hormones diminish, muscles relax, and you'll feel less tense, proponents say.

"I've seen people under stress whose hands are 63°F even after an hour in a warm room," Dr. Fahrion says. "By warming your hands, you're actually changing your chemistry into a more relaxed state."

To try it, sit in a comfortable chair and wrap your hands around a thermometer so that your fingertips are touching (see the illustration on page 604). Rest your hands in your lap and focus your mind on any sensation that you feel in your fingers. Do you feel a tingling or pulsing in your fingertips? That's a sign that your hands are warming. Take an occasional glance at the thermometer with the intention to warm, but don't strive to raise your hand temperature. That will occur naturally. If you get distracted, refocus your attention on your hands.

The goal is to raise your finger temperature to 97°F and hold it there for about ten minutes. As you become more accustomed to the sensations in your hands, you should be able to do this exercise without using the thermometer, Dr. Fahrion says.

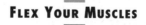

USE TENSION TO RELIEVE TENSION

When you feel under stress, your muscles naturally contract and create tension. So what can relieve that? Believe it or not, more tension, say proponents of a technique called progressive relaxation.

By systematically tightening and releasing muscles, progressive relaxation can prevent stress from overwhelming you, proponents say.

"Progressive relaxation is extremely useful, particularly if my muscles feel tense and seem incapable of relaxing," Dr. Fiore says.

Tensing taut muscles might seem strange, but Dr. Fiore says that the additional exercise actually increases blood flow to the muscles and helps them unwind faster than if you try to relax them.

Developed in the 1920s by Edmund Jacobson, a Chicago physician, progressive relaxation is considered an excellent technique for beginners because it is practical and doesn't depend on imagination. Research suggests that it can help alleviate insomnia, headaches and digestive ailments such as irritable bowel syndrome. Experts say that it can also help relieve muscle spasms, back pain and high blood pressure.

There are many methods of progressive relaxation, but Dr. Davis suggests this approach: Clench your right fist as tightly as you can. Keep it clenched for about ten seconds, then release the tension immediately and completely, as though you were turning off a switch. All of the tension should drain out of your body. Feel the looseness in your right hand and notice how much more relaxed it feels than when you tensed it. Do the same thing with your left hand; then clench both fists at the same time. Bend your elbows and tense your arms. Release and let your arms hang at your sides. Continue this process by tensing and relaxing your shoulders and neck, then wrinkling and relaxing your forehead and brows. Then squeeze your eyes and clench your jaw before moving on to tense and then relax your stomach, lower back, buttocks, thighs, calves and feet.

FLEX YOUR MUSCLES

Like flossing your teeth, rotating your tires or starting a diet, stretching is something you always vow to do . . . tomorrow. But it isn't something that you should put off, researchers say, because stretching can soothe the stressed-out beast within.

"Gentle stretching fosters relaxation," says Charles Carlson, Ph.D., professor of psychology at the University of Kentucky in Lexington. "Physiologically, if you gently stretch the muscle, it will relax. Stretching also gives you something to focus your attention on, which enables you to quiet your mind."

Gentle stretching is particularly good for people who have chronic muscle pain, such as in the neck or shoulders, and have difficulty doing muscle-tensing exercises such as progressive relaxation.

"Asking a person who has a painful muscle to tense it only creates more pain," Dr. Carlson says. "Our approach minimizes muscle tension."

Stretching should always be done slowly and without pain, Dr. Carlson says. Avoid overstretching or bouncing your muscles. While you're doing a stretching sequence, think about how your tension feels, so you'll come to know when you need to stretch to release it. In any case, do a stretching sequence at least once a day. For instructions on how to do such a sequence, see the illustrations that begin on page 602.

SOUND THERAPY

Music to Your Ears, Health to Your Body

Close your eyes for a minute and listen to the world around you. What do you hear? Car horns, jackhammers and blaring stereos? Or gentle raindrops, laughing children and the soothing strings of a symphony orchestra?

It may make a difference. Sound therapists say that what you hear can help—or hurt—your health. "I believe that sound, especially music, can be a great healer," says Steven Halpern, Ph.D., composer, researcher and author of *Sound Health: The Music and Sounds That Make Us Whole.* "Sound can relax you. When applied the right way, it can help release energy and help your body heal itself."

Therapists are using sound, especially music, to help people with a wide variety of medical problems, from Alzheimer's disease to tooth pain. Medical doctors know about the power of sound, too. They use high-tech devices such as ultrasound machines to help heal soft-tissue injuries and to take diagnostic photographs of fetuses in their mothers' wombs. And researchers have released a number of studies that verify music's ability to ease pain, improve memory and reduce stress.

So how can you take advantage of sound therapy? Well, chances are that you're already using it. Three in four people who responded to a *Prevention* magazine health survey said they listen to music to ease tension and stress. And of those, 82 percent reported that it brings significant relief.

Experts say people can harness the healing power of sound in many ways. You can listen to music that quiets your mind and relaxes your body. Or walk through a forest and soak up the sounds of nature. Stroll along the beach and listen to the waves lapping the shore. Sing to yourself, play an instrument or learn toning, where you make a series of elongated vowel sounds to ease tension and energize your body. (For more information on how to do toning, see "Hum Yourself to Health.")

"The rewards of sound are great," Dr. Halpern says. "The more we learn about it, the more we see its potential as a natural healer. And one of the best parts is that it's something that people can learn to do for themselves."

A HISTORY OF HARMONY

Mankind has long recognized the power of sound. About 2,500 years ago, the Greek mathematician and philosopher Pythagoras developed "prescriptions" of music for his students. He told them which sounds would help them work, relax, sleep and wake up better. The Bible tells of David, the famed harp player whose music eased the madness of King Saul. Charles Darwin believed that prehistoric humans originally used musical sounds as mating calls.

Unfortunately, no one knows exactly what is behind sound's power. "We're

HUM YOURSELF TO HEALTH

If you want to give sound therapy a try, start with the handiest and most versatile of all instruments: your vocal chords.

"I do not believe in putting sound into another person's body when his own voice can massage his own body from within," says Don G. Campbell, director of the Institute for Music, Health and Education in Boulder, Colorado, and the author of *Music: Physician for Times to Come.* "The sounds you can make with your own voice can be the most powerful healer of all."

Campbell recommends a process called toning, which involves making elongated vowel sounds. The vibrations from the tones can help relax you, ease stress and balance the mind and body, Campbell says.

In his book *The Roar of Silence: The Healing Power of Breath, Tone and Music,* Campbell outlines simple exercises that he says can show the relaxing power of toning.

Start by sitting in a comfortable chair. The first thing you have to do, Campbell says, is ask the left, rational side of your brain, the side that controls thought and that may find this exercise new and challenging, permission to experiment with tone. Ask your brain to explore the vowel sounds for ten minutes.

Now close your eyes and focus on listening. Take a deep, easy breath and start humming "a soft and resonant sound," Campbell says. There is no need to worry whether the sound is high or low or whether it is beautiful. Gradually begin to sense the vibration of the sound in your chest and head.

Campbell suggests that you allow the sound to naturally rise and fall without effort. Place your hands on your cheeks and let them feel the sound. Listen with your hands, not with your ears. Continue toning with your hands, feeling your face and skull for five minutes.

Then relax your hands and tone on just one sound, such as *ah*, for another five minutes, keeping your eyes closed. When you are finished, just notice the relaxation that has come to your mind, body and breath.

aware of many of the effects that sound can have on the body," Dr. Halpern says. "But no one can really, really say how sound therapy helps heal the body."

All sound, whether it comes from a shiny brass trumpet or a rusty car muffler, travels in waves of energy. These waves have a number of variables that give a sound its unique quality. Among others, there are velocity, or the speed at which the waves travel; frequency, which is the number of waves per second that an object produces; and intensity, which is a measure of a sound's loudness.

Our body's main sound sensor is the ear. The skin, bones, fluid and nerves in the ear help collect sound waves and send impulses to the brain. The brain reacts to these impulses and sends out directions that help control heart rate, breathing rate and other bodily functions.

Dr. Halpern says sound can have a great effect on your heartbeat. "Your heart will speed up or slow down to match the rhythm of a sound," he says. "If you're listening to music with a fast drumbeat, your heart will speed up. And if you're listening to a slower piece, your heart will beat slower to match it." Dr. Halpern calls this process entrainment and says you can test it yourself by listening to various pieces of music, fast and slow, and then taking your own pulse.

Sounds can also affect your breathing, blood pressure and muscle tension and perhaps cause the release of painkilling, mood-changing chemicals called endorphins, Dr. Halpern says. All of these factors may combine to create a state of total relaxation, he says, reducing stress and giving the body a chance to heal itself.

One theory holds that vibrations from sound waves can also have a direct impact on individual body parts. Science has long known that every atom vibrates, emitting sound waves even though they're far too faint for us to hear. Since body parts are made up of atoms, they all produce sound waves. Some therapists believe that these sound waves are altered when disease or stress hits—and they also believe that directing sound waves at the body or its parts can restore natural rhythms and encourage and support healing. This technique, called cymatic therapy, is used in the United States by holistic practitioners, including acupuncturists, osteopaths and others.

Finally, there's the theory that sound waves can balance energy centers, or chakras, in the body and promote health. Eastern philosophy holds that the body has seven chakras, which control function and energy flow in different organs of the body. Dr. Halpern believes that the chakras vibrate at specific frequencies that relate to the notes on a music scale. When there are disruptions to the chakras caused by stress, disease or other factors, the frequencies are thrown off. By applying specific sounds or music to the body, the chakras can be returned to normal, and the body will heal itself, he says.

SOUND THERAPY

THE SCIENCE OF SOUND

Though researchers are still fuzzy on how sound therapy works, there's plenty of scientific proof that it can be effective for everything from reducing stress to boosting your brainpower. Many studies, for example, have shown that music can reduce pain and ease anxiety during surgical procedures. German researchers found that patients having gastroscopies, during which a doctor runs a snakelike scope down the patient's throat to look at the stomach, had lower levels of stress hormones in their bloodstreams when they listened to the music of their choice during the procedures. Doctors at the Bethesda Naval Medical Center in Maryland found that men who listened to music during sigmoidoscopies reported feeling more relaxed during the sometimes uncomfortable examination of the colon, which requires a tube to be passed through the anus.

Dentists have long known the value of sound. Back in 1960, a Boston dentist, Wallace Gardner, D.M.D., wrote that music completely relieved pain in about 65 percent of the 1,000 patients he tested, while another 25 percent had enough reduced pain that they didn't need anesthesia. Some researchers speculate that distraction plays a big role in pain relief, since the music takes the patient's mind off the procedure. Others point to endorphins, claiming that music's ability to make the body release these natural painkillers is the key to easing discomfort.

Music may make you smarter, too—at least temporarily. A study from the University of California, Irvine, found that college students who listened to Mozart for 10 minutes scored higher on intelligence tests than they did after listening to relaxation tapes or sitting in silence for the same amount of time. The 36 students in the study scored an average of eight to nine points higher on tests taken immediately after listening to the music. Unfortunately, the effect lasted only 10 to 15 minutes, after which the scores returned to normal.

Sound therapy could also help people improve the quality of their workouts. A study from Louisiana State University in Shreveport concluded that listening to slow easy-listening music lowered the heart rates and allowed for longer training sessions in a group of 24 young adults. Listening to hard-driving rock music had the opposite effect; heart rates increased and workouts were shorter when the subjects tuned in to rock 'n' roll. The study's author, B. Don Franks, Ph.D., professor in the university's Department of Kinesiology, says the soft music may make the exercise seem less difficult and allow people to work out longer.

Many doctors use music with patients they have trouble communicating with, such as autistic children, older people with Alzheimer's disease and victims of head trauma. Studies report that music can help make contact with these people when traditional therapy and verbal communication fail. For example: A six-month study from Indiana University of Pennsylvania looked at 60 elderly patients with Alzheimer's disease and found that those who listened to big band music during their daily recreation periods were more alert and happier and could recall more from the past than those who didn't listen to music.

A new branch of sound therapy, called music thanatology, seeks to ease the emotional and physical suffering of terminally ill patients. The creator of music thanatology, Therese Schroeder-Sheker, uses harp and vocal music similar to that which medieval monks used to comfort people who were dying.

SOUND ADVICE

A trained sound therapist uses a wide range of tools, including musical instruments, tapes, tuning forks, machines that release sound waves at specific frequencies and even his own voice, to help heal the body. Many hospitals, nursing homes and rehabilitation centers offer group therapy sessions as part of their treatment programs.

If you want to find a private music therapist, be sure to check for proper credentials, says Al Bumanis, director of public relations for the National Association for Music Therapy. A qualified therapist may be called either a registered music therapist (R.M.T.) or a certified music therapist (C.M.T.). Both require an undergraduate degree in music therapy from an approved program and successful completion of a clinical internship.

A therapist can also complete continuing education requirements every five years or take a test from the Certification Board for Music Therapists. Those who complete these requirements are called board-certified and are up-to-date on the trends in the field, Bumanis says. To find a music therapist in your area, contact either the National Association for Music Therapy or the American Association for Music Therapy (refer to the resource list on page 642).

Expect to spend about $50 per hour for a session with a private therapist, Bumanis says.

If you'd like to try sound therapy on your own, experts say there are some techniques that you can use at home. Most involve using recorded music to relax or invigorate your body and mind. Part II of this book offers suggestions on pieces of music that may help you handle specific health conditions. It's important to pick music that's right for you, Dr. Halpern says. "Everyone has a different reaction to a piece of music. One person could tell you that a song helped relax him, but if it had violins in it and you don't like violins, it's not going to help you at all. It's going to feel like someone dragging fingernails

SAILING AWAY TO KEY LARGO

When it comes to relaxing music, the key is largo. That's music played at a slow tempo, called largo, which can reduce your heart and breathing rates, calm your body and help it heal itself, says Janalea Hoffman, R.M.T, a composer and music therapist based in Kansas City, Missouri.

Look for music that is played at 60 beats per minute or less. Most music is faster than that and won't help slow your heartbeat, Hoffman says. "What you are looking for is the largo section of each piece. That's the part with a beat that works." These composers are among those who have largo sections in many of their compositions: Johann Sebastian Bach, Antonio Vivaldi, George Frideric Handel and Georg Philipp Telemann. Most records, tapes and CDs list the different sections of each piece, in order, on their covers. The problem is that these slow sections last only a few minutes.

For longer listening, you will find lots of specially made tapes in music stores and can order even more from other sources. For information on mail order, refer to the resource list on page 642.

Experts recommend many of these tapes for the health conditions listed in Part II of this book. Hoffman has produced several tapes with the precise beat that can slow your heartbeat and calm your jangled nerves: *Musical Massage, Musical Biofeedback, Musical Acupuncture, Musical Hypnosis* and *Deep Daydreams*.

In addition, the following compositions are suggested by Steven Halpern, Ph.D., composer, researcher and author of *Sound Health: The Music and Sounds That Make Us Whole: Seapeace* by Georgia Kelly; *Spectrum Suite, Inner Peace* and *Comfort Zone*, all by Dr. Halpern; *Kuthumi* by Joel Andrews; *Dolphin Dreams* by Jonathan Goldman; *Inside* by Paul Horn; *Velvet Dreams* by Daniel Kobialka; *Light from Assisi* by Richard Shulman; *Angels of Compassion* by Iasos; and *Silk Road* by Kitaro. Dr. Halpern also suggests listening to any recordings of Gregorian chants and to *Relax with the Classics* by the Lind Institute. For information on mail-ordering any of these works, refer to the resource list on page 642.

across a blackboard." (For more information on selecting music for sound therapy, see "Sailing Away to Key Largo.")

You'll have to experiment to find out what makes you feel best. Classical music is often a good choice for music therapy, but some experts warn that it's

TURNING DOWN THE VOLUME OF LIFE

Sound may be a great healer, but noise sure isn't. Jets roaring overhead, music pounding through your apartment walls, your 20-year-old refrigerator chugging in the kitchen, even a computer or television screen whining at a frequency you can barely hear may be causing health problems, experts say.

"Noise is a hazard," says Steven Halpern, Ph.D., composer, researcher and author of *Sound Health: The Music and Sounds That Make Us Whole.* "And the scary part is that it doesn't even have to be at the point where it's hurting your ears. Even if your hearing isn't affected, the rest of you may be."

Evidence is mounting that noise pollution may be linked to high blood pressure, stress, lack of concentration, irritability and more. The case is growing so strong that former U.S. Surgeon General William H. Stewart says that "calling noise a nuisance is like calling smog an inconvenience."

Excessive noise may increase your risk of high blood pressure and other cardiovascular problems by as much as 10 percent, according to Shirley Thompson, Ph.D., associate professor of epidemiology at the University of South Carolina School of Public Health in Columbia. The reason for this isn't fully understood, but some researchers believe unpleasant sounds may trigger your body's fight-or-flight response, says Redford B. Williams, M.D., professor of psychiatry and director of the Behavioral Medicine Research Center at Duke University Medical Center in Durham, North Carolina.

When your body senses danger, it produces adrenaline and the hormone norepinephrine, which can speed up your heart and send more blood to your muscles. If you don't do anything with all of this extra body energy, it can strain your blood vessels and possibly cause high blood pressure in the long run, Dr. Williams says.

Women may be at even greater risk than men. That's because they can hear higher frequencies, such as those coming from computers and television sets, says Caroline Dow, Ph.D., associate professor of communication at the University of Evansville in Indiana. She studied 100 college-age

not perfect. "It wasn't written specifically for music therapy," explains Janalea Hoffman, R.M.T., a composer and music therapist based in Kansas City, Missouri. "Baroque music has a beat that's slow enough to slow down your heartbeat. But the beat changes during the piece, sometimes faster and sometimes women and found that those exposed to high-frequency computer noise scored 8.5 percent worse on a standardized test than women who didn't have to contend with the sound.

So how do you nix all of this extra noise? Try wearing soft-foam earplugs that are designed to reduce sound by at least 20 decibels, says Ernest A. Peterson, Ph.D., professor emeritus at the University of Miami School of Medicine. The federal Occupational Safety and Health Administration requires workers to wear ear protection if they are exposed to noise at 89 decibels or more. For comparison, you're exposed to between 42 and 49 decibels sitting in your living room holding a conversation—and to about 130 decibels or above at a rock concert. Earplugs are available in most drugstores and shouldn't cost more than a few dollars.

You can also reduce noise in your home with a few simple tricks. Use a rake instead of a leaf blower. Let your hair dry naturally once in a while instead of using a blow-dryer. Put appliances such as washing machines on rubber cushions, which help absorb the sound. And try adding carpets and drapes, which tend to muffle sounds that rattle off bare walls and floors.

If you can't eliminate a sound, you can at least try to mask it with a more pleasant sound. Try some soft, soothing music, says psychotherapist and stress management expert Emmett Miller, M.D., of Menlo Park, California. Play it just loud enough to block whatever other sounds you hear. Or try seeking out the sounds of nature, even if you have to buy a tape that mimics rainfall on a roof or a rushing mountain stream.

One final alternative is a white noise machine, a gadget that emits sounds designed to nullify other background noise. You can put one anywhere in your house or office or carry it on the road if you have to sleep or work in a noisy environment. Dr. Halpern says these machines usually cost between $50 and $150 and are available in many stereo shops and department stores.

"It's better to eliminate the source of the noise," he says. "But if that's not possible, I'd rather listen to the white noise than to something more annoying."

slower. And that may make it harder for your heart to react."

Many composers now write music specifically for therapeutic use. Much of it falls into a category called New Age. This music has a carefully timed beat and a sequence of tones that is supposed to stimulate relaxation. Music stores usually carry a selection of New Age recordings, some of which are tailored for relaxation, improved concentration, weight loss and other purposes.

Popular music can be relaxing to some people, too. But Dr. Halpern says research shows that the typical backbeat of rock 'n' roll music might actually weaken muscle strength while people are listening to it. "Many times people will listen to music and think it's relaxing them. But what it's really doing is just distracting them," he says. "They're not getting any physical benefit. They're just trying to block out whatever is making them tense."

The best way to see if you're relaxed is to check your pulse and breathing rate, Hoffman says. "If you want, you can measure them before and after you listen to music. If they're slower after the music than before, you're getting relaxation."

Finally, experts say you should seek out natural sounds, such as leaves rustling in the breeze or wind whipping through a stand of pine trees. As humans evolved, they became accustomed to these sounds, Dr. Halpern says. "These are the sounds that soothe us, that bring us back into balance. These are what the body is designed to hear. They can help make us well." Whenever possible, he says, it's a good idea to escape the whirring computers and growling lawn mowers of everyday life and listen to the sounds of natural silence. "Just find a quiet place and take a walk. Your health will be better for it," Dr. Halpern says.

VITAMIN AND MINERAL THERAPY

Pills That Can Ease Your Ills

The keys to a longer and healthier life, we're told, are simple enough: Just eat right, exercise regularly, manage stress and get enough sleep. The tough part is practicing what's preached.

Take food, for instance. The National Cancer Institute in Rockville, Maryland, recommends eating five servings of fruits and vegetables a day to reduce your risk of certain cancers, but fewer than 10 percent of us follow that advice. And by not making the right food choices, we might be eating our way toward cancer rather than away from it. Meanwhile, most of us don't get enough exercise to stay healthy. And stress management? It's hard enough to manage the kids, the job and the checkbook. And let's not even begin to discuss coping with a lack of sleep.

Sigh! It can be hard to swallow all of this advice for better health. But there's something that can make it go down a little easier: vitamin and mineral supplements.

CHEAP, SAFE AND PROVEN

Nearly half of all Americans—about 100 million people—use supplements at least occasionally. About half of them pop vitamin pills daily, spending nearly $4 billion a year in the process. It seems like money well-spent: Growing evidence suggests that high doses of certain nutrients can help slow the natural aging process and stave off heart disease, stroke, certain types of cancer and other diseases.

In foods, there are hundreds of nutrient compounds called phytochemicals, many of which have beneficial effects on health. For example, some of the phytochemicals in vegetables are thought by researchers to ward off cancer but are not available in supplements. That makes eating a healthy diet important.

But many nutrients are found only in very low amounts in the foods we eat every day. And some nutrients, such as folic acid, are better absorbed in the form that is used in supplements.

"There is overwhelming evidence that supplements have beneficial effects on a person's health, because they offer much higher doses of key nutrients than you find in food—sometimes amounts that you could never get from diet alone," says Richard Anderson, Ph.D., lead scientist for the nutrient requirements and functions laboratory at the U.S. Department of Agriculture Human Nutrition Research Center in Beltsville, Maryland.

"Unless you're consuming 4,000 to 5,000 calories of healthy foods a day—about twice the amount of the typical American—you're not even getting the Recommended Dietary Allowances (RDAs) for several trace minerals, let alone amounts that can help prevent and treat disease."

Supplements can also be fairly inexpensive. If you shop carefully, for as little as nine cents a day you can gulp down a brand-name multivitamin/mineral supplement that provides all of the essential nutrients you'd get from a whole day of healthy eating. Add another nine cents, and you can take enough of vitamins C and E in supplements to possibly protect you from cancer and heart disease. For a little more, you can take a calcium supplement to prevent osteoporosis. That's less than the cost of a single apple in some places. Of course, some supplements cost more, but generally, for less than a dollar a day you can get more essential vitamins and minerals than you'd get from an entire day of healthy eating. Look for a natural supplement that's free of food colorings, sweeteners and other additives.

And supplements are generally safe, especially if they are not grossly abused. "It's true that a few supplements, most notably vitamins A and D, can cause some problems if taken in extremely large doses for extended periods of time," says Michael Janson, M.D., director of the Center for Preventive Medicine in Barnstable, Massachusetts, and an officer of the American College for Advancement in Medicine. "But we're talking about extremely large doses taken daily for a year or two." These are amounts that may be as much as 50 times above the RDAs and even 10 or more times higher than the megadoses suggested on a short-term therapeutic basis to relieve a specific medical problem. (For more information about possible side effects of supplements, see "Watch What You're Taking.")

FROM HUMBLE BEGINNINGS

Vitamins and minerals—or rather, the foods containing these nutrients—have been used as therapy for thousands of years. The ancient Egyptians ate the livers of roosters and oxen to cure night blindness due to vitamin A deficiency and sea sponge, a natural source of iodine, to treat goiters.

It wasn't until around 1906 that vitamins were first discovered. What triggered the search for vitamins was the fact that fat, protein and carbohydrates were found to be insufficient to support life. "It became clear that there was something else in food that was needed for survival, and the search was on. The 'something else' turned out to be vitamins," says Annette Dickinson, Ph.D., director of scientific and regulatory affairs for the Council for Responsible Nutrition in Washington, D.C., a research and lobbying group for the supplement industry.

Scientists went to work isolating the nutrient compounds from foods through complex chemical procedures. In 1912, the term *vitamine* was coined (for "vital amine," amine being a kind of chemical structure; a few years later, the *e* was dropped when it was learned that some vitamins had different chemical structures and were not amines). By 1925, vitamin supplements were on the market

WATCH WHAT YOU'RE TAKING

Of course, too much of a good thing can be bad—and very dangerous. Some vitamins shouldn't be taken in supplement form unless you are under a doctor's care for a specific problem. Vitamins A and D, niacin and iron can all have adverse effects, resulting in problems such as liver damage, heart disease, loss of nerve function and increased risk of cancer.

But even the supplements you're encouraged to take in large doses can have some side effects, albeit less serious ones. "If you take enough magnesium, you can get diarrhea," says Michael Janson, M.D., director of the Center for Preventive Medicine in Barnstable, Massachusetts, and an officer of the American College for Advancement in Medicine. "And overloading on B_6 can cause restless sleep, because it promotes heavy dreaming."

Overdoing other B vitamins or a B-complex mixture can leave your urine a bright yellow color that's neither serious nor dangerous. And too much vitamin C can cause loose bowels or diarrhea in some people. "But usually," says Dr. Janson, "these side effects occur in extremely large doses—sometimes 100 times above the Recommended Dietary Allowance and well beyond what most people would ever take."

Another problem: Some nutrients may "block out" each other. "You should never take extra zinc without taking additional copper, because zinc will overwhelm the copper and induce a marginal deficiency," says Richard Anderson, Ph.D., lead scientist for the nutrient requirements and functions laboratory at the U.S. Department of Agriculture Human Nutrition Research Center in Beltsville, Maryland. "So if you're going to take a zinc supplement separate from a multivitamin/mineral supplement, be sure to take about three milligrams of copper as well."

to a sufficient-enough degree that national magazines were tracking their sales, just like those of the automobile industry.

From 1906 through the 1940s, there was a lot of research going on with vitamins and supplements, and the actual vitamins were named alphabetically in the order they were discovered: The first vitamin isolated was called A, the next was called B, then C and so on, says Dr. Dickinson. "It took about 20 or 30 years to separate the compounds that were really vitamins from those that were something else." And by that time, some letters were discarded, and others were filled in—one reason why there are eight B vitamins.

VITAMINS VERSUS MINERALS

There are at least 13 vitamins and 15 minerals considered essential for good health. (To find out which nutrients these are, see "Getting What You Need" on page 142.) Vitamins are organic compounds, meaning that they contain carbon, which is found only in living things. Minerals are simpler, nonorganic compounds and are usually found in smaller amounts in foods. Along with essential fatty aids and amino acids, vitamins and minerals are among the almost 50 known essential nutrients we need for a healthy life, says Dr. Janson.

Four of those vitamins—A, D, E and K—are fat-soluble, meaning that excess amounts may be stored in the body. The others—C and the eight B vitamins—are water-soluble, so excess amounts are simply urinated away.

Minerals, most of which were identified years after the initial research into vitamins, are also classified in two categories: major minerals, or macronutrients, such as calcium, magnesium and potassium, which are found in relatively high concentrations in food; and trace minerals, or micronutrients, such chromium, copper, iron and zinc, which are usually found in only minute amounts.

All of these nutrients are crucial to the preservation of life. Whether from food or supplements, vitamins and minerals play a role in cell building and in the health of every organ in your body as well as of your bones, immunity and nervous system. And while they don't supply energy—you get that from carbohydrates, protein and fat—they do release energy from food so that your body can use it.

"Every cell in your body needs every vitamin, but not every cell utilizes them in the same way or needs the same amounts," says Dr. Janson. "Because of that, it's hard to say which vitamins or minerals are most important."

A RADICAL SOLUTION

On the front line, at least when it comes to fending off today's most common health concerns, are the so-called antioxidants: vitamins C and E and beta-carotene (a form of vitamin A). When taken in large-enough doses, these vitamins are believed to offer protection against 60 age-related afflictions, from cancer and cataracts to heart disease and high cholesterol.

How? By stopping toxic molecules called free radicals. Caused by radiation, cigarette smoke, car exhaust and other pollutants, free radicals eat away at healthy cells and turn them defective, similar to the way cancer cells run amok. Over time, the damage done by free radicals can cause the development of cancer, turn innocuous cholesterol into sticky plaque that clogs arteries and accelerate the natural aging process and the disease that it brings.

But researchers say that the best defense against free radicals is to get plenty of antioxidant vitamins, which stop free radicals from overtaking healthy cells. "Because of this, it's hard to think of anyone in our society who couldn't benefit from taking vitamin supplements, especially those containing plenty of antioxidants," says Michael A. Klaper, M.D., a nutritional medicine specialist in Pompano Beach, Florida, and director of the Institute of Nutritional Education and Research, an organization based in Manhattan Beach, California, that teaches doctors about nutrition and its relationship to disease.

"We live in a far different world than our parents did. The sunshine is more oxidizing because of the thinning ozone layer. We add more chlorine to the water, so it is more oxidizing. Frying, barbecuing and adding preservatives and coloring make our foods more oxidizing. And the sad fact is, unless you're lucky enough to run the local organic food co-op and live in a really clean area, you may not be getting the protection you need from diet alone."

WHO BENEFITS MOST?

Your vitamin and mineral needs vary at different stages of your life, often because of the changing way your body absorbs nutrients. Infants, for instance, absorb about 70 percent of the calcium they consume; adults take in only about 30 percent. That's why supplements become even more important as you age.

"The elderly could definitely benefit from supplementation, because once you're in your sixties, food intake typically drops, and you're not as active as you used to be," says Judith S. Stern, R.D., Sc.D., professor of nutrition and internal medicine at the University of California, Davis.

Even if you manage to stay active, you can benefit from supplements. "Moderate exercise enhances immunity, but if you're running more than 30 miles a week or doing a lot of other types of exercise, you can actually hurt immunity and be more prone to viruses," says Kenneth H. Cooper, M.D., founder and president of the Cooper Aerobics Center in Dallas. "So if you exercise a lot, you should definitely take vitamin supplements rich in antioxidants." His recommendation: 1,000 milligrams of vitamin C, 400 international units (IU) of vitamin E in the natural alpha-tocopherol form and 15 milligrams (25,000 IU) of beta-carotene each day.

Others who may be in special need of vitamin and mineral supplements, according to Dr. Stern: women of childbearing age; women who are pregnant or nursing; dieters, especially when they consume fewer than 1,200 calories a day; people preparing for or recovering from surgery; those who drink alcoholic beverages frequently; smokers; people who travel a lot and may not be able to eat a variety of foods; people who live in smoggy climates; and, possibly, strict vegetarians.

BEYOND THE RDA

Why do so many of us need nutritional boosts from a pill or tablet—or from a few of them? Because so many of us base our nutritional needs on the RDAs, first established by the Food and Nutrition Board in 1941 and updated periodically ever since.

RDAs are across-the-board guidelines for everyone from infants to adults and do not take into account special nutritional needs. The general nature of RDAs may leave us shy of the nutrients we need, which is why, some experts say, we're a society nagged by so many health problems, from immune disorders such as colds and slow-healing cuts to more serious conditions such as arthritis and heart disease.

"The RDA is really a useless guideline for today, because it was designed to prevent deficiency diseases such as scurvy and beriberi—problems we don't see in this country," says Dr. Janson. "The RDA is not a useful guideline for achieving optimal health and treating disease, especially in today's society."

Changes in food labeling have added another number: the Daily Value, or DV. Like the RDA, the DV is a recommendation for how much of a specific nutrient you need in your daily diet to maintain adequate nutrition. On food labels, the percent DV tells you the percentage of your daily nutrient needs provided by one serving of that food, based on a diet of 2,000 calories per day. Multivitamin/mineral supplements are also labeled with the percent DV. Neither DVs nor RDAs are necessarily a true measure of what you may need to treat or to protect yourself from disease.

For that, experts say, you need to go beyond RDAs—often way beyond. "Generally, I'd say that vitamins in amounts well above the RDAs are safe for most people," says Gladys Block, Ph.D., professor of public health and nutrition and epidemiology at the University of California, Berkeley, and an authority on vitamin therapy. In fact, experts say, the biggest benefits of some nutrients seem to occur when taken in large doses.

"Take vitamin C, for example," says Alan Gaby, M.D., a physician specializing in preventive and nutritional medicine in Baltimore and president of the American Holistic Medical Association. Vitamin C's RDA is 60 milligrams a day, approximately the amount you'd get in a glass of citrus fruit juice or ½ cup of broccoli.

"You could get as much as 500 milligrams if you eat a diet really high in fruits and vegetables, but that would be pushing it," he says. "Yet most of the studies show that vitamin C does the most good—functioning as an antihistamine, killing viruses, boosting immunity and protecting against cancer, diabetes and other diseases—in dosages that range anywhere from 500 to 10,000 milligrams, which you could never achieve with food."

Dr. Block has reviewed more than 100 studies examining the relationship between vitamin C and cancer. In virtually every study, the nutrient had a protective effect. In most studies, people with high intakes of fruits and vegetables containing vitamin C had a lower risk of cancer.

Same goes for beta-carotene, which converts into vitamin A in the body when needed. It's safer to take in supplement form than vitamin A because it derives from plant sources and excess amounts are excreted (whereas fat-soluble vitamin A comes from animal sources, and excess amounts are stored in your body). Studies show that people who take this antioxidant vitamin in supplement form—it's also found in carrots, squash, melons and other yellow-orange fruits and vegetables—cut their risk of heart attack and stroke in half compared with those who don't.

And when taken in doses five to ten times what's typically recommended, which is about six milligrams (10,000 IU), beta-carotene has been shown to greatly reduce precancerous lesions of the mouth, says cancer researcher Harinder Garewal, M.D., Ph.D., of the University of Arizona Cancer Center in Tucson.

Meanwhile, vitamin E has been found to help protect against heart disease, but only when taken in amounts at least seven times above the RDA of ten milligrams alpha-tocopherol equivalents (15 IU) for men and eight milligrams alpha-tocopherol equivalents (12 IU) for women—amounts hard to achieve through diet. (You'd have to eat four large mangoes or 12 apples just to get the RDA.) "Studies show it takes even more, between 400 and 800 IU, to relieve fibrocystic breast disease," adds Dr. Gaby. "It would be impossible to get that much vitamin E from foods alone."

THE MIGHTY MINERALS

While antioxidants get most of the headlines, they're not the only super supplements. "There is a lot of exciting research being done with minerals right now," says Dr. Anderson. And as with antioxidants, it seems that big benefits come in dosages you can't normally get through foods alone.

"One thing I've been working on is chromium, a trace mineral that has been shown to reduce risk factors for diabetes and cardiovascular disease in some people," he says. "It improves glucose and insulin and lowers cholesterol and triglycerides, a form of blood fat that has been linked to an increased risk of heart disease. Give someone the recommended 50 micrograms, and he'll get along fine. But if you want protection against diabetes, you need about 400 micrograms; if you want to protect against heart disease, you need 400 micrograms. And research also shows that copper and magnesium can protect against heart disease—but only in amounts that you rarely get from food."

Other experts say that zinc, a mineral best known for healing wounds and building tissue, may be even more important than antioxidants for warding off infections and keeping the immune system strong. In fact, one of the hottest remedies for fighting colds is zinc gluconate lozenges; they kill many of the germs that cause sore throat and other symptoms associated with the common cold.

Zinc's RDA is 15 milligrams for men and 12 milligrams for women, but most people get only between 8 and 10 milligrams—"and even less if they're vegetarian," says Ananda Prasad, M.D., Ph.D., professor of medicine at Wayne State University in Detroit and a leading expert on zinc. What should they get? "I'd say about 30 milligrams a day—more if they're having a specific skin problem or another condition," adds Dr. Janson. "As long as it is properly balanced with 2 to 3 milligrams of copper." This is because zinc and copper interfere with each other's absorption, says Dr. Janson. Too much of one can cause a deficiency of the other, so they should always be supplemented together. Check with your doctor before regularly taking doses of zinc picolinate over 15 milligrams a day.

Selenium is a mineral with antioxidant qualities that may also strengthen immunity. Research shows it protects against heart disease and cancer, alleviates arthritis symptoms and can even improve mood. The RDA is 70 micrograms for men and 55 micrograms for women; Dr. Janson recommends taking up to six times that amount each day to reap these rewards.

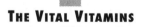

The Vital Vitamins

On the vitamin side, B_6 is another nutrient that is essential to strong immunity. It also offers relief from carpal tunnel syndrome, prevents kidney stones and relieves premenstrual syndrome.

And vitamin B_6 becomes even more important as you age. Elderly people seem to metabolize it less effectively than younger people, says Simin Meydani, Ph.D., chief of the nutritional immunology laboratory at the U.S. Department of Agriculture Human Nutrition Research Center on Aging at Tufts University in Boston. This could lead to a B_6 deficiency, and such a deficiency can hurt immunity.

Dr. Janson recommends taking 50 to 100 milligrams of vitamin B_6 daily, well above the RDA of 2 milligrams for men and 1.6 milligrams for women.

The bottom line: No matter what your age, gender, lifestyle or exercise habits, most people can benefit from supplementing their diets with vitamins and minerals, experts say.

"You can't replace a healthy diet with vitamin and mineral supplements; you still need to eat as well as possible," says Dr. Janson. "But you can make up for some of the fault of a poor diet with them—and most of us have fault with our diets."

Like diet, exercise and stress management, supplements are only part of a total health plan—not magic pills that can make up for all of your other bad habits. "No matter how much I tell my patients to eat a better diet, a lot would rather take the pills, because it's easier," says Dr. Janson. "Sorry, but supplements are only a part."

But they can make a big difference, he adds. "If you are healthy now and feel good, your energy levels are high, you have no problems with physical stamina when doing exercise and your mental processes are clear, then I don't think you should expect immediately obvious effects from taking supplements—other than to maintain that state for many more years than if you didn't take them."

GETTING WHAT YOU NEED

Here's how much you need every day of the most essential vitamins and minerals, along with where to find them and what they do for your body.

Nutrient	RDA for Men	RDA for Women	DV
VITAMINS			
Vitamin A	1,000 mcg. RE or 5,000 IU	800 mcg. RE or 4,000 IU (1,300 mcg. RE or 6,500 IU if nursing)	5,000 IU
B Vitamins			
Thiamin	1.5 mg.	1.1 mg. (1.5 mg. if pregnant; 1.6 mg. if nursing)	1.5 mg.
Riboflavin	1.7 mg.	1.3 mg. (1.6 mg. if pregnant; 1.8 mg. if nursing)	1.7 mg.
Niacin	19 mg.	15 mg. (17 mg. if pregnant; 20 mg. if nursing)	20 mg.
Vitamin B$_6$	2.0 mg.	1.6 mg. (2.2 mg. if pregnant; 2.1 mg. if nursing)	2.0 mg.
Folate (folic acid)	200 mcg.	180 mcg. (400 mcg. if pregnant; 280 mcg. if nursing)	0.4 mg. (400 mcg.)

BENEFIT	FOOD SOURCES
Needed for normal vision in dim light; maintains normal structure and function of mucous membranes; aids growth of bones, teeth and skin	Carrots, pumpkin, sweet potatoes, spinach, butternut squash, tuna, cantaloupe, mangoes, apricots, broccoli, watermelon
Carbohydrate metabolism; maintains healthy nervous system	Pork, wheat germ, pasta, peanuts, legumes, watermelon, oranges, brown rice, oatmeal, eggs
Fat, protein and carbohydrate metabolism; healthy skin	Milk, cottage cheese, avocados, tangerines, prunes, asparagus, broccoli, mushrooms, beef, salmon, turkey
Fat, protein and carbohydrate metabolism; nervous system function; needed for oxygen use by cells	Meats, poultry, fish, peanut butter, legumes, soybeans, whole-grain cereals and breads, broccoli, asparagus, baked potatoes
Protein metabolism; needed for normal growth	Fish, soybeans, avocados, lima beans, chicken, bananas, cauli-flower, green peppers, potatoes, spinach, raisins
Red blood cell development; tissue growth and repair	Legumes, poultry, tuna, wheat germ, mushrooms, oranges, asparagus, broccoli, spinach, bananas, strawberries, cantaloupe

(continued)

GETTING WHAT YOU NEED—Continued

Nutrient	RDA for Men	RDA for Women	DV
B Vitamins—Continued			
Vitamin B$_{12}$	2.0 mcg.	2.0 mcg. (2.2 mcg. if pregnant; 2.6 mcg. if nursing)	6.0 mcg.
Biotin	30–100 mcg.★	30–100 mcg.★	0.3 mg. (300 mcg.)
Pantothenic acid	4–7 mg.★	4–7 mg.★	10 mg.
Vitamin C	60 mg.	60 mg. (70 mg. if pregnant; 95 mg. if nursing)	60 mg.
Vitamin D	5 mcg.	5 mcg. (10 mcg. if pregnant or nursing)	400 IU (10 mcg.)
Vitamin E	10 mg. alpha-TE or 15 IU	8 mg. alpha-TE or 12 IU (10 mg. alpha-TE or 15 IU if pregnant; 12 mg. alpha-TE or 18 IU if nursing)	30 IU
Vitamin K	80 mcg.	65 mcg.	None

BENEFIT	FOOD SOURCES
Needed for new tissue growth, red blood cells, nervous system and skin	Salmon, eggs, cheese, swordfish, tuna, clams, crab, mussels, oysters
Fat, protein and carbohydrate metabolism	Peanut butter, eggs, oatmeal, wheat germ, poultry, cauliflower, nuts, legumes
Fat, protein and carbohydrate metabolism	Fish, whole-grain cereals, mushrooms, avocados, broccoli, peanuts, cashews, lentils, soybeans, eggs
Builds collagen; maintains healthy gums, teeth and blood vessels	Oranges, grapefruit, bell peppers, strawberries, tomatoes, spinach, cabbage, melons, broccoli, kiwifruit, raspberries
Calcium absorption; growth of bones and teeth	Sunlight, eggs, milk, butter, tuna, salmon, cereals, baked goods (if fortified flour is used)
Protects cells from damage	Nut and vegetable oils, wheat germ, mangoes, blackberries, apples, broccoli, peanuts, spinach, whole-wheat breads
Blood clotting	Spinach, broccoli, brussels sprouts, cabbage, parsley, eggs, dairy products, carrots, avocados, tomatoes

(continued)

GETTING WHAT YOU NEED—Continued

Nutrient	RDA for Men	RDA for Women	DV
MINERALS			
Calcium	800 mg.	800 mg. (1,200 mg. if pregnant or nursing)	1 g. (1,000 mg.)
Chloride	750 mg.[†]	750 mg.[†]	None
Chromium	50–200 mcg.[*]	50–200 mcg.[*]	None
Copper	1.5–3.0 mg.[*]	1.5–3.0 mg.[*]	2.0 mg.
Fluoride	1.5–4.0 mg.[*]	1.5–4.0 mg.[*]	None
Iodine	150 mcg.	150 mcg. (175 mcg. if pregnant; 200 mcg. if nursing)	150 mcg.
Iron	10 mg.	15 mg. (30 mg. if pregnant)	18 mg.
Magnesium	350 mg.	280 mg. (320 mg. if pregnant; 355 mg. if nursing)	400 mg.

BENEFIT	FOOD SOURCES
Strong bones and teeth; muscle and nerve function; blood clotting	Milk, cheese, yogurt, salmon and sardines with bones, broccoli, green beans, almonds, turnip greens, fortified orange juice
Aids digestion; works with sodium to maintain fluid balance	Foods with salt
Carbohydrate metabolism	Whole grains, broccoli, grape juice, orange juice, brown sugar, meats, black pepper, brewer's yeast, cheese
Blood cell and connective tissue formation	Oysters and other shellfish, nuts, cherries, cocoa, mushrooms, gelatin, whole-grain cereals, eggs, fish, legumes
Strengthens tooth enamel	Fluoridated water, fish, tea
Maintains proper thyroid function	Spinach, lobster, shrimp, oysters, milk, iodized salt
Carries oxygen in blood; energy metabolism	Clams, asparagus, meats, chicken, prunes, raisins, spinach, pumpkin seeds, soybeans, tofu
Aids nerve and muscle function; strong bones	Molasses, nuts, spinach, wheat germ, pumpkin seeds, seafood, dairy products, baked potatoes, broccoli, bananas

(continued)

VITAMIN AND MINERAL THERAPY

GETTING WHAT YOU NEED—Continued

Nutrient	RDA for Men	RDA for Women	DV
Manganese	2.0–5.0 mg.★	2.0–5.0 mg.★	None
Molybdenum	75–250 mcg.★	75–250 mcg.★	None
Phosphorus	800 mg.	800 mg. (1,200 mg. if pregnant or nursing)	1 g. (1,000 mg.)
Potassium	2,000 mg.†	2,000 mg.†	3,500 mg.
Selenium	70 mcg.	55 mcg. (65 mcg. if pregnant; 75 mcg. if nursing)	None
Sodium	500 mg.†	500 mg.†	2,400 mg.
Zinc	15 mg.	12 mg. (15 mg. if pregnant; 19 mg. if nursing)	15 mg.

★Value is the Estimated Safe and Adequate Daily Intake.
 There is no RDA for this nutrient.

VITAMIN AND MINERAL THERAPY

BENEFIT	FOOD SOURCES
Bone and connective tissue formation; fat and carbohydrate metabolism	Nuts, whole-grain cereals, legumes, tea, dried fruits, spinach and other green leafy vegetables
Nitrogen metabolism	Legumes, meats, whole-grain cereals, breads, milk and milk products
Energy metabolism; teams up with calcium for strong bones and teeth	Meats, fish, poultry, eggs, dairy products, cereals
Controls acid balance in the body; works with sodium to maintain fluid balance	Baked potatoes, avocados, dried fruits, yogurt, cantaloupe, spinach, bananas, mushrooms, milk, tomatoes
Helps vitamin E protect cells and body tissue	Meats, whole-grain cereals, dairy products, fish, shellfish, mushrooms, Brazil nuts
Fluid balance; nervous system function	Salt, processed foods, soy sauce, seasonings
Wound healing; growth; appetite; sperm production	Oysters, lean beef, wheat germ, seafood, lima beans, legumes, nuts, poultry, dairy products

†Value is the Estimated Minimum Requirement. There is no RDA for this nutrient.

YOGA

Stretching Your Natural Defenses

What could be more natural than taking a deep, easy breath? Or stretching gently from head to toe? Or lounging in bed on Saturday morning, letting thoughts of the past week drift quietly in and out of your mind?

Simple as it sounds, that's yoga. It's not about body-wrenching positions or secret Eastern philosophy. It's about gently bringing your body and mind back in touch with each other—and giving yourself a chance to heal.

"One of the big benefits of yoga is that it releases built-up tension and stress, which burrow into the muscles of the body," says yoga instructor Lilias Folan, whose television shows "Lilias, Yoga and You" and "Lilias!" have appeared on public television for more than two decades. "Spending time on the body is the key to being a healthy, contented human being."

In many ways, yoga is the most basic of natural remedies. You don't need anything but a quiet, comfortable place and a few minutes each day to practice breathing, stretching and meditation. Experts say yoga offers specific exercises and techniques that you can do by yourself to help with a variety of ailments.

Yoga can become a calming, friendly addition to your hectic daily routine. "You'll soon begin to enjoy the stillness. You'll welcome it, instead of trying to shut quiet and calm out of your life," says Folan, creator of the audiotape series *Rest, Relax and Sleep*, used by hospitals and wellness programs.

"In these ways, it can help you become a happier and healthier person."

LIMBS OF THE TREE

The term *yoga* comes from the Sanskrit word *yuj*, meaning "to yoke." The purpose of yoga is to yoke—to join or balance—the mind, body and breath. Too often, Folan says, we view the three as separate parts of us, unconnected and unrelated. "But they're intimately connected," she says. "A change in one will reflect in the others. When the mind is disturbed, the breath and body are affected. When the body is active, the mind and breath change right along with it. You can quiet the mind by quieting the breath; you can quiet your breathing by slowing down your activity." Proper yoga poses, or asanas, will bring about this desired balance, she says.

No one knows exactly how long people have been practicing yoga. The

150

earliest mentions of it come from small stone symbols in India that are thought to date from 3000 B.C.—nearly 5,000 years ago. About 2,300 years ago, the sage Patanjali compiled this passed-down knowledge in the Yoga Sutras, which include the eight steps that lead to spiritual enlightenment.

Some of the steps, which include poses and yoga breathing techniques (called pranayama), form what is known as hatha yoga. These, plus meditation, are the parts of yoga best known in the Western world. Other steps include moral codes such as dedication to nonviolence and severe simplicity.

How does yoga heal? Classic texts say that it works by increasing the body's stores of prana, or vital energy. If prana is blocked by stress, emotional troubles, poor diet or other factors, your body is left vulnerable to sickness and disease.

Western experts believe yoga heals in two ways. The first is through relaxation. "I really feel that the most powerful healer of all is deep relaxation," says yoga teacher Judith Lasater, P.T., Ph.D., author of *Rest and Renew: Quiet Yoga Poses to Reduce Stress and Tension*. "Yoga allows everything to relax. That aids your muscular system, your circulatory system and other parts of you that suffer from the effects of stress."

Yoga poses also help cleanse organs through what Dr. Lasater calls squeezing and soaking. Moving your body into different poses forces blood out of vital organs, allowing fresh blood to take its place. This gives your organs more nutrients, making them stronger and more resistant to disease. And as you practice pranayama, you change your normal patterns of breathing, which in turn calms your state of mind, reducing the disturbances and impurities in your body.

Dr. Lasater and other experts say they have witnessed firsthand how powerful yoga can be. They say they've seen improvements in conditions such as infertility, arthritis, high cholesterol, back pain and many more. Scientific research is proving many of these claims. For example, researchers in Britain studied yoga's effects on 18 people with mild asthma, who ranged in age from 19 to 54. The result: All 18 reported more improvement in their conditions when they used yoga-style breathing. The researchers also found that the people had greater resistance to the effects of histamine, a body chemical that can trigger an asthma attack, while they were doing their breathing exercises.

Yoga can apparently lift your spirits and reduce stress, too. Scientists at the City University of New York in New York City studied 63 students who had volunteered to take a beginner yoga class. The students reported feeling less anxious, tense, depressed, angry and fatigued immediately after class. And the results began to kick in after the very first class.

The news on other health problems remains mixed. A study from Holland, for instance, found that relaxation therapy that included yoga had no significant effect on lowering blood pressure. But individual cases still show promise. U.S. government researchers report that a 46-year-old air force pilot with high blood pressure lowered his readings from 138/92 to 122/82 in six weeks after stopping traditional medication and starting a relaxation program that included daily yoga practice.

BREATHING IT IN

Daily yoga routines come in four parts: breathing, relaxation, meditation and poses. Together, Folan says, they relax the body and focus and clear the mind, giving you more energy and vigor with a sense of inner contentment and peace.

Experts say your routine should last at least a half-hour and should begin with breathing. Deep breathing draws energy into your body, provides you with precious oxygen and calms your muscles and organs, according to Alice Christensen, founder and executive director of the American Yoga Association.

Unfortunately, most of us take very shallow breaths, not allowing our lungs to expand and soak up oxygen. The proper way to breathe is by using the diaphragm, the thin muscle underneath your lungs. When the diaphragm flexes, it pulls down and opens the lower lobes of your lungs, allowing more air inside. Christensen calls this type of breathing the belly breath because your belly, not your chest, expands as air enters the lungs.

The belly breath is simple to learn. Start by sitting comfortably in a chair or on the floor. If you sit on the floor, sit on one or more firm cushions so that your hips tilt slightly forward, to reduce the strain on your lower back. Place one hand on your stomach. Then breathe out slowly through your nose, contracting your stomach muscles and lightly pushing on your stomach. To breathe in, relax your stomach muscles, arch your back slightly and let the air flow in your nose. You should feel your hand push out as your belly expands.

Breathe slowly and evenly, taking at least three seconds to inhale and three to exhale. Try to make the two parts equal. You'll find yourself taking deeper, slower breaths without even trying. After you get the hang of it, you can remove your hand from your belly.

"This is the way to breathe all of the time," Christensen says. "Chest breathing comes from stress; it's a reaction to stress. But breathing from the belly is a natural way to relax and spread more oxygen to your entire body."

Yoga offers many different advanced breathing techniques: some designed to clear the sinuses, some to go with meditation and others to strengthen stomach and chest muscles. The best overall stress reducer is called the complete breath. Christensen says this is the one you should practice for a few minutes each day as part of your yoga routine.

The complete breath starts like the belly breath, except your hands are in a different position. Place them on either side of your lower rib cage, with your fingers touching slightly. Begin breathing from your abdomen, letting the air fill your lower lungs. Now let the breath begin to fill the lower part of your chest. Try to make your ribs expand sideways as your lungs fill; you should feel your fingers spreading apart as your chest grows. Keep drawing in more air, working toward the top of your lungs. Straighten your shoulders and arch your back, letting the air "top off" your lungs. Be careful not to breathe so deeply that you feel straining in your stomach or chest muscles.

The entire inhalation should last up to ten seconds, and the exhalation should last about as long. Always breathe through your nose, because this helps you control your breath better. Do the complete breath for at least five minutes at the start of your yoga routine—but don't stop there. Christensen recommends doing it any time during the day that you feel high stress.

Fill Your Mind with Empty

You can't be relaxed if your mind is racing, worrying about clients at work, leaky plumbing at home and spats with your spouse. That's why yoga experts say you need to set aside a few minutes a day to think about absolutely nothing.

Meditation helps you focus on what's important and lets you explore yourself. And that can be very healing, says Folan.

Relaxation gently guides you into meditation. Anyone can do it, provided he has a warm, quiet room with few outside interruptions. "Meditation is something you do by yourself without children or pets in the room. No telephones," Folan says. "Eventually, you'll be able to stay centered and calm when there are distractions. And when you get off base, you'll know how to return to the center through the use of your breathing and relaxation techniques."

In advanced meditation, people usually sit upright in one of several poses. But the American Yoga Association offers a simple meditation program that you can do on your back in a position called the corpse pose (see the illustration on page 612). Christensen says this position allows you to relax completely, since there's no pressure on any of your limbs.

Find a dimly lit, warm room with no drafts. Place a mat or blanket on the floor and lie on it faceup. Don't use a pillow unless your doctor says you need to keep your head raised for medical reasons. Relax your arms at your sides, with your palms facing the ceiling. Straighten and relax your legs. If you have back pain, you can bend your knees to take the strain off of your lower back (or put a small cushion under your thighs).

Now spend about five minutes unwinding. Focus your mind on different body parts, feeling them release their tension. Begin with the face, then move to the shoulders, arms, hands and chest, focusing on your heart and lungs. No-

(continued on page 156)

FINDING A CLASS ACT

If you want to learn more about yoga, experts suggest taking a group class. Locating a class is easy; almost every fitness club, YM/YWCA and community center offers one, and hundreds of yoga centers across America advertise both short- and long-term instruction. There are also many excellent home videos to practice with in your own home.

But sometimes all of those possibilities can make it hard to choose. "Yoga has become the fitness of the '90s," says Los Angeles yoga therapist Larry Payne, Ph.D., creator of the videotape *Healthy Back, Healthy Mind.* "So you are seeing tremendous growth in the number and types of teachers. To pick the one that's right for you takes some thought and sometimes a little trial and error."

The majority of American yoga classes focus on hatha yoga, which emphasizes the familiar yoga poses along with breathing and meditation. Within hatha yoga, however, teachers stress different things: Some focus more on demanding physical poses, while others concentrate on relaxation and contemplation.

Dr. Payne says instructors often come from "schools" of yoga and are influenced by the methods of particular teachers. If you want a physical class, look for these names: B. K. S. Iyengar, the Astanga yoga of Pattabi Jois, Bikram Choudhuri. Those seeking more emphasis on breathing, moderate poses and meditation should look for these names: T. K. V. Desikachar, A. G. Mohan, Vishnu Devananda, Satchidananda.

If you are using yoga therapeutically, it is important that you meet with a qualified yoga teacher, go to yoga classes or have a private consultation before you practice a yoga routine on your own. You can learn which poses (asanas) to add to your basic routine and which ones to avoid. Your teacher can guide you through the correct positions and teach you the basics of breathing, relaxation and meditation. Choose a qualified yoga teacher the way you would any health professional: Ask family and friends who have done yoga, and ask the teachers about their credentials.

Unfortunately, yoga has no standard certification process or training guidelines. So you're going to have to ask a lot of questions before settling on someone. When you're looking for a good instructor, experts say you should follow these tips.

Look for a student/teacher. Ask if the instructor has a teacher of his own. Does the instructor practice yoga daily? "You want a dedicated teacher—someone who is always learning more," says Alice Christensen, founder and executive director of the American Yoga Association.

Sample a class. Before you sign up for a long-term course, ask if you can sit in on one or two sessions. "This will give you a good idea of what the teacher is all about," says Judith Lasater, P.T., Ph.D., a yoga teacher and author of *Rest and Renew: Quiet Yoga Poses to Reduce Stress and Tension.* "Good teachers don't mind letting you take an introductory class. If they do mind, it may be a bad sign. They may just be trying to lock you in to a long-term commitment."

Don't overpay. Group classes shouldn't cost more than $10 to $15 per session, Dr. Payne says. Individual instruction usually costs more.

Avoid pain. Yoga should never hurt. And you shouldn't take any verbal abuse from a teacher, either, Dr. Lasater says. "You need someone who respects your boundaries, both physically and mentally." Make sure the teacher doesn't try to compare one student with another. "You should never feel like you're competing against someone," Dr. Payne says.

Relax and enjoy. "At the end of the session, you should feel very good," says yoga instructor Lilias Folan, whose television shows "Lilias, Yoga and You" and "Lilias!" have appeared on public television for more than two decades. "I hope a student leaves class uplifted, hopeful. Your muscles shouldn't be shaking. That's the mark of a good class. If you find a teacher who helps you feel that way, stick with him."

Watch for hidden agendas. Hatha yoga does not attempt to force any spiritual beliefs on the people who practice it. While it is true that yoga emerged as a set of practices in an Indian religious context, "it's not wedded to any particular spiritual tradition," says Folan, creator of the audiotape series *Rest, Relax and Sleep.* "Yoga is here to assist you in whatever pathway you choose in life. It is a vehicle for growth and development with emphasis on doing and practicing, not blindly believing." But some instructors may incorporate religious philosophy into their classes. Most will tell you this up front, and if it makes you uncomfortable, don't stay. Christensen says you should be wary of any instructor who tries to get you to use a religious chant or phrase as part of meditation.

tice how your breathing becomes slower and deeper. Then move on to your stomach and other organs in your abdomen. Finally, work down to your hips, legs and feet. Christensen then suggests going back to your face to make sure that it is still calm and relaxed.

Once you've scanned your body, it's time to begin meditation. It can help to start by silently repeating a mantra, a phrase that focuses your attention. Christensen suggest the word *om*, pronounced "ohm." Repeat this silently for about a minute to help draw attention from your body to your mind.

Now lie quietly. As thoughts enter your mind, observe them—but don't dwell on them. This is the tricky part about meditation. We're used to thinking about things, not thinking about nothing. Try to gently move your thoughts to the edge of your mind, but don't force them. Just let them drift away.

What you're trying to find is stillness. Your mind should be quiet, concentrating, focused. You may not reach this point the first time you meditate. And if it doesn't last long, don't fret. "If you can get one to two minutes of absolute silence, give yourself an A," Christensen says.

Meditate for ten minutes or so—more if you have the time. Then bring yourself back slowly, repeating the mantra again for about a minute. Don't set an alarm, because that will jar you when it sounds.

Everyone has a different experience meditating. Some people feel their bodies go heavy, and others, light. Some fall asleep once in a while. Whatever happens, enjoy it. You're beginning to learn how to relax, the first step in letting your body and mind heal themselves.

THE POSE THAT REFRESHES

The fourth part of your daily yoga routine is the physical one, the poses. There are dozens and dozens of them, and they have changed little over the centuries. Experts say the poses work in many ways. Some stretch and strengthen muscles. Others improve posture and the skeletal system. Still others compress and relax organs and nerves. Together, the poses are a powerful weapon against disease, making your body more resistant, resilient and ready to heal itself.

Below is the Daily Routine of 16 expert-recommended poses, along with brief descriptions of the health benefits that experts say you might expect from them. Step-by-step instructions for each pose start on page 606. Be sure to check with your doctor before attempting these poses, especially if you have special medical needs or a chronic medical condition or if you are pregnant.

Christensen suggests picking three or four poses per day and alternating them every day to give your body a complete workout. Perform them in the order listed.

YOGA

Throughout this book, yoga experts recommend combinations of these poses to deal with specific diseases and conditions. Those listed under specific diseases are in addition to your daily yoga routine, which should include breathing, relaxation, meditation and poses.

You should start slowly and work up to any difficult poses, according to Nancy Ford-Kohne, founder-director of the Yoga and Health Studies Center in Alexandria, Virginia. Some, such as the cobra and the spine twist, should be avoided if there are severe back problems. Add them when the back heals or is less stressed.

Always wind down and relax, ending with the corpse pose and five to ten minutes of relaxation exercises. And while attention to breath takes place throughout any yoga practice, Ford-Kohne suggests thinking to yourself "Inhale energy and healing, exhale fatigue and stress" or whatever is adversely affecting your well-being.

To get started, find a comfortable, warm place with a level floor. Wear loose clothing. And go gently—never push your body until it hurts. "The old saying 'No pain, no gain' doesn't apply to yoga," Folan says. "Yoga should make you feel good."

1. *Mountain pose.* An easy standing pose that may help people with osteoporosis.
2. *Standing sun pose.* This pose may help relieve constipation and bladder problems, loosen hips and shoulders and improve nerve function.
3. *Tree pose.* A standing pose that tones your legs and improves balance, concentration and breathing.
4. *Dancer pose.* A standing pose that can improve balance, open nasal passages, stretch and strengthen hips and thighs and help beat fatigue. Use care if you have a lower back problem.
5. *Windmill pose.* If you tilt along with this standing pose, you may help loosen your hips and lower back and improve breathing. Use care if you have a lower back problem.
6. *Corpse pose.* The ultimate relaxation pose. As its name suggests, you lie still and let everything go loose. Experts say this may help with back pain, stress and even high blood pressure. Use this rest pose whenever you need it, and always end your routine with a few minutes in the corpse pose.
7. *Knee squeeze.* A simple pose, done while lying on the floor, that can relieve gas, increase circulation in your head and neck, ease lower back pain and strengthen stomach muscles.
8. *Spine twist.* Sit and turn for this pose, which may help constipation and

bladder problems, loosen hips and shoulders and improve nerve function. Use extreme caution if you have spinal disk problems.

9. ***Head-to-knee.*** This seated stretch can help improve the function of your internal organs.

10. ***Seated sun pose.*** Another seated pose, this one can help with digestion and possibly with impotence as well as strengthen the legs and spine.

11. ***Baby pose.*** This kneeling pose limbers your lower back, improves digestion and strengthens and relieves stiffness in the knees, ankles and hips. If you have arthritic knees, this pose can be done in a chair.

12. ***Easy bridge pose.*** This pose, adapted from a more difficult pose, can help with back pain and fatigue, improve circulation to your head and face, bolster your endocrine system and maybe help with high blood pressure. Do not do this pose during the second half of pregnancy.

13. ***Half boat pose.*** An easier version of the boat pose described below. Use this until you've worked your way to the full pose.

14. ***Boat pose.*** Done while lying on your stomach, this pose strengthens your back muscles and spinal column, aids digestion and helps vital organs function better.

15. ***Cobra pose.*** This snakelike pose helps strengthen your entire body, aids digestion, makes your spine more flexible and might even help improve eyesight. Women should not do this during menstrual periods. No one should do this within several weeks of surgery or if they have open wounds.

16. ***Lion pose.*** A simple breathing exercise that relaxes facial muscles and eases tension.

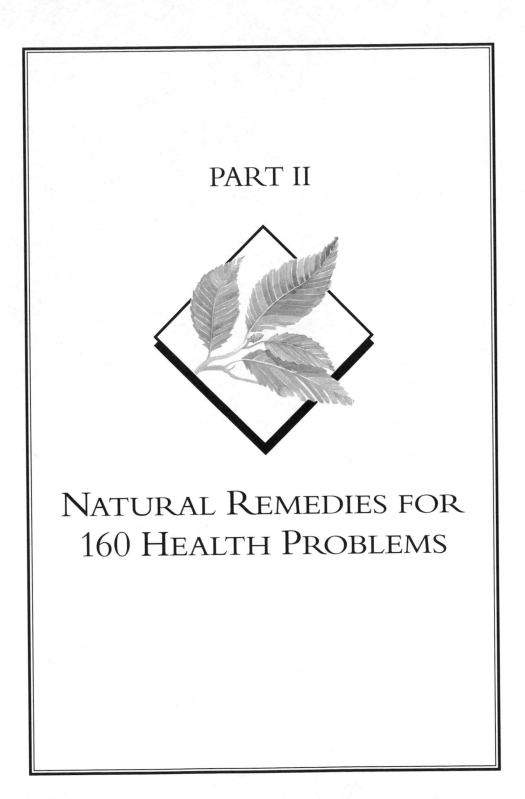

PART II

Natural Remedies for 160 Health Problems

ACNE

Once viewed as the bane of burger-eating, cola-guzzling teenagers, acne also affects plenty of adults as well.

In spite of what your friends have told you, breakouts aren't the product of poor hygiene or poor diet. At the root of the problem is an over-production of sebum, a waxy substance that clogs the pores and leads to black-heads, whiteheads and pimples. In teenagers, this overload of sebum is caused by the hormone explosion known as puberty. In adults, it can result from heredity, stress and women's monthly hormone fluctuations.

So what can you do when your skin won't act its age? Treat it with kid gloves. That means no harsh soaps or frenzied scrubbing. Women should avoid oil-based cosmetics, which can clog pores and encourage breakouts. The natural remedies in this chapter—used in conjunction with everyday hygiene and with your dermatologist's approval—may help prevent or relieve acne, according to some health professionals.

SEE YOUR MEDICAL DOCTOR WHEN . . .

- Your skin becomes severely inflamed, with a reddish or purplish cast.
- You've tried over-the-counter medicines and they aren't helping.
- Your pimples are forming scars after they heal.

ACUPRESSURE

Acupressure can improve the appearance of your skin, says Michael Reed Gach, Ph.D., director of the Acupressure Institute in Berkeley, California, and author of *Acupressure's Potent Points*. According to Chinese medicine, the stomach meridian is one of several energy pathways that govern skin function. Press both St 2 points, which are situated one finger-width below the lower ridge of each eye socket, in line with the center of the iris and in an indentation of the cheek, says Dr. Gach. (To help locate the points, please see the illustration on page 564.) Hold the points for one minute. Dr. Gach says to do this three times a day for clearer, more radiant skin.

AROMATHERAPY

Tea tree essential oil is a natural antiseptic that is gentle to the skin and speeds the healing of blemishes, says Los Angeles aromatherapist Michael Scholes, of Aromatherapy Seminars, an organization that trains professionals and others in the use of essential oils. He suggests applying a single drop of tea tree oil directly to the blemish after cleansing.

For information on preparing and administering essential oils, including cautions about their use, see page 19. For information on purchasing essential oils, refer to the resource list on page 633.

AYURVEDA

Angry-looking red pimples filled with a yellowish discharge are a sign of excess pitta dosha, says Vasant Lad, B.A.M.S., M.A.Sc., director of the Ayurvedic Institute in Albuquerque, New Mexico. (For more information about the Ayurvedic doshas, see "All about Vata, Pitta and Kapha" on page 28.) To control acne, he suggests adopting a diet that includes plenty of bland foods such as oatmeal, applesauce and basmati rice and eliminates fried foods, spicy foods and citrus fruits.

Dr. Lad also recommends this daily routine for cleansing your face: First, wash your face with chick-pea paste, made by mixing one teaspoon of chick-pea flour (available in some health food stores and from Indian grocers) with a little water. Dry with a clean towel. Then apply a paste made by mixing one teaspoon of almond powder (you can make your own by grinding peeled almonds in a coffee grinder) with a cup of goat's milk (available in most health food stores). Let this almond-paste mask dry on your face for a few minutes before washing it off.

If you live near an Indian grocery store, Dr. Lad says to look for a sandalwood-turmeric cream that you can apply after removing the mask; follow the label directions when applying the cream. A word of caution from Dr. Lad: It may be best to use sandalwood-turmeric cream at night, because it can color your skin a faint yellow. He suggests testing it first to see how it looks. Any discoloration should wash off in about two weeks. Or, he says, you can ask for a cream that is made with white turmeric; it won't stain at all.

Dr. Lad also recommends drinking cumin/coriander/fennel tea. He says to combine just under ½ teaspoon of each of the three herbs (you should have about 1 teaspoon of the herbs when they're combined), put them in a tea ball and steep them for ten minutes in a cup of hot water. Then strain until the water is clear of the herbs and drink this tea after breakfast, lunch and dinner.

He also suggests drinking "blue" water. "Fill a clear bottle with water and cover it with blue plastic wrap," Dr. Lad says. "Put the bottle in the sunlight for two hours, then drink the water, one cup daily in the morning." He adds that the unused portion can be sealed and stored in the refrigerator for two to three days.

FOOD THERAPY

Acne may be caused by consuming the wrong foods, says Elson Haas, M.D., director of the Preventive Medical Center of Marin in San Rafael, California, and author of *Staying Healthy with Nutrition*. He recommends following his three-week detoxification diet (see "Detoxing Your Ills" on page 48).

"For some people, acne may be triggered because they're sensitive to sugar, wheat, chocolate—foods that are more acid irritating in the body," he says. "What happens is these foods can cause more mucus and pus in the hair follicles, clogging up pores. Other times, acne may be the result of intestinal yeast, and when you give up cheeses, baked goods, sugar and other yeast-producing foods, the skin clears up."

Dr. Haas also recommends eating foods high in beta-carotene, such as carrots, pumpkin, cantaloupe and other yellow-orange fruits and vegetables.

HERBAL THERAPY

Take black currant seed oil or evening primrose oil, both of which are available in capsule form in most health food stores, says Barre, Vermont, herbalist Rosemary Gladstar, author of *Herbal Healing for Women* and other books about herbs. The standard adult dosage for both of these herbs is three 500-milligram capsules a day, according to Gladstar. She suggests taking this dosage every day for three months or until your acne clears up, whichever comes first. Black currant seed oil is less expensive than evening primrose oil and works just as well, she says.

HOMEOPATHY

In severe cases, acne should be treated by a medical doctor or homeopath on an individual basis, says Maesimund Panos, M.D., a homeopathic physician in Tipp City, Ohio, and co-author with Jane Heimlich of *Homeopathic Medicine at Home*. For an occasional mild outbreak, however, she recommends trying these remedies.

If you have itchy acne, restless sleep and unpleasant dreams, try taking Kali bromatum 6X three times daily until you notice improvement, says Dr. Panos. A similar dosage of Sulphur may subdue acne for a person who sweats profusely, has rough, hard skin and is frequently constipated, she says. If you have pus-filled pimples, Dr. Panos suggests a 6X dose of Antimonium tartaricum, taken three times daily until you notice improvement.

All of these remedies are available in many health food stores. To purchase the remedies by mail, refer to the resource list on page 637.

IMAGERY

In his book *Healing Visualizations*, Gerald Epstein, M.D., a New York City psychiatrist, suggests that you close your eyes, breathe out three times and imagine yourself standing in a large, open field of green grass on a perfect day. Envision stretching up toward the sun. Notice that your arms are becoming very long as you reach, palms up, into the sky. The sun's rays seep into your palms and circulate through your palms and fingers and beyond the fingertips so that there is a ray beyond each fingertip. If you are right-handed, see a small hand at the end of each ray at the fingertips of your right hand and five small eyes at the end of each ray at the fingertips of your left hand (if you're left-handed, reverse the order).

Turn the five small hands and the eyes to the area where the acne is located. Using the eyes to emit light so that you can see what you are doing, take a golden fine-bristle brush in one of your small hands. Carefully cleanse and scrape the acne pustules in the entire area. With another small hand, shine a blue laser light directly on the cleansed area and watch the skin healing. Realize as you do this that your acne is permanently clearing up. Use a third small hand to apply a salve of blue sky and sunshine to the area to keep the skin dry and clean. Open your eyes.

Dr. Epstein says to practice this imagery three times a day, three to five minutes each session, for three cycles of 21 days on and 7 days off.

JUICE THERAPY

"Acne is a signal that the organs of excretion aren't functioning optimally," says Elaine Gillaspie, N.D., a naturopathic physician in Portland, Oregon. She recommends stimulating the liver with a blend of one part beet juice, three parts carrot juice and two parts water to help clear the complexion from the inside out.

For more information on juicing techniques, see page 93.

REFLEXOLOGY

Try working the liver, adrenal gland, kidney, intestine, thyroid gland and diaphragm reflex points on your hands or feet, says St. Petersburg, Florida, reflexologist Dwight Byers, author of *Better Health with Foot Reflexology*.

To help you locate these points, consult the hand and foot reflex charts beginning on page 582. For instructions on how to work the points, see "Your Reflexology Session" on page 110.

VITAMIN AND MINERAL THERAPY

Use the food sensitivity diet (see "Food Sensitivity: How to Discover the 'Healthy' Foods That Can Cause Disease" on page 52) to eliminate any foods

that might have a role in causing the problem, suggests David Edelberg, M.D., an internist and medical director of the American Holistic Center/Chicago. He also says people with acne may want to take the following vitamin and mineral regimen to help control outbreaks: 30 milligrams of zinc picolinate twice a day; 2 milligrams of copper a day; 400 international units (IU) of vitamin E twice a day; and 150,000 IU of vitamin A a day for three months, then reducing the dose to 10,000 IU a day.

YOGA

A series of five yoga poses can help increase blood flow to your face, flushing away toxins and providing nutrients to your skin, according to Alice Christensen, founder and executive director of the American Yoga Association. She suggests a daily routine of these poses: standing sun (page 607), knee squeeze (page 612), seated sun (page 616), baby (page 618) and cobra (page 622).

ALLERGIES

Imagine owning a car alarm that's a tad too sensitive, letting out a piercing shriek at the slightest provocation. If you're one of the 50 million Americans with respiratory allergies, you have a similar problem with your immune system: It treats harmless dust, pollen and pet hair as if they were the enemy.

If you're allergic, it takes just a tiny particle of the right allergen to put your panicky immune system on the defensive. Your body strikes back by releasing a rush of histamine, the chemical that causes that familiar swelling and running in your nose, eyes and sinuses. Allergy shots and antihistamines can control your symptoms, but there are other things you can do as well. The natural remedies in this chapter—in conjunction with medical care and used with your doctor's approval—may help prevent or relieve allergic problems, according to some health professionals.

SEE YOUR MEDICAL DOCTOR WHEN . . .

- You have new symptoms that include hives or wheezing, alone or with severe chest congestion that makes breathing difficult.

ALLERGIES

ACUPRESSURE

To relieve hay fever and allergic sneezing and itching, press point LI 4, situated in the webbing between your thumb and index finger, close to the bone at the base of the index finger, says Michael Reed Gach, Ph.D., director of the Acupressure Institute in Berkeley, California, and author of *Acupressure's Potent Points.* (To help you locate this point, please see the illustration on page 565.) Hold this point with your thumb on top of the webbing and your index finger underneath, then squeeze into the webbing, angling the pressure toward the bone that connects the index finger to the hand. Work on one hand, then on the other. Hold firmly for about one minute per hand while breathing slowly and deeply.

This is not recommended for pregnant women, because pressing this point can cause contractions of the uterus, says Dr. Gach.

AROMATHERAPY

For quick relief of the watery eyes and runny nose of hay fever, Victoria Edwards, an aromatherapist in Fair Oaks, California, suggests mixing one drop each of cypress and hyssop essential oils in the palm of your hand. Apply the mixture to the back of your tongue with your fingertip. Edwards says to use the remedy every few hours whenever hay fever symptoms are bothering you. "It doesn't taste very good, but it helps clear your head immediately, and the effects last from one to two hours," she says.

For information on preparing and administering essential oils, including cautions about their use, see page 19. For information on purchasing essential oils, refer to the resource list on page 633.

AYURVEDA

Kapha types are most apt to suffer seasonal allergies such as hay fever, with symptoms that include nasal congestion, coughing and sneezing, says Vasant Lad, B.A.M.S., M.A.Sc., director of the Ayurvedic Institute in Albuquerque, New Mexico. (For more information about the doshas of Ayurveda, see "All about Vata, Pitta and Kapha" on page 28.) To prevent attacks, Dr. Lad recommends lubricating the nasal passages with warm ghee, or clarified butter. Using an eyedropper or the tip of your little finger, put about three drops in each nostril three times a day, morning, midday and evening. This will make it hard for allergens to penetrate the nasal passages, Dr. Lad says. (For a recipe for ghee, see "How to Make Ghee" on page 26.)

You can also try taking ½ teaspoon of the Indian herbal formula sitopaladi after lunch and dinner with a little honey, he says. Sitopaladi is available from some Indian grocers and by mail order (refer to the resource list on page 634).

FOOD THERAPY

Some allergies may be caused by congestion from eating the wrong foods, says Elson Haas, M.D., director of the Preventive Medical Center of Marin in San Rafael, California, and author of *Staying Healthy with Nutrition*. He suggests his three-week detoxification diet (see "Detoxing Your Ills" on page 48).

HOMEOPATHY

"Acute hay fever is commonly treated with homeopathy," according to Judyth Reichenberg-Ullman, N.D., a naturopathic physician in Edmonds, Washington, and co-author of *The Patient's Guide to Homeopathic Medicine*. If you are sneezing a lot and have itchy, watery eyes and a runny nose, Dr. Reichenberg-Ullman suggests trying Allium cepa 30C once or twice daily until you begin to feel better. The same dose of Sabadilla can help people who have violent sneezing attacks in addition to other hay fever symptoms, she says.

For people whose prime symptom is watery, burning eyes, take Euphrasia 30C once or twice a day, advises Dr. Reichenberg-Ullman. If one of these remedies doesn't seem to help within seven days, she says to consult your medical doctor or homeopath.

All of these remedies are available in many health food stores. To purchase the remedies by mail, refer to the resource list on page 637.

HYDROTHERAPY

A vitamin C bath can be effective for easing the symptoms of an allergy attack, suggests Agatha Thrash, M.D., a medical pathologist and co-founder and co-director of Uchee Pines Institute, a natural healing center in Seale, Alabama. Add three tablespoons of ascorbic acid powder (available in most health food stores) to a warm bath. You can stay in the bath for up to two hours.

REFLEXOLOGY

Focus on the following reflex point on your hands or feet, says Rebecca Dioda, a reflexologist with the Morris Institute of Natural Therapeutics, a holistic health education center in Denville, New Jersey: adrenal gland, reproductive system, solar plexus, ileocecal valve and any organ showing allergy symptoms (lungs or nose, for example).

To help you locate these points, consult the hand and foot reflex charts beginning on page 582. For instructions on how to work the points, see "Your Reflexology Session" on page 110.

VITAMIN AND MINERAL THERAPY

Some people with allergies might get relief by taking 5,000 international units of vitamin A daily, suggests Richard Gerson, Ph.D., author of *The Right Vitamins*. He also advises getting more essential fatty acids, such as those found in flaxseed oil. Flaxseed oil is available in both liquid and capsule form in most health food stores; Dr. Gerson suggests that you follow the dosage recommendations on the labels of flaxseed oil products.

YOGA

Daily yoga practice can help bring allergies under control, according to Alice Christensen, founder and executive director of the American Yoga Association. She says allergies are caused by both physical and psychological problems, which is why they tend to emerge after illness or periods of extreme stress.

As part of your daily routine, she says, be sure to include these poses: standing sun (page 607), knee squeeze (page 612), seated sun (page 616), boat (page 621) and cobra (page 622). (You should practice the half boat pose, shown on page 620, for about one week before attempting the boat pose.) She also recommends that you include the complete breath exercise (see page 152) to strengthen the muscles that help you breathe and meditation (see page 153) to help relieve allergy-related problems such as poor sleep.

In addition to the exercises above, you can try a *neti*, or daily nasal wash, says Stephen A. Nezezon, M.D., yoga teacher and staff physician at the Himalayan International Institute of Yoga Science and Philosophy in Honesdale, Pennsylvania. The wash will remove pollen from your sinuses and toughen your mucosal membranes, he says. Here are Dr. Nezezon's instructions: Fill a four-ounce paper cup halfway with warm water, and then add ½ teaspoon of salt. Put a crease in the lip of the cup so that it forms a spout. Slightly tilt your head back and to the left. Then slowly pour the water into your right nostril. The water will flow out of your left nostril or down the back of your throat if your left nostril is clogged. Spit out the water if it goes down your throat, or wipe the water from your face if it flows out of your left nostril. Fill the cup again, then repeat the procedure on the other side, pouring the water into your left nostril and tilting your head back and to the right so that the water flows out of your right nostril.

SEE ALSO Food Allergies; Lactose Intolerance

ANEMIA

If you're like most people who beat up on the snooze button each morning, an earlier bedtime is the way to end your energy crisis. But if no amount of rest helps, it may not be sleep that your body is craving. You may have a form of anemia.

Anemia saps your energy by depriving your cells of oxygen. This happens when your blood has too few red blood cells or too little hemoglobin, a protein in red blood cells that transports oxygen through the bloodstream. Anemia can be a symptom of many different serious problems, including cancer. But millions of Americans suffer from iron deficiency anemia, which is less serious and is usually caused by blood loss from an injury, an ulcer, hemmorhoids, excess menstruation or the demands of pregnancy. According to the Recommended Dietary Allowances, women need 15 milligrams of iron a day, while men need 10.

And there's another, less common form of anemia, nutritional deficiency anemia, that can be caused by a lack of folate and vitamin B_{12}. You'll need to see your doctor to determine the cause of your anemia and the proper course of action.

The natural remedies in this chapter—in conjunction with medical care and used with your doctor's approval—may provide some relief from iron deficiency and nutritional deficiency anemia, according to some health professionals.

SEE YOUR MEDICAL DOCTOR WHEN . . .

- You are unable to do your usual physical activities.
- You feel the blahs for more than five days.
- Your skin is pale and you feel weak, tired and out of breath.
- Your tongue is slick or smooth.
- You experience fatigue upon exertion.
- Your skin is jaundiced.
- You have bleeding under your skin and you bruise in response to the slightest trauma.

AYURVEDA

Add up to one teaspoon of turmeric to a cup of plain yogurt, says Vasant Lad, B.A.M.S., M.A.Sc., director of the Ayurvedic Institute in Albuquerque, New Mexico. He says to eat this mixture on an empty stomach in the morning or afternoon but not after sunset. Do this daily until symptoms subside, he advises.

FOOD THERAPY

Anemia can result from an iron deficiency or from a deficiency of vitamin B_{12} and folate, says Julian Whitaker, M.D., founder and president of the Whitaker Wellness Center in Newport Beach, California. "The first thing you have to do is determine which form of anemia you have."

After you've seen your doctor for an initial diagnosis, Dr. Whitaker says to eat more of the foods rich in the nutrients you need. Dark green leafy vegetables are good sources of absorbable iron, says Dr. Whitaker. He also recommends salmon and mackerel as good sources of vitamin B_{12} and black-eyed peas, beans and lentils for folate. (For more good food sources of these nutrients, see "Getting What You Need" on page 142.)

JUICE THERAPY

Juices can help correct nutritional imbalances that lead to anemia, says Cherie Calbom, M.S., a certified nutritionist in Kirkland, Washington, and co-author of *Juicing for Life*. Focus on vegetables high in iron, such as parsley and beet greens, says Calbom. She recommends blending these iron-rich juices with juices high in vitamin C for maximum iron absorption. "Broccoli, kale and parsley work just as well as the more familiar sources of vitamin C, such as peppers, strawberries and citrus," says Calbom.

Juicing also aids against folate deficiency anemia, adds Calbom. "I tell people with this problem to include asparagus, spinach or kale in their daily juicing." For information on juicing techniques, see page 93.

REFLEXOLOGY

When working on your hands or feet, focus on the spleen and liver reflex points, says St. Petersburg, Florida, reflexologist Dwight Byers, author of *Better Health with Foot Reflexology*.

To help you locate these points, consult the hand and foot reflex charts beginning on page 582. For instructions on how to work the points, see "Your Reflexology Session" on page 110.

VITAMIN AND MINERAL THERAPY

For nutritional deficiency anemia, take one milligram of vitamin B_{12} and 400 micrograms of folic acid daily, advises Julian Whitaker, M.D., founder and president of the Whitaker Wellness Center in Newport Beach, California. For iron deficiency anemia, he says that any multivitamin/mineral supplement containing iron can help.

ANGER

Hell, wrote Jean-Paul Sartre, is other people. And he didn't even know your boss, your in-laws or that infuriating talk show host with the wrong opinion on everything.

Then there are your teenage son's new earring and the neighbor who lets her poodle yap all night. Be aware, though, that the longer the list of things that drive you up a wall, the more likely it is that you'll suffer health consequences.

Research shows that carrying around a load of anger can hurt. One study of couples with high blood pressure found that a heated ten-minute argument caused a jump in pressure for both partners. And for those who are susceptible, anger can also bring on asthma symptoms and angina attacks. The remedies in this chapter—used with your doctor's approval—may help reduce everyday anger, according to some health professionals.

SEE YOUR MEDICAL DOCTOR WHEN . . .

- You experience difficulty breathing or sudden breathlessness while angry.
- You have chest pain or painful breathing.
- You hurt yourself or another person.
- Your angry behavior persists for long periods or interrupts family life.
- You get into frequent fights.

AROMATHERAPY

"Rose is a classic remedy for anger," says Los Angeles aromatic consultant John Steele. "We associate it so strongly with beauty and love that it's almost impossible to stay angry once we catch a whiff of the fragrance." It can be inhaled directly from the bottle or dabbed on the pulse points of the wrist, says Steele. If you're in a pinch, he recommends putting a couple of drops of the essential oil on a handkerchief and inhaling. But a more economical way to use this expensive oil is in a candle diffuser. "Without a doubt, the oil goes further in a diffuser, and you can share it with whomever happens to be in the room," says Steele.

For information on preparing and administering essential oils, including cautions about their use, see page 19. For information on purchasing essential oils, refer to the resource list on page 633.

AYURVEDA

"Anger is a psychological reaction to excess pitta dosha," says Vasant Lad, B.A.M.S., M.A.Sc., director of the Ayurvedic Institute in Albuquerque, New

Mexico. (For more information about the Ayurvedic doshas, see "All about Vata, Pitta and Kapha" on page 28.) The first step toward controlling anger, he says, is to follow a diet that emphasizes simple, bland foods and eliminates hot, spicy dishes.

If chronic anger persists, Dr. Lad suggests using cooling oils to calm your emotions. Every morning, apply a drop of sandalwood essential oil to the area in the middle of your forehead, to the throat, to the breastbone, to the navel, to the temples and to the wrists. Before going to bed, rub one teaspoon of coconut oil on your scalp and on the soles of your feet, then take a warm shower before retiring. Sandalwood essential oil and coconut oil are available in most health food stores.

When you're in the grip of sudden anger, Dr. Lad recommends steeping ½ teaspoon of chamomile (available in most health food stores) and one tablespoon of finely chopped cilantro leaves in hot water for ten minutes. Allow the tea to cool, strain and sip it slowly.

Certain forms of *pranayama*, a yogic breathing exercise, can dissipate anger, says Dr. Lad. "Whenever you're angry, make a tube of your tongue and breathe deeply through the tongue opening down into the belly," says Dr. Lad. "Hold the breath in your lower belly for up to a half-minute and then exhale through the nose." He recommends repeating this breathing pattern for a total of 12 to 24 breaths, twice daily.

Dr. Lad also suggests putting a cotton ball in the right nostril and breathing only through the left nostril for about 1 hour. Or he says to try plugging your right ear with cotton and hearing only through the left ear for between 6 and 12 hours. According to Dr. Lad, these techniques will help open up channels to the right brain and cool down anger.

FLOWER REMEDY/ESSENCE THERAPY

"Children who have temper tantrums can really benefit from a blend of Impatiens and Crab Apple," says Eve Campanelli, Ph.D., a holistic family practitioner in Beverly Hills, California. "Adults who experience dark, brooding, cynical anger are usually reacting to hopelessness and frustration, so I give them Gentian."

Flower remedies are available in some health food stores and through mail order (refer to the resource list on page 635). For information on preparing and administering flower remedies, see page 37.

FOOD THERAPY

Try not to overeat, and especially don't overdo it on sugar, says Elson Haas, M.D., director of the Preventive Medical Center of Marin in San Rafael, California and author of *Staying Healthy with Nutrition*. "Any sugar overload can lead to anger, because as your blood sugar shifts, you go from being up and happy to down and irritable. The key is to reduce the sugar in your diet." But reducing everything in your diet can also minimize food-related anger bursts. When you overeat, he says, you become bloated and full of gas. "That causes some people to feel agitated, frustrated and angry. Smaller meals can solve that. Also, avoid mixing too many foods per meal, which may not digest well and may cause gas."

HOMEOPATHY

"If you feel more irritable than normal, one remedy you can try is Nux vomica," says Stephen Messer, N.D., dean of the National Center for Homeopathy's summer school and a naturopathic physician in Eugene, Oregon. He suggests taking Nux vomica 6C every four hours until you begin feeling less hostile.

Nux vomica is available in many health food stores. To purchase homeopathic remedies by mail, refer to the resource list on page 637.

IMAGERY

Close your eyes and imagine looking at yourself in a mirror. You'll probably realize that you look terrible when you're angry, and you don't want to look like that. That may help calm you down, according to Dennis Gersten, M.D., a San Diego psychiatrist and publisher of *Atlantis*, a bi-monthly imagery newsletter.

On the other hand, if you tend to suppress your anger, imagine that you're in a room with the person you're angry with, Dr. Gersten says. Let yourself go and really chew him out as loud as you'd like. Then imagine that there are three buckets in front of you. One is filled with water, the second is filled with honey, and the third holds confetti. Dump the buckets on the head of the person in any order you'd like until you feel that the person has been punished enough. Then stop, let go of your anger and chuckle.

MASSAGE

A 15-minute Hellerwork self-massage (page 575) can ease or prevent the tension that people hold in their bodies when they get angry, says Dan Bienenfeld, a certified Hellerwork practitioner, a massage therapist and director of the Los Angeles Healing Arts Center.

RELAXATION AND MEDITATION

Anger often dissipates after just 20 minutes of quiet meditation, says Sundar Ramaswami, Ph.D., a clinical psychologist at the F. S. Dubois Community Mental Health Center in Stamford, Connecticut. To give meditation a try, see page 117.

SOUND THERAPY

It really is true: Music can soothe the savage breast. So try listening to at least 20 to 30 minutes of relaxing music when you're feeling angry, says Steven Halpern, Ph.D., composer, researcher and author of *Sound Health: The Music and Sounds That Make Us Whole*. To get started, turn on the music, then sit or lie comfortably, close your eyes and take a deep breath. Dr. Halpern suggests that you wear headphones to focus your full attention and avoid distraction. He recommends, however, that you keep the speakers playing, so your body absorbs the sound energy. While the music plays, let your breath slow down and become steady. Listen not just to the notes but to the silence between the notes. Dr. Halpern says this will keep you from analyzing the music, which will allow it to relax you.

For suggested pieces to relax by, see "Sailing Away to Key Largo" on page 129. Many of these pieces are available in music stores. For mail-order information, refer to the resource list on page 642.

VITAMIN AND MINERAL THERAPY

"Both calcium and magnesium have a calming effect, so if you're not eating a lot of foods rich in these nutrients, perhaps a supplement might be advised," says Elson Haas, M.D., director of the Preventive Medical Center of Marin in San Rafael, California, and author of *Staying Healthy with Nutrition*. You can get these nutrients in many multivitamin/mineral supplements, he says. For information on foods rich in calcium and magnesium, refer to "Getting What You Need" on page 142.

YOGA

Daily practice of the complete breath exercise and meditation will help soothe hostility, says Alice Christensen, founder and executive director of the American Yoga Association. Fear is the true cause of hostility, Christensen says, and spending 5 minutes doing the complete breath exercise (see page 152) and 15 to 20 minutes doing meditation (see page 153) will help you deal with that fear. You can add a second period of meditation during the day if you have time.

SEE ALSO Irritability; Type A Personality

ANGINA

It's not a heart attack," you tell yourself. Maybe not—but whatever it is, it's grabbing your chest like a massive fist and squeezing hard enough to get juice from a golf ball.

If you're one of the three million Americans who have experienced the terror of an angina attack, you probably remember it as the longest ten minutes of your life. Angina is the heart's not-too-subtle way of telling you that it isn't getting enough oxygen.

If you've ever suffered an angina attack, it's crucial that you see your medical doctor. But—in conjunction with your medical treatment and with your doctor's approval—the natural remedies in this chapter may help decrease angina pain and possibly prevent future attacks, according to some health professionals.

SEE YOUR MEDICAL DOCTOR WHEN . . .

- You're beginning to get angina pain after moderate exercise or physical exertion, even though you used to be able to function at that level with no problem.
- You're experiencing pain with even less activity than before.
- You used to have pain only after exerting yourself but now experience pain even when you're resting.

FOOD THERAPY

"The most powerful treatment seems to be a very low fat vegetarian diet," says Julian Whitaker, M.D., founder and president of the Whitaker Wellness Center in Newport Beach, California. He says to be sure to include plenty of dark green leafy vegetables, such as spinach, kale, mustard greens and turnip greens. "They're good sources of magnesium, which relaxes the heart muscle and establishes function, so the heart can perform better," says Dr. Whitaker. (For other good sources of magnesium, see "Getting What You Need" on page 142.)

Studies by cardiologist Dean Ornish, M.D., director of the Preventive Medicine Research Institute in Sausalito, California, and the author of *Dr. Dean Ornish's Program for Reversing Heart Disease*, found that when people follow a diet that includes no animal sources except for skim milk, egg whites and low-fat yogurt, angina pain diminishes in just a few weeks.

JUICE THERAPY

Those prone to angina attacks may benefit from regular doses of cantaloupe juice, suggests Michael Murray, N.D., a naturopathic physician and author of *The Complete Book of Juicing*. Cantaloupe contains the compound adenosine, which is used in heart patients to thin the blood and prevent angina attacks, according to Dr. Murray. Along with proper medical treatment, he recommends drinking two eight-ounce glasses of canteloupe juice a day.

For more information about juicing techniques, see page 93.

REFLEXOLOGY

Try working these reflexes on your hands or feet, suggests Laura Norman, a New York City reflexologist and author of *Feet First: A Guide to Foot Reflexology*: solar plexus; diaphragm and chest; lung, heart and shoulder; arm; neck; thoracic and cervical spine; intestine, with emphasis on sigmoid colon; and adrenal gland.

To help you locate these points, consult the hand and foot reflex charts beginning on page 582. For instructions on how to work the points, see "Your Reflexology Session" on page 110.

RELAXATION AND MEDITATION

Progressive relaxation, meditation and other relaxation techniques, used in conjunction with medication and with the knowledge and approval of your doctor, may help prevent angina, says Robert S. Eliot, M.D., director of the Institute of Stress Medicine in Jackson Hole, Wyoming, and author of *From Stress to Strength: How to Lighten Your Load and Save Your Life*. "Relaxation techniques may raise the threshold so that it takes more anxiety to provoke angina," Dr. Eliot says. "Secondly, if an individual practices a relaxation technique, he may be less likely to have a severe case of angina." For more on progressive relaxation, see page 122. To try a simple meditation, see page 117. Dr. Eliot suggests practicing either of these techniques twice a day, preferably before breakfast and before dinner, for 10 to 20 minutes a session.

SOUND THERAPY

Listening to at least 10 to 20 minutes of relaxing music each day can help ease the pain of angina for some people, says Steven Halpern, Ph.D., composer, researcher and author of *Sound Health: The Music and Sounds That Make Us Whole*. To get started, turn on the music, then sit or lie comfortably, close your eyes and take a deep breath. Dr. Halpern suggests that you wear headphones to focus your full attention and avoid distraction. He recommends, however, that you keep the speakers playing, so your body absorbs the sound energy. While the music plays, let your breath slow down and become steady. Listen not just to the notes but to the silence between the notes. Dr. Halpern says this will keep you from analyzing the music, which will allow it to relax you.

For suggested pieces to relax by, see "Sailing Away to Key Largo" on page 129. Many of these pieces are available in music stores. For mail-order information, refer to the resource list on page 642.

VITAMIN AND MINERAL THERAPY

"I recommend that people with angina take the following supplements each day to help control pain: 5,000 milligrams of vitamin C, 3,000 milligrams of the amino acid lysine and 800 milligrams of elemental magnesium," says Julian Whitaker, M.D., founder and director of the Whitaker Wellness Center in Newport Beach, California.

ANXIETY

Worry is a fact of life. But if you're so stressed out that you often break out in a cold sweat, your pulse races and your blood pressure goes through the roof, you may have crossed the border into the hair-raising world of anxiety.

Anxiety is often vague and undirected, a sinking feeling that something terrible is about to happen. Unlike concrete fears (of illness or losing a job, for example), anxiety often stems from what used to be called borrowed trouble. Anxious people imagine worst-case scenarios and spend lots of time dreading things that may never happen. For persistent anxiety, seek professional counseling. But the natural remedies below—used in conjunction with medical care and with your doctor's approval—may also reduce or relieve the problem, according to some health professionals.

SEE YOUR MEDICAL DOCTOR WHEN . . .

- You experience panic attacks, which are short, unexplained periods of intense fear or discomfort.

- Your anxiety causes chronic physical symptoms, including headaches, dizziness, breathlessness, chest pains or stomach or intestinal problems.
- Your anxiety causes you to avoid certain people, places or situations.

ACUPRESSURE

"Find point P 6, approximately two thumb-widths from the bottom of your palm," says Cindy Banker, co-founder of the New England Shiatsu Center in Boston and education director for the American Oriental Bodywork Therapy Association. (For help in locating this point, refer to the illustration on page 564.) "Press firmly on this spot and take a few deep, full breaths. You may feel some relief right away."

Hold your thumb, says Wayne Hackett, a Jin Shin Jyutsu teacher in Boulder, Colorado. Do it gently and intently, he advises, but keep doing it until you feel your body start to relax. The Jin Shin Jyutsu philosophy connects emotions with each finger of the hand, and worry is the province of the thumb.

You can also press the spot between your eyebrows at the center of your forehead, according to Hackett. He explains that pressing this spot helps disperse anxious thoughts. Then try holding your middle toe, the point where the stomach meridian ends. "Holding your toe helps bring energy from your head down through the body," Hackett says, reducing anxiety.

AROMATHERAPY

Soothing oils such as lavender, geranium, ylang-ylang, bergamot and melissa are great for calming frazzled nerves, particularly when they're used together, says Los Angeles aromatic consultant John Steele. He suggests mixing together two, three or four of these oils in equal parts and storing the blend in a five-milliliter bottle. Then whenever you feel anxious, he says, you can: Use 50 drops of this blend in a diffuser or an aroma lamp; add 6 drops to a hot bath (stirring gently to disperse); or make a massage oil by adding 10 drops of the blend to one ounce of carrier oil such as almond or olive. (Carrier oils are available in most health food stores.)

For information on preparing and administering essential oils, including cautions about their use, see page 19. For information on purchasing essential oils, refer to the resource list on page 633.

FLOWER REMEDY/ESSENCE THERAPY

Choosing the proper flower remedy to treat any physical or emotional problem depends upon identifying the exact feeling underlying the problem, says herbalist Leslie J. Kaslof, author of *The Traditional Flower Remedies of Dr. Edward Bach*. For those who worry excessively about the well-being of others, Kaslof recommends Red Chestnut. People who suffer from a vague sense of foreboding, a persistent feeling that something bad is about to happen, should try Aspen, he says.

Flower remedies are available in some health food stores and through mail order (refer to the resource list on page 635). For information on preparing and administering flower remedies, see page 37.

FOOD THERAPY

What you don't eat may be even more important than what you do eat, says Julian Whitaker, M.D., founder and president of the Whitaker Wellness Center in Newport Beach, California. He recommends avoiding alcohol, caffeine and sugar, because they tend to worsen anxiety. If you can't avoid them, he suggests that you at least cut down.

HERBAL THERAPY

For a soothing tea, Mary Bove, L.M., N.D., a naturopathic physician and director of the Brattleboro Naturopathic Clinic in Vermont, suggests blending lavender, oats, linden flower, catnip and lemon balm. (Although oats are usually thought of as a food, they also have a medicinal effect, and herbalists recommend them for a variety of health problems.) Look for these dried herbs in most health food stores. Dr. Bove says to buy ½ ounce of each of the dried herbs in cut form, then mix them together. To make a day's supply of tea, according to Dr. Bove, use four tablespoons of this herbal blend per quart of boiling water. Pour the water over the herbs and steep for about ten minutes. Strain until only liquid remains, then drink the tea while it's warm. She says this can be sweetened, if preferred. She suggests drinking a cup after each meal and up to six cups a day if necessary.

HOMEOPATHY

A dose of Ignatia 6X every 15 minutes may help you reduce fear and anxiety, according to Maesimund Panos, M.D., a homeopathic physician in Tipp City, Ohio, and co-author with Jane Heimlich of *Homeopathic Medicine at Home*. However, she says not to exceed four doses, since excessive repetition of Ignatia can actually trigger anxiety.

"Gelsemium is another excellent remedy that can help you deal with stage fright or anticipation of an ordeal such as an important business conference,"

Dr. Panos says. "If you have anxiety accompanied by diarrhea, that's a sure sign for Gelsemium." As with Ignatia, she recommends taking a dose of Gelsemium 6X every 15 minutes until you begin to feel calmer, not to exceed four doses.

Gelsemium and Ignatia can be purchased in many health food stores. To purchase homeopathic remedies by mail, refer to the resource list on page 637.

HYDROTHERAPY

The neutral bath has a balancing effect on anxious or irritable people, according to Charles Thomas, Ph.D., co-author of *Hydrotherapy: Simple Treatments for Common Ailments* and a physical therapist at the Desert Springs Therapy Center in Desert Hot Springs, California. His instructions for a neutral bath: Fill your bathtub with water slightly cooler than body temperature, around 94° to 97°F, according to Dr. Thomas. (You can check the temperature of the water with a regular thermometer.) Submerging as much of your body as possible, stay in the bath for at least 20 minutes, adding water as needed to maintain the temperature of the bath.

IMAGERY

"For quick anxiety relief, imagine that you're lying on a beach. As each wave splashes on the beach, it rolls up to your neck, and as it recedes, it pulls more and more tension and fear out of your body," says Dennis Gersten, M.D., a San Diego psychiatrist and publisher of *Atlantis*, a bi-monthly imagery newsletter.

As an alternative, picture that each thought you have is enclosed in a helium balloon tied with a string. If you have an anxious thought, just untie the string and watch the balloon float out of your mind and up into the sky until it disappears on the horizon, Dr. Gersten says.

MASSAGE

You can soothe anxiety with a 15-minute Hellerwork self-massage, says Dan Bienenfeld, a certified Hellerwork practitioner, a massage therapist and director of the Los Angeles Healing Arts Center. The massage (page 575) will ease tightness in the muscles that often tense up when you're nervous or anxious, he says.

REFLEXOLOGY

Be sure to work the diaphragm reflex on your feet, in addition to the spine and the pituitary, parathyroid, thyroid and adrenal gland reflex points, says St.

Petersburg, Florida, reflexologist Dwight Byers, author of *Better Health with Foot Reflexology*.

To help you locate these points, consult the foot reflex chart on page 592. For instructions on how to work the points, see "Your Reflexology Session" on page 110.

RELAXATION AND MEDITATION

Any of the relaxation and meditation techniques mentioned in this book, such as mindfulness meditation, autogenics, progressive relaxation and stretching, will relieve anxiety, says Sundar Ramaswami, Ph.D., a clinical psychologist at F. S. Dubois Community Mental Health Center in Stamford, Connecticut. It's a matter of finding the one that works best for you. For a brief description of each of these techniques and how to do them, see page 113.

SOUND THERAPY

Listening to music with a slow, steady beat may reduce your heart rate and help you calm down, says Janalea Hoffman, R.M.T., a composer and music therapist based in Kansas City, Missouri. Whenever you feel anxious, Hoffman suggests sitting quietly in a comfortable chair and listening to the music for 20 to 30 minutes or until the anxiety has passed. Hoffman suggests her own tape, *Musical Biofeedback*; for other selections, see "Sailing Away to Key Largo" on page 129. For information on ordering these and other tapes, refer to the resource list on page 642.

VITAMIN AND MINERAL THERAPY

An amino acid available in supplement form in most health food stores can help those prone to anxiety, says Julian Whitaker, M.D., founder and president of the Whitaker Wellness Center in Newport Beach, California. "It's called GABA (gamma-aminobutyric acid), and I recommend taking 750 milligrams three times a day, after meals." He says that GABA has a calming effect.

YOGA

A daily yoga session combining the complete breath exercise (see page 152), meditation (see page 153) and poses can help quell anxiety, says Alice Christensen, founder and executive director of the American Yoga Association. We become anxious when we start feeling like victims in life, Christensen says, and practicing yoga helps us build the inner strength to combat that mind-set.

For the poses, Christensen suggests choosing three or four from the Daily Routine that begins on page 606. She says to be sure to vary the poses from day to day to keep your interest high and to strengthen different parts of your body

SEE ALSO Panic Attacks; Phobias

ARTHRITIS

Arthritis is actually a number of different diseases affecting the joints. The most common form is osteoarthritis, which affects almost 16 million Americans, most of them over age 45. Osteoarthritis usually strikes weight-bearing joints such as the ankles, knees and hips but can also affect the fingers, wrists, elbows, spine and neck. The pain is caused by the gradual breakdown of cartilage, the dense, spongy material that cushions the joints.

Another common form of the disease is rheumatoid arthritis, which affects about two million Americans. Rheumatoid arthritis may strike in a person's twenties, attacking the lining of the joints and causing pain and severe inflammation.

If you suspect that you have arthritis, see a doctor. But the natural remedies below—in conjunction with medical care and used with your doctor's approval—may also help relieve the pain of arthritis, according to some health professionals.

SEE YOUR MEDICAL DOCTOR WHEN . . .

- Your joints are stiff in the morning but loosen up later in the day.
- Your stiffness lasts for more than six weeks.
- You have severe joint pain that doesn't respond to heat, ice packs or aspirin.
- Your joint is hot, red, swollen and very painful.
- You experience stiffness after an injury to the joint.
- Your joints remain swollen even after you take aspirin or ibuprofen.
- You have chills or fever as well as swollen joints.
- You have already been diagnosed with arthritis but notice a new or different type of swelling in your joints.

ACUPRESSURE

Stiff, achy joints can be relieved with daily acupressure treatments, says Michael Reed Gach, Ph.D., author of *Arthritis Relief at Your Fingertips* and *Acu-*

pressure's Potent Points and director of the Acupressure Institute in Berkeley, California. To soothe discomfort in the neck and lessen the general irritability that arthritis pain can cause, use your thumbs to press both GB 20 points, situated below the base of the skull, two inches out from the middle of your neck. (To help locate these points, refer to the illustration on page 565.) Press for one minute, suggests Dr. Gach.

"This is not a quick fix," he says. "Work on these points regularly, several times each day, in combination with other therapies. The GB 20 point is a good overall pain-relieving point and is one of the 12 anti-inflammatory points."

AROMATHERAPY

When arthritis acts up, a blend of aromatic oils massaged into sore joints will help, according to Judith Jackson, a Greenwich, Connecticut, aromatherapist and author of *Scentual Touch: A Personal Guide to Aromatherapy*. Jackson's arthritis "recipe" calls for six drops each of rosemary and chamomile essential oils added to four ounces of a carrier oil such as almond, avocado, soybean or sesame. (Carrier oils are available in most health food stores.) For extra relief, she advises that you add ten drops each of rosemary and chamomile to a warm bath and soak for ten minutes.

For information on preparing and administering essential oils, including cautions about their use, see page 19. For information on purchasing essential oils, refer to the resource list on page 633.

AYURVEDA

"Arthritis takes many different forms," says David Frawley, O.M.D., director of the American Institute of Vedic Studies in Santa Fe, New Mexico. "In Ayurveda, we're concerned with underlying energetic imbalances. Is the condition affected by heat or cold, dampness or dryness? An obese person with swollen joints, for instance, will be treated quite differently than a thin person with dry skin and brittle bones."

Although long-term treatments differ, Dr. Frawley says the following remedies can soothe the pain of periodic attacks for most people. To nourish tissue, loosen stiff joints and relieve pain, he suggests rubbing warmed sesame oil (available in most health food stores) onto affected areas once or twice a day, then taking a hot shower about 20 to 60 minutes afterward to heat the oil and drive it into the pores. Also, add hot or spicy herbs such as cayenne, cinnamon and dried ginger to foods, he says.

For rheumatoid arthritis, Vasant Lad, B.A.M.S., M.A.Sc., director of the Ayurvedic Institute in Albuquerque, New Mexico, recommends taking ¼ teaspoon of yogaraj guggulu three times daily, with a little warm water. This ancient herbal preparation is available by mail order (refer to the resource list on page 634). You can also add one tablespoon of castor oil to a cup of ginger tea and drink it before going to bed, he says. Ginger tea is available in tea bag form in most health food stores.

FLOWER REMEDY/ESSENCE THERAPY

"In people with arthritis, the whole system becomes slightly acidic, which many alternative practitioners believe is the result of hidden, unexpressed anger," says Eve Campanelli, Ph.D., a holistic family practitioner in Beverly Hills, California. "A combination of the remedies Holly and Vine can help even out this type of personality."

Flower remedies are available in some health food stores and through mail order (refer to the resource list on page 635). For information on preparing and administering flower remedies, see page 37.

FOOD THERAPY

Many studies have shown that a vegetarian diet is very beneficial in helping to lessen or even eliminate arthritis pain, says Neal Barnard, M.D., president of the Physicians Committee for Responsible Medicine in Washington, D.C., and author of *Food for Life* and other books on the healing aspects of food. "We don't know exactly why, but when we take patients off animal food sources, in many cases their arthritis will go into complete remission. This applies particularly to dairy as well as to meats."

HOMEOPATHY

Rhus toxicodendron will help relieve painful joints accompanied by stiffness in the neck and in the small of the back that is worse in cold weather and better on warm, dry days and after exercise, says Cynthia Mervis Watson, M.D., a family practice physician specializing in homeopathic and herbal therapies in Santa Monica, California. She suggests taking a 30C dose once a day or a 12C dose twice daily. A similar dosage of Bryonia will help if you have stiff and painful joints that are hot and swollen and feel worse with motion, adds Dr. Watson. And she says that a 30C dose of Cimicifuga is a good remedy if you have an uneasy, restless feeling and achy muscles that are worse with cold and in the morning. Dr. Watson recommends taking any of these remedies in the indicated dosage until you begin to feel better.

Rhus toxicodendron, Bryonia and Cimicifuga can be purchased in many health food stores. To purchase homeopathic remedies by mail, refer to the resource list on page 637.

HYDROTHERAPY

After you've seen a doctor for an initial diagnosis, hydrotherapy treatments are very helpful in managing chronic conditions such as osteoarthritis and rheumatoid arthritis, says John Abruzzo, M.D., professor of medicine and director of the Rheumatology and Osteoporosis Center at Thomas Jefferson University Hospital in Philadelphia. "Generally speaking, osteoarthritis patients get better results with moist, warm treatments, such as moist heat packs, than with dry applications, such as electric heating pads," says Dr. Abruzzo. Using a warm compress for 10 to 20 minutes every four hours helps relieve stiffness and dull, penetrating pain, according to Dr. Abruzzo. Wading, swimming or exercising in a pool heated to 85°F can also be very effective. But remember, the affected part of the body should be immersed in the water.

To treat sharper, more intense pain, Dr. Abruzzo suggests a cold, wet compress or an ice pack wrapped in a plastic bag and placed over a towel on the skin. He says to use the cold treatment for 10 to 20 minutes every four hours. "Never use cold treatments for more than 20 minutes at a time, because they can damage the skin," he says. And if pain lessens after using cold treatments for a day or two, switch to hot compresses, he adds.

IMAGERY

Picture your joint pain, giving it a size, shape and color. Reach out and touch it. Is it rough or smooth? Now transform this object into liquid and let it flow down your leg and out the bottom of your foot. Watch it trickling out of your room, out of your house and into the nearest creek or river and then floating out to the ocean until it disappears in the crashing waves, says Dennis Gersten, M.D., a San Diego psychiatrist and publisher of *Atlantis*, a bi-monthly imagery newsletter. "I've seen that imagery work wonders," Dr. Gersten says. He suggests using it for 10 to 20 minutes twice a day.

JUICE THERAPY

Black cherry juice is good for arthritis, says Eve Campanelli, Ph.D., a holistic family practitioner in Beverly Hills, California. She estimates that around 85 percent of her patients with arthritis get at least partial relief from drinking two glasses of this juice twice a day (each glass contains four ounces of juice diluted with four ounces of water). "Fresh is always best, but even black cherry juice from concentrate seems to benefit arthritis," she says. She adds that you can discontinue this treatment once the pain clears up.

"People with rheumatoid arthritis should include in their daily diets juices high in the anti-inflammatory nutrients," says Cherie Calbom, M.S., a certified nutritionist in Kirkland, Washington, and co-author of *Juicing for Life*. She says that these nutrients include beta-carotene (found in parsley, broccoli and spinach) and copper (found in carrots, apples and ginger). Calbom has also seen rheumatoid arthritis improve with a glass or two a day of pineapple juice. "It's the only known source of the enzyme bromelain, which has strong anti-inflammatory properties," she says.

Calbom also cautions that certain juices may cause adverse reactions in people with osteoarthritis. "Avoid citrus fruits, and be careful with vegetables from the nightshade family, including potatoes, tomatoes, peppers and egg-plant," says Calbom. "Citrus seems to promote swelling, and nightshades contain psyllium alkaloids, which cause problems for some people."

For more information about juicing techniques, see page 93.

MASSAGE

If you have osteoarthritis, gentle massage can help ease the pain, says Elliot Greene, past president of the American Massage Therapy Association. Start by putting a little vegetable oil or massage oil on your fingertips, so they glide more easily over your skin. Then work slowly around the affected joint, making small, gentle circles with your fingertips. It's best to avoid massage directly on the joint; stay just above and below it with your fingertips. Work on the area around the joint for three to five minutes each day.

Gentle massage may also help reduce swelling in rheumatoid arthritis, says Greene. He suggests using the effleurage stroke (page 570) to work the muscle and tissue around the joint with your fingertips. Make sure you use oil or cream on your fingers to make the massage more gentle. Greene says to work the area for five to ten minutes a day.

REFLEXOLOGY

Although arthritis affects specific joints, you may get relief by working reflexology points for a number of organs, say Kevin and Barbara Kunz, reflexology researchers in Sante Fe, New Mexico, and authors of *Hand and Foot Reflexology*. They recommend using the golf ball technique (page 588) that corresponds to the brain, liver and kidney points on your hands. They also say to work these points on your hands: solar plexus, uterus/prostate, ovary/testicle, pancreas and adrenal, pituitary and thyroid gland.

To help you locate these points, consult the hand reflex chart on page 582. For instructions on how to work the points, see "Your Reflexology Session" on page 110.

ARTHRITIS

RELAXATION AND MEDITATION

Practicing stretch-based relaxation for 20 minutes twice a day can help manage the pain, says Charles Carlson, Ph.D., professor of psychology at the University of Kentucky in Lexington. See page 602 for a stretch-based relaxation sequence.

A daily ten-minute session of thermal biofeedback may also be helpful, says Steven Fahrion, Ph.D., director of research at the Life Sciences Institute of Mind-Body Health in Topeka, Kansas. For more on thermal biofeedback, see page 121.

VITAMIN AND MINERAL THERAPY

For osteoarthritis, David Edelberg, M.D., an internist and medical director of the American Holistic Center/Chicago, suggests using the food sensitivity diet (see "Food Sensitivity: How to Discover the 'Healthy' Foods That Can Cause Disease" on page 52) to eliminate any foods that might have a role in causing the problem. He also says that people with osteoarthritis may want to use the following supplemental regimen to help relieve pain: 500 milligrams of glucosamine sulfate three times a day (Dr. Edelberg says to be patient, because this supplement takes about a month to work); 400 international units of vitamin E twice a day; 200 micrograms of selenium twice a day; and 1,000 milligrams of vitamin C twice a day. Glucosamine sulfate is available in most health food stores.

For rheumatoid arthritis, Dr. Edelberg also suggests the food sensitivity diet. And he says a person with rheumatoid arthritis may want to try the following combination of supplements: 250 milligrams of zinc picolinate twice a day; 1 milligram of copper twice a day; 200 micrograms of selenium twice a day; two to three capsules of bromelain (a digestive enzyme) three times a day, between meals; and one borage oil capsule twice a day. Bromelain and borage oil capsules are available in most health food stores.

YOGA

If arthritis affects your hands and fingers, a series of six exercises done once a day can help loosen things up, says yoga teacher Rosalind Widdowson in her book *The Joy of Yoga*. The exercises, called curling, contracting, fanning, fish, deer and peacock's tail, are shown on page 625.

SEE ALSO Gout; Joint Pain

ASTHMA

I t's the most vital thing that you do each day, yet you don't even think about it. Unless you're one of the 12 million Americans with asthma—then you don't take breathing for granted.

Asthma's wheezing, coughing and tightness in the chest are caused by an inflammation of the bronchioles, the tubes that carry air within the lungs. During an asthma attack, this swelling worsens, and the bronchial tubes narrow. Asthma can also make mucus glands work overtime, producing a thick, sticky fluid that congests the airways.

Asthma attacks are often triggered by allergies. Strong emotions such as fear and anxiety can also kick off an attack. See a doctor if you think you have asthma. But the natural remedies in this chapter—in conjunction with medical care and used with your doctor's approval—may provide relief, according to some health professionals.

SEE YOUR MEDICAL DOCTOR WHEN . . .

- You need to use medication more frequently or in larger doses.
- You have severe difficulty breathing or are experiencing an asthma attack that you cannot control.

ACUPRESSURE

A couple of minutes of firm pressure on the upper chest can help relieve asthma and breathing problems, says Michael Reed Gach, Ph.D., director of the Acupressure Institute in Berkeley, California, and author of *Acupressure's Potent Points*. He suggests pressing the Lu 1 points to breathe easier. To find these points, also named Letting Go, make fists in front of your chest with your thumbs pointing up, says Dr. Gach. Place your thumbs on the outer portion of your chest, pressing on the muscles that run horizontally below your collarbone. You'll find a sensitive, knotted spot on each side of your chest. Underneath each spot is Lu 1. (If you have difficulty locating these points, see the illustration on page 564.) Dr. Gach says to let your head hang forward, then breathe slowly and deeply as you press the points with your thumbs for two minutes.

Dr. Gach says that pressing the Lu 1 points is helpful for prevention as well as relief of asthma attacks. But he adds this caution: Never discontinue any prescribed asthma medication without the approval of your doctor.

You can also press the B 13 points, called the Lung Associated points, according to Dr. Gach. Each point is situated one finger-width below the upper tip of the shoulder blade, between the spine and the shoulder blade. (See the illustration on page 565.) Try using tennis balls to press these hard-to-reach points, suggests Dr. Gach. Lie on your back with your knees bent, placing a pillow under your head for comfort, if you wish. Raise your shoulders slightly while you reach behind your back with your hands to position the tennis balls. Now cross your arms over your body and breathe deeply, letting your weight sink into the floor. Let the tennis balls press into your shoulder muscles for a few minutes or for as long as it feels comfortable, says Dr. Gach.

AROMATHERAPY

To treat her own asthma, San Francisco herbalist Jeanne Rose mixes four parts eucalyptus, two parts lavender, two parts myrrh and three parts Roman chamomile essential oils. "I store the mixture in its own bottle and use it in a diffuser or siphon some off, mix it with olive oil (available in most health food stores) and use it as a chest rub at bedtime," says Rose, chairperson of the National Association for Holistic Aromatherapy and author of *Aromatherapy: Applications and Inhalations*. Ten drops of the essential oil blend mixed with 90 drops (about ⅛ ounce) of olive oil makes an excellent rub, she says.

Because people with asthma are prone to allergies, they should exercise caution when using unfamiliar oils in a diffuser, explains Rose. She suggests backing away from the diffuser after turning it on, than gradually moving closer to make sure the fragrance isn't irritating.

For information on preparing and administering essential oils, including cautions about their use, see page 19. For information on purchasing essential oils, refer to the resource list on page 633.

AYURVEDA

To relieve discomfort, try drinking a tea made by stirring 1 teaspoon of cinnamon and ¼ teaspoon of trikatu into one cup of hot water, says Vasant Lad, B.A.M.S., M.A.Sc., director of the Ayurvedic Institute in Albuquerque, New Mexico. (Trikatu is a blend of ginger and peppers available from Ayurvedic practitioners and in some health food stores. You can also purchase it by mail order; refer to the resource list on page 634.) Steep for ten minutes and then add 1 teaspoon of honey; drink twice daily, he suggests.

Mustard also helps, according to Dr. Lad. For bronchial asthma, take one teaspoon of brown mustard oil (available in Indian pharmacies and by mail order; refer to the resource list on page 634), mix it with one teaspoon of raw sugar and eat this mixture two or three times a day, preferably before each meal, he says. Rubbing brown mustard oil on the chest as needed is also beneficial, he adds.

FLOWER REMEDY/ESSENCE THERAPY

When you feel an asthma attack coming on, Eve Campanelli, Ph.D., a holistic family practitioner in Beverly Hills, California, recommends the emergency stress relief formula: Place four drops of the formula under the tongue, or add four drops to one-fourth of a glass of water and sip slowly. Used in conjunction with your usual medical treatment, the formula has a calming effect that may ease breathing, according to Dr. Campanelli.

Sold under brand names such as Calming Essence, Rescue Remedy and Five-Flower Formula, the emergency stress relief formula is available in most health food stores and through mail order (see the resource list on page 635). For more information on preparing and administering the formula, see page 40.

HOMEOPATHY

Although treating asthma usually requires professional care, a few homeopathic remedies may temporarily relieve your symptoms while you wait to see your medical doctor or homeopath, according to Maesimund Panos, M.D., a homeopathic physician in Tipp City, Ohio, and co-author with Jane Heimlich of *Homeopathic Medicine at Home*. If your asthma attack occurs soon after midnight and you feel anxious and restless, or if you feel uncomfortable and suffocating when you lie down, Dr. Panos says to try a dose of Arsenicum 6X every 15 minutes. But do not exceed four doses, she cautions.

If you feel worse in the evening or after eating or talking, or if the attack occurs after a long, spasmodic coughing spell accompanied by gagging and vomiting, Dr. Panos suggests trying up to four doses of Carbo vegetabilis 6X, taken every 15 minutes. She adds that a similar dosage of Ipecacuanha will help if you have a sudden wheezing and coughing attack that makes you feel as if there were a weight on your chest suffocating you.

Arsenicum, Carbo vegetabilis and Ipecacuanha can be purchased in many health food stores. To purchase homeopathic remedies by mail, refer to the resource list on page 637.

IMAGERY

When asthma strikes, close your eyes, breathe out three times and imagine yourself standing next to a pine tree, writes New York City psychiatrist Gerald Epstein, M.D., in his book *Healing Visualizations*. Breathe in the aromatic fragrance of the pine. As you breathe out, feel the exhalation spread throughout your body down to the soles of your feet. Envision each breath leaving your body as gray smoke that will be buried deep in the earth. After three to five minutes of this exercise, open your eyes and breathe easily.

JUICE THERAPY

Because they contain compounds that relax the bronchial muscles and prevent spasms, onions have long been used in the treatment of asthma, writes Michael Murray, N.D., a naturopathic physician, in *The Complete Book of Juicing*. Dr. Murray suggests blending two ounces of onion juice with two ounces of carrot juice and two ounces of parsley juice, then drinking this blend twice each day. Use this remedy in conjunction with proper medical treatment, he adds.

For more information about juicing techniques, see page 93.

REFLEXOLOGY

Relaxing the lungs and solar plexus are vital to dealing with asthma, say Kevin and Barbara Kunz, reflexology researchers in Sante Fe, New Mexico, and authors of *Hand and Foot Reflexology*. To do this with reflexology, they suggest using the golf ball technique (page 588) that corresponds to those reflex points on both hands. They also recommend working these reflexes on your hands: brain, uterus/prostate, ovary/testicle, pancreas and adrenal, pituitary and thyroid gland.

To help you locate these points, consult the hand reflex chart on page 582. For instructions on how to work the points, see "Your Reflexology Session" on page 110.

RELAXATION AND MEDITATION

Autogenics can help relieve bronchial asthma, according to Martha Davis, Ph.D., Elizabeth Robbins Eshelman and Matthew McKay, Ph.D., in *The Relaxation and Stress Reduction Workbook*. Practice two-minute sessions of the autogenic technique described on page 120 ten times daily, suggests Martin Shaffer, Ph.D., executive director of the Stress Management Institute in San Francisco and author of *Life after Stress*.

VITAMIN AND MINERAL THERAPY

Use the food sensitivity diet (see "Food Sensitivity: How to Discover the 'Healthy' Foods That Can Cause Disease" on page 52) to eliminate any foods

that might have a role in causing the problem, suggests David Edelberg, M.D., an internist and the medical director of the American Holistic Center/Chicago. He also says people with asthma may want to use the following nutritional regimen to help control the condition: 50 milligrams of vitamin B_6 three times a day; 3,000 milligrams of vitamin C twice a day (he says to reduce the dose if diarrhea develops); 400 milligrams of magnesium aspartate twice a day; 500 milligrams of N–acetylcysteine twice a day; and 333 milligrams of quercetin twice a day. N–acetylcysteine and quercetin are available in most health food stores.

YOGA

Yoga breathing exercises are a powerful tool against asthma, according to Alice Christensen, founder and executive director of the American Yoga Association. She says that they strengthen and relax the muscles that you use to breathe, which reduces nerve activity in your airways, helping them constrict less during an asthma attack.

The complete breath (see page 152) is one of the best breathing exercises for asthma, says Christensen. She suggests doing the exercise for at least five minutes daily, which will help you breathe more deeply and slowly all day long. She adds that several poses, performed daily, will also help with asthma, including the standing sun (page 607), knee squeeze (page 612), seated sun (page 616) and cobra (page 622).

ATHLETE'S FOOT

Don't let the name fool you: Even confirmed couch potatoes aren't immune to athlete's foot. While the fungus that causes athlete's foot loves warm, damp environments such as locker rooms, it'll hang out just about anywhere.

Itchy, flaky skin, especially between the toes, is the most common symptom. If left untreated, the fungus can cause the skin to blister and crack and may even spread to other parts of the body.

Athlete's foot is easier to prevent than it is to treat, so avoid going barefoot at the gym, in hotel rooms and anywhere else that other people's feet have been. Keep your feet as clean and dry as possible by wearing cotton socks and using an absorbent dusting powder, especially between the toes. And—used with your doctor's approval—the remedies below may help relieve the symptoms of athlete's foot and perhaps prevent future occurrences of the problem, according to some health professionals.

SEE YOUR MEDICAL DOCTOR WHEN . . .

- You notice swelling in your foot or leg and you develop a fever.
- You notice that pus has accumulated in the blisters or cracks in your skin.
- Your athlete's foot interferes with normal activity.

AROMATHERAPY

"Tea tree oil is a natural antiseptic and is great for all kinds of infections, including athlete's foot," says San Francisco herbalist Jeanne Rose, chairperson of the National Association for Holistic Aromatherapy and author of *Aromatherapy: Applications and Inhalations*. She recommends drying the skin thoroughly with a hair dryer after showering, then applying enough undiluted tea tree essential oil to cover the affected area (usually about four to ten drops).

For information on preparing and administering essential oils, including cautions about their use, see page 19. For information on purchasing essential oils, refer to the resource list on page 633.

AYURVEDA

"This problem is most common in kapha-pitta people who sweat a lot," says Vasant Lad, B.A.M.S., M.A.Sc., director of the Ayurvedic Institute in Albuquerque, New Mexico. (For more information about the doshas of Ayurveda, see "All about Vata, Pitta and Kapha" on page 28.) To treat athlete's foot, he says, first clean the affected area with tea tree oil, which is sold in most health food stores. Then mix 1 teaspoon of aloe vera gel (also available in most health food stores) with ½ teaspoon of turmeric and apply this mixture topically every day, in the morning and before bedtime, he says. If you still have symptoms after two weeks but they're less severe, Dr. Lad suggests applying the mixture at least once a day for another week. He says you can continue this treatment cycle for as long as necessary. And he adds this word of caution: Turmeric stains, so wear old socks when you're taking this treatment and keep your socks on in bed to avoid staining your sheets. Any discoloration of the skin should wash off in about two weeks, he says.

FOOD THERAPY

"Put chopped garlic in your socks before bedtime and then wear them overnight," advises Julian Whitaker, M.D., founder and president of the Whitaker Wellness Center in Newport Beach, California. "Raw garlic is a powerful antibiotic and helps reduce the fungus that causes athlete's foot." He also recommends that you avoid yeast products such as breads and other baked goods, along with vinegar and alcohol, if you're prone to athlete's foot. "People with high yeast intakes are more likely to get athlete's foot," says Dr. Whitaker.

HOMEOPATHY

Wash your feet thoroughly with mild soap and warm water, then apply a Calendula ointment, suggests Maesimund Panos, M.D., a homeopathic physician in Tipp City, Ohio, and co-author with Jane Heimlich of *Homeopathic Medicine at Home*. Do this in the morning and before bedtime until you notice improvement, she says.

Calendula ointment can be purchased in many health food stores. To purchase homeopathic remedies by mail, refer to the resource list on page 637.

BACKACHE

B end over to tie a shoelace—*pop*! Lift a heavy box without bending your knees—*sproing*! Slip on an unseen patch of ice—*crunch*!

Almost no one escapes occasional back pain. It's the price we pay for walking on two legs instead of four. Fortunately, 70 to 90 percent of backaches go away by themselves or with home treatment. The natural remedies in this chapter—in conjunction with medical care and used with your doctor's approval—may help relieve back pain, according to some health professionals.

SEE YOUR MEDICAL DOCTOR WHEN . . .

- Your back pain lasts for more than three days.
- Your pain shoots down your leg to your knee or foot.
- You feel numbness in your legs.
- You have a fever, stomach cramps or chest pain along with the backache.

ACUPRESSURE

Pressing the B 54 acupressure points, which are behind your knees, may help move pain and pressure away from your back, according to Michael Reed Gach, Ph.D., director of the Acupressure Institute in Berkeley, California, and author of *Accupressure's Potent Points*. "They open a pathway for energy to flow out of the back," he explains. To press these points (to help locate them, see the illustration on page 565), Dr. Gach says to lie on your back with your legs up and your knees bent. Place your fingertips in the center of the crease behind each knee. Holding on to these points, gently rock your legs back and forth for one minute as you breathe deeply. When you're done, says Dr. Gach, let your feet rest flat on the floor, with your knees bent, and relax. Repeat this exercise three times a day, he adds.

AROMATHERAPY

For severe backaches, Los Angeles aromatic consultant John Steele offers the following soothing massage oil: Mix together 4 drops of blue chamomile, 4 drops of birch, 4 drops of rosemary, coriander or eucalyptus, 4 drops of ginger or black pepper and 14 drops of lavender essential oils. Then add this solution to ½ ounce of any carrier oil, available in most health food stores.

BACKACHE

For a minor ache, Steele says to use the following mixture: two drops of blue chamomile, two drops of birch, two drops of rosemary, coriander or eucalyptus, two drops of ginger or black pepper and two drops of lavender in ½ ounce of carrier oil.

Steele suggests using either of these mixtures daily as needed, rubbing it into the affected area after a hot bath, when muscles are relaxed and pores are open.

For information on preparing and administering essential oils, including cautions about their use, see page 19. For information on purchasing essential oils, refer to the resource list on page 633.

AYURVEDA

For relief of minor backaches, make a paste using ginger powder and water, and apply it to the place on your back that hurts, says Vasant Lad, B.A.M.S., M.A.Sc., director of the Ayurvedic Institute in Albuquerque, New Mexico. Give the paste a little time to sink in, he says, then after 10 to 15 minutes, wash it off and ask a friend to rub your back with eucalyptus oil (available in most health food stores). Dr. Lad cautions that this treatment is not good for red, inflamed conditions.

HOMEOPATHY

To lessen back pain, try one of the following 6C or 12C remedies three or four times a day until you begin to notice improvement, says Chris Meletis, N.D., a naturopathic physician and medicinary director at the National College of Naturopathic Medicine in Portland, Oregon. If you feel bruised and sore and don't want to be touched, and if the pain is better while you're lying down, Dr. Meletis recommends Arnica. Aesculus may help, he says, if your lower back gives out, accompanied by dull pain that is worse after walking or stooping. For a painful, stiff neck that feels worse with motion, cold and weather changes and better with rest, he says to try Bryonia. Rhus toxicodendron may help if your back symptoms make you restless and you can't get comfortable in any position, especially if you have stiffness in the small of your back that is worse with motion, he says.

All of these remedies are available in many health food stores. To purchase homeopathic remedies by mail, refer to the resource list on page 637.

HYDROTHERAPY

Those prone to chronic backaches may benefit from alternating hot and cold showers, according to Agatha Thrash, M.D., a medical pathologist and co-founder and co-director of Uchee Pines Institute, a natural healing center in

BACKACHE

Seale, Alabama. She says to begin with a hot jet or strong spray aimed at the back for one to four minutes, followed by a cold jet or strong spray for 5 to 30 seconds. Depending how much time you have available, you can repeat this treatment as often as once every hour, says Dr. Thrash.

IMAGERY

Imagine that you're carrying a 100-pound bag on your back. Drop the bag, open it and examine the contents. There may be a lot of stuff in that bag—anger, frustration, depression, painful memories—that you can throw away to lighten your load, says Dennis Gersten, M.D., a San Diego psychiatrist and publisher of *Atlantis*, a bi-monthly imagery newsletter. He suggests doing this exercise once a day for several minutes every time you have a bout of back pain.

JUICE THERAPY

Drink ½ to 1 cup of fresh grape juice daily, apart from meals, suggests John Peterson, M.D., an Ayurvedic practitioner in Muncie, Indiana. He says that grape juice made from dark grapes is the most effective. Keep the juice at room temperature, he says, and do not mix it with other juices. Or if it's too sweet for your taste, he recommends mixing it with plain water. He advises drinking the juice once a day, preferably before a meal, as a preventive.

For information on juicing techniques, see page 93.

MASSAGE

It's tough to reach your own back for a massage, so try using tennis balls to do the job, says Ed Moore, a certified massage therapist who has worked with the U.S. Olympic cycling team.

First, says Moore, take a hot bath or shower, followed by some gentle stretching. Then before you begin the massage, slide two tennis balls into a sock, tying off the open end of the sock so that the balls are touching each other, says Moore. Now lie on your back on the floor. Have the socks at hand and place them under the small of your back, one ball on each side of your spine. Moore says to take a deep breath and let your body relax into the balls. Rock your hips gently from side to side. Then adjust your body slightly so that the balls move up your back a few inches. Hold that position briefly, then take a deep breath. Wait until you feel a sense of softening or melting into the balls before you move them farther up your back, says Moore.

Moore recommends taking about 10 to 15 minutes to work the balls up and down your back. If you have a particularly sore area on your back, he says that you can spend extra time with the balls touching that spot.

BACKACHE

REFLEXOLOGY

Focus on these reflexes when working on your hands and feet, suggests New York City reflexologist Laura Norman, author of *Feet First: A Guide to Foot Reflexology*: solar plexus, diaphragm, spine, shoulder, arm, neck, hip, knee, leg and sciatic nerve.

To help you locate these points, consult the hand and foot reflex charts beginning on page 582. For instructions on how to work the points, see "Your Reflexology Session" on page 110.

RELAXATION AND MEDITATION

A ten-minute session of thermal biofeedback may help relieve back pain, says Steven Fahrion, Ph.D., director of research at the Life Sciences Institute of Mind-Body Health in Topeka, Kansas. To learn how to do it, see page 121.

YOGA

To strengthen your back, the American Yoga Association recommends doing the easy bridge pose as part of your daily yoga routine. According to the association, this pose (page 619) helps your back gradually become more flexible, making it less likely to be strained in the future. *Note:* Do not do the easy bridge pose during the second half of pregnancy.

Doing the corpse pose every day, with either straight or bent legs, is another effective yoga remedy for minor back pain, according to Los Angeles yoga therapist Larry Payne, Ph.D., creator of the videotape *Healthy Back, Healthy Mind.* Relax into the pose (page 612) for about five to ten minutes, emphasizing the exhalation as you focus on your breathing. Because the corpse pose is great for relaxation, it can help soothe sore muscles, Dr. Payne says.

You should also practice meditation each day while lying flat on your back, says Alice Christensen, founder and executive director of the American Yoga Association. Place pillows under your knees and thighs to ease pressure on your back. For information on how to meditate, see page 153.

SEE ALSO Sciatica

BAD BREATH

Are your friends doing the limbo lean every time you open your mouth? Are your three favorite food groups Garlic, Onions and Chili Powder? Well, your diet certainly sounds tasty. But bad breath may be a problem. Lots of things can cause it—spicy foods, medication, tobacco and coffee, to name a few. One of the most likely culprits is gum disease caused by bacteria buildup in your mouth.

The natural remedies in this chapter, used with your doctor's approval, could help freshen things up, according to some health professionals. But if bad breath persists, it could be a sign of something serious, such as tonsillitis, liver or kidney problems or diabetes. In that case, see your doctor for a diagnosis.

SEE YOUR MEDICAL DOCTOR WHEN . . .

- Your bad breath lingers for more than a day and there's no reason for it, such as spicy foods or tobacco use.

AROMATHERAPY

A drop of pure peppermint essential oil on the tongue is a quick breath freshener, says Victoria Edwards, an aromatherapist in Fair Oaks, California.

For information on preparing and administering essential oils, including cautions about their use, see page 19. For information on purchasing essential oils, refer to the resource list on page 633.

AYURVEDA

"Chew a few fennel seeds," says Vasant Lad, B.A.M.S., M.A.Sc., director of the Ayurvedic Institute in Albuquerque, New Mexico. Fennel's clean licorice taste will freshen breath, according to Dr. Lad.

FOOD THERAPY

"Bad breath is mostly caused by fermentation in the intestinal tract," says Elson Haas, M.D., director of the Preventive Medical Center of Marin in San Rafael, California, and author of *Staying Healthy with Nutrition*. "People who have a lot of yeast in their intestinal tracts, which ferments foods such as cheeses and baked goods, are especially prone." While Dr. Haas thinks it's wise to limit those foods, as well as sugar, alcohol, vinegar and other fermented fare, he also recommends upping your intake of fresh fruits and vegetables. Besides having a high water content, which can help overcome bad breath caused by dry mouth, these foods have a cleansing effect in the intestinal tract, says Dr. Haas.

HERBAL THERAPY

Carry fennel seeds, anise seeds or cloves to chew on after meals or whenever you feel your breath needs sweetening, says Varro E. Tyler, Ph.D., professor of pharmacognosy at Purdue University in West Lafayette, Indiana. He suggests chewing two or three fennel or anise seeds or one clove as needed.

HOMEOPATHY

"If you can smell someone's bad breath from across the room, that's usually a sign that he needs Mercurius," says Richard D. Fischer, D.D.S., a dentist and homeopath in Annandale, Virginia, and president of the International Academy of Oral Medicine and Toxicology. Take a 30X dose of Mercurius three or four times a day for three to four days to curb offending breath, he advises. In addition, he says to gargle at least once a day with a solution of 20 drops of Calendula tincture diluted in eight ounces of water.

Mercurius and Calendula can be purchased in many health food stores. To purchase homeopathic remedies by mail, refer to the resource list on page 637.

HYDROTHERAPY

Avoid bad breath by drinking lots of water and peppermint tea, both spiked with a pinch of anise, caraway or cinnamon, suggests Agatha Thrash, M.D., a medical pathologist and co-founder and co-director of Uchee Pines Institute, a natural healing center in Seale, Alabama. Peppermint tea is available in tea bag form in most health food stores.

REFLEXOLOGY

Be sure to hit the reflex points for the stomach, liver and intestine and all of the points on the sides and bottom of each big toe when working your feet, says St. Petersburg, Florida, reflexologist Dwight Byers, author of *Better Health with Foot Reflexology*. (To work your big toes, use whichever technique you find most comfortable.)

To help you locate these points, consult the foot reflex chart on page 592. For instructions on how to work the points, see "Your Reflexology Session" on page 110.

YOGA

Daily practice of the head-to-knee pose may help, says Stephen A. Nezezon, M.D., yoga teacher and staff physician at the Himalayan International Institute of Yoga Science and Philosophy in Honesdale, Pennsylvania. This pose (page 616) can improve liver function, which can have a direct effect on your breath, says Dr. Nezezon.

BITES AND STINGS

Meandering through a meadow? Waltzing through the woods? "Bee" careful! There's a whole battalion of bugs out there waiting to sting, bite, chomp and clamp your tender skin.

The best way to handle bites and stings is to avoid them in the first place. Experts say that when venturing into the outdoors, you should wear white or khaki-colored clothing (including socks and long pants), use insect repellent, avoid sweet-scented fragrances, never mess around with a beehive and always check yourself for hangers-on such as ticks after you go back inside. But even when that doesn't work, most insect bites are just minor annoyances. You'll get an itch, a bump and maybe a burning sensation. The natural remedies in this chapter, used with the approval of your doctor, may provide relief, according to some health professionals.

SEE YOUR MEDICAL DOCTOR WHEN . . .

- You're bitten by an animal.
- You develop a fever after being bitten.
- You have difficulty breathing or feel severe pain after a bite or sting.

AROMATHERAPY

For quick relief from insect bites, apply one drop of pure lavender, tea tree, helichrysum (also called immortelle or everlast) or blue chamomile essential oil directly to the affected area, suggests Los Angeles aromatic consultant John Steele. The oil can be reapplied every ten minutes until you feel better, he says.

For information on preparing and administering essential oils, including cautions about their use, see page 19. For information on purchasing essential oils, refer to the resource list on page 633.

AYURVEDA

Neem powder, made from extracts from India's neem tree and available from Ayurvedic practitioners, can be applied as a plaster to soothe insect bites, according to Vasant Lad, B.A.M.S., M.A.Sc., director of the Ayurvedic Institute in Albuquerque, New Mexico. To make the plaster, Dr. Lad says to take enough neem powder to just cover the area of the bite, then add warm water to make a thick paste. He suggests applying the plaster to the skin twice a day, letting it dry for 10 to 20 minutes each time.

But you can keep the bugs from biting in the first place, says Dr. Lad, by rubbing neem oil (also available from Ayurvedic practitioners) on exposed skin before going outside. According to Dr. Lad, neem contains a compound called salannin that repels insects as effectively as the synthetic chemical DEET—but without DEET's toxic effects on humans. Do not use pure neem tree oil, he cautions, since it's too strong for this use.

You can also soothe insect bites by drinking fresh cilantro juice and applying the cilantro pulp to the skin, says Dr. Lad. Here's how he says to prepare the juice and pulp: Chop 1 cup of fresh cilantro leaves and mix with ⅓ cup of water in a blender. Strain this mixture through cheesecloth, saving the pulp to apply directly to the affected area of the skin. Dr. Lad suggests spreading the pulp on the bite once or twice a day and to drink the juice two tablespoons at a time, three times a day. Keep the juice refrigerated; you should have enough for three to four days.

FLOWER REMEDY/ESSENCE THERAPY

Try the emergency stress relief formula, sold under brand names such as Calming Essence, Rescue Remedy and Five-Flower Formula, says Leslie J. Kaslof, an herbalist and author of *The Traditional Flower Remedies of Dr. Edward Bach*. He suggests using the formula topically on minor insect bites to relieve pain, swelling and itching. Also, he says, the formula may be helpful in relieving mild allergic reactions to insect bites and stings. He recommends taking four drops under the tongue as needed to calm and relax.

Kaslof cautions, however, that the formula is not a replacement for emergency medical intervention or doctor-recommended treatment for allergic reactions. If you have a history of allergic reactions to insect bites and stings, he says, you must consult your doctor before using the emergency stress relief formula.

The emergency stress relief formula is available in most health food stores and through mail order (refer to the resource list on page 635). For more information on preparing and administering the formula, see page 40.

FOOD THERAPY

"A compress made from meat tenderizer breaks down the venom and can take the sting out of bites and stings," says Elson Haas, M.D., director of the Preventive Medical Center of Marin in San Rafael, California, and author of *Staying Healthy with Nutrition.* That's because most insect bites and stings, as well as jellyfish stings, are protein-based, and meat tenderizer breaks down protein— as long as the tenderizer contains either papain or bromelain, the active protein-busting ingredients. Dr. Haas says to mix a thick paste of water and powdered meat tenderizer and apply it directly on the skin; relief will come within a minute. (Bromelain can cause dermatitis in some people, so don't apply any more if the skin begins to look red and inflamed.)

HERBAL THERAPY

Here's a natural insect repellent from Barre, Vermont, herbalist Rosemary Gladstar, author of *Herbal Healing for Women* and several other books on herbs: Combine one part bay leaf, four parts pennyroyal, two parts rosemary and one part eucalyptus in a jar with a tight-fitting lid. Add enough olive oil to cover the herbs, then top off with another inch or two. Close the jar and place it on a sunny windowsill or in a sunny spot outside for two weeks. (You can do this even during colder months, says Gladstar, since oil usually won't freeze.) Then strain the mixture so that there's only liquid left. (For extra scent, add a drop or two of eucalyptus essential oil to the liquid.)

Gladstar recommends using this herbal repellent just as you would a store-bought product, spreading it evenly and lightly on your skin (but avoiding the eyes). And she says that this herbal repellent is safe to use even on children's skin and that it works as well as store-bought chemical varieties.

All of these herbs and oils are available in most health food stores.

HOMEOPATHY

To reduce the swelling and pain of bites that have the sensation of coldness and that are better when you apply cold, take a 6C or 12C dose of Ledum or apply Ledum tincture on the bite with a cotton swab every two to three hours as needed until you feel relief, says Mitchell Fleisher, M.D., a family practice physician and homeopath in Colleen, Virginia. Taking Apis mellifica in 6C or 12C potency is another good remedy, he says, particularly for bites that are burning or stinging, are worse with heat and better with ice packs and cause hivelike reactions on the skin.

Dr. Fleisher suggests taking one dose of Ledum or Apis mellifica every 15 minutes for up to four doses. If you're still experiencing pain, he says, take one 30C dose. If there is still no improvement, consult a medical doctor or homeopath, he says.

Ledum and Apis mellifica can be purchased in many health food stores. To purchase homeopathic remedies by mail, refer to the resource list on page 637.

HYDROTHERAPY

To relieve the discomfort of insect bites, make up a thin paste of water, apple cider vinegar and fuller's earth (available in most health food stores) and apply to the bite for a few minutes, suggests Agatha Thrash, M.D., a medical pathologist and co-founder and co-director of Uchee Pines Institute, a natural healing center in Seale, Alabama. Rinse with warm water.

SEE ALSO Lyme Disease

BOILS

R ub yourself the wrong way, and a boil is the price you might pay. These painful oversize pimples have less to do with personal hygiene than you might think. They're usually caused when friction (from ill-fitting undergarments or a tight shirt collar) or a scratch allows bacteria under your skin.

The bacteria, *Staphylococcus aureus*, settle in a hair follicle or an oil gland, where they are attacked by your immune system. The result is a red, pus-filled nodule. In time, the boil will be absorbed by your body or will erupt and drain.

Boils are usually harmless, but it's not a good idea to squeeze one. The natural remedies in this chapter, used with the approval of your doctor, may provide relief, according to some health professionals.

SEE YOUR MEDICAL DOCTOR WHEN . . .

• You develop recurrent boils.
• You develop a fever, feel chills or have swollen lymph nodes or glands.

BOILS

AROMATHERAPY

Tea tree essential oil is a great natural antiseptic that speeds the healing of virtually any kind of skin irritation, says San Francisco herbalist Jeanne Rose, chairperson of the National Association for Holistic Aromatherapy and author of *Aromatherapy: Applications and Inhalations*. She suggests applying a single drop of tea tree oil directly to the boil after bathing until the boil goes away.

For information on preparing and administering essential oils, including cautions about their use, see page 19. For information on purchasing essential oils, refer to the resource list on page 633.

AYURVEDA

Here's how to bring a boil to a head, according to Vasant Lad, B.A.M.S., M.A.Sc., director of the Ayurvedic Institute in Albuquerque, New Mexico: Apply a paste made from ½ teaspoon each of ginger powder and turmeric and enough warm water to mix. Rub the paste directly on the affected area, cover with gauze and leave in place for a half-hour. Repeat as necessary until the boil breaks and begins to heal. Turmeric can stain skin and clothes, cautions Dr. Lad, so be sure to wear old garments when using this remedy. Any skin discoloration should wash off in two weeks, he adds.

FOOD THERAPY

"Eat foods that are rich in vitamin A and zinc, because these nutrients aid in skin healing and repair and can help relieve boils," says Allan Magaziner, D.O., a nutritional medicine specialist and head of the Magaziner Medical Center in Cherry Hill, New Jersey. "Good sources of vitamin A include any fruit or vegetable that has a yellow or orange color—squash, yams, sweet potatoes and carrots. Zinc is found in oysters, sunflower seeds and pumpkin seeds. Vitamin A is also found in dark green leafy vegetables such as spinach and kale." (For more information on food sources of vitamin A and zinc, refer to "Getting What You Need" on page 142.)

HOMEOPATHY

"If you have a boil that comes on quite suddenly, is very bright red and inflamed and is hot and very painful to the touch, then Belladonna is a good remedy choice for you," says Mitchell Fleisher, M.D., a family practice physician and homeopath in Colleen, Virginia. "If it's a boil that comes on more slowly, looks more darkish blue than red and is extremely painful to touch and you feel quite chilled, then try Hepar sulphuris. Take a 6C or 12C dose of the indicated remedy every three to four hours as needed until you feel relief." If the swelling and inflammation go down within 12 to 24 hours, then you're on the right track; otherwise, seek professional medical care, says John G. Collins, N.D., a naturopathic physician and associate professor at the National College of Naturopathic Medicine in Portland, Oregon.

Belladonna and Hepar sulphuris can be purchased in many health food stores. To purchase homeopathic remedies by mail, refer to the resource list on page 637.

HYDROTHERAPY

Alternating hot and cold compresses speeds the healing of a boil by increasing the flow of blood to the affected area, says Agatha Thrash, M.D., a medical pathologist and co-founder and co-director of Uchee Pines Institute, a natural healing center in Seale, Alabama. Her instructions: Soak a washcloth in comfortably hot water and hold it against the boil, refreshing the heat as necessary to keep the cloth hot. After three to five minutes, apply a cold compress for 30 to 60 seconds. Dr. Thrash says to repeat this treatment three times daily until the boil comes to a head or goes away.

JUICE THERAPY

Like many other skin ailments, boils result from a buildup of toxins in the system, according to Eve Campanelli, Ph.D., a holistic family practitioner in Beverly Hills, California. To stimulate the liver and speed up the elimination of wastes, Dr. Campanelli recommends drinking a blend of 8 ounces of carrot juice, 1 ounce of beet juice, 4 ounces of celery juice and ½ to 1 ounce of parsley juice. "A large glass each morning and a smaller glass in the afternoon is an effective and a very nutritious way to get the liver moving," says Dr. Campanelli.

For more information on juicing techniques, see page 93.

VITAMIN AND MINERAL THERAPY

To relieve a boil, take 10,000 international units of vitamin A and 15 to 20 milligrams of zinc, advises Allan Magaziner, D.O., a nutritional medicine specialist and head of the Magaziner Medical Center in Cherry Hill, New Jersey. If you're prone to boils, keep taking these nutrients, but cut the dosage in half after the boil disappears, he says. And if boils aren't a chronic problem for you, he advises that you stop taking the supplements after the boil has cleared up.

BREASTFEEDING PROBLEMS

When things go right, breastfeeding can do a lot for a mother and child. The baby gets top-quality, natural nutrition. The mother bonds with her child in a very intimate way. And they're both healthier.

Studies show that breastfeeding can boost a baby's immune system and protect against future diseases. For the mom, it conserves the body's iron stores and helps protect against bone loss and breast cancer. And there are even more immediate advantages: After a pregnancy, it can help a mother's uterus return to normal size more quickly and help her get down to her prepregnancy weight faster.

Of course, things don't always go right. Nipples can get sore. Milk ducts can become plugged. Breasts can produce too much or too little milk. The natural remedies in this chapter—in conjunction with medical care and used with the approval of your doctor—may provide relief from breastfeeding problems, according to some health professionals.

SEE YOUR MEDICAL DOCTOR WHEN . . .

- Your breasts become inflamed.
- You develop flulike symptoms, including a fever, when trying to breastfeed.

ACUPRESSURE

For lactation problems, gradually press both St 16 points on your upper chest for a couple of minutes three times a day, recommends Michael Reed Gach, Ph.D., director of the Acupressure Institute in Berkeley, California, and author of *Acupressure's Potent Points.* The points are located directly above the breast tissue in line with the nipples, between the third and fourth ribs. (For help in locating these points, refer to the illustration on page 564.)

AROMATHERAPY

Start each day by slowly sipping an eight-ounce glass of water spiked with a drop of fennel essential oil, recommends San Francisco herbalist Jeanne Rose, chairperson of the National Association for Holistic Aromatherapy and author of *Aromatherapy: Applications and Inhalations.* "At night, after nursing, you can also rub the breasts with a fennel massage oil," says Rose. "Use one drop of fennel oil in a teaspoon of olive oil." (Olive oil is available in most health food stores.)

For information on preparing and administering essential oils, including cautions about their use, see page 19. For information on purchasing essential oils, refer to the resource list on page 633.

AYURVEDA

If your breast milk is scanty, try this mixture of almond milk and herbs, says Vasant Lad, B.A.M.S., M.A.Sc., director of the Ayurvedic Institute in Albuquerque, New Mexico. He says to soak ten shelled almonds in water overnight. Then peel them, put them in a blender, add a cup of hot water or hot milk and puree them. Pour the almond milk into a glass and stir in a pinch each of ginger powder, cardamom and saffron and a teaspoon of date sugar (available in most health food stores) or honey. Dr. Lad says to drink this twice a day, morning and evening, to help strengthen the quality and quantity of your breast milk.

If you have too much milk, Dr. Lad recommends pumping the excess and massaging painful breasts as needed with warm castor oil. He also suggests that women with pitta or kapha doshas drink three to four cups of pomegranate juice daily to regulate lactation. (Vata women should avoid pomegranate juice, says Dr. Lad, since it can aggravate that dosha.) Pomegranate juice is available in most health food stores. (For more information about the doshas of Ayurveda, see "All about Vata, Pitta and Kapha" on page 28.)

If a baby is not nursing well, he may be allergic to something the mother is eating, Dr. Lad says. All nursing mothers should avoid eating meats, canned foods and hot, spicy dishes, says Dr. Lad. "Avoid beans, too," he advises. "They cause colic." The best diet for a nursing mother is a simple, bland vegetarian menu. Dr. Lad adds that you can also "take the baby to an Ayurvedic practitioner, find out the baby's prakruti and follow that diet." (For more information on prakruti, see page 30.)

FLOWER REMEDY/ESSENCE THERAPY

Women who have difficulty breastfeeding may be experiencing some ambivalence about the process, says Patricia Kaminski, co-director of the Flower Essence Society, a Nevada City, California, organization that studies and promotes the therapeutic use of flower remedies/essences.

"Women who find breastfeeding embarrassing or repulsive on some deep level may benefit from the essence of Alpine Lily," she says. "Mariposa Lily is good for women who are just very anxious and need a little help bonding with their babies."

For mothers whose milk is insufficient, the essence Mugwort may stimulate the flow, adds Kaminski.

Flower essences are available in some health food stores and through mail order (refer to the resource list on page 635). For information on preparing and administering flower essences, see page 37.

FOOD THERAPY

Eat more nuts, seeds and whole grains, because they're rich in essential fatty acids and the vitamins and minerals that can relieve the pain of breastfeeding problems, says Julian Whitaker, M.D., founder and president of the Whitaker Wellness Center in Newport Beach, California. "You might also want to avoid cruciferous vegetables," he says. "Some babies won't drink milk from mothers who eat a lot of cruciferous vegetables."

HERBAL THERAPY

Fennel is a well-known folk remedy that can help first-time mothers in-crease their milk production, says San Francisco herbalist Jeanne Rose, author of *Jeanne Rose's Modern Herbal* and several other herb books. "We don't really know why it works—it may stimulate hormone production—but it does help get the milk flowing." She recommends starting each day by drinking a cup of fennel seed tea. You can make the tea yourself, she says, by simmering one tea-spoon of fennel seeds in one cup of hot water for three to ten minutes. Strain out the seeds, then drink a cup of the tea (first letting it cool to a drinkable temperature, of course).

HOMEOPATHY

If you're eating right and getting enough rest but you're still having difficul-ties producing milk, worry, anxiety and stress may be compounding your dilemma, according to Maesimund Panos, M.D., a homeopathic physician in Tipp City, Ohio, and co-author with Jane Heimlich of *Homeopathic Medicine at Home*. To relieve stress-related breastfeeding problems, Dr. Panos advises taking two tablets of Ignatia 6X three times a day until your milk production begins to increase. If stress isn't a problem, she suggests trying Calcarea phosphorica in the same dosage. You should notice a boost in your output in a few days, she says.

If you suspect that you have a plugged milk duct or an inflamed breast, see your doctor. But you can also try Phytolacca 6X three or four times a day until you begin to notice improvement, Dr. Panos says.

Ignatia, Calcarea phosphorica and Phytolacca can be purchased in many health food stores. To purchase homeopathic remedies by mail, refer to the re-source list on page 637.

IMAGERY

Think about picking up your baby and cuddling him in your arms. Then picture your child easily taking hold of one of your breasts and putting enough of the nipple in his mouth so that it's comfortable. See your baby sucking firmly without any problems. Envision your breast milk spurting into your child's mouth with every suck. Look into your baby's eyes and see absolute contentment, says Barbara L. Rees, R.N., Ph.D., an imagery expert and professor of nursing at the University of New Mexico College of Nursing in Albuquerque. She suggests doing this exercise for about 10 to 15 minutes every day.

MASSAGE

A three-part massage of the breasts can help relieve soreness and engorgement, says Elaine Stillerman, L.M.T., a New York City massage therapist and author of *Mother Massage: A Handbook for Relieving the Discomforts of Pregnancy*. Here's how she says to do the massage: Rub a small amount of massage oil or cream between both hands to warm it. Then rub either one or both breasts. Make large circles around the outside of the breast, but avoid directly touching your nipple or areola. Do this for several minutes. Now massage one breast at a time, using the fingertips of one hand to make small circles all around the outside of the breast. After several minutes, repeat the same stroke on the other breast. Then place both hands flat on either side of the areola, with your thumbs pointing toward your head and your fingers pointing toward your waist. Slowly slide your hands away from the areola until you reach the edge of the breast. Be sure to avoid the sensitive areola region. Turn your hands slightly to cover a different portion of the breast and repeat. Do this for one to two minutes, then massage the other breast. Stillerman recommends massaging yourself once a day when your breasts are sore or engorged.

VITAMIN AND MINERAL THERAPY

To heal nipples that are sore from breastfeeding, you can prick a vitamin E capsule with a pin and rub the liquid over tender areas, suggests Julian Whitaker, M.D., founder and president of the Whitaker Wellness Center in Newport Beach, California. "It's very soothing, and the vitamin helps heal any skin cracking you may have." Clean off any excess liquid vitamin E before the next feeding.

BRITTLE NAILS

Y**ou** inherited your father's dazzling green eyes, your mother's perfect nose and your grandmother's gentle disposition. Unfortunately, your nails look like you picked up your grandpa's bad habit of whacking his fingers with a hammer.

As with the color of your hair, the thickness and strength of your nails can be strongly influenced by your genes. Of course, you may not be helping matters. Do you use your nails as staple removers? Do you pick or bite at them constantly? Maybe you're exposing your nails to harsh chemicals or using too much nail polish remover, both of which deprive your nails of moisture. The natural remedies in this chapter, used with the approval of your doctor, may help improve the strength and appearance of your nails, according to some health professionals.

SEE YOUR MEDICAL DOCTOR WHEN . . .

• You notice long-lasting and unexplained changes in the color or shape of your nails that are unrelated to an injury.

AROMATHERAPY

Brittle nails benefit from a warm fragrant oil soak, according to Greenwich, Connecticut, aromatherapist Judith Jackson, author of *Scentual Touch: A Personal Guide to Aromatherapy*. Add six drops of lavender, six drops of bay and six drops of sandalwood essential oils to six ounces of warm sesame oil or soy oil, suggests Jackson. (Both sesame oil and soy oil are available in most health food stores.) She says to soak for 15 minutes once or twice a week.

For information on preparing and administering essential oils, including cautions about their use, see page 19. For information on purchasing essential oils, refer to the resource list on page 633.

AYURVEDA

Toxins in the colon may prevent the absorption of minerals that are essential to nourish bones and nails, says Vasant Lad, B.A.M.S., M.A.Sc., director of the Ayurvedic Institute in Albuquerque, New Mexico. To restore brittle nails to health, Dr. Lad recommends cleansing the colon with triphala, a traditional Ayurvedic remedy that combines the fruits of three trees native to India. You can find triphala in some health food stores, often in capsule form, according to

Dr. Lad. He says to follow the label directions for daily use. Dr. Lad says you can also obtain triphala powder in Indian pharmacies or by mail order (refer to the resource list on page 634).

FOOD THERAPY

Eat more cold water fish such as salmon, mackerel and herring, advises Julian Whitaker, M.D., founder and president of the Whitaker Wellness Center in Newport Beach, California. "It's rich in omega-6 fatty acids, which can strengthen nails." Dr. Whitaker also recommends cauliflower, soybeans, peanuts, walnuts and lentils, which are all rich in biotin, a B vitamin that he says can prevent the splitting and cracking that are associated with brittle nails. (For other food sources of biotin, see "Getting What You Need" on page 142.)

HOMEOPATHY

Take one of the following remedies in a 6C dose three times a day until improvement is noted, says Chris Meletis, N.D., a naturopathic physician and medicinary director at the National College of Naturopathic Medicine in Portland, Oregon. To strengthen brittle nails that are accompanied by dry, rough hair, especially if you dread cold air and drafts and feel better in the summer and with heat, try Psorinum, says Dr. Meletis. He adds that Graphites may be helpful if you have brittle nails along with dry, hard, rough skin, numerous cracks in your skin and a tendency for even small wounds to become infected.

Psorinum and Graphites are available in many health food stores. To purchase homeopathic remedies by mail, refer to the resource list on page 637.

VITAMIN AND MINERAL THERAPY

Get the essential fatty acids that strengthen nails by taking flaxseed oil, says Julian Whitaker, M.D., founder and president of the Whitaker Wellness Center in Newport Beach, California. It comes in capsule or liquid form, and Dr. Whitaker says to follow the dosage recommendations on the label. Flaxseed oil is available in most health food stores.

YOGA

Brittle nails are sometimes the result of bad digestion and may be helped with a daily exercise called the stomach lift, says Stephen A. Nezezon, M.D., yoga teacher and staff physician at the Himalayan International Institute of Yoga Science and Philosophy in Honesdale, Pennsylvania.

Here's how Dr. Nezezon says to perform the exercise: Start by standing with your feet about two feet apart. Keep your back straight and bend forward slightly at the waist. Place your left palm on your left thigh, just above the knee, and your right palm in the same place on your right thigh. Breathe out all the way, then bend your neck forward so that your chin tucks into your throat.

Now, says Dr. Nezezon, you're ready for the stomach lift itself. Without breathing, suck in your stomach muscles as if you were trying to touch your belly button to your backbone. Hold this as long as possible, then relax and breathe. Stand up straight. Repeat this three times.

Because of its impact on the circulatory system, Dr. Nezezon says not to do this exercise during menstruation or pregnancy, after surgery, if you are bleeding or if you have heart disease or high blood pressure.

BRONCHITIS

It starts with a tiny tickle deep in your chest. It turns into a painful hack that rattles your collarbone, turns your face three shades of red and leaves you gasping for air. The worst part? The coughs just keep coming.

More than seven million Americans suffer from chronic bronchitis, an inflammation of the bronchial tubes, the larger passages of your lungs that deliver oxygen to your body. Bronchitis can be caused by viruses, bacteria, dust, car exhaust or tobacco smoke.

Some types of bronchitis are short-lived, lasting maybe one to two weeks. But others linger for months. The natural remedies in this chapter—in conjunction with medical care and used with your doctor's approval—may provide relief from the symptoms of bronchitis, according to some health professionals.

SEE YOUR MEDICAL DOCTOR WHEN . . .

- Your cough lingers for more than one week.
- You cough up blood at any time.
- You run a fever that's over 101°F or that lasts for more than three days.

AROMATHERAPY

An inhalation of cool eucalyptus is wonderful for inflamed lungs, says Victoria Edwards, an aromatherapist in Fair Oaks, California. She suggests putting three drops of eucalyptus essential oil on a hot, wet washcloth and holding the cloth over your face for three to four minutes every few hours (be sure to keep your eyes closed). "You can also put a couple of drops in your hand, rub your palms together and inhale it right from your hands," says Edwards.

For information on preparing and administering essential oils, including cautions about their use, see page 19. For information on purchasing essential oils, refer to the resource list on page 633.

FOOD THERAPY

"Think cayenne pepper when you have bronchitis," says Julian Whitaker, M.D., founder and president of the Whitaker Wellness Center in Newport Beach, California. "Cayenne helps break up the congestion and may help you get quicker relief. And stay away from dairy products. They are mucus producing and may aggravate your condition."

Also, you ought to take some advice from Mom, says Allan Magaziner, D.O., a nutritional medicine specialist and head of the Magaziner Medical Center in Cherry Hill, New Jersey. "Drinking chicken soup is an excellent way to break up congestion," he says. "Another food you should eat when you have bronchitis is garlic, which has natural antiviral and antibacterial qualities. Also, try to eat plenty of fruits and vegetables, since they're high in vitamin C, which stimulates white blood cells, so you get over the infection quicker." (For other food sources of vitamin C, see "Getting What You Need" on page 142.)

HERBAL THERAPY

Thyme, the popular kitchen herb, can help relieve bronchial spasms, says Varro E. Tyler, Ph.D., professor of pharmacognosy at Purdue University in West Lafayette, Indiana. He says to make a tea by steeping one teaspoon of dried thyme in a cup of hot water for five to ten minutes, then straining the mixture so that there's no dried thyme in it. He suggests drinking a cup of tea three times daily, adding a little honey to sweeten.

Dr. Tyler says you might also try taking echinacea tincture, available in most health food stores. One manufacturer of this tincture recommends 15 to 30 drops between two and five times a day, says Dr. Tyler; he suggests you follow the label directions for dosage. This herb boosts immune system functioning and will help you fight off a virus, he explains.

HYDROTHERAPY

To loosen chest congestion, try hot compresses, suggests Charles Thomas, Ph.D., a physical therapist at Desert Springs Therapy Center in Desert Hot

Springs, California, and co-author of *Hydrotherapy: Simple Treatments for Common Ailments*. Here are Dr. Thomas's instructions for making and using a compress: Fold a large bath towel lengthwise, twist it as if you were wringing it out and dip the center third into almost-boiling water. Pull the ends apart as hard as you can to remove most of the water, then lay the hot towel over a dry one on your chest. Leave in place for about five minutes, and repeat for three changes of the hot towel. Repeat the entire procedure every two hours, suggests Dr. Thomas.

IMAGERY

In your mind, see yourself as a tiny person who can go on a trip down into your lungs. On this journey, you carry a bucket and a special backpack that holds all of the supplies you need to clean up your respiratory system. Take in a deep breath and begin your trip, writes Barbara Dossey, R.N., co-author of *Rituals of Healing: Using Imagery for Health and Wellness*. Move with the cool air through your nose, down the back of your throat and into the windpipe. Here, two large airways branch off to the left and right. Choose one of the airways and follow it down into your lungs.

Notice the condition of the walls of your breathing passages. If you see inflammation, redness or roughness, imagine painting those walls with a cool, relaxing blue-green solution. If you see any airways that are constricted, caress the surrounding muscles, so they'll relax. If you find mucus or phlegm, mop it up with a sponge and squeeze it into the bucket you are carrying with you. As your journey ends and you retrace your steps through your respiratory system, feel your body clear any remaining phlegm from your throat with a gentle cough. Feel a sensation of warmth and relaxation in your chest.

Dossey says to practice this imagery twice a day for 15 to 20 minutes each time until the condition clears.

JUICE THERAPY

"Juices rich in the antioxidant nutrients beta-carotene and vitamin C strengthen the immune system," says Cherie Calbom, M.S., a certified nutritionist in Kirkland, Washington, and co-author of *Juicing for Life*. "But because sugar—even fruit sugar—has been shown to depress the immune system, I tell people to get their vitamins from vegetable juices rather than from fruit juices when they're fighting infections." To prepare Calbom's antioxidant-rich Garden Salad Special, juice three broccoli florets and a clove of garlic with four or five carrots, two celery stalks and half of a green pepper. To shore up the immune system, drink this blend or other fresh juices several times a day, says Calbom.

For more information on juicing techniques, see page 93.

MASSAGE

Massaging your chest and back can help break up congestion in your lungs, says Vincent Iuppo, N.D., massage therapist, naturopathic physician and director of the Morris Institute of Natural Therapeutics, a holistic health education center in Denville, New Jersey.

Here's how Dr. Iuppo says to perform the massage: Take off your shirt, then lightly oil your hands with vegetable oil or massage oil. Sit in a comfortable chair or lie on a bed. Then lightly stroke your entire chest for several minutes using the effleurage stroke (page 570).

Then switch to your fingertips and make gentle, slow circles over your entire chest. Do this for several minutes. If you have a partner, let that person rub your upper back using the same strokes.

Dr. Iuppo says this massage may cause some discomfort in the early stages of bronchitis. He suggests doing this routine at least once a day—twice, if you can tolerate it—until the infection clears.

REFLEXOLOGY

Using the corresponding golf ball technique (page 588), work the adrenal gland, lung and solar plexus points on both hands, say Kevin and Barbara Kunz, reflexology researchers in Santa Fe, New Mexico, and authors of *Hand and Foot Reflexology*. They also suggest working the lung and solar plexus points on your feet.

To help you locate these points, consult the hand and foot reflex charts beginning on page 582. For instructions on how to work the points, see "Your Reflexology Session" on page 110.

VITAMIN AND MINERAL THERAPY

"Bronchitis is an inflammation of the bronchial tubes, so you might benefit from taking more vitamins A and C, which can help heal that inflammation," says Richard Gerson, Ph.D., author of *The Right Vitamins*. "My advice: Take 5,000 international units of vitamin A and at least 1,000 milligrams of vitamin C when you have bronchitis." Once you recover, he adds, a daily vitamin C supplement of at least 500 milligrams may prevent new cases.

"Another thing that helps you get over bronchitis more quickly is a cayenne pepper supplement, which is available in most health food stores," adds Julian Whitaker, M.D., founder and president of the Whitaker Wellness Center in Newport Beach, California. "I recommend one capsule a day containing between 40,000 and 80,000 heat units."

BRUISES

You look great in purple shirts, purple suits and purple socks. Purple skin, though, is quite another matter.

Bruises may look nasty and hurt like crazy, but they're really no big deal. Any time you bump into something sharp or take a fall, you're likely to develop one. They get their telltale color from blood that pools under the skin after you break a blood vessel.

We're more likely to develop bruises as we get older, since our skin grows thinner and less able to absorb punishment. Too much exposure to the sun weakens skin, too. And some types of medication can make you bruise more easily.

The natural remedies in this chapter, used with your doctor's approval, may help reduce the pain and discomfort of a bruise and speed the healing process, according to some health professionals.

SEE YOUR MEDICAL DOCTOR WHEN . . .

• You develop unexplained bruises.
• You notice more serious bruising than usual.

AROMATHERAPY

Treat bruises with compresses soaked in cool water that has been spiked with four drops of the essential oil helichrysum (also known as immortelle or everlast), recommends Los Angeles aromatic consultant John Steele. "Helichrysum reduces swelling, controls bleeding under the skin and has anti-inflammatory properties," says Steele. Lavender oil can be substituted for the helichrysum, he adds. He says to use the compresses once or twice a day, leaving them in place for about ten minutes each time.

For severe bruises, apply several drops of undiluted helichrysum directly to the bruise several times a day, suggests Steele. He says to follow this with a cold water compress containing eight to ten drops of helichrysum, leaving the compress on for about ten minutes. Finally, he says, wrap ice cubes in a towel and apply to the bruise. Yarrow, hyssop or lavender essential oil can be substituted for helichrysum, Steele says.

For information on preparing and administering essential oils, including cautions about their use, see page 19. For information on purchasing essential oils, refer to the resource list on page 633.

FOOD THERAPY

Eat more peppers, citrus fruits or any other food that's rich in vitamin C, advises Elson Haas, M.D., director of the Preventive Medical Center of Marin in San Rafael, California, and author of *Staying Healthy with Nutrition*. Vitamin C builds collagen—skin tissue—around blood vessels in the skin, he explains. The quicker collagen is formed, the shorter the healing time of bruises. (For more food sources of vitamin C, see "Getting What You Need" on page 142.)

HERBAL THERAPY

Try a cream or tincture made from arnica to help heal a bruise, suggests Varro E. Tyler, Ph.D., professor of pharmacognosy at Purdue University in West Lafayette, Indiana. (These products are available in most health food stores.) According to Dr. Tyler, the dried flower heads of this plant contain chemical compounds that promote healing. For best results, he says, apply the cream or tincture directly to the injured area three or four times a day.

HOMEOPATHY

A dose of Arnica montana is the first remedy most homeopaths would suggest to heal a bruise, says Mitchell Fleisher, M.D., a family practice physician and homeopath in Colleen, Virginia. He suggests taking a 6C dose four to six times a day, a 12C dose three or four times a day or a 30C dose once or twice a day until you begin to see improvement (usually in about two to three days).

If you have a deep bruise in the pelvic area or in the breast, try a 6C dose of Bellis perennis every 20 minutes until you see your doctor, says John G. Collins, N.D., a naturopathic physician and associate professor at the National College of Naturopathic Medicine in Portland, Oregon. If the bruise is not serious, he says, you can continue taking this remedy four times a day for no longer than four days, decreasing the dosage as the bruise begins to heal.

Arnica montana and Bellis perennis can be purchased in many health food stores. To purchase homeopathic remedies by mail, refer to the resource list on page 637.

HYDROTHERAPY

Clean the bruise with soap and water, then apply a warm compress, suggests Agatha Thrash, M.D., a medical pathologist and co-founder and co-director of Uchee Pines Institute, a natural healing center in Seale, Alabama. Applying a sage tea compress for an hour to overnight speeds the healing of many bruises, according to Dr. Thrash.

To make the compress, Varro E. Tyler, Ph.D., professor of pharmacognosy at Purdue University in West Lafayette, Indiana, suggests soaking gauze in a strong sage tea (available in most health food stores). Wring out the compress and apply it to the bruise, leaving it in place until it cools down. Then resoak the gauze and reapply it to the bruise. Dr. Tyler says to repeat the application for 30 minutes, three times a day.

VITAMIN AND MINERAL THERAPY

"To speed up the healing process, I recommend taking 5,000 milligrams of vitamin C at the earliest sign of a bruise," says Richard Gerson, Ph.D., author of *The Right Vitamins*. Daily supplements of 400 international units of vitamin E and 10,000 international units of vitamin A can also help rebuild skin tissue and heal the bruise, says Elson Haas, M.D., director of the Preventive Medical Center of Marin in San Rafael, California, and author of *Staying Healthy with Nutrition*.

BURNOUT

Seventy-hour workweeks. Crazy commutes. Piles of unpaid bills. Endless family demands.

Can't we just jump off the world and let it spin without us for a while?

Life in the fast lane often comes with a built-in speeding ticket: burnout. It's a state of mental and physical exhaustion that can lead to negative feelings about your job, your life and yourself. Reducing stress is key to dealing with burnout. And the natural remedies in this chapter, used with the approval of your doctor, may help relieve some of the symptoms of burnout, according to some health professionals.

SEE YOUR MEDICAL DOCTOR WHEN . . .

- You experience any signs of depression for longer than two weeks, including pervasive sadness, insomnia, weight loss and/or a decline in appetite, inability to concentrate and thoughts of suicide.
- You experience physical symptoms that persist, such as stomach upset, headaches and back pain.
- You have distinct episodes of feeling panicky, including a racing heartbeat, unusual sweating and light-headedness.
- You start using alcohol excessively or abusing drugs.

FLOWER REMEDY/ ESSENCE THERAPY

For anyone suffering from profound mental or physical exhaustion, the flower remedy Olive can be quite potent, says Patricia Kaminski, co-director of the Flower Essence Society, a Nevada City, California, organization that studies and promotes the therapeutic use of flower remedies/essences. "Burned-out people can also feel tiredness that comes and goes—it disappears when they're happy but comes back when they have to do something they don't want to do." In such cases, when burnout stems from mental resistance to a particular situation or task, Kaminski recommends the remedy Hornbeam.

Regardless of what's causing it, mental exhaustion also responds well to the essence of the Aloe Vera flower, according to Kaminski. "It heals mental burnout the same way the juice from the leaves heals burned skin."

Flower remedies/essences are available in some health food stores and through mail order (refer to the resource list on page 635). For information on preparing and administering flower remedies/essences, see page 37.

FOOD THERAPY

"When you're really burned out, I suggest you get plenty of ginseng to give you more energy," says Julian Whitaker, M.D., founder and president of the Whitaker Wellness Center in Newport Beach, California. "You can buy it as an herb and cook with it or drink it as a tea. Be sure to look for the standardized percentage of ginsenosides, the active ingredient. You'll want something that's over 10 percent ginsenosides." Dr. Whitaker recommends using one to two teaspoons of dried ginseng in your cooking for at least one or two meals a day. It's available in most health food stores.

IMAGERY

Imagine that you have fallen into a pit of quicksand. The more you struggle to get out, the more you're sinking into it. So you remain perfectly still, says Dennis Gersten, M.D., a San Diego psychiatrist and publisher of *Atlantis*, a bimonthly imagery newsletter. Now picture people or images, such as your messy desk, that are contributing to your sense of burnout. See these people or objects surrounding the pit of quicksand. Realize that they are unable or unwilling to help you. In fact, they are part of your problem. Imagine grabbing hold of a jungle vine and use it to pull yourself out of the pit.

When you're out of danger, take a moment to talk to the people and images surrounding the pit. Express your anger or frustration or any other emotions that you feel.

BURNOUT

Once you have done that, walk away and down a path until you come to a barrier blocking your way. This barrier is a symbol of burnout. It could be a wall, gate, fallen tree or other roadblock. Touch the image and tell it how you feel about it. Spend some time talking to the image and find out how it feels about you. Is it trying to protect you in some way? Now that you've listened to its concerns, see if the image will agree to allow you to climb over it or to transform itself into something more positive, something that will help you overcome your burnout.

Dr. Gersten recommends practicing this imagery once or twice a day, ten minutes each time.

RELAXATION AND MEDITATION

Frequent meditation is key to beating burnout, according to Alice Christensen, founder and executive director of the American Yoga Association. Christensen recommends spending 10 to 20 minutes meditating at your desk at work each day. And she also suggests meditating yourself to sleep at night while you're lying in bed. The result, she says, will be bursts of creative energy that will help see you through the day.

For instructions on meditation techniques, see page 117; for yoga meditation, see page 153.

SOUND THERAPY

If burnout is hurting your creativity, listening to the right music may help return the spark, says Barbara Anne Scarantino in her book *Music Power: Creative Living through the Joys of Music*. Here are some of the pieces she suggests: *Scheherazade* by Nikolay Rimsky-Korsakov, the soundtrack from *Gone with the Wind* by Max Steiner, *Fresh Aire VI* by Mannheim Steamroller, *Chariots of Fire* by Vangelis, *Nutcracker Suite* by Pyotr Ilich Tchaikovsky, *Rhapsody in Blue* by George Gershwin, the soundtrack to *The Color Purple* by Quincy Jones and music by the late German composer Richard Wagner. These are available from music stores.

SEE ALSO Stress

BURNS

Just had to peek at that pot roast, didn't you? Yep, you opened the oven and lifted the tinfoil—and the baking dish stung your hand like a hornet. Now you have a throbbing little burn, and supper is going to have to wait.

There are three types of burns. First-degree burns look like red patches on your skin and can be painful. Second-degree burns cause blisters and hurt even more. Third-degree burns, the most serious, leave your skin charred or waxy. They hurt very little, since they usually cause damage to the nerve endings that send pain impulses to your brain. Don't mess with third-degree burns; seek emergency help immediately. The natural remedies in this chapter—used in conjunction with medical care and with the approval of your doctor—may help relieve the discomfort of minor burns, according to some health professionals.

SEE YOUR MEDICAL DOCTOR WHEN . . .

- You get any third-degree burn.
- You get a first- or second-degree burn that covers a large area of skin and is extremely painful.
- Your burn becomes infected; watch for blisters that fill with a brownish or greenish fluid.

AROMATHERAPY

In the 1920s, the founder of modern aromatherapy, French chemist René-Maurice Gattefossé, discovered the burn-healing power of lavender quite by accident. After burning his hand in a laboratory accident, he quickly dunked it in pure lavender oil and was surprised by how quickly the skin healed. Use a few drops of undiluted lavender directly on the burn, recommends Los Angeles aromatherapist Michael Scholes, of Aromatherapy Seminars, an organization that trains professionals and others in the use of essential oils.

For information on preparing and administering essential oils, including cautions about their use, see page 19. For information on purchasing essential oils, refer to the resource list on page 633.

AYURVEDA

Add a pinch of turmeric to fresh aloe vera gel (available in most health food stores) and apply the paste to the burned area, then cover the area with gauze, says Vasant Lad, B.A.M.S., M.A.Sc., director of the Ayurvedic Institute in Albuquerque, New Mexico. Wash off and reapply the paste two to four times a day, re-covering the area each time, until the burn heals. Turmeric can stain the skin, warns Dr. Lad, but any discoloration should wash off in about two weeks.

Dr. Lad also suggests using fresh cilantro juice on a burn. To make the juice, he says, put cilantro leaves and water in a blender, using enough of each ingredient to make a puree that will cover the burned area. Dr. Lad suggests applying this mixture two teaspoons at a time, three times a day, directly to the burned skin, covering the area with gauze. Continue the treatment as necessary, he says.

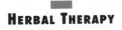

FOOD THERAPY

Milk is great for minor (first-degree) burns—but place it on the burn rather than drink it, says Stephen M. Purcell, D.O., chairman of the Department of Dermatology at Philadelphia College of Osteopathic Medicine. He recommends that you soak the burned area in whole milk for 15 minutes or so or apply a milk-soaked washcloth. He says to repeat either treatment every two to six hours as needed for pain. Just be sure to rinse your skin (and the washcloth) afterward, says Dr. Purcell, because the milk will smell bad as it warms up.

HERBAL THERAPY

Try fresh aloe vera for burns, says Varro E. Tyler, Ph.D., professor of pharmacognosy at Purdue University in West Lafayette, Indiana. Studies show that aloe vera helps new cells form and hastens healing, according to Dr. Tyler. He suggests keeping a plant on a sunny windowsill for treating minor (first-degree) burns. To use, he says, cut open one of the plant's fleshy leaves and squeeze out the clear gel, applying it directly to the affected area three or four times a day. Aloe vera heals best in the open air, so leave the burn uncovered, he adds.

HOMEOPATHY

"There are great remedies for burns," says Mitchell Fleisher, M.D., a family practice physician and homeopath in Colleen, Virginia. To treat a minor (first-degree) burn, he recommends that you put 20 drops of Calendula tincture in four ounces of water and bathe the skin with it four to six times a day until the pain goes away or the burn heals. He says you can also use Urtica urens as a tincture in the same way as Calendula or you can take 6C or 12C tablets every two to three hours as needed to relieve the pain. If it's a stinging, swollen burn, Dr. Fleisher says to try a 6C or 12C dose of Apis every two to three hours until the pain goes away.

If you have a second-degree burn, a burn that has blistered and is extremely painful, you should seek medical attention immediately. But as additional therapy, Dr. Fleisher recommends taking a 12C or 30C dose of Causticum or

Cantharis once every 30 to 60 minutes until the pain is relieved.

All of these remedies can be purchased in many health food stores. To purchase homeopathic remedies by mail, refer to the resource list on page 637.

HYDROTHERAPY

For minor (first-degree) burns, hold the area under cold water until the pain subsides, suggests Charles Thomas, Ph.D., a physical therapist at Desert Springs Therapy Center in Desert Hot Springs, California, and co-author of *Hydrotherapy: Simple Treatments for Common Ailments*. Then, he says, switch to slightly warmer water (a little cooler than body temperature) and keep the burned area in the water until there's no pain when you take it out of the water. After this treatment, apply a little aloe vera gel, suggests Dr. Thomas. Aloe vera gel is available in most health food stores.

VITAMIN AND MINERAL THERAPY

"Any healing tissue can benefit from 10,000 international units of vitamin A twice daily, 15 milligrams of zinc once daily and a minimum of 500 milligrams of vitamin C two or three times daily," says Elson Haas, M.D., director of the Preventive Medical Center of Marin in San Rafael, California, and author of *Staying Healthy with Nutrition*. He recommends continuing the supplements for a full three weeks after you get the burn, even if it heals sooner, so your skin has the vitamins it needs to rebuild properly.

SEE ALSO Sunburn

BURSITIS AND TENDINITIS

The exercise program is going great, and it's time to turn things up a notch. Just take it slowly. Packing 50 more pounds on the barbell, pushing an extra 30 minutes on the stair-climber or adding ten laps to your daily walk can bring on a case of the "itises"—bursitis and tendinitis, that is.

Bursitis occurs when you irritate the bursae, which are fluid-filled sacs that reduce friction in your joints. Tendinitis is an inflammation of the tendons, which connect your muscles to your bones. If you lift something that's too heavy or repeat an awkward motion over and over, you'll get a painful reminder in the form of sore, swollen joints.

BURSITIS AND TENDINITIS

Tendinitis and bursitis can improve with a little rest, but unless you change your exercise habits, they could turn into chronic conditions. The natural remedies in this chapter—used in conjunction with medical care and with your doctor's approval—may help relieve the symptoms of bursitis and tendinitis, according to some health professionals.

SEE YOUR MEDICAL DOCTOR WHEN . . .

- Your pain is getting worse and interferes with your ability to do whatever it is you want to do.
- Your pain has lasted a long time.
- Your joints are tender, warm and red and you suspect an infection.

FOOD THERAPY

"Barley green is a good anti-inflammatory agent, so I'd suggest sprinkling some on a salad," says Julian Whitaker, M.D., founder and president of the Whitaker Wellness Center in Newport Beach, California. You can buy barley green in most health food stores, he says.

"Also, eat a lot of pineapple when bursitis bothers you," he adds. "Pineapple is rich in bromelain, a natural anti-inflammatory that speeds healing."

HOMEOPATHY

"If your joint is stiff and painful when you first move it and better the more you use it, and if it is better in warmth and worse in cold, then you might consider taking a 6C or 12C dose of Rhus toxicodendron every three to four hours until you feel relief," says Mitchell Fleisher, M.D., a family practice physician and homeopath in Colleen, Virginia. If the joint pain is worse with the least motion or touch, better with resting and applied pressure and better in cold and worse in warmth, then he suggests trying a similar dosage of Bryonia.

Rhus toxicodendron and Bryonia can be purchased in many health food stores. To purchase homeopathic remedies by mail, refer to the resource list on page 637.

HYDROTHERAPY

Cold treatments usually work best against the intense pain of bursitis or tendinitis, says John Abruzzo, M.D., professor of medicine and director of the Rheumatology and Osteoporosis Center at Thomas Jefferson University Hospital in Philadelphia. He recommends that you use a cold, wet compress or an ice pack wrapped in a plastic bag and placed over a towel on the skin. You should feel relief within 10 to 20 minutes, says Dr. Abruzzo. He suggests repeating the treatment every four hours as needed for pain relief. He also adds this word of caution: Never use cold treatments for more than 20 minutes at a time, because they can damage the skin.

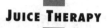

JUICE THERAPY

Black cherry juice is a popular folk remedy for arthritis that may also relieve bursitis and tendinitis, says Eve Campanelli, Ph.D., a holistic family practitioner in Beverly Hills, California. Dr. Campanelli recommends drinking two eight-ounce glasses a day, either fresh or from concentrate. (To make it fresh, she suggests a half-and-half mixture of four ounces of black cherry juice and four ounces of water.) Discontinue the treatment once the pain clears up, she says.

For more information on juicing techniques, see page 93.

MASSAGE

Gently stroking the muscles near the affected joint can ease both bursitis and tendinitis, says Vincent Iuppo, N.D., a massage therapist, a naturopathic physician and director of the Morris Institute of Natural Therapeutics, a holistic health education center in Denville, New Jersey.

Here's the massage that Dr. Iuppo recommends: Lubricate your hands with vegetable oil or massage oil. (Scented oils can make the massage more pleasurable, Dr. Iuppo says.) Place your hands on the "belly" of the muscle you want to massage (the belly is the thickest part of the muscle). Use the effleurage stroke (page 570) to warm up the muscle for several minutes, then switch to the friction stroke (page 570) for another five minutes or so. Do not massage directly on the joint, because that could cause more pain and inflammation, says Dr. Iuppo. He suggests massaging the area for 10 to 15 minutes every day until the pain clears up or to help prevent flare-ups.

REFLEXOLOGY

When working on your hands or feet, focus on the reflex that matches the part of the body where the pain is flaring up, says St. Petersburg, Florida, reflexologist Dwight Byers, author of *Better Health with Foot Reflexology*. For example, Dr. Byers says to work on the shoulder reflex if you have bursitis in your shoulder.

To help you locate reflex points, consult the hand and foot reflex charts beginning on page 582. For instructions on how to work the points, see "Your Reflexology Session" on page 110.

CAFFEINE DEPENDENCY

If you can't imagine morning without a cup of hot coffee, you're not alone: About 75 percent of Americans use caffeine to clear out the cobwebs and jump-start their bodies. Whether they guzzle coffee, tea or cola, sip cocoa or nibble on chocolate bars, most people are well-acquainted with the quick energy boost that comes from caffeine.

What's wrong with that? Nothing—until the caffeine leaves your body about six to eight hours after your last fix. Then you're fighting the urge to nod off.

While the obvious way to avoid this crash-and-burn syndrome is to cut out caffeine completely, going cold turkey can leave you shaky, exhausted and irritable, all classic symptoms of caffeine withdrawal. The natural remedies in this chapter, used with your doctor's approval, may help you reduce your dependency on caffeine, according to some health professionals.

SEE YOUR MEDICAL DOCTOR WHEN . . .

- You are unable to reduce your need for caffeine.
- You are troubled by persistent problems of stomach upset, such as nausea and bloating.
- You are constantly nervous or irritable.
- You have chronic insomnia.
- Your heartbeat is often rapid or irregular.
- You experience frequent headaches or ringing in the ears or see flashing zigzag lights.
- You are often dizzy.

FLOWER REMEDY/ESSENCE THERAPY

You can learn to cope without coffee, says Patricia Kaminski, co-director of the Flower Essence Society, a Nevada City, California, organization that studies and promotes the therapeutic use of flower remedies/essences. She advises nocturnal types to take four drops of the flower essence Morning Glory four times a day, with one dose first thing in the morning and the last dose right before bedtime. Over time, she says, this will help you readjust your internal clock, so you start the day feeling energized, not traumatized.

Flower essences are available in some health food stores and through mail order (refer to the resource list on page 635). For more information on preparing and administering flower essences, see page 37.

FOOD THERAPY

To free your body of caffeine, Elson Haas, M.D., director of the Preventive Medical Center of Marin in San Rafael, California, and author of *Staying Healthy with Nutrition*, recommends that you follow his three-week detoxification diet (see "Detoxing Your Ills" on page 48).

SOUND THERAPY

Relaxation is one of the keys to beating caffeine dependency, and listening to the right music for 20 to 30 minutes each day can help you relax, according to Steven Halpern, Ph.D., composer, researcher and author of *Sound Health: The Music and Sounds That Make Us Whole*. To get started, says Dr. Halpern, turn on the music, then sit or lie comfortably, close your eyes and take a deep breath. He suggests that you wear headphones to focus your full attention and avoid distraction. He recommends, however, that you keep the speakers playing, so your body absorbs the sound energy. While the music plays, let your breath slow down and become steady. Listen not just to the notes but to the silence between the notes. Dr. Halpern says this will keep you from analyzing the music, which will allow it to relax you.

For suggested pieces to relax by, see "Sailing Away to Key Largo" on page 129. Many of these are available in music stores. For information on ordering any of the works, refer to the resource list on page 642.

YOGA

It's easier to give up your caffeine habit if you're willing to pick up a yoga habit, according to Alice Christensen, founder and executive director of the American Yoga Association. Fifteen to 20 minutes of meditation daily, combined with your choice of three or four yoga poses, will give you energy bursts to replace the caffeine jolts you've come to depend on, she says.

For instruction on meditation, see page 153; choose your poses from the Daily Routine, which begins on page 606.

CALLUSES AND CORNS

The perfect style, the perfect color, and at half-price, they're a steal. They're also a half-size too small. But you can take it, right?

Wrong. You'll pay the price later in calluses, lumpy accumulations of dead skin cells caused by constant friction between your feet and your shoes. You can get calluses on your hands and fingers as well. A callus isn't very attractive, but it isn't painful, either, unless one on your foot develops a hard core and becomes a corn.

Corns usually appear on the outside of the little toe or on the upper surfaces of the other toes and can make a five-minute walk feel like a marathon. Some people also get soft corns, which form between the toes when they're squeezed together so tightly that their bones rub against each other.

The best way to prevent any foot problem is by choosing shoes that fit. But the natural remedies in this chapter, used with the approval of your doctor, may help relieve calluses and corns, according to some health professionals.

SEE YOUR MEDICAL DOCTOR WHEN . . .

- Your callus is red and feels hot to the touch.
- Your callus cracks and bleeds or has a bluish tint.
- You have diabetes and your foot problems don't improve with home remedies. Any cut or break in the skin of your feet should be examined by a physician.

AYURVEDA

Here's a remedy from Vasant Lad, B.A.M.S., M.A.Sc., director of the Ayurvedic Institute in Albuquerque, New Mexico: First, clean the area with tea tree oil. Then apply a paste made by mixing 1 teaspoon of aloe vera gel with ½ teaspoon of turmeric. Once the paste is applied, cover the area with a bandage. The treatment works best at night when you're off your feet, according to Dr. Lad. (Since turmeric can stain skin and clothing, he suggests putting on old socks after you've applied this remedy. Any skin discoloration should wash off in about two weeks.)

In the morning, says Dr. Lad, remove the bandage and soak your foot in a bucket of warm water for ten minutes. Then rub mustard oil deeply into the corn or callus. Continue this treatment for several days, and eventually, the corn or callus will fall off, says Dr. Lad.

Both tea tree oil and aloe vera gel are available in most health food stores. Mustard oil is available in Indian pharmacies and by mail order (refer to the resource list on page 634).

FOOD THERAPY

To remove corns and calluses, try this home remedy suggested by Julian Whitaker, M.D., founder and president of the Whitaker Wellness Center in Newport Beach, California. "Mix one teaspoon of lemon juice, one teaspoon of dried chamomile tea and one garlic clove that has been crushed. Rub this mixture directly on the corn one or more times a day." This kitchen-created remedy helps dissolve corns and calluses for quicker relief, says Dr. Whitaker. Dried chamomile tea is available in most health food stores.

HOMEOPATHY

Try a 6C dose of one of the following remedies three times a day until you see improvement, says Chris Meletis, N.D., a naturopathic physician and medicinary director at the National College of Naturopathic Medicine in Portland, Oregon. According to Dr. Meletis, Ranunculus bulbosus works when you have hard skin that is very sensitive, often with burning and intense itching. For painful calluses on your toes and fingers that are worse on your right side, worse with heat and better with cold, he says to use Lycopodium. Ranunculus sceleratus may help if you have a piercing pain, with burning and soreness that are worse when you let your feet hang down, he says.

All of these remedies are available in many health food stores. To purchase homeopathic remedies by mail, refer to the resource list on page 637.

SEE ALSO Foot Pain

CANKER SORES

O ut of sight, out of mind. Tucked away inside your mouth, some canker sores are easy to ignore. But bite into the wrong food—usually something acidic, such as an orange or a tomato—and these small, round ulcers make their presence known in the most painful way possible. Other sores can hurt because they're in areas that brush against your teeth. *Yeeowch!*

White or yellow in color and surrounded by red halos, canker sores often pop up when you're under stress or after you've eaten an irritating food (pineapple, nuts and chocolate are common culprits). Experts believe canker sores are contagious; if you've recently kissed someone who has one, you'll soon find out if the experts are right. The natural remedies in this chapter, used with the approval of your doctor, may help relieve the symptoms of canker sores or may prevent sores from recurring, according to some health professionals.

SEE YOUR MEDICAL DOCTOR WHEN . . .

- Your sore persists for more than two weeks.
- You get sores once a week or more, especially when they appear in bunches.

FOOD THERAPY

Eat more yogurt, says Julian Whitaker, M.D., founder and president of the Whitaker Wellness Center in Newport Beach, California. Dr. Whitaker says the active acidophilus cultures in yogurt can both prevent and heal canker sores. If you're prone to canker sores, he recommends eating at least four tablespoons of yogurt daily to prevent outbreaks. To heal an outbreak, he recommends eating at least one eight-ounce container a day.

HERBAL THERAPY

Gargle with calendula tea or goldenseal tea to help canker sores heal, says Varro E. Tyler, Ph.D., professor of pharmacognosy at Purdue University in West Lafayette, Indiana. He says to make the tea by pouring a cup of boiling water over one to two teaspoons of the dried herb (both are available in most health food stores). Let this mixture steep for ten minutes, says Dr. Tyler, then strain it so that there is no herb left in the liquid and use it as a mouthwash three or four times daily.

HOMEOPATHY

Take a 30X dose of homeopathic Borax every one to two hours until the pain is relieved, says Richard D. Fischer, D.D.S., a dentist and homeopath in Annandale, Virginia, and president of the International Academy of Oral Medicine and Toxicology.

Borax can be purchased in many health food stores. To purchase homeopathic remedies by mail, refer to the resource list on page 637.

IMAGERY

Visualize a soothing light shining on your sore. For the next five minutes, see the light slowly penetrate the sore and begin healing it from the bottom up (that's how canker sores heal naturally). Do this twice a day until the sore has healed, says Dennis Gersten, M.D., a San Diego psychiatrist and publisher of *Atlantis*, a bi-monthly imagery newsletter.

JUICE THERAPY

"Frequent canker sores can signal that you're not getting enough iron or folate," says Cherie Calbom, M.S., a certified nutritionist in Kirkland, Washington, and co-author of *Juicing for Life*. She recommends a daily dose of her nutrient-rich Folic Acid Special juice: Bunch up two kale leaves and a small handful each of parsley and spinach. Process the greens with four or five carrots, using the carrots to push the greens through the juicer. "This is also a good source of beta-carotene, which has been shown to heal mouth sores," says Calbom.

For more information about juicing techniques, see page 93.

VITAMIN AND MINERAL THERAPY

Take 1,000 milligrams of the amino acid lysine at each meal during an outbreak and then 500 milligrams at each meal for a week afterward, says Richard D. Fischer, D.D.S., a dentist and homeopath in Annandale, Virginia, and president of the International Academy of Oral Medicine and Toxicology. "Another thing that works for some people is to take a vitamin E capsule, poke a hole in it and then rub the liquid directly on the sore," he says. He suggests using the vitamin E three times a day during an outbreak until the sore heals.

You can also take between 4,000 and 5,000 milligrams of vitamin C daily during outbreaks and at least 500 milligrams daily as a way of preventing canker sores, says Julian Whitaker, M.D., founder and president of the Whitaker Wellness Center in Newport Beach, California.

CATARACTS

You stop driving at night because the glare of the headlights makes it hard to see. You need a stronger light for reading or sewing, but no matter how bright the light, your vision seems dim, like a television screen that needs adjusting.

There's no magic knob you can turn to brighten things up if you have cataracts, a vision problem that affects half of all Americans between ages 65 and 74. With cataracts, the lens of the eye gradually yellows and loses its transparency, causing dim or blurry vision.

While cataracts coincide with aging, the more likely cause, researchers believe, is accumulated exposure to ultraviolet light.

Some cataracts are severe enough to cause blindness and must be surgically removed. Others are so mild that stronger glasses are enough. If you suspect you have a cataract, see your doctor for a diagnosis. But the natural remedies in this chapter—used in conjunction with medical care and with your doctor's approval—may help prevent or slow the development of cataracts, according to some health professionals.

SEE YOUR MEDICAL DOCTOR WHEN . . .

- Your vision becomes cloudy or blurred.
- You have problems driving at night because headlights seem too bright.
- You find that glare from the sun bothers you.
- You notice changes in the way you see colors.

AYURVEDA

To prevent cataracts from worsening, wash your eyes in triphala tea, says Vasant Lad, B.A.M.S., M.A.Sc., director of the Ayurvedic Institute in Albuquerque, New Mexico. (Triphala is a powder made from the fruits of three Indian trees and is available in Indian pharmacies and some health food stores. To order by mail, please refer to the resource list on page 634.)

Here's how Dr. Lad says to use the tea: Boil one teaspoon of triphala in a cup of water for three minutes. Allow the tea to cool, then gently—without disturbing the sediment—strain it through a double layer of cheesecloth. Make sure no particles of powder remain in the strained tea. Then put the tea in an eye cup (available in most pharmacies) and use it as an eyewash, exposing the open eye once or twice to the tea.

Wash your eyes with triphala tea every day, up to three times a day, suggests Dr. Lad. He says your eyes will be soothed, strengthened and cleansed. But, he cautions, this treatment is not a substitute for medical care; you should be sure to consult with your doctor before trying it.

FOOD THERAPY

Vegetables rich in the antioxidant nutrients beta-carotene and vitamins C and E—any yellow, orange or dark green leafy vegetable—help prevent the oxidation process that can contribute to and worsen cataracts, says Jay Cohen, O.D., associate professor in the State University College of Optometry in New York City. (For more food sources of vitamin C and vitamin E, see "Getting What You Need" on page 142.)

IMAGERY

Picture yourself standing under a large waterfall. Imagine that you can remove the lens from your eye and see it in your hand, suggests Gerald Epstein, M.D., a New York City psychiatrist and author of *Healing Visualizations*. Notice that the lens appears cloudy, so wash it thoroughly in the clean, clear water.

See and sense that the cataract is dissolving. Breathe out once. Before replacing the lens, let a holy person (if you are religious) or someone you love put some saliva onto the lens and into the empty space where the lens was, so it will stay clear and clean. Now replace the lens, knowing that it has cleared up. Open your eyes.

Dr. Epstein recommends practicing this imagery every two hours while awake, three minutes a session, for 21 days. Take 7 days off, then repeat for another 21 days, followed by another 7-day rest period and one more 21-day cycle.

JUICE THERAPY

Juices rich in beta-carotene and vitamin C can help slow the development of cataracts, according to Cherie Calbom, M.S., a certified nutritionist in Kirkland, Washington, and co-author of *Juicing for Life*. "These nutrients protect the eye from free radical damage caused by exposure to the sun," says Calbom. To prepare her Eye Therapy Express juice, Calbom says to bunch two endive leaves and a handful of parsley, then juice them along with two celery stalks and four or five carrots. Drinking this juice every day won't cure cataracts, but it will help protect your eyes from further damage, according to Calbom.

For information on juicing techniques, see page 93.

CATARACTS

REFLEXOLOGY

Focus on these reflexes on your feet, recommends New York City reflexologist Laura Norman, author of *Feet First: A Guide to Foot Reflexology*: eye, ear, neck, cervical spine, kidney and all of the points on the tops and bottoms of the toes, with emphasis on the pituitary and thyroid gland. (To work the toes, use whichever technique you find most comfortable.)

To help you locate these points, consult the foot reflex chart on page 592. For instructions on how to work the points, see "Your Reflexology Session" on page 110.

VITAMIN AND MINERAL THERAPY

Antioxidants are recommended by Jay Cohen, O.D., associate professor in the State University of New York College of Optometry in New York City, as a way to minimize the oxidation damage that experts say is responsible for cataracts. He says to make sure you're getting 500 milligrams of vitamin C, up to 400 international units of vitamin E and up to 15 milligrams (25,000 international units) of beta-carotene daily, whether through a multivitamin/mineral supplement or additional pills.

SEE ALSO Vision Problems

CHRONIC FATIGUE SYNDROME

To the average overworked, overstressed American, chronic fatigue syndrome (CFS) doesn't sound like a disease. It sounds like reality.

But people with CFS aren't just tired. Their exhaustion is so severe and persistent that normal activity is impossible. Chronic fatigue won't go away after a good night's sleep.

Other symptoms of CFS include fever, sore throat, muscle pain, sore lymph nodes and depression. Some patients also report dizziness, poor memory and difficulty concentrating.

Scientists still don't know what causes CFS. Because the disease appears to weaken the immune system, many researchers suspect a virus that impairs immune reponse. The natural remedies in this chapter—used in conjunction with medical care and with your doctor's approval—may help treat the symptoms and underlying causes of CFS, according to some health professionals.

SEE YOUR MEDICAL DOCTOR WHEN . . .

- You suffer unexplained tiredness that lasts for at least two weeks.
- You notice other symptoms such as muscle aches, pain, fever, nausea and depression.

ACUPRESSURE

Boost your physical condition to cope with the tired, weak feeling of CFS by stimulating point CV 6, says Michael Reed Gach, Ph.D., director of the Acupressure Institute in Berkeley, California, and author of *Acupressure's Potent Points*. CV 6 is also called the Sea of Energy and is situated three finger-widths below the navel. (For help in locating this point, refer to the illustration on page 564.) Dr. Gach says to close your eyes and relax, breathe deeply and hold the point for two minutes. Pressing this point can also alleviate the dizziness and confusion sometimes experienced with this condition, he says.

FOOD THERAPY

"CFS appears to be, at least partially, a cellular injury affecting many tissues and organs. A good place to start is to clean out the liver," says Michael A.

Klaper, M.D., a nutritional medicine specialist in Pompano Beach, Florida, and director of the Institute of Nutritional Education and Research, an organization based in Manhattan Beach, California, that teaches doctors about nutrition and its relationship to disease. "Get on a lean, clean, vegetable-based diet with little or no saturated fat. And increase your intake of magnesium-rich foods and essential fatty acids, such as those you get from nuts and grains." (For good food sources of magnesium, see "Getting What You Need" on page 142.)

"What you put in your body makes all the difference in how well your immune system functions," says Cherie Calbom, M.S., a certified nutritionist in Kirkland, Washington, and co-author of *Juicing for Life*. Calbom speaks from experience. She and her husband fought CFS and won, a recovery she credits largely to dietary changes and fresh juices. She advises people with CFS to cut out caffeine, junk foods and foods made with refined flour (whole-grain breads are fine).

So what's left to eat? "Raw, unprocessed fruits, vegetables, whole grains, nuts, seeds, lean protein and juices," says Calbom. "They're loaded with nutrients that build the immune system. And by eliminating processed foods from your diet, you may discover hidden food allergies, which are common in people with CFS."

Calbom's CFS diet is made up of 50 to 75 percent raw foods. "Make half of that amount raw fruits, vegetables and salads and the other half raw juices," she suggests.

Finally, Calbom advises CFS patients to limit or eliminate sugar, honey, corn syrup and even sugar substitutes. "Sugar weakens the immune system and encourages the buildup of bacteria in the system, which is why so many people with CFS are prone to yeast infections and candidiasis," says Calbom. "Even fruit juices should be taken in moderation, and some patients can't handle them at all. If you stick to vegetables and vegetable juices for the first month or two and introduce fruits gradually, you'll be able to tell if they make your symptoms worse."

HYDROTHERAPY

At Uchee Pines Institute, a natural healing center in Seale, Alabama, co-founder and co-director Agatha Thrash, M.D., a medical pathologist, treats CFS with a three-pronged approach of strict diet, gentle exercise and a 15-day regimen of therapeutic baths. By elevating the body temperature to 102°F for at least five minutes every day, the baths increase the number and activity of white blood cells, jump-starting the depressed immune system of the CFS patient, Dr. Thrash says.

Here are Dr. Thrash's instructions for preparing the bath: Fill a bathtub halfway with comfortably warm water. Sit in the tub and immediately finish filling it with water that's as hot as you can tolerate. Keep a basin of cold water within easy reach, so you can sponge off your face periodically. After soaking for about 10 minutes, begin taking your temperature at regular intervals. Once your body temperature reaches 102°F, usually within 20 to 25 minutes, stay in the tub for as long as you're comfortable—up to another 45 minutes—adding hot water as necessary to keep your temperature at 102°.

While the 15-day regimen brings results in some patients, others find that their symptoms return when the series is finished. In such cases, start another 15-day series of baths, suggests Dr. Thrash.

In addition to the baths, Dr. Thrash recommends a vegetarian diet made up of whole grains, nuts, seeds and fresh fruits and vegetables; no meats, eggs or dairy products should be eaten. Dr. Thrash also advises her patients to take a daily walk at a comfortable pace, increasing the speed and distance as they become stronger.

IMAGERY

Close your eyes, breathe out three times and go inside your body, suggests New York City psychiatrist Gerald Epstein, M.D., in his book *Healing Visualizations*. Imagine yourself playing a flute while riding a polo pony and carrying a polo mallet in your saddle. Coax the viruses out of your organs by playing music, then kill them with the mallet. Then open your eyes.

Dr. Epstein suggests that you practice this imagery three times daily, three minutes a session, for nine cycles of 21 days on and 7 days off.

SOUND THERAPY

Listening to relaxing music for 20 to 30 minutes each day can ease stress and help build resistance to chronic fatigue, says Steven Halpern, Ph.D., composer, researcher and author of *Sound Health: The Music and Sounds That Make Us Whole*. To get started, he says, turn on the music, then sit or lie comfortably, close your eyes and take a deep breath. Dr. Halpern suggests that you wear headphones to focus your full attention and avoid distraction. He recommends, however, that you keep the speakers playing, so your body absorbs the sound energy. While the music plays, let your breath slow down and become steady. Listen not just to the notes but to the silence between the notes. Dr. Halpern says this will keep you from analyzing the music, which will allow it to relax you.

For suggested pieces to relax by, see "Sailing Away to Key Largo" on page 129. Dr. Halpern especially recommends *Spectrum Suite* because, he says, it helps activate the body's natural ability to balance and heal itself. Many of the works are available in music stores. For mail-order information, refer to the resource list on page 642.

VITAMIN AND MINERAL THERAPY

Flaxseed oil is an essential fatty acid that could help people with CFS, says Michael A. Klaper, M.D., a nutritional medicine specialist in Pompano Beach, Florida, and director of the Institute of Nutritional Education and Research, an organization based in Manhattan Beach, California, that teaches doctors about nutrition and its relationship to disease. His advice: Take up to two teaspoons a day, along with a magnesium supplement of 400 milligrams. Flaxseed oil is available in liquid and capsule form in most health food stores. If you choose to take the capsules, Dr. Klaper suggests following the label directions for dosage, but keep in mind that about three capsules equals one teaspoon of the liquid.

Use the food sensitivity diet (see "Food Sensitivity: How to Discover the 'Healthy' Foods That Can Cause Disease" on page 52) to eliminate any foods that might have a role in causing chronic fatigue, suggests David Edelberg, M.D., an internist and medical director of the American Holistic Center/Chicago. He also says people with chronic fatigue may want to use the following nutritional regimen to help control the problem: one tablet of multi-amino acids three times a day; 2,000 milligrams of vitamin C twice a day; and 400 milligrams of magnesium aspartate a day. Multi-amino acids are available in most health food stores.

YOGA

Yoga gives more energy than it takes, so it's a perfect way to combat CFS, according to Alice Christensen, founder and executive director of the American Yoga Association. She recommends a daily routine that combines 5 minutes of the complete breath exercise (see page 152), 10 to 20 minutes of meditation (see page 153) and your choice of three or four yoga poses from the Daily Routine, which begins on page 606. The poses will push more oxygen through your system and release muscle tension, according to Christensen. And, she says, the meditation will teach you how to conserve energy and build self-confidence.

SEE ALSO Drowsiness; Fatigue

COLDS

We depend on other people for advice and companionship, laughter and support.

But if we hang around them long enough, they'll probably share something else: microscopic critters that, when coughed, sneezed or sniffled into our air space, can lead to acute rhinitis, or the common cold.

Caused by any of about 20 different viruses, colds are easier to get than knock knock jokes and easier still to give away.

While colds are usually no big deal, persistent symptoms can signal a more serious problem such as bronchitis or a sinus infection. The common cold, however, will usually run its course in 7 to 14 days. The natural remedies in this chapter, used with your doctor's approval, may help prevent a cold or relieve its symptoms, according to some health professionals.

SEE YOUR MEDICAL DOCTOR WHEN . . .

- You have trouble swallowing.
- You have no appetite.
- You cough up large amounts of sputum.
- Your sputum is bloody or greenish in color.
- You experience wheezing or shortness of breath.
- You have acute, burning pain in your ears, sinuses or chest.
- You have either a very high fever (over 103°F) or a moderately high fever (over 101°) that lasts for more than three days. Children with high fevers should see a doctor within 24 hours.

ACUPRESSURE

"Acupressure helps your body expel cold viruses more quickly, and it can provide relief from congestion and muscle aches," says Harriet Beinfield, L.Ac., co-author of *Between Heaven and Earth: A Guide to Chinese Medicine* and an acupuncturist at Chinese Medicine Works, a clinic and herb shop in San Francisco.

For a cold with a dry cough and fever, Beinfield suggests using pressure points in the depressions directly below the protrusions on the left and right sides of the collarbone (K 27), underneath the base of the skull, two inches out from the middle of your neck (GB 20), and at the outer edge of each elbow crease (LI 11). (To help locate these points, refer to the illustrations beginning on page 564.) To work these points, follow this sequence recommended by Michael Reed Gach, Ph.D., director of the Acupressure Institute in Berkeley, California, and author of *Acupressure's Potent Points*: Starting with K 27, press both points for one minute while breathing slowly and deeply. Move to GB 20 and press both points with the thumbs for one minute. Then move to LI 11, stimulating one of the points with the middle finger of your opposite hand for one minute before switching hands. Then return to K 27 and repeat the entire sequence. This should be done at least three times a day for maximum relief.

For sniffly, sneezy cold symptoms, Dr. Gach recommends one minute of pressure each on points in the webbing between the thumb and index finger (LI 4), on the face just beside the nostrils (LI 20) and in the upper ridges of the eye sockets, close to the bridge of the nose (B 2). (To help locate these points, refer to the illustrations beginning on page 564.) Dr. Gach cautions pregnant women to avoid pressure point LI 4, because stimulating this point can activate uterine contractions.

AROMATHERAPY

At the first sign of a cold, Los Angeles aromatic consultant John Steele turns on his aromatic diffuser. "Scenting a room with the right essences can alleviate the symptoms of a cold," says Steele. He favors exotic essences such as ravensare and niaouli for their natural anti-infectious and antiviral properties. Because these oils have strong, slightly medicinal smells, Steele often blends them with a sweeter-smelling oil such as rosewood, lemon, eucalyptus, pine or fir, all of which have an antiseptic effect. "The most important thing is to start using aromatics as soon as you start feeling run-down," says Steele. "In my experience, there is a very narrow window during which you can head off a cold before it starts."

For information on preparing and administering essential oils, including cautions about their use, see page 19. For information on purchasing essential oils, refer to the resource list on page 633.

AYURVEDA

Colds are a kapha-vata disorder, says Vasant Lad, B.A.M.S., M.A.Sc., director of the Ayurvedic Institute in Albuquerque, New Mexico. (For more information about the doshas of Ayurveda, see "All about Vata, Pitta and Kapha" on page 28.) He explains that you develop a cold when your body has an excess of kapha's cool, moist characteristics, causing a stuffy or runny nose and lots of sneezing. And, he says, excess vata energy reduces *agni*, or gastric fire, so you get the chills. But, according to Dr. Lad, ginger can reduce excess kapha and restore agni, making it "the best medicine for colds and flus."

Here is Dr. Lad's recipe for ginger tea: Add just under ½ teaspoon each of ginger powder, fennel seeds and cinnamon and a pinch of clove powder to one cup of hot water. Let the herbs steep for about ten minutes, then strain them out of the tea before drinking. Drink as much of the tea as you wish, Dr. Lad says.

Because aspirin and ginger are both blood thinners, Dr. Lad recommends drinking ginger tea at least two hours before or after you take a dose of aspirin.

FOOD THERAPY

Grapefruit is a great food for fighting a cold, says Paul Yanick, Ph.D., a research scientist in Milford, Pennsylvania. One reason is that it's high in vitamin C, according to Dr. Yanick. A lesser-known reason, he says, is that grapefruit helps detoxify the liver. "The liver is your front line to the immune system, and when immunity is impaired, you need something that's alkaline and not acidic to detoxify it," he says. All citrus fruits become alkaline when metabolized in the body, he explains, but oranges and other citrus fruits are too sweet to promote proper liver drainage, so you get much better detoxification from grapefruit. He recommends eating one or more grapefruit and their white bitter pulp each day to prevent colds and to build immunity.

HERBAL THERAPY

Garlic can help prevent colds and help reduce symptoms because it contains a potent antibiotic called allicin, which is released when cloves of garlic are chopped, crushed or chewed, says Varro E. Tyler, Ph.D., professor of pharmacognosy at Purdue University in West Lafayette, Indiana. You can add raw garlic to foods as a preventive measure, according to Dr. Tyler, or you can buy garlic supplements, which are available in most health food stores (and in many drugstores, too). He says the best supplemental form is enteric-coated capsules, which are easier for the body to absorb. He recommends that you follow label directions for dosage; a typical dosage is 300 milligrams daily for as long as symptoms persist, he adds.

HOMEOPATHY

If you have sinus congestion, a thick green nasal discharge, sensitivity to touch and pain in your cheekbones or on the bridge of your nose, then try a 30C dose of Kali bichromicum once or twice daily until you begin to feel better, says Judyth Reichenberg-Ullman, N.D., a naturopathic physician in Edmonds, Washington, and co-author of *The Patient's Guide to Homeopathic Medicine*. If you feel warm, feel better in fresh air, don't feel thirsty and are unusually emotional, try a 30C dose of Pulsatilla once or twice a day, she says. If you have a chest cold with a cough, are irritable and are thirsty to the point of gulping water, and if your sinuses feel raw, Dr. Reichenberg-Ullman recommends a 30C dose of Bryonia three times a day. On the other hand, if you feel restless, anxious, irritable and chilly, are thirsty but drink in sips and have a watery, burning nasal discharge, she advises taking a 30C dose of Arsenicum once or twice a day.

All of these homeopathic remedies are available in many health food stores. To purchase the remedies by mail, refer to the resource list on page 637.

HYDROTHERAPY

Hot baths and drinking plenty of water are two of the best and simplest water treatments for a cold, according to Charles Thomas, Ph.D., a physical therapist at Desert Springs Therapy Center in Desert Hot Springs, California, and co-author of *Hydrotherapy: Simple Treatments for Common Ailments*. Here's what he recommends: Fill your tub with comfortably hot water (about 102° to 104°F—you can use a regular thermometer to check) and submerge as much of your body as possible. Soak for about 15 minutes. Towel off, jump into a prewarmed bed and rest for at least one hour or longer (be sure to keep yourself warm, with your arms and legs well-covered). Dr. Thomas says to use this treatment one to three times every day until your symptoms subside.

Herbal steam treatments are a soothing way to treat the head congestion that can come with a cold, says Barre, Vermont, herbalist Rosemary Gladstar, author of *Herbal Healing for Women* and other books about herbs. Her advice: Heat a large pot of water to boiling. Then remove it from the heat source and drip a few drops of essential oil into it. (You can buy essential oils in most health food stores. Eucalyptus, sage and balsam are particularly good for cold congestion, Gladstar says.) Drape a bath towel over your head and breathe deeply for five to ten minutes. Do this two or three times a day until your symptoms subside.

JUICE THERAPY

"Fresh pineapple juice is wonderful for colds," says Eve Campanelli, Ph.D., a holistic family practitioner in Beverly Hills, California. "It's less allergenic than citrus and less acidic in the stomach, and it actually contains more vitamin C. It also breaks down mucus better." To treat a cold, she recommends drinking four to six ounces of juice (diluted with the same amount of water) at least four times a day.

For more information on juicing techniques, see page 93.

REFLEXOLOGY

Use the corresponding golf ball technique (page 588) to work the adrenal gland, head, throat and chest reflex points on both hands, say Kevin and Barbara Kunz, reflexology researchers in Sante Fe, New Mexico, and authors of *Hand and Foot Reflexology*. They also suggest working the head, throat and chest points on both feet.

To help you locate these points, consult the hand and foot reflex charts beginning on page 582. For instructions on how to work the points, see "Your Reflexology Session" on page 110.

SOUND THERAPY

Stress can lower your immune system and make you prone to colds, says Steven Halpern, Ph.D., composer, researcher and author of *Sound Health: The Music and Sounds That Make Us Whole*. To combat stress, he recommends spending at least 20 minutes each day listening to music that will relax you. To get started, he says, turn on the music, then sit or lie comfortably, close your eyes and take a deep breath. Dr. Halpern suggests that you wear headphones to focus your full attention and avoid distraction. He recommends, however, that you keep the speakers playing, so your body absorbs the sound energy. While the music plays, let your breath slow down and become steady. Listen not just to the notes but to the silence between the notes. This will keep you from analyzing the music, which will allow it to relax you.

Of the sources listed in "Sailing Away to Key Largo" on page 129, Dr. Halpern recommends *Seapeace*, *Spectrum Suite*, *Inner Peace*, *Comfort Zone* and any recording of Gregorian chants. Many of these are available in music stores. For mail-order information, refer to the resource list on page 642.

VITAMIN AND MINERAL THERAPY

A person with a cold may want to use the following vitamin, mineral and herbal supplements to help shorten the duration of the cold and reduce the severity of symptoms, says David Edelberg, M.D., an internist and medical director of the American Holistic Center/Chicago: 50,000 international units of vitamin A three times a day for no more than five days; 2,000 milligrams of vitamin C three times a day for no more than five days; two capsules of garlic three times a day; two capsules of echinacea three times a day (or, as a tincture, 15 drops four times a day); and 15 drops of lomatium tincture three times a day. For a sore throat, Dr. Edelberg says to try one zinc lozenge dissolved in the mouth every two to three hours or as needed. And to clear up nasal congestion, he suggests using steam inhalation (see "Hydrotherapy at Home" on page 78), adding eucalyptus oil to the water.

Garlic supplements, echinacea (in capsule and tincture form), lomatium tincture and eucalyptus oil are available in most health food stores.

YOGA

You can greatly reduce your chances of catching a cold if you do a yoga nasal wash, called *neti*, once a day, says Stephen A. Nezezon, M.D., yoga teacher and staff physician at the Himalayan International Institute of Yoga Science and Philosophy in Honesdale, Pennsylvania. Here's what Dr. Nezezon recommends: Start by filling a four-ounce paper cup halfway with warm water, then add ½ teaspoon of salt. Put a small crease in the lip of the cup so that it forms a spout. Slightly tilt your head back and to the left. Then slowly pour the water into your right nostril. The water will flow out of your left nostril or down the back of your throat if your left nostril is clogged. Spit out the water if it goes down your throat, or wipe the water from your face with a hand towel if it flows out of your left nostril. Fill the cup again, then repeat the procedure on the other side, pouring the water into your left nostril and tilting your head back and to the right so that the water flows out of your right nostril.

SEE ALSO Coughing; Fever; Sore Throat

COLD SORES

They're more conspicuous than painful. Short of wearing a pair of candy store wax lips or growing the quickest moustache on record, there's really no way to hide the angry red cold sore that has popped up on your lip. Cold sores, also known as fever blisters, are small red lesions that appear on the lips, the nostrils and sometimes the gums or the roof of the mouth. Cold sores are caused by the herpes simplex virus known as type 1 (as opposed to the type 2 virus, which causes genital herpes). The virus is so contagious that about 90 percent of all Americans are exposed to it by age five. Once you're infected, the virus lies dormant in your body until a cold or fever triggers a flare-up.

Sunshine and extreme temperatures can also bring on a cold sore, so wear a lip balm containing sunscreen, and protect your nose and mouth from the cold with a scarf. The natural remedies in this chapter—used in conjunction with medical care and with your doctor's approval—may help prevent cold sores or speed their healing, according to some health professionals.

SEE YOUR MEDICAL DOCTOR WHEN . . .

- You get four or more cold sores a year.
- You experience fever, swollen glands or flulike symptoms with a cold sore.
- Your cold sore is so painful that you have trouble eating or carrying out normal activities.

AROMATHERAPY

To help speed the healing of cold sores, Los Angeles aromatherapist Michael Scholes, of Aromatherapy Seminars, an organization that trains professionals and others in the use of essential oils, suggests the following essential oils: tea tree, bergamot, geranium, rose and melissa. He says to apply a single drop of any one of these oils first thing in the morning and again at bedtime.

For information on preparing and administering essential oils, including cautions about their use, see page 19. For information on purchasing essential oils, refer to the resource list on page 633.

FOOD THERAPY

Eat more yogurt, recommends registered pharmacist Earl Mindell, R.Ph., Ph.D., professor of nutrition at Pacific Western University in Los Angeles and author of *Earl Mindell's Food as Medicine* and other books on nutrition. "The acidophilus in the live cultures acts as a natural antibiotic to the virus that causes cold sores," he says.

Dr. Mindell also points out that certain foods may trigger cold sores because they contain arginine, an amino acid that the herpes virus needs to thrive. Arginine-rich foods include cola, chocolate, peanuts and cashews, gelatin, beer and peas. So if you're prone to cold sores, Dr. Mindell advises that you limit your intake of these foods—and eliminate them completely during an outbreak.

HERBAL THERAPY

Europeans depend on lemon balm ointment to treat cold sores caused by the herpes simplex virus, says Varro E. Tyler, Ph.D., professor of pharmacognosy at Purdue University in West Lafayette, Indiana. The leaves and flower tops of this fragrant plant have antibacterial and antiviral properties, according to Dr. Tyler. You can't ordinarily buy the ointment that Europeans use in the United States, he explains, but you can get similar results by treating cold sores with a wash made from strong lemon balm tea.

To make the tea, says Dr. Tyler, pour ½ cup of boiling water over two to three teaspoons of finely cut dried leaves, available in most health food stores. Let the mixture steep for 20 to 30 minutes, he says, then strain the solution so that there's no dried herb left in the tea and let the tea cool. To apply, Dr. Tyler suggests dipping a clean cotton cloth into the tea and dabbing it on the cold sore three or four times daily.

HOMEOPATHY

Use a damp cotton swab to apply two or three drops of a 10 percent tincture of Calendula to the sore as needed, says Mitchell Fleisher, M.D., a family practice physician and homeopath in Colleen, Virginia.

Calendula is available in many health food stores. To purchase homeopathic remedies by mail, refer to the resource list on page 637.

HYDROTHERAPY

As soon as you feel a cold sore emerging, rub an ice cube over the area for ten minutes three times a day, suggests Agatha Thrash, M.D., a medical pathologist and co-founder and co-director of Uchee Pines Institute, a natural healing center in Seale, Alabama. If you treat the cold sore early on, you may be able to prevent it from erupting, according to Dr. Thrash.

COLD SORES

IMAGERY

You can speed the healing of a cold sore if you imagine that a soothing light penetrates the sore and heals it from the bottom up (that's how cold sores heal naturally), says Dennis Gersten, M.D., a San Diego psychiatrist and publisher of *Atlantis*, a bi-monthly imagery newsletter. He suggests doing this for five minutes twice a day until the sore heals.

SOUND THERAPY

Because stress can lead to cold sores, try listening to 20 to 30 minutes of relaxing music every day, says Steven Halpern, Ph.D., composer, researcher and author of *Sound Health: The Music and Sounds That Make Us Whole.* To get started, turn on the music, then sit or lie comfortably, close your eyes and take a deep breath. Dr. Halpern suggests that you wear headphones to focus your full attention and avoid distraction. He recommends, however, that you keep the speakers playing, so your body absorbs the sound energy. While the music plays, let your breath slow down and become steady. Listen not just to the notes but to the silence between the notes. Dr. Halpern says this will keep you from analyzing the music, which will allow it to relax you.

For suggested pieces to relax by, see "Sailing Away to Key Largo" on page 129. Dr. Halpern especially recommends *Spectrum Suite* because, he says, it helps activate the body's natural ability to balance and heal itself. Many of the pieces are available in music stores. For mail-order information, refer to the resource list on page 642.

VITAMIN AND MINERAL THERAPY

If you get three or more cold sores a year, you might benefit from a daily supplement of lysine, an amino acid that counteracts arginine, an amino acid that the herpes virus needs to thrive, says Richard D. Fischer, D.D.S., president of the International Academy of Oral Medicine and Toxicology and a dentist in Annandale, Virginia. "I recommend taking two 500-milligram tablets with each meal during an outbreak and then dropping down to one 500-milligram tablet per meal after your cold sore heals as a preventive measure," says Dr. Fischer.

YOGA

Cold sores often arise during stressful times, says Stephen A. Nezezon, M.D., yoga teacher and staff physician at the Himalayan International Institute of Yoga Science and Philosophy in Honesdale, Pennsylvania. To lower stress, you can do a daily routine of breathing exercises, meditation and poses, suggests Dr. Nezezon.

Do the complete breath exercise (see page 152) whenever you're feeling stress, whether it's at the office, in the car or at home, suggests Alice Christensen, founder and executive director of the American Yoga Association. Daily meditation (see page 153) helps clear your mind and teaches you to relax at will, she says. For the poses, choose three or four from the Daily Routine, which begins on page 606. Make sure to vary the poses every day rather than doing the same three or four day after day; this will keep your interest high and strengthen different parts of your body, according to Christensen. Dr. Nezezon says you should include at least one relaxation pose, such as the corpse (page 612), knee squeeze (page 612) or baby (page 618), in your routine.

CONJUNCTIVITIS

It's as much a childhood rite of passage as lost baby teeth. But while an outbreak of conjunctivitis, or pinkeye, can whip through a second-grade classroom like nobody's business, kids aren't the only ones who fall victim to it.

Conjunctivitis is an inflammation of the delicate membrane that lines the eyelid and covers the eyeball, causing redness and irritation. While similar symptoms can be triggered by an allergy or injury to the eye, most cases are caused by a bacterial or viral infection, which is highly contagious.

Conjunctivitis usually goes away on its own in about a week. The real trick is to avoid passing it from one family member to the next. Wash your hands often with an antibacterial soap and keep them away from your eyes. And if you're a contact wearer, be sure not to wear them during an outbreak of conjunctivitis. The natural remedies in this chapter—used in conjunction with medical care and with your doctor's approval—may help ease the symptoms of conjunctivitis, according to some health professionals.

SEE YOUR MEDICAL DOCTOR WHEN . . .

- Your eye has been injured and is red.
- Your vision changes.
- Your eyes give off a greenish or yellow discharge.
- You show no improvement within five days.

HOMEOPATHY

Try Apis, a honeybee venom extract that is particularly good for swollen eyes that sting and burn, says Judyth Reichenberg-Ullman, N.D., a naturopathic physician in Edmonds, Washington, and co-author of *The Patient's Guide to Homeopathic Medicine*. She recommends taking a 30C dose once or twice a day until you begin to feel better. She also says that holding a cold washcloth to the eyes for ten minutes after taking Apis may help reduce the swelling.

Apis is available in many health food stores. To purchase homeopathic remedies by mail, refer to the resource list on page 637.

HYDROTHERAPY

Rinse your eyes with an eyewash made from a teaspoon of salt and a pint of boiled water and cooled before being put in the eyes, writes Charles Thomas, Ph.D., co-author of *Hydrotherapy: Simple Treatments for Common Ailments* and a physical therapist at Desert Springs Therapy Center in Desert Hot Springs, California. He suggests repeating this treatment every few hours.

Dr. Thomas also recommends another treatment: alternating hot and cold compresses to the eye area, with three to four minutes of the hot application, followed by 20 to 30 seconds of cold. He says you can use the compresses one to three times a day either by themselves or as part of a treatment program that includes the eyewash.

IMAGERY

Close your eyes, breathe out three times and imagine yourself standing in a large, open field of green grass on a beautiful day, writes New York City psychiatrist Gerald Epstein, M.D., in his book *Healing Visualizations*. Envision stretching up toward the sun. Notice that your arms are becoming very long as you reach, palms up, into the sky. The sun's rays seep into your palms and circulate through the palms and fingers and beyond the fingertips so that there is a ray beyond each fingertip. If you are right-handed, see a small hand at the end of each ray of the fingertips of your right hand and five small eyes at the end of each ray of the fingertips of your left hand (if you're left-handed, reverse the order).

Turn these small eyes and hands toward your eyelid. Use the small eyes to help you see what the small hands are doing. Take a golden feather in one of your small hands and clean out all of the redness and inflammation from the conjunctiva, the delicate membrane lining the eyelid. With another small hand, shine a blue laser light along the conjunctiva that you've just cleansed. Picture the conjunctiva healing. Open your eyes and breathe out.

Do this exercise three times daily, one to two minutes a session, for 21 days, says Dr. Epstein.

REFLEXOLOGY

Work the eye, neck and kidney reflexes on your hands or feet, says St. Petersburg, Florida, reflexologist Dwight Byers, author of *Better Health with Foot Reflexology*. Byers also recommends working all of the points on the sides and bottoms of the toes on both feet, using whichever technique you find most comfortable.

To help you locate these points, consult the hand and foot reflex charts beginning on page 582. For instructions on how to work the points, see "Your Reflexology Session" on page 110.

CONSTIPATION

Judging from the number of laxative commercials on television, Americans must be in the throes of an epidemic.

Nobody needs to tell you what constipation is. Besides the obvious, there are headaches, abdominal pain and a full, bloated feeling to suffer through. While many people don't have bowel movements every day, having fewer than three a week or passing small, hard stools usually signals a problem.

While constipation is rarely serious, it usually means you've been depriving your body of essential stuff such as water, dietary fiber and adequate exercise. A long-term solution to constipation can be as simple as a daily walk and a few dietary changes. The natural remedies in this chapter, used with your doctor's approval, may help prevent or relieve constipation, according to some health professionals.

SEE YOUR MEDICAL DOCTOR WHEN . . .

- Your symptoms last for more than three weeks in spite of extra fiber, fluids and exercise.
- You notice blood in your stool.
- Your constipation is accompanied by severe abdominal pain.

CONSTIPATION

ACUPRESSURE

When proper eating and exercise fail to relieve constipation, try these acupressure points to relax the abdomen, reduce discomfort and encourage regular bowel movements, says Michael Reed Gach, Ph.D., director of the Acupressure Institute in Berkeley, California, and author of *Acupressure's Potent Points*. While lying down comfortably, press CV 6, the Sea of Energy point, which is found three finger-widths below the navel. Close your eyes and breathe deeply as you use all of your fingertips to apply gradual pressure. Dr. Gach suggests pressing the point for two minutes.

You can also press each LI 11 point, situated at the outer edge of the elbow crease, says Dr. Gach. He recommends holding one LI 11 point for a half-minute, then switching to the other side. Repeat this remedy three times a day, he adds.

For help in locating the CV 6 and LI 11 points, refer to the illustrations beginning on page 564.

AROMATHERAPY

Try a gentle abdominal massage to stimulate elimination, says Greenwich, Connecticut, aromatherapist Judith Jackson in her book *Scentual Touch: A Personal Guide to Aromatherapy*. She says to add six drops each of rosemary and thyme essential oils to one ounce of a carrier oil such as olive or almond. (Carrier oils are available in most health food stores.) Massage the stomach area up the right side, across the top and down the left in a circular motion, she suggests.

For information on preparing and administering essential oils, including cautions about their use, see page 19. For information on purchasing essential oils, refer to the resource list on page 633.

AYURVEDA

There are three types of constipation: mild, medium and hard, says Vasant Lad, B.A.M.S., M.A.Sc., director of the Ayurvedic Institute in Albuquerque, New Mexico. According to Dr. Lad, each type of constipation corresponds to one of the Ayurvedic doshas. (For more information about the doshas, see "All about Vata, Pitta and Kapha" on page 28.)

Pitta constipation is usually mild and is easily cured by increasing physical exercise and adding more fiber to the diet, explains Dr. Lad.

Medium, or kapha, constipation is a little more intense, says Dr. Lad, but usually responds to the use of this mild laxative: Stir a teaspoonful of ghee, or clarified butter (see "How to Make Ghee" on page 26 for the recipe), into a glass of warm milk and drink at bedtime. Senna leaf tea is another remedy for medium constipation, he adds. (You can find senna leaf tea in most health food stores.)

For hard or chronic constipation, which Ayurveda says is caused by a low gastric fire (*agni*) and an excess of vata dosha, the most reliable long-term cure is triphala, says Dr. Lad. One of the best-known and most popular Ayurvedic herbal remedies, triphala combines the fruits of three tropical trees: amalaki, haritaki and bibhitaki. Together, these herbs stimulate digestion and aid elimination, according to Dr. Lad.

To use triphala, says Dr. Lad, mix ½ teaspoon of the powder with one cup of warm water and drink it a half-hour before bedtime. He says not to eat after drinking the tea. Used regularly, triphala will cure constipation and keep it from returning—or it can be used regularly to prevent constipation and keep your digestive system running smoothly, says Dr. Lad. Triphala is available in Indian pharmacies and some health food stores; to order by mail, refer to the resource list on page 634.

FOOD THERAPY

"A high-fiber diet is the answer for constipation," says Julian Whitaker, M.D., founder and president of the Whitaker Wellness Center in Newport Beach, California. Most Americans eat only between 11 and 18 grams of fiber a day, he explains, but experts say that if you're constipated, you should shoot for more than 35 grams, the amount you'd get from eating five servings of fresh fruits and vegetables as well as a heaping serving of high-fiber cereal, such as oat or wheat bran, each day. Most fruits are high in fiber, as are prunes, whole grains such as rice and oatmeal and legumes such as lentils and garbanzo beans.

Chronic constipation may be caused by congestion in the elimination system, says Elson Haas, M.D., director of the Preventive Medical Center of Marin in San Rafael, California, and author of *Staying Healthy with Nutrition*. He recommends unclogging your system with his three-week detoxification diet (see "Detoxing Your Ills" on page 48).

HERBAL THERAPY

Cascara sagrada, prepared from the bark of a small tree native to the Pacific Northwest, is the best herbal remedy for constipation, says Varro E. Tyler, Ph.D., professor of pharmacognosy at Purdue University in West Lafayette, Indiana. You can find the most effective form of the herb, cascara aromatic fluid extract, in most health food stores. The average dosage is one gram (about ½ teaspoon) daily, says Dr. Tyler. He suggests following label directions for dosage.

HOMEOPATHY

If you have hemorrhoids and develop constipation along with a full feeling in your stomach or abdominal cramping that is temporarily relieved by passing gas, try Graphites, suggests Cynthia Mervis Watson, M.D., a family practice physician specializing in homeopathic and herbal therapies in Santa Monica, California. If you alternate between feeling constipated and having diarrhea and suspect that it may be caused by anxiety or medication, Dr. Watson suggests Nux vomica. And if your belly is bloated, your stools are hard and dry, you have a painful anus after defecating and you feel depressed and run-down, try Natrum muriaticum, she says. For each of these remedies, Dr. Watson says to take either a 6X dose three or four times a day or one 30C dose once a day.

Graphites, Nux vomica and Natrum muriaticum are available in many health food stores. To purchase homeopathic remedies by mail, refer to the resource list on page 637.

HYDROTHERAPY

Constipation is often a sign that you're not drinking enough water, says Agatha Thrash, M.D., a medical pathologist and co-founder and co-director of Uchee Pines Institute, a natural healing center in Seale, Alabama. Along with proper diet and exercise, drinking 8 to 12 eight-ounce glasses of water a day is often enough to cure constipation for life, according to Dr. Thrash.

When constipation does occur, Dr. Thrash often recommends a hot enema to stimulate the bowel reflex. (For instructions, see "How to Perform an Enema" on page 76.) She cautions that children under ten years of age should not be given more than one enema a day, since water can be absorbed and can cause blood sodium to drop dangerously low (a condition called hyponatremia).

JUICE THERAPY

Start the day with an eight- to ten-ounce blend of equal parts apple, fresh ginger, beet and carrot juices or an eight-ounce blend of equal parts apple and pear juices (dilute with a little water if it's too sweet), says Cherie Calbom, M.S., a certified nutritionist in Kirkland, Washington, and co-author of *Juicing for Life.* "Apple juice contains sorbitol, a natural sugar with laxative properties," explains Calbom.

And because a folate deficiency can aggravate constipation, Calbom also recommends eating or juicing dark green leafy vegetables such as parsley, spinach and asparagus, all excellent sources of this nutrient.

For more information on juicing techniques, see page 93.

MASSAGE

In her book *The Magic of Massage*, massage therapist Ouida West recommends the leg rub (page 578) to relieve constipation. West recommends doing the massage before attempting a bowel movement as well as once in the morning and once in the evening. Be sure to massage up the thigh, from the knee to the hip.

You can also use Swedish massage, says Elliot Greene, past president of the American Massage Therapy Association. Lightly lubricate your hands with vegetable oil. Then lie on your back and begin massaging your abdominal area. Using your palms or fingertips, press in lightly and stroke down the left side of your abdomen (toward your feet). Then move your hands to the right side of your abdomen, just below the ribs, and stroke across your abdomen to the left. Finally, starting on the right side just below navel level, stroke upward along the abdomen (toward your head). Do this for five to ten minutes.

REFLEXOLOGY

Use the corresponding golf ball technique (page 588) to work the adrenal gland and digestive system points on both hands, say Kevin and Barbara Kunz, reflexology researchers in Santa Fe, New Mexico, and authors of *Hand and Foot Reflexology*. Since constipation can be triggered by tension and lower back stress, they also suggest working the lower back and tailbone points on both feet and the solar plexus points on both hands.

To help you locate these points, consult the hand and foot reflex charts beginning on page 582. For instructions on how to work the points, see "Your Reflexology Session" on page 110.

RELAXATION AND MEDITATION

When you feel constipated, try doing autogenics for 15 minutes two or three times a day, suggests Martin Shaffer, Ph.D., executive director of the Stress Management Institute in San Francisco and author of *Life after Stress*. Practicing this relaxation technique longer but less frequently than what is normally recommended (two minutes, ten times a day) has a powerful physiological effect on the digestive system and may get your bowels moving quickly, he explains. To learn how to do autogenics, see page 120.

SOUND THERAPY

Some people find relief from constipation by listening to relaxation tapes, says Janalea Hoffman, R.M.T., a composer and music therapist based in Kansas

City, Missouri. Slow, steady music helps release tension that can subconsciously lead to constipation, according to Hoffman. She suggests her own tape, called *Musical Acupuncture*. For other selections, see "Sailing Away to Key Largo" on page 129. Many of these pieces are available in music stores. For mail-order information, refer to the resource list on page 642.

VITAMIN AND MINERAL THERAPY

The nutrients vitamin C and magnesium can help keep you regular, says Julian Whitaker, M.D., founder and president of the Whitaker Wellness Center in Newport Beach, California. "In fact, in Germany, they actually sell powdered vitamin C as a laxative," he says. His advice: Take at least 500 milligrams of vitamin C and 400 milligrams of magnesium in supplement form every day to prevent constipation. When constipation occurs, he says to increase the dosages for both nutrients by 100-milligram increments each day until you get relief, up to a maximum of 5,000 milligrams of vitamin C and 1,000 milligrams of magnesium. Go back to the preventive dosages once the problem has cleared, he says. If you develop diarrhea, he adds, decrease the amount of vitamin C to 500 milligrams.

YOGA

The spine twist (page 614) can help with constipation, says Stephen A. Nezezon, M.D., yoga teacher and staff physician at the Himalayan International Institute of Yoga Science and Philosophy in Honesdale, Pennsylvania. He says to try to practice the pose every day if you frequently have problems with constipation.

COUGHING

While a person hacking away doesn't sound particularly healthy, coughing is actually quite beneficial. It is the body's instinctive, highly effective way of keeping the lungs and airways clear.
Coughing flushes out mucus when we've caught colds and helps us catch our breath when food or drink takes a wrong turn. There's also the famous, dangerous "smoker's cough," a seemingly inevitable consequence of years on the pack that can signal serious problems. The natural remedies in this chapter—used in conjunction with medical care and with your doctor's approval—may help relieve coughing and its symptoms, according to some health professionals.

SEE YOUR MEDICAL DOCTOR WHEN . . .

- Your cough is accompanied by shortness of breath.
- You cough up phlegm tinged with blood.
- Your phlegm is very thick and won't come up easily.
- You develop a persistent, hacking cough on top of another illness.
- Your cough lasts for more than one week.

ACUPRESSURE

Acupressure on the chest can help relax the body and relieve coughing, says Michael Reed Gach, Ph.D., director of the Acupressure Institute in Berkeley, California, and author of *Acupressure's Potent Points*. With the middle fingers of both hands, press the K 27 points, situated in the depressions directly below the protrusions on the left and right sides of the collarbone. (For help in locating these points, refer to the illustration on page 564.) Dr. Gach says to continue pressing for a few minutes until the cough subsides.

AYURVEDA

For a cough with a hoarse voice, mix ¼ teaspoon of black pepper into 1 teaspoon of ghee, or clarified butter, and take the mixture on a full stomach, says Vasant Lad, B.A.M.S., M.A.Sc., director of the Ayurvedic Institute in Albuquerque, New Mexico. (See "How to Make Ghee" on page 26 for the recipe for ghee.) For a cough without hoarseness, Dr. Lad says to mix ¼ teaspoon of black pepper with 1 teaspoon of honey, also taking the mixture on a full stomach. Take the appropriate mixture three times a day for three to five days.

Pepper may not seem like a throat-soothing remedy, but when it's mixed with ghee, Dr. Lad says it helps coat the throat and restore balance to the lungs. Black pepper is also pungent and heating, he says, helping rid the body of mucus. (Taken more frequently or in larger amounts, however, it may actually increase mucus instead, according to Dr. Lad.) And, he explains, pepper increases pitta energy, which helps push out hoarseness and cough. (See "All about Vata, Pitta and Kapha" on page 28 for information about the doshas of Ayurveda.)

HERBAL THERAPY

Most cough drops contain oils from herbs, including eucalyptus, peppermint, anise and fennel, says Varro E. Tyler, Ph.D., professor of pharmacognosy at Purdue University in West Lafayette, Indiana. According to Dr. Tyler, these herbs stop coughing by increasing the production of saliva, which makes you swallow more frequently, suppressing the cough reflex. He says you can get similar results by drinking a tea made from one of these herbs, which you can purchase in most health food stores. To make a tea, steep one to two teaspoons of the herb in a cup of boiling water for 3 to 15 minutes, depending on the part of the plant you're using. (For roots, steep 15 minutes; for seeds, steep 10 to 15 minutes; and for leaves, steep 3 to 10 minutes.) Then strain the mixture to remove the dried herb, let the tea cool to a drinkable temperature and drink. Dr. Tyler says you can drink three to four cups a day of any of these teas, sipping it slowly throughout the day at 15- to 30-minute intervals. If you're using a tea bag, follow the dosage recommendations on the product.

Slippery elm is another anti-cough herb, says Dr. Tyler, but it stops the cough reflex by forming a protective and soothing layer around the irritated mucous membranes of your throat. You can find slippery elm teas and lozenges in most health food stores. Dr. Tyler recommends following the dosage recommendations on the label of the product you buy.

A few other anti-cough herbs are what herbalists call expectorants—that is, the herbs thin the cough-causing mucus, so you can expectorate (spit, to us nonherbalists) it out any way you choose. Horehound is probably the most effective and best tasting of these herbs, according to Dr. Tyler, and many people use horehound hard candies as cough lozenges. You can also find horehound tea bags in most health food stores.

HOMEOPATHY

Go for a combination remedy called Chestal, suggests Mitchell Fleisher, M.D., a family practitioner and homeopath in Colleen, Virginia. "It's a good combination remedy to try because all of the remedies in it are well-indicated for a typical cough," he explains. He says to take Chestal according to the directions on the product label.

Or try one of the following 30C remedies that best fits your individual symptoms, says Judyth Reichenberg-Ullman, N.D., a naturopathic physician in Edmonds, Washington, and co-author of *The Patient's Guide to Homeopathic Medicine.* If you have a dry, raspy cough that is worsened by talking or drinking cold beverages, Dr. Reichenberg-Ullman suggests taking Spongia tosta once or twice daily until you begin to feel better. She says Drosera, also taken once or twice daily, is another good remedy that can relieve a gagging, spasmodic cough that is worsened by eating or drinking. And if you have a cough that causes a tickle in your throat and seems to get worse when you lie down, she recommends trying Rumex once or twice daily.

All of these homeopathic remedies are available in many health food stores. To purchase the remedies by mail, refer to the resource list on page 637.

HYDROTHERAPY

Inhaling steam relieves throat irritation and loosens mucus in the lungs, according to Charles Thomas, Ph.D., a physical therapist at the Desert Springs Therapy Center in Desert Hot Springs, California, and co-author of *Hydrotherapy: Simple Treatments for Common Ailments.* Here's his recommendation for a steam treatment that you should do two to four times a day until your cough subsides: Begin with a pot full of boiling water. Take the pot off the stove and let it cool, so no active boiling is taking place (if the water is actively boiling, you can scald your face and respiratory tract). Hold your face about a foot away from the pot, and cover your head and shoulders with a towel to trap the steam. Inhale for up to 30 minutes. You can also add a few drops of eucalyptus oil to the water for a soothing effect, according to Dr. Thomas. Eucalyptus oil is available in most health food stores.

CUTS, SCRAPES AND SCRATCHES

If you're like most people, your knees are covered with faded reminders of those early years of living dangerously.

Most of us eventually outgrow the habit of falling on our knees or elbows or faces. But with adulthood comes access to all manner of sharp objects, from razors to steak knives. So unless you're highly coordinated and very careful, odds are good that you'll have to contend with the occasional flesh wound. The natural remedies in this chapter, used with the approval of your doctor, may relieve pain and help your wound heal faster, according to some health professionals.

SEE YOUR MEDICAL DOCTOR WHEN . . .

- The cut is very dirty and you have trouble getting it clean.
- Blood is spurting out of the wound. You may have cut an artery.
- The wound is on the face or anywhere else you want to avoid a permanent scar.
- The cut is large and open. You may need stitches.
- You see pus forming on or around the wound.
- The wound develops red streaks or a red area that extends more than a finger-width beyond the edge of the cut.

AROMATHERAPY

Lavender, a multipurpose first-aid oil, helps heal virtually any kind of superficial wound, says Los Angeles aromatherapist Michael Scholes, of Aromatherapy Seminars, an organization that trains professionals and others in the use of essential oils. He recommends applying a drop or two of lavender directly to the skin after the wound is cleaned.

For information on preparing and administering essential oils, including cautions about their use, see page 19. For information on purchasing essential oils, refer to the resource list on page 633.

FOOD THERAPY

"For quicker relief of minor scrapes and scratches, put some cayenne pepper on them—but not on open wounds," advises Julian Whitaker, M.D., founder and president of the Whitaker Wellness Center in Newport Beach, California. According to Dr. Whitaker, cayenne contains capsaicin, the active ingredient that puts the hot in hot peppers and that helps speed healing and block pain messages to the brain. He recommends dabbing a little cayenne pepper on the scrape, then wiping it off when the pain is lessened. Cayenne pepper could cause pain on open wounds, he cautions.

For open wounds or skin ulcerations, Dr. Whitaker suggests sprinkling on granulated sugar to help kill bacteria and speed healing. He says to smear a ring of petroleum jelly around the edges of the wound to hold the sugar in place, then put a little sugar directly on the wound. Cover the area with a bandage, he says, and be sure to change the bandage once or twice a day.

Herbal Therapy

Keep an aloe vera plant on your windowsill—it's a living first-aid kit, says Varro E. Tyler, Ph.D., professor of pharmacognosy at Purdue University in West Lafayette, Indiana. When you get a cut, scratch or scrape, suggests Dr. Tyler, just break off one of the plant's fleshy leaves, squeeze out a little of the cool, colorless gel from the center of the leaf and apply it directly to the affected area. Reapply three or four times a day for maximum healing, he says. He adds that aloe vera seals off the injury, relieves pain and helps cuts and scrapes heal more quickly.

Homeopathy

Cleanse the wound with soap and water, then apply Calendula ointment, says Mitchell Fleisher, M.D., a family practice physician and homeopath in Colleen, Virginia. "If it's a painful scrape or abrasion, what I find works excellently is to wash the wound well with a mixture of 20 drops of Calendula tincture and 20 drops of Hypericum tincture diluted in four ounces of water," he says. Then apply a sterile dressing moistened with this mixture two or three times a day until the wound has healed, says Dr. Fleisher.

These homeopathic remedies are available in many health food stores. To purchase the remedies by mail, refer to the resource list on page 637.

DANDRUFF

You've tried washing your hair and not washing it. You've tried blow-drying and not blow-drying. You've tried every shampoo, conditioner, oil treatment, comb, brush and miracle salve known to man. And you still can't wear your favorite black blazer because of that stubborn dandruff.

It seems like such a simple problem to solve. After all, dandruff is nothing more than skin cells flaking off your scalp. Still, the condition has long defied treatment. Researchers believe dandruff may be caused by a yeastlike fungus on your scalp, though they haven't figured out a foolproof way to beat it. For now, most experts suggest shampoos that contain zinc pyrithione or selenium sulfide. And the natural remedies in this chapter, used with your doctor's approval, may help prevent or relieve dandruff, according to some health professionals.

SEE YOUR MEDICAL DOCTOR WHEN . . .

- You have severe dandruff despite using a dandruff shampoo.
- You have red patches on your scalp, especially along the neckline.
- You notice yellowish crusting on your head.

AROMATHERAPY

In her book *Aromatherapy: Applications and Inhalations*, San Francisco herbalist Jeanne Rose, chairperson of the National Association for Holistic Aromatherapy, suggests an aromatic formula to treat dandruff. After using a dandruff shampoo, she says, let your hair dry thoroughly and pour a few drops each of rosemary and lemon essential oils into your palms. Massage the oils into your scalp and brush your hair with a soft brush, she says.

For information on preparing and administering essential oils, including cautions about their use, see page 19. For information on purchasing essential oils, refer to the resource list on page 633.

AYURVEDA

Dandruff may be a sign that circulation is blocked, says David Frawley, O.M.D., director of the American Institute of Vedic Studies in Santa Fe, New Mexico. He recommends massaging the scalp with sesame oil (available in most health food stores) for five to ten minutes once a week, applying the oil before your evening shower and then washing it out in the shower.

The herb fenugreek is also an Ayurvedic remedy for dandruff, according to Dr. Frawley. He suggests using it in cooking or taking a teaspoonful daily, mixed with honey. Fenugreek works best for people with vata or kapha doshas, he explains, and is less effective for pittas. (For more information about the Ayurvedic doshas, see "All about Vata, Pitta and Kapha" on page 28.)

FOOD THERAPY

"Dandruff is not something you should treat with shampoo. You should treat it with diet," says Michael A. Klaper, M.D., a nutritional medicine specialist in Pompano Beach, Florida, and director of the Institute of Nutritional Education and Research, an organization based in Manhattan Beach, California, that teaches physicians about nutrition and its relationship to disease. "Part of the reason dandruff occurs is that skin oils in the scalp are thick and acidic, largely from a diet of saturated fat," Dr. Klaper explains. "Thick secretions of skin and dried oil flake off—that's what dandruff is. But if you get a person to clean up his diet by eliminating the junk food, animal fats and heavy plant oils such as palm and coconut and to eat more of the good fats that are found in nuts and seeds, dandruff often improves greatly or disappears."

HOMEOPATHY

Several homeopathic remedies can help you shake off dandruff, according to Andrew Lockie, M.D., author of *The Family Guide to Homeopathy*. In his book, Dr. Lockie suggests taking one of the following 6C remedies three times a day for up to two weeks. If your dandruff is thick, you scratch your head a lot at night, your scalp burns and washing your hair makes your scalp even drier, try Sulphur, he says. If there are moist, smelly spots behind your ears, your itching is worsened by heat and you feel as if there were insect bites along the hairline of your forehead, he says Oleander may be the remedy for you. He also says that Sepia will help soothe a scalp that is moist, greasy and sensitive near the hair roots.

Sulphur, Oleander and Sepia are available in many health food stores. To purchase homeopathic remedies by mail, refer to the resource list on page 637.

VITAMIN AND MINERAL THERAPY

To help stop dandruff, try supplementing your diet with flaxseed oil, says Michael A. Klaper, M.D., a nutritional medicine specialist in Pompano Beach, Florida, and director of the Institute of Nutritional Education and Research, an organization based in Manhattan Beach, California, that teaches doctors about nutrition and its relationship to disease. Adding flaxseed oil to your diet can cut down on skin oil secretions, which flake and cause dandruff, he says. He recommends taking one to two teaspoons a day of flaxseed oil. Flaxseed oil is also sold in capsule form, and about three capsules equals one teaspoon of the liquid. Both forms can be found in most health food stores.

DEPRESSION

There's a big difference between sadness and depression. Everyone feels sad now and then, such as when the family dog dies or a romantic relationship falls apart.

But depression is far more serious. It's a clinical psychological condition marked by extreme feelings of dejection, lack of confidence and melancholy. Unlike sadness or temporary feelings of grief, depression lingers. Depression also takes a financial toll, costing $44 billion a year in treatment and lost productivity.

Experts believe that one in ten men and one in four women will suffer from severe depression at some point in their lives. Drugs and psychotherapy may be the treatments you're most familiar with. But the natural remedies in this chapter—used in conjunction with medical care and with your doctor's approval—may help relieve some of the symptoms of depression, according to some health professionals.

SEE YOUR MEDICAL DOCTOR WHEN . . .

- You experience at least four of these symptoms for at least two weeks.

  Feelings of guilt, worthlessness and/or helplessness
  Thoughts of death or suicide
  Restlessness or irritability
  Difficulty concentrating, remembering or making decisions
  Decreased energy or fatigue
  Loss of interest in ordinary activities, including sex
  Persistent sadness, anxiousness or emptiness
  Sleep problems, including insomnia, oversleeping or waking up
    too early
  Changes in appetite or weight gain/loss
  Feelings of hopelessness or pessimism

DEPRESSION

ACUPRESSURE

Acupressure can help calm and balance your emotions during times of distress, says Michael Reed Gach, Ph.D., director of the Acupressure Institute in Berkeley, California, and author of *Acupressure's Potent Points*. He suggests pressing the B 38 points, located between the shoulder blades and the spine, at the level of the heart. (For help in locating these points, refer to the illustration on page 565.) To apply pressure on these points, Dr. Gach says to lie on your back, placing two tennis balls on the floor underneath your upper back between your shoulder blades. (If you wish, place a thick towel, folded in half, over the tennis balls, he says.) Then close your eyes and breathe deeply for a few minutes.

AROMATHERAPY

Inhaling an uplifting scent is a wonderful therapy, says Los Angeles aromatic consultant John Steele. He recommends floral oils such as rose, jasmine, neroli, melissa and ylang ylang and citrus oils such as grapefruit, lime, mandarin and bergamot. "Choose one that appeals to you," Steele says. "If you have a bad association with a particular fragrance, it may only make matters worse." He suggests inhaling the fragrance directly from the bottle, adding three or four drops of your favorite to a tissue or handkerchief and inhaling or adding six to ten drops to a warm bath. For a massage, he says, use ten drops of any one of these oils.

For information on preparing and administering essential oils, including cautions about their use, see page 19. For information on purchasing essential oils, refer to the resource list on page 633.

AYURVEDA

Vata depression is associated with fear and anxiety; pitta, with fear of failure, losing control or making mistakes; and kapha, with fatigue and weight gain, says Vasant Lad, B.A.M.S., M.A.Sc., director of the Ayurvedic Institute in Albuquerque, New Mexico. Pitta types are also most susceptible to seasonal affective disorder, he says. (For more information on the Ayurvedic doshas, turn to "All about Vata, Pitta and Kapha" on page 28.) In each case, the first step in healing the depression is to modify the diet to reduce the aggravated dosha, says Dr. Lad. (See page 30 for information on dosha diets.)

For vata depression, Dr. Lab says to rub sesame oil (available in most health food stores) on the scalp and into the soles of the feet for five minutes before your morning shower, washing it off in the shower. He also suggests putting three to five drops of brahmi ghee in each nostril with an eyedropper twice a day—once in the morning and again in the evening. (Brahmi ghee, an Ayurvedic food and medicine, is available by mail order; refer to the resource list on page 634.) He also recommends sipping ginger tea or gotu kola tea (available in tea bag form in most health food stores) during the day. Exercise helps too, he adds. "Take a walk through a garden," he says, "and look at the flowers."

For pitta depression, Dr. Lad recommends a different type of oil—coconut or sunflower (which are also available in most health food stores). He says to rub it into the scalp and the soles of the feet for five minutes before your morning shower, washing it off in the shower. The teas he recommends for this type of depression are gotu kola and ginkgo (also available in tea bag form in most health food stores); he says to drink them twice a day. He also suggests yoga meditation for this depression (see page 153 for information on yoga meditation techniques).

For kapha depression, Dr. Lad recommends regular exercise, eating light foods and engaging in mental activity or yoga meditation.

If your depression does not respond to these remedies within a few days, Dr. Lad says you should see your doctor.

FLOWER REMEDY/ESSENCE THERAPY

Flower remedies are useful in dealing with a number of conditions often associated with mild depression, says herbalist Leslie J. Kaslof, author of *The Traditional Flower Remedies of Dr. Edward Bach*. "Mustard is wonderful for people experiencing gloom and despair," Kaslof says. "Wild Rose is more beneficial for people who have lost interest in life, who have become apathetic and have stopped caring about anything—something many mildly depressed people experience."

For depression that results from difficulty in adjusting to change, try the Bach flower remedy Walnut, suggests Eve Campanelli, Ph.D., a holistic family practitioner in Beverly Hills, California. "Los Angeles is full of comic screenwriters who are very depressed, and they find Walnut especially helpful."

Flower remedies are available in some health food stores and through mail order (refer to the resource list on page 635). For information on preparing and administering flower remedies, see page 37.

FOOD THERAPY

The first step is to eliminate sugar, processed foods, caffeinated foods and alcohol, all of which can worsen depression because of their effects on the body's biochemistry, says David Edelberg, M.D., an internist and medical director of the American Holistic Center/Chicago. He also suggests using the food sensitivity diet (see "Food Sensitivity: How to Discover the 'Healthy' Foods That

Can Cause Disease" on page 52) to eliminate any foods that might have a role in causing depression. And he recommends an herbal supplement: one capsule of Saint-John's-wort, three times a day, which he says can help boost mood. Saint-John's-wort is available in most health food stores.

"I would suggest eating more foods that are high in protein—things such as turkey, chicken and fish," says Allan Magaziner, D.O., a nutritional medicine specialist and head of the Magaziner Medical Center in Cherry Hill, New Jersey. "These foods contain high levels of compounds that help produce neurotransmitters, which can elevate mood and increase energy."

HERBAL THERAPY

Saint-John's-wort is widely used in Europe as a natural alternative to antidepressant drugs, says Varro E. Tyler, Ph.D., professor of pharmacognosy at Purdue University in West Lafayette, Indiana. (Scientific studies on animals show that ingredients in the herb can stimulate brain cells.) To make a medicinal tea using Saint-John's-wort (which you can find in most health food stores), Dr. Tyler says to pour one cup of boiling water over one to two heaping teaspoons of the dried herb. Allow the mixture to steep for ten minutes, strain out the dried herb, let the tea cool to a drinkable temperature, then drink a cup or two daily, he suggests.

Results are gradual, says Dr. Tyler; it may take four to six weeks before you notice a positive change in your mood. And he adds this note of caution: Some fair-skinned people become sensitive to the sun's ultraviolet rays when they take Saint-John's-wort. They should avoid all unnecessary sun exposure when using this remedy, he says, and if they must be out in the sun, they should be sure to use a sunblock on all exposed areas.

HOMEOPATHY

In his book *The Family Guide to Homeopathy*, Andrew Lockie, M.D., suggests taking a 6C dose of one of following remedies three times daily for up to 14 days to treat mild depression.

If you feel restless, chilly and exhausted and are obsessively neat and tidy, try Arsenicum, says Dr. Lockie. He advises taking Pulsatilla if you burst into tears with little provocation or if you crave a lot of reassurance and attention. If you feel irritable and find fault with everyone around you, Dr. Lockie says to try Nux vomica. If you feel irritable, weepy and chilly and your sex drive has disappeared, take Sepia, he says.

All of these remedies are available in many health food stores. To purchase the remedies by mail, refer to the resource list on page 637.

DEPRESSION

IMAGERY

If you're mildly depressed, doing an imagery exercise called the trapeze of hope may help brighten your outlook, says Elizabeth Ann Barrett, R.N., Ph.D., professor and coordinator of the Center for Nursing Research at Hunter College of the City University of New York in New York City.

Imagine that you are a trapeze artist standing high in the air on a platform. Now see yourself swinging from the left on a trapeze bar. From the right, see another trapeze bar swinging toward you. Keep swinging and building up your momentum. When you're ready, let go of the old bar, and reach out and catch the new one. See yourself landing safely on the other platform. Grab a golden rope and lower yourself to the ground. Tie the golden rope around yourself and someone you love. Now see both of you standing in a golden light.

Dr. Barrett suggests practicing this imagery first thing in the morning, then up to twice more at any time during the day as needed. Do this for 21 days in a row, she says, then discontinue the imagery for one week. Then repeat the cycle, if necessary.

REFLEXOLOGY

To deal with depression, New York City reflexologist Laura Norman, author of *Feet First: A Guide to Foot Reflexology*, recommends a two-part session for your hands or feet. On one day, she says, work the solar plexus, diaphragm, chest, lung, shoulder, arm, neck, heart, pancreas and thyroid, parathyroid and adrenal gland reflex points as well as all of the points on the tops and bottoms of the toes, paying special attention to the brain and pituitary gland. (To work the toes, use whichever technique you find most comfortable.) Also work the hypothalamus points on the feet. The next day, she says, switch to the shoulder/arm, neck and throat points. Also work the breast/chest and thymus points on the feet.

To help you locate these points, consult the hand and foot reflex charts beginning on page 582. For instructions on how to work the points, see "Your Reflexology Session" on page 110.

RELAXATION AND MEDITATION

To overcome the blues, try a daily ten-minute session of thermal biofeedback, suggests Steven Fahrion, Ph.D., director of research at the Life Sciences Institute of Mind-Body Health in Topeka, Kansas.

"To fight off depression, you need to do something that is active and that gives you a sense of control," Dr. Fahrion says. "Using the thermal technique is something concrete. You can see yourself making progress, and you get a sense of accomplishment from it." To learn more about it, see page 121.

SOUND THERAPY

Slow, relaxing music helps some people deal with the root causes of their depression, such as anger, frustration, sadness or anxiety, says Janalea Hoffman, R.M.T., a composer and music therapist based in Kansas City, Missouri. Listening to the music for at least 20 minutes each day can help slow down your heart rate and other body functions and can help you focus on your feelings, she says. Hoffman says you can try her tape, called *Deep Daydreams*. For other selections, see "Sailing Away to Key Largo" on page 129. Many of these are available from music stores. For mail-order information, refer to the resource list on page 642.

YOGA

Meditation and yoga poses can help you attack the main source of depression: the feeling that you can't handle the demands of your life, says Alice Christensen, founder and executive director of the American Yoga Association. She recommends a daily yoga routine that includes 30 minutes of meditation (see page 153) and at least 20 minutes of poses, focusing on these four: dancer (page 609), windmill (page 610), knee squeeze (page 612) and lion (page 623). These poses help improve blood circulation, she explains, making it easier to break through the lethargy that often accompanies depression.

SEE ALSO Grief

DERMATITIS AND ECZEMA

Is it too much to ask? Jeez, it's not as if you wanted skin like a fashion model's. All you're seeking is relief—from the scaly sores, the redness, the flaking and especially all of that itching.

Dermatitis is a broad term that refers to any inflammation of the skin. Poison ivy and similar rashes are known as contact dermatitis, caused by touching something that irritates a patch of skin. Reactions to internal medication can cause red, scaly skin and sometimes even hair loss.

But the broadest category is known as atopic dermatitis, or eczema. It's a chronic condition that can be triggered by allergic reactions to foods, pollen, dry air or any number of other factors. The problem can flare up any time, without notice, and the causes can be hard to pinpoint. The natural remedies in this chapter—used in conjunction with medical care and with your doctor's approval—may help relieve some of the symptoms of dermatitis and eczema, according to some health professionals.

SEE YOUR MEDICAL DOCTOR WHEN . . .

- Your dermatitis or eczema is persistent.
- Your dermatitis or eczema is widespread.
- Your skin is oozing, smelly and crusted, indicating infection.

ACUPRESSURE

Stimulating the Sea of Vitality trigger points can fortify the body's entire system and improve skin conditions, says Michael Reed Gach, Ph.D., director of the Acupressure Institute in Berkeley, California, and author of *Acupressure's Potent Points*. He says to press and briskly rub the B 23 and B 47 points, situated on the lower back on the left and right sides of the spine, in line with the navel. The B 47 points can be found four finger-widths away from the spine at waist level. To locate the B 23 points, move two additional finger-widths closer to your spine. (For help in locating these points, refer to the illustration on page 565.) Dr. Gach says to work all of these points simultaneously by making loose fists and rubbing the points with the backs of your hands for one minute. Repeat this treatment several times a day, he adds.

"Pressing these points can help when used in combination with other therapies, especially a healthy diet, deep breathing and stretching exercises," says Dr. Gach. If you have a weak back, he adds, press these points lightly, and be sure not to press directly on the disks or vertebrae.

AROMATHERAPY

To soothe inflamed, itchy skin, try the essential oil Roman chamomile, suggests Fair Oaks, California, aromatherapist Victoria Edwards. She says to add five drops to a warm (not hot) bath, soak for ten minutes and apply a soothing body oil. For a body oil, Edwards suggests a blend of five drops of Roman chamomile, five drops of neroli, ten drops of lavender and five drops of bergamot essential oils in two ounces of a carrier oil such as olive or almond. (Carrier oils are available in most health food stores.)

For information on preparing and administering essential oils, including cautions about their use, see page 19. For information on purchasing essential oils, refer to the resource list on page 633.

FOOD THERAPY

"As with other skin conditions, the cause may be a nutritional deficiency, where you're not getting enough of the necessary vitamins, minerals and essential fatty acids," says Elson Haas, M.D., director of the Preventive Medical Center of Marin in San Rafael, California, and author of *Staying Healthy with Nutrition*. To heal dermatitis and eczema, he recommends following his three-week detoxification diet (see "Detoxing Your Ills" on page 48).

HOMEOPATHY

Homeopathy can offer relief from dermatitis and eczema symptoms, says Chris Meletis, N.D., a naturopathic physician and medicinary director at the National College of Naturopathic Medicine in Portland, Oregon. He recommends taking one of the following remedies twice a day for 30 days.

If your skin is irritated, especially in the folds of the elbows and knees, try Psorinum 12C, according to Dr. Meletis. He says Calcarea carbonica 30C can be helpful when you have itchy crusts of eczema that seem to heal slowly and are better in dry weather and worse with cold and if the sores are on your scalp and face. If eruptions are behind your ears and on your scalp, Graphites 12C will often help, he says, especially if you also have a honey-colored discharge and moderate itching. If you don't see improvement in 30 days, Dr. Meletis recommends seeing your medical doctor or homeopath.

All of these remedies are available in many health food stores. To purchase homeopathic remedies by mail, refer to the resource list on page 637.

HYDROTHERAPY

A baking soda bath soothes the itch of dermatitis and eczema, according to medical pathologist Agatha Thrash, M.D., co-founder and co-director of Uchee

Pines Institute, a natural healing center in Seale, Alabama. Add one cup of baking soda to a tub filled with lukewarm water (94° to 98°F—use a regular thermometer to check) and soak for 30 to 60 minutes, using a cup to pour the water over any part of the body that isn't submerged. Pat dry. Dr. Thrash says to use this treatment once or twice a day for as long as itching is a problem.

JUICE THERAPY

"Dermatitis and eczema are both symptoms that mean the body isn't eliminating toxins efficiently," says Elaine Gillaspie, N.D., a naturopathic physician in Portland, Oregon. "These toxins end up coming out through the skin." To get elimination back on track, Dr. Gillaspie recommends stimulating the liver daily with an eight-ounce blend of one part beet juice, one part water and two parts carrot juice.

For information on juicing techniques, see page 93.

VITAMIN AND MINERAL THERAPY

Use the food sensitivity diet (see "Food Sensitivity: How to Discover the 'Healthy' Foods That Can Cause Disease" on page 52) to eliminate any foods that might have a role in causing eczema, suggests David Edelberg, M.D., an internist and medical director of the American Holistic Center/Chicago. He also says people with eczema may want to use the following nutritional regimen to help control outbreaks: 50,000 international units (IU) of vitamin A a day for three weeks, then reducing the dose to 10,000 IU a day; one tablespoon of flaxseed oil a day; 400 IU of vitamin E a day; and one milligram of copper a day. Flaxseed oil is available in most health food stores.

YOGA

Eczema can flare up when you're under stress, says Stephen A. Nezezon, M.D., yoga teacher and staff physician at the Himalayan International Institute of Yoga Science and Philosophy in Honesdale, Pennsylvania. To lower stress, Dr. Nezezon recommends trying a daily routine of breathing exercises, meditation and yoga poses.

Do the complete breath exercise (see page 152) whenever you're feeling stress, whether it's at the office, in the car or at home, recommends Alice Christensen, founder and executive director of the American Yoga Association. Daily meditation (see page 153) helps clear your mind and teaches you to relax at will, she says. For the yoga poses, choose three or four from the Daily Routine, which begins on page 606. Christensen suggests varying the poses every day to keep your interest high and to strengthen different parts of your body.

Dr. Nezezon says you should include at least one relaxation pose, such as the corpse (page 612), knee squeeze (page 612) or baby (page 618), in your daily yoga routine.

SEE ALSO Psoriasis

DIABETES

You top off the tank with premium and slide behind the wheel. Time for a little pleasure drive. Too bad you forgot the keys.

It's the same way with diabetes. Your body, an amazing machine, uses a form of sugar called glucose to fire its engine. Your body makes glucose from foods, then sends it into your bloodstream, where it's available for use by every cell.

But without the right key—insulin—none of the cells can open up and take the energy. As a result, glucose levels build in the bloodstream, with dangerous consequences. Few people with diabetes need daily insulin injections.

People with Type II or non-insulin-dependent diabetes are at higher risk of vision and kidney problems, heart disease and nerve damage. More than 90 percent of the time, lifestyle changes such as losing weight, cutting back on fat and getting daily exercise can help keep your blood sugar levels in line. If you have diabetes, follow your doctor's advice. But the natural remedies in this chapter—used in conjunction with medical care and with your doctor's approval—may help stabilize blood sugar levels, according to some health professionals.

SEE YOUR MEDICAL DOCTOR WHEN . . .

- You notice frequent urination.
- You have extreme hunger and/or thirst.
- You have unusual weight loss.
- You suffer from extreme fatigue.
- You are more irritable than usual.
- You have blurred vision.
- Your cuts and bruises are slow to heal.
- You have tingling or numbness in your hands or feet.
- You have recurring skin, gum or bladder infections.

FOOD THERAPY

Limit or eliminate meats, cheeses and other foods from animal sources, says Neal Barnard, M.D., president of the Physicians Committee for Responsible Medicine in Washington, D.C., and author of *Food for Life* and other books on the healing aspects of food. The reason: They tend to be high in fat, which Dr. Barnard says can interfere with insulin's action and raise body weight, cholesterol and blood pressure—all additional risk factors for those with Type I and Type II diabetes.

REFLEXOLOGY

Be sure to work the reflex points on the hands and feet for the liver, pancreas and pituitary and adrenal glands, says St. Petersburg, Florida, reflexologist Dwight Byers, author of *Better Health with Foot Reflexology*.

To help you locate these points, consult the hand and foot reflex charts beginning on page 582. For instructions on how to work the points, see "Your Reflexology Session" on page 110.

RELAXATION AND MEDITATION

Thermal biofeedback may increase blood flow and circulation and reduce your need for insulin, says Steven Fahrion, Ph.D., director of research at the Life Sciences Institute of Mind-Body Health in Topeka, Kansas. To learn more about it, see page 121. Practice it at least once a day for ten minutes, Dr. Fahrion suggests.

VITAMIN AND MINERAL THERAPY

A person with diabetes may want to use the following vitamin and mineral regimen to help control the disease, says David Edelberg, M.D., an internist and medical director of the American Holistic Center/Chicago: 1,000 milligrams of vitamin C three times a day; 400 international units of vitamin E twice a day; 200 micrograms of chromium twice a day; 50 milligrams of vitamin B_6 twice a day; 30 milligrams of niacin three times a day; and 250 milligrams of niacinamide once a day. Niacinamide is available in most health food stores.

YOGA

Yogic exercises can help with diabetes, say Dr. Robin Monro, Dr. R. Nagarathna and Dr. H. R. Nagendra in their book *Yoga for Common Ailments*. When practiced as part of a daily yoga routine of breathing exercises (see page

DIARRHEA

152), meditation (see page 153) and poses (see the Daily Routine beginning on page 606), these exercises enhance digestion and help the pancreas and liver function more normally, regulating blood sugar levels, according to the authors.

Here are their instructions for performing these two exercises: Stand with your feet spread shoulder-width apart. Bend forward, with your hands on your knees. Then exhale through your mouth. When your breath is gone, close your throat so that no air will enter your lungs. Now expand your chest, as if breathing, and suck in your abdominal muscles tightly, forming a hollow space. As you do so, try to relax your muscles. Stay in this position until you need to breathe, then relax and inhale slowly. Now go into abdominal pumping. Release the muscles so that your stomach returns to its normal position, then suck in the abdominal muscles again. Pump your abdomen in and out until you need to breathe. Release slowly and breathe normally. Repeat the entire exercise three times, say the authors.

Because of the impact of these exercises on the circulatory system, the authors recommend not doing them during menstruation or pregnancy, after surgery, if you are bleeding or if you have heart disease or high blood pressure.

DIARRHEA

They told you not to drink the water. But you have one of those heavy-duty cast-iron bellies. You know, the kind that can handle a hundred jalapeños without a whimper. What harm could a glass of *agua* do?

Plenty, as it turns out. Diarrhea is a surefire vacation wrecker—and an occasional nuisance at home as well. More than 50 things can cause it, the most common of which are parasites and bacterial and viral infections. The constant trips to the bathroom are your body's way of flushing the offenders out of your system. Bouts of diarrhea may also occur after you eat more fruits, vegetables or other fiber than your digestive tract is used to or if you have chronic bowel or colon disease. The natural remedies in this chapter—used in conjunction with medical care and with the approval of your doctor—may help shorten a bout of diarrhea and relieve some of its symptoms, according to some health professionals.

SEE YOUR MEDICAL DOCTOR WHEN . . .

- Your bout lasts for more than two days.
- You see blood in your stool.

- You have a fever, nausea or vomiting.
- You suffer from dehydration, whose symptoms include excessive thirst, dry lips and reduced urination.
- You are unable to keep down liquids.

AYURVEDA

Pitta personalities are more prone than others to diarrhea, although anyone can have trouble with it, says Vasant Lad, B.A.M.S., M.A.Sc., director of the Ayurvedic Institute in Albuquerque, New Mexico. But whether you're pitta, vata or kapha, a bout of diarrhea indicates that your pitta energy, which helps you digest properly, is out of balance, says Dr. Lad. (For more information about the Ayurvedic doshas, see "All about Vata, Pitta and Kapha" on page 28.)

To relieve diarrhea, Dr. Lad says to eat a bland diet. He also recommends drinking pomegranate juice laced with a pinch of nutmeg and a pinch of ginger powder. (Pomegranate juice is available in most health food stores.)

This recipe for applesauce will also help soothe your digestive tract, says Dr. Lad: Cook a couple of apples, mash them into pulp and add a pinch of nutmeg, a pinch of saffron and one teaspoon of ghee, or clarified butter (see "How to Make Ghee" on page 26 for the recipe).

To avoid dehydration during a bout of diarrhea, Dr. Lad suggests drinking water with honey. He says to add one teaspoon of honey, one teaspoon of lime juice and a pinch of salt to a pint of warm or room temperature water and sip it throughout the day.

FOOD THERAPY

"What I have people do is eat brown rice with bananas but mix the rice with more water than usual," says Elson Haas, M.D., director of the Preventive Medical Center of Marin in San Rafael, California, and author of *Staying Healthy with Nutrition*. His recipe: Cook one cup of rice in three cups of water, then mix in one banana. "The rice acts as a bulking agent and is gentle enough on your system. Eat a few bowlfuls of rice for a day or so, and the diarrhea should improve."

HERBAL THERAPY

Blackberry tea should do the trick, says Varro E. Tyler, Ph.D., professor of pharmacognosy at Purdue University in West Lafayette, Indiana. Blackberry leaves contain tannins, chemical compounds that reduce intestinal inflammation, according to Dr. Tyler. He says to make the tea by steeping one to two teaspoons of the dried herb (available in most health food stores) in a cup of water for ten minutes.

You can also buy packaged blackberry tea in most health food stores. If you do buy the tea, Dr. Tyler says to make sure it is prepared from blackberry leaves. There are many blackberry-flavored black teas on the market; read the label closely.

Drink up to six cups of blackberry tea daily to control diarrhea, suggests Dr. Tyler. If the problem lasts for more than two days, see a doctor, he adds.

HOMEOPATHY

"Podophyllum can be a very helpful remedy for traveler's diarrhea," says Judyth Reichenberg-Ullman, N.D., a naturopathic physician in Edmonds, Washington, and co-author of *The Patient's Guide to Homeopathic Medicine*. She suggests trying Podophyllum in a 30C dose once or twice a day if you have cramping or explosive gas in addition to diarrhea. Arsenicum 30C is another common remedy, which she says is good for diarrhea that also causes exhaustion, restlessness or chills. If you have nausea, vomiting and green stool, she recommends a 30C dose of Ipecacuanha once or twice a day. If you don't feel better within 48 hours, Dr. Reichenberg-Ullman says to discontinue the remedy and see a health professional.

Podophyllum, Arsenicum and Ipecacuanha are available in many health food stores. To purchase homeopathic remedies by mail, refer to the resource list on page 637.

HYDROTHERAPY

"I tell people never to travel anywhere without activated charcoal. It has saved many a vacation," says Agatha Thrash, M.D., a medical pathologist and co-founder and co-director of Uchee Pines Institute, a natural healing center in Seale, Alabama. Of course, you can use this remedy at home, too. Here are Dr. Thrash's instructions: Put two to three tablespoons of activated charcoal powder in the bottom of a large glass and add a small amount of water (bottled may be best if you're traveling). Stir slowly with a long-handled spoon to keep the fine powder from flying everywhere, suggests Dr. Thrash. Fill the glass the rest of the way with water and drink with a straw. Dr. Thrash says to use this remedy with each loose stool or at the first sign of queasiness. "It's the safest, simplest and best treatment for diarrhea there is," she says. Activated charcoal is available in most health food stores and some pharmacies.

REFLEXOLOGY

Try working these spots on your feet, says St. Petersburg, Florida, reflexologist Dwight Byers, author of *Better Health with Foot Reflexology*: ascending colon, transverse colon, diaphragm, liver and adrenal gland.

To help you locate these points, consult the foot reflex chart on page 592. For instructions on how to work the points, see "Your Reflexology Session" on page 110.

RELAXATION AND MEDITATION

Autogenics can help relieve diarrhea caused by anxiety, according to Martha Davis, Ph.D., Elizabeth Robbins Eshelman and Matthew McKay, Ph.D., in *The Relaxation and Stress Reduction Workbook*. So when diarrhea strikes, do ten two-minute sessions of this technique daily until you feel better, suggests Martin Shaffer, Ph.D., executive director of the Stress Management Institute in San Francisco and author of *Life after Stress*. To learn how it's done, see page 120. If symptoms persist, see your doctor.

DIVERTICULAR DISEASE

Through your colon all things must pass. If they don't, you get constipated. And if that happens too often, you may develop diverticular disease.

Diverticula are small pouches that can form in the lining and walls of your colon. When this happens, you have diverticulosis. While the condition is often harmless, sometimes irritants can get trapped in the diverticula and cause an infection. The result is a more serious condition called diverticulitis. The natural remedies in this chapter—used in conjunction with medical care and with your doctor's approval—may help relieve some of the symptoms of diverticular disease, according to some health professionals.

SEE YOUR MEDICAL DOCTOR WHEN . . .

- You have a fever and feel severe pain in the lower left part of your abdomen.

FOOD THERAPY

"A high-fiber diet, along with drinking plenty of water, is the best treatment because it speeds the time it takes for food to move through your bowels," says Julian Whitaker, M.D., founder and president of the Whitaker Wellness Center in Newport Beach, California. People with diverticular disease should consume 30 to 40 grams of fiber a day, he says, about three times the amount eaten by the typical American. "Oat bran is an excellent fiber," explains Dr. Whitaker. "And be sure to have at least five servings of fresh fruits and vegetables each day."

JUICE THERAPY

Many people with intestinal problems are deficient in vitamin K, found in dark green lettuce and cruciferous vegetables such as broccoli and kale, says Cherie Calbom, M.S., a certified nutritionist in Kirkland, Washington, and co-author of *Juicing for Life*. She also advises those with diverticular disease to load up on beta-carotene, which is believed to help heal damaged intestinal tissue.

Juice blends such as Calbom's Alkaline Cocktail provide a healthy dose of both nutrients. To prepare, says Calbom, juice three carrots, three celery ribs and one-fourth of a head of cabbage. Drink this blend once a day, she adds.

For information on juicing techniques, see page 93.

REFLEXOLOGY

Focus on these reflexes on the feet, suggests New York City reflexologist Laura Norman, author of *Feet First: A Guide to Foot Reflexology*: solar plexus, diaphragm, lower spine, intestine (with emphasis on the sigmoid colon), liver, gallbladder and adrenal gland.

To help you locate these points, consult the foot reflex chart on page 592. For instructions on how to work the points, see "Your Reflexology Session" on page 110.

DIZZINESS

When you were little, being dizzy was fun. Remember how you used to roll down that big hill at the playground, end over end over end, then stand up and watch the world spin around?

Unfortunately, for an estimated one in five people, bouts of dizziness are more than just child's play. Lots of things can cause dizziness, including a bump on the head, the jarring motion of running, an infection, low blood pressure or conditions such as Ménière's disease. If you have recurring dizziness, it's best to see a doctor. But the natural remedies in this chapter—used in conjunction with medical care and with the approval of your doctor—may help relieve dizziness, according to some health professionals.

SEE YOUR MEDICAL DOCTOR WHEN . . .

- Your dizziness comes without warning, along with numbness, chest pain, rapid heartbeat or blurred vision.
- Your dizziness accompanies a change in your ability to speak.
- You have ringing in your ears or deafness after an attack of dizziness.

ACUPRESSURE

You can stop the spinning by pressing both St 36 points, situated four finger-widths below each kneecap, in the indentation at the front of the shinbone, says Glenn S. Rothfeld, M.D., clinical instructor at Tufts University School of Medicine in Boston and a family practitioner in Arlington, Massachusetts. These points are on the stomach meridian, and according to Dr. Rothfeld, pressing them "deepens your connection to nourishment, to the earth. When you're dizzy, you need this kind of centering." (For help in locating these points, refer to the illustration on page 564.)

Here's how Dr. Rothfeld says to press these points: Sitting down with your knees bent, press the point on each shinbone with the thumb or forefinger of the same or the opposite hand. Begin gently and gradually increase the pressure. Hold for about two minutes and gradually release. If you wish, you may hold the points longer or repeat the treatment if you begin to feel dizzy again.

FLOWER REMEDY/ESSENCE THERAPY

For occasional mild dizziness that's related to balance problems, the flower remedy Scleranthus may be helpful, according to Leslie J. Kaslof, an herbalist and author of *The Traditional Flower Remedies of Dr. Edward Bach.*

For best results, combine Scleranthus and the emergency stress relief formula (sold under brand names such as Calming Essence, Rescue Remedy and Five-Flower Formula) together in one bottle and take them as one remedy, says Kaslof. He suggests taking two to four drops under the tongue, holding them in your mouth for a minute before swallowing. He also says you can apply this combination directly to the temples and the inside of the belly button.

Both Scleranthus and the emergency stress relief formula are available in some health food stores and through mail order (refer to the resource list on page 635). For more information on preparing and administering flower remedies, see page 37.

HERBAL THERAPY

A reduced flow of blood to the brain is a common cause of dizziness, and scientific research shows that the herb ginkgo improves blood flow to the brain, according to Varro E. Tyler, Ph.D., professor of pharmacognosy at Purdue University in West Lafayette, Indiana. He suggests taking ginkgo in supplemental form, following the dosage recommendations on the product label. These supplements are available in most health food stores.

IMAGERY

In his book *Healing Visualizations*, Gerald Epstein, M.D., a New York City psychiatrist, suggests that you close your eyes, take three very slow, deep breaths and imagine yourself as a tightrope walker standing on a stationary platform high in the air. On this platform, you have a balancing pole, bicycle or parasol. Before crossing the wire, envision yourself reaching the other side. Then start your crossing, knowing that as you do it successfully, your dizziness will disappear. When you reach the other side of the wire, put down your balancing pole, bicycle or parasol, then climb down the ladder to the ground. When you reach the ground, your dizziness should be just a memory.

Dr. Epstein says to do this imagery as needed every ten minutes, one to two minutes each time, until your dizziness vanishes.

REFLEXOLOGY

Work the ear, cervical spine and neck reflexes on both feet, says St. Petersburg, Florida, reflexologist Dwight Byers, author of *Better Health with Foot Reflexology*. To help you locate these points, consult the foot reflex chart on page 592. For instructions on how to work the points, see "Your Reflexology Session" on page 110.

DROWSINESS

Zzzzzzzzzz...huh, what?
Catch yourself napping a lot lately? Even when you're awake, do you feel sluggish and dull? Lots of things may make you drowsy. Over-the-counter and prescription medications, especially antihistamines, can do it. So can poor sleep habits or sleep-related problems such as apnea. Even being out of shape or working under high stress can cause fatigue and make you feel sleepy. But the natural remedies in this chapter—used in conjunction with medical care and with the approval of your doctor—may help relieve drowsiness, according to some health professionals.

SEE YOUR MEDICAL DOCTOR WHEN . . .

- You become sleepy so fast that you collapse.
- You snore frequently or have problems with interrupted sleep.
- You put yourself or other people at risk because of your drowsiness, such as when you drive a car.
- You have repeated drowsy periods over a week or more but are getting enough sleep (six to eight hours nightly).

AROMATHERAPY

To help her stay awake on long car trips, Victoria Edwards, a Fair Oaks, California, aromatherapist, uses the essential oils rosemary and basil. "I put a drop or two of each oil on a napkin or tissue and let it sit on the dashboard," says Edwards. "The warmth of the sun or the car heater diffuses the fragrance, which is a great mental stimulant."

For information on preparing and administering essential oils, including cautions about their use, see page 19. For information on purchasing essential oils, refer to the resource list on page 633.

HYDROTHERAPY

Wake up with a cold mitten friction rub, suggests Agatha Thrash, M.D., a medical pathologist and co-founder and co-director of Uchee Pines Institute, a natural healing center in Seale, Alabama. Dip a towel or washcloth into cold (50° to 60°F) water, curl one hand into a fist and wrap the cloth around it. Use your fist to rub your other arm in a vigorous circular motion, beginning with the fingers and finishing at the shoulder. Dip the cloth in the cold water again and repeat. The skin should be pink. Dry your arm with a towel using the same vigorous circular movement, then repeat the process on your other arm and on your legs, feet, chest and abdomen.

"If this doesn't make you more alert, I don't know what will," says Dr. Thrash. "If you do it properly, it's also good exercise."

MASSAGE

Give yourself a vigorous ten-minute whole-body massage, and you'll feel more perky, says Vincent Iuppo, N.D., massage therapist, naturopathic physician and director of the Morris Institute of Natural Therapeutics, a holistic health education center in Denville, New Jersey. Obviously, you can't reach every part of your body, but every little bit helps.

Start by lightly lubricating your hands with vegetable oil or massage oil. You can rub your legs and arms with the effleurage (page 570), tapotement (page 571) and vibration (page 571) strokes. Work from your feet to your hips. Then rub your abdomen and chest with gliding, circular strokes. Work each arm by running your hand vigorously from your wrist to your elbow, then from your elbow to your shoulder. Do this on both sides of your body. Also take time to vigorously rub your shoulder and neck muscles.

SOUND THERAPY

Music can snap you out of a drowsy state and activate your body, says Don G. Campbell, director of the Institute for Music, Health and Education in Boulder, Colorado, and author of *Music: Physician for Times to Come*. He suggests listening to any of these pieces when you're feeling drowsy: *Well-Tempered Klavier* by Johann Sebastian Bach, the soundtrack from the movie *Flashdance*, *Saving the Wildlife* by Mannheim Steamroller, the soundtrack from the movie *The Sting*, marches by John Philip Sousa and *Not Live from New York* by the Cambridge Buskers.

Many of the selections above are available in music stores. For mail-order information, refer to the resource list on page 642.

VITAMIN AND MINERAL THERAPY

Drowsiness can be caused by a deficiency of biotin, a B vitamin, says Richard Gerson, Ph.D., author of *The Right Vitamins*. If you've ruled out other possible causes of drowsiness, he suggests taking a biotin supplement of 150 to 300 micrograms each day until the drowsiness goes away.

SEE ALSO Chronic Fatigue Syndrome; Fatigue

DRY HAIR AND SKIN

D on't take this personally, but you're all wet. Well, more than half wet anyway. Water makes up 60 percent of the average adult's body weight and more than 70 percent of non–fat tissue such as skin.

No wonder you can feel so dried out. Radiator heat, blow–dryers, deodorant soap and dehumidifiers can all rob you of the moisture you desperately need. That can leave your hair brittle and strawlike and your skin flaky and dry. The natural remedies in this chapter, used with your doctor's approval, may help relieve dry hair and skin, according to some health professionals.

SEE YOUR MEDICAL DOCTOR WHEN . . .

- You have redness, oozing, crusting or other signs of irritation.

AROMATHERAPY

To help chronically dry skin retain more of its natural moisture, Fair Oaks, California, aromatherapist Victoria Edwards recommends this fragrant face and body oil: Add ten drops each of the essential oils lavender, Roman chamomile, neroli, rosemary and carrot seed to two ounces of a carrier oil such as almond, olive or sesame. (Carrier oils are available in most health food stores.) Apply the oil once a day after your bath or shower, while your skin is still slightly damp, says Edwards.

To make dry hair silky and manageable, add six drops each of lavender, bay and sandalwood essential oils to six ounces of warm sesame or soy oil, suggests Greenwich, Connecticut, aromatherapist Judith Jackson, author of *Scentual Touch: A Personal Guide to Aromatherapy*. (Soy oil is also available in most health food stores.) To apply the oil, says Jackson, part your hair into one-inch sections and apply the mixture to the scalp with a wad of cotton. Wrap your head in a towel and let the oils penetrate for about 15 minutes, then shampoo twice, she says.

For information on preparing and administering essential oils, including cautions about their use, see page 19. For information on purchasing essential oils, refer to the resource list on page 633.

FOOD THERAPY

"Eat fish at least twice a week," suggests registered pharmacist Earl Mindell, R.Ph., Ph.D., professor of nutrition at Pacific Western University in

Los Angeles and author of *Earl Mindell's Food as Medicine* and other books on nutrition. The oil in salmon, herring and other cold water fish is rich in omega-3 fatty acids, which help replenish lost moisture in dry skin and hair, according to Dr. Mindell.

Up to two tablespoons of flaxseed oil a day can also help replenish hair and skin oils, says Julian Whitaker, M.D., founder and president of the Whitaker Wellness Center in Newport Beach, California. It has a nutty-buttery taste, so you can use it as a topping on popcorn, potatoes or other foods you might otherwise flavor with butter, he says. Flaxseed oil is available in most health food stores.

REFLEXOLOGY

To deal with dry skin, pay special attention to the thyroid and adrenal gland reflexes on your hands or feet, says St. Petersburg, Florida, reflexologist Dwight Byers, author of *Better Health with Foot Reflexology*.

To help you locate these points, consult the hand and foot reflex charts beginning on page 582. For instructions on how to work the points, see "Your Reflexology Session" on page 110.

EARACHE

An earache is often a symptom of a cold, the flu or another infection. It usually results when the eustachian tube, which leads from the back of the throat to the middle ear, gets plugged with microbes. An earache can also occur when hair and other objects get stuck in the ear. The natural remedies in this chapter—used in conjunction with medical care and with the approval of your doctor—may help prevent or relieve an earache, according to some health professionals.

SEE YOUR MEDICAL DOCTOR WHEN . . .

- Your earache lasts for more than a week or continues to hurt three days after taking antibiotics.
- Your ear hurts when you chew.
- You have sudden or severe ear pain without an accompanying cold or sore throat.

EARACHE

AYURVEDA

Acute ear infections require professional medical attention, says David Frawley, O.M.D., director of the American Institute of Vedic Studies in Santa Fe, New Mexico. But people who have chronic problems with ear infections can try some preventive measures. First, simplify your diet, says Dr. Frawley: Cut back on sweets, fats and dairy products, and use ginger and cloves to spice foods.

The herb gotu kola reduces the likelihood of ear infections (and, as an added benefit, improves hearing), according to Dr. Frawley. You can purchase gotu kola in capsule form in most health food stores. Dr. Frawley says to take two 500-milligram capsules in the morning and two in the evening. You can also buy gotu kola powder (it's also available in most health food stores) and take ¼ teaspoon, mixed with honey, twice daily, says Dr. Frawley.

FOOD THERAPY

"Eating one or two cloves of raw garlic each day may help end chronic episodes of earache," says Julian Whitaker, M.D., founder and president of the Whitaker Wellness Center in Newport Beach, California. "It has natural antiviral and antibiotic qualities that kill many of the germs that cause earaches."

But be careful: Eating raw garlic can cause gastrointestinal upset, says registered pharmacist Earl Mindell, R.Ph., Ph.D., professor of nutrition at Pacific Western University in Los Angeles and author of *Earl Mindell's Food as Medicine* and other books on nutrition. If you find you have trouble tolerating raw garlic, try taking garlic supplements instead. Dr. Mindell suggests taking one capsule with each meal. Garlic supplements are available in most health food stores and many drugstores.

HOMEOPATHY

If you develop an earache accompanied by a yellowish green, creamy discharge from the ear after having had a cold for several days, you have no thirst and you desire company and sympathy, try taking a 6C or 12C dose of Pulsatilla, says Mitchell Fleisher, M.D., a family practice physician and homeopath in Colleen, Virginia. He suggests a similar dose of Mercurius if you have an earache accompanied by a high fever, thick, greenish nasal or ear discharge, salivation, foul breath and irritability. If you develop a very painful earache during the night, the ear is very sensitive to touch and to cold and you feel very chilly, Dr. Fleisher recommends a 6C or 12C dose of Hepar sulphuris. If the earache develops suddenly with a fever and a hot, red ear, he says to try a dose of Belladonna 30C. If there is no response after four doses of the indicated remedy in 24 hours, Dr. Fleisher advises that you contact your homeopath or medical doctor.

All of these remedies are available in many health food stores. To purchase the remedies by mail, refer to the resource list on page 637.

HYDROTHERAPY

Hot compresses on the ears, combined with a hot foot bath, are the treatment of choice for earaches, according to Charles Thomas, Ph.D., co-author of *Hydrotherapy: Simple Treatments for Common Ailments* and a physical therapist at the Desert Springs Therapy Center in Desert Hot Springs, California. Soak your feet in a tub of hot water for anywhere from 10 to 30 minutes, adding water as needed to keep the water comfortably hot. While you're soaking, apply a hot compress from ear to ear, covering the throat. Leave it in place for about 5 minutes. Apply another hot compress for 5 minutes and continue with a new compress every 3 to 5 minutes until the ache is relieved or for a maximum of 30 minutes. If the pain persists, repeat the entire procedure two or three times a day.

REFLEXOLOGY

Pay special attention to the ear, throat and neck reflexes on your feet, says St. Petersburg, Florida, reflexologist Dwight Byers, author of *Better Health with Foot Reflexology*. He also recommends working all of the points on the sides and bottoms of the toes on both feet, using whichever technique you find most comfortable.

To help you locate these points, consult the foot reflex chart on page 592. For instructions on how to work the points, see "Your Reflexology Session" on page 110.

EARWAX

Earwax may not be much to look at, but that's the beauty of it. When you see that disgusting speck of yellowish, brown or orange glob on your pillow or washcloth, you know it's doing its job—that is, preventing dust, infection and bugs from doing some real damage by getting inside your ears.

The problem occurs when earwax doesn't exit. Earwax can get all jammed up, which can be annoying, uncomfortable and itchy and can completely block the ear canal, producing noticeable hearing loss. Earwax buildup is usually the result of sticking cotton swabs, fingers and other things in your ear, which shoves earwax deeper into the ear canal. Some people have this buildup because their ear canals have gentle bends to them, making it harder for earwax to flow out. The natural remedy in this chapter—used in conjunction with medical care and with the approval of your doctor—may help relieve excess earwax, according to one health professional.

SEE YOUR MEDICAL DOCTOR WHEN ...

- You are experiencing itching, pain or hearing loss.
- You have discharge from your ear.

HOMEOPATHY

Taking a 6C dose of Causticum four times daily for up to seven days may help reduce your earwax production and relieve intermittent hearing loss, writes Andrew Lockie, M.D., in his book *The Family Guide to Homeopathy*.

Causticum is available in many health food stores. To purchase homeopathic remedies by mail, refer to the resource list on page 637.

EATING DISORDERS

An eating disorder is usually more about emotions than about appetite. Trying to suppress feelings of stress, depression or anger can trigger a distorted attitude toward food or a significant change in eating habits. But no matter the problem—whether it's compulsive overeating or purposeful starvation, hoarding food in unusual ways or purging yourself after a meal—the final course is usually a hefty serving of guilt. Women under age 25 are particularly susceptible.

While doctors say that understanding and resolving feelings about yourself and your situation are the best ways to stop an eating disorder, here's some immediate help. The natural remedy in this chapter—used in conjunction with medical care and with your doctor's approval—may assist in overcoming this disorder, according to one health professional.

SEE YOUR MEDICAL DOCTOR WHEN...

- You are eating to the point of, or even after, feeling uncomfortably full.
- You go on eating binges at least twice a week in which you consume about 2,000 calories per sitting.
- You have lost a lot of body weight yet continue to view yourself as "fat."
- You purposely avoid or skip meals, even when you're hungry.
- You force yourself to vomit after consuming food in an effort to lose weight.

RELAXATION AND MEDITATION

Meditation is one of the best ways a person can overcome a binge/purge eating disorder, according to Alice Christensen, founder and executive director of the American Yoga Association. Daily meditation, lasting 20 to 30 minutes, can help you find the inner strength you need to resist binges. Christensen says you can meditate for brief periods during the day—even for a few minutes, if that's all of the time you have—to help stem the craving to overeat. For instructions on meditation, see page 117.

ENDOMETRIOSIS

For many women, menstruation is just a monthly occurrence. But when you have endometriosis, monthly cramps don't just cramp your style: Your period may be punctuated with severe lower back pain, tenderness and swelling in your abdomen. There may even be discomfort during sex or while you're going to the bathroom. Sometimes there can be difficulty conceiving.

Each month, the tissue lining your uterus thickens with blood to form a nourishing nest in preparation for a fetus. When conception doesn't occur, this lining, called the endometrium, sheds through your vagina, and you menstruate. But with endometriosis, this tissue is outside the uterus—attached to the ovaries, fallopian tubes, bladder or colon—and causing misery because it's in the wrong place.

Doctors aren't sure what causes endometriosis, but pregnancy (when possible) and breastfeeding can temporarily end the symptoms. And the natural remedies in this chapter—in conjunction with medical care and used with your doctor's approval—may help relieve the symptoms of endometriosis, according to some health professionals.

SEE YOUR MEDICAL DOCTOR WHEN...

- You have sudden sharp pain in your pelvic area around the time of your period that lasts for more than two days.
- You feel pain or burning while having a bowel movement.
- You have blood in your urine or stool.
- You have pain during sex.
- You are having trouble conceiving.

FLOWER REMEDY/ESSENCE THERAPY

"Many women with endometriosis have a tendency to bottle up destructive emotions such as anger," says Susan Lange, O.M.D., of the Meridian Center for Personal and Environmental Health in Santa Monica, California. "The essence Sticky Monkey Flower helps them release these feelings, which is very therapeutic." The California Pitcher Plant also has an unblocking effect and may help some women with endometriosis, according to Dr. Lange.

Flower essences are available in some health food stores and through mail order (refer to the resource list on page 635). For information on preparing and administering flower essences, see page 37.

FOOD THERAPY

Fish that are rich in omega-3 fatty acids—mackerel, salmon, anchovies, tuna, whitefish, herring and sardines—help by suppressing the production of prostaglandins, the hormones that cause the cramping that can accompany endometriosis, according to Camran Nezhat, M.D., director of the Fertility and Endoscopy Center and Center for Special Pelvic Surgery in Atlanta.

The three-week detoxification diet (see "Detoxing Your Ills" on page 48) may also benefit some women with endometriosis, says Elson Haas, M.D., director of the Preventive Medical Center of Marin in San Rafael, California, and author of *Staying Healthy with Nutrition.*

HOMEOPATHY

If you are anxious and weepy and have pain in your ovaries that spreads down to your thighs, try a 6X dose of Lilium tigrum three times a day or a 30C dose once or twice a day until you feel better, suggests Cynthia Mervis Watson, M.D., a family practice physician specializing in homeopathic and herbal therapies in Santa Monica, California. She says that the same dosage of Sepia may help other women, particularly pale-skinned brunettes who have premenstrual syndrome, with outbursts of anger and pain during intercourse or menstruation. Belladonna, in a 6X dose three times a day or a 30C dose once or twice daily, may relieve endometriosis, says Dr. Watson, especially if you feel hot and flushed, feel restless and anxious, develop sudden pain during menstruation that spreads into your legs and have a blood flow that is bright red and profuse.

Lilium tigrum, Sepia and Belladonna are available in many health food stores. To purchase homeopathic remedies by mail, refer to the resource list on page 637.

HYDROTHERAPY

Taken three times a week, the contrast sitz bath is very effective at relieving the discomfort of endometriosis, says Tori Hudson, N.D., a naturopathic physician and professor at the National College of Naturopathic Medicine in Portland, Oregon. "This improves circulation in the pelvis and reduces pain and irritation," says Dr. Hudson. For instructions on preparing a contrast sitz bath, see "Hydrotherapy at Home" on page 78.

JUICE THERAPY

Try any fresh fruit juice, but dark grape, mango, papaya and pineapple juices are best, says John Peterson, M.D., an Ayurvedic practitioner in Muncie, Indiana. He recommends drinking as much as you want of the juice daily, apart from meals. Drink the juice at room temperature and do not blend the juice of your choice with other fruit or vegetable juices.

For information on juicing techniques, see page 93.

VITAMIN AND MINERAL THERAPY

Omega-3 fatty acids suppress production of prostaglandins, the hormones that cause cramping, says Elson Haas, M.D., director of the Preventive Medical Center of Marin in San Rafael, California, and author of *Staying Healthy with Nutrition*. To get these acids, he recommends fish oil capsules, taken according to the dosage on the label. Fish oil capsules are available in most health food stores.

Flaxseed oil contains another essential fatty acid that may help, says Dr. Haas. Flaxseed oil is available in liquid and capsule form in most health food stores; Dr. Haas says to take a daily dose of either one teaspoon of the liquid or two to three capsules.

Some women benefit from the following daily supplement regimen, according to Susan Lark, M.D., author of *Fibroid Tumors and Endometriosis*: between 400 and 2,000 international units (IU) of vitamin E (women with diabetes or high blood pressure should take only 100 IU); 3 milligrams (5,000 IU) of beta-carotene; 300 milligrams of vitamin B_6 and 50 milligrams of B-complex vitamins; up to 4,000 milligrams of vitamin C; and 800 milligrams of bioflavonoids. The doses recommended for vitamin E, vitamin C, vitamin B_6 and the B-complex vitamins are higher than the Recommended Dietary Allowances, says Dr. Lark, and should not be taken for longer than three months without the advice of a doctor.

EYESTRAIN

From that first bleary squint at the alarm clock to the last nodding glimpses of the late show, your baby blues prove all day why the eyes have it—tough, that is.

The human eye can see up to 60 "pictures" a second, and many of these sights can lead to sore eyes. A spreadsheet or even the morning's headlines can tax eye muscles, leaving your peepers pooped. But eyestrain does more than make your eyes sting, blur and water; the pain can also spread to your head, neck or back.

Sound familiar? It ought to. Just about everyone gets eyestrain at least occasionally, especially if you are over age 40 and use a computer, watch television, drive a car or live in a smoggy environment. The natural remedies in this chapter—in conjunction with medical care and used with your doctor's approval—may help relieve eyestrain, according to some health professionals.

SEE YOUR MEDICAL DOCTOR WHEN . . .

- Your eyes remain red for longer than two days or for longer than two hours after contact lenses are removed.
- You also experience piercing or throbbing pain, blurred vision or sensitivity to light.
- Your eyestrain is the result of a blow or something embedded in your eye.

ACUPRESSURE

With both thumbs, press the B 2 points, located on the upper ridges of your eye sockets close to the bridge of your nose, recommends Michael Reed Gach, Ph.D., director of the Acupressure Institute in Berkeley, California, and author of *Acupressure's Potent Points*. (To help locate these points, refer to the illustration on page 564.) Press upward into the indentations of the eye sockets and hold for two minutes while you concentrate on slow, deep breathing, suggests Dr. Gach. He says to be sure to wash your hands carefully before putting them near your eyes.

FOOD THERAPY

Eat more fruits and vegetables, especially those rich in the antioxidant vitamin C, says Jay Cohen, O.D., associate professor at the State University of New

York College of Optometry in New York City. "Getting more vitamin C is a good idea for overall eye health and particularly for eyestrain," he explains. "Vitamin C deficiency may make the eyes a little more sensitive, so you're more prone to eyestrain. You could probably get the vitamin C you need from fruits and vegetables, as opposed to needing a supplement." (For good food sources of vitamin C, see "Getting What You Need" on page 142.)

Also, some people place slices of raw cucumber over their (closed) eyes to relieve eyestrain. "I'm sure it helps," adds Dr. Cohen, "but probably not any better than a cold compress."

HOMEOPATHY

"If you've been reading a lot or spending a lot of time staring at a computer screen, you have a headache and your eyes hurt a bit, then Ruta graveolens is a good remedy to try," says Stephen Messer, N.D., dean of the National Center for Homeopathy's summer school and a naturopathic physician in Eugene, Oregon. He suggests taking a 6C dose three times daily for up to two days.

Ruta graveolens is available in many health food stores. To purchase homeopathic remedies by mail, refer to the resource list on page 637.

MASSAGE

Here's a quick massage for any time you feel eyestrain, from *Massageworks* by D. Baloti Lawrence and Lewis Harrison.

Quickly rub the palms of your hands together until you feel them heat up. Then gently press your left palm over your closed left eye and your right palm over your closed right eye. Hold for a count of 12.

In her book *The Magic of Massage*, massage therapist Ouida West offers another massage technique for eyestrain. Place your right thumb on the orbital bone above your right eye. This bone is located directly beneath the eyebrow. The tip of the thumb should be pointing toward the nose at the inside corner of the eye, and the back of your hand should be facing your forehead. Place your left thumb on the left orbital bone. Now gently press your thumbs upward against the orbital bones and hold for three to five seconds.

West also suggests applying pressure to the orbital bones located below the eyes. Place the fingertips of your right hand on the bony ridge underneath your right eye. Do the same for your left eye. Gently press against the bones for three to five seconds, then release. Never press directly against your eyes; press only against the bones.

REFLEXOLOGY

You should work these reflexes on your feet thoroughly, according to New York City reflexologist Laura Norman, author of *Feet First: A Guide to Foot Reflexology*: helper to inner ear, helper to eye, kidney and cervical spine, along with all of the points on the tops and bottoms of the toes, paying extra attention to the brain zones. (To work the toes, use whichever technique you find most comfortable.)

To help you locate these points, consult the foot reflex chart on page 592. For instructions on how to work the points, see "Your Reflexology Session" on page 110.

VITAMIN AND MINERAL THERAPY

Deficiencies in the B vitamins may lead to eyestrain, says Jay Cohen, O.D., associate professor at the State University of New York College of Optometry in New York City. "A Japanese study found that people who get eyestrain from working on computers benefit from injections of vitamin B_{12}," he says. In fact, he points out, one sign of a deficiency in the B vitamins is red, irritated eyes. While Dr. Cohen doesn't recommend taking large doses of any individual B vitamin, he does advise a B-complex supplement containing the Recommended Dietary Allowances for the essential B vitamins (thiamin, riboflavin, niacin, vitamin B_6, vitamin B_{12} and pantothenic acid).

YOGA

In addition to the palm-rubbing massage described above, try splashing water on your eyes after every meal, says Stephen A. Nezezon, M.D., yoga teacher and staff physician at the Himalayan International Institute of Yoga Science and Philosophy in Honesdale, Pennsylvania.

SEE ALSO Vision Problems

FATIGUE

Y ou're tired. Again. Still.

It's called fatigue, and all of us have had a go-around with it at one time or another.

The usual Rx is a little R and R. But if you have caught up with your rest and relaxation and are still feeling so low that the blues could be your autobiographical anthem, maybe that burned-out feeling isn't the result of burning the candle at both ends. Fatigue can be an early warning sign of any number of diseases, so take note and see a doctor. And the natural remedies in this chapter—in conjunction with medical care and used with your doctor's approval—may also help relieve fatigue, according to some health professionals.

SEE YOUR MEDICAL DOCTOR WHEN . . .

- You feel lethargic and a loss of energy that lasts two weeks or longer for no apparent reason.
- Your fatigue is accompanied by muscle aches, nausea, fever, depression or mood swings.

AROMATHERAPY

Place a drop each of rosemary (or geranium) and basil essential oils on a tissue and inhale whenever you need a quick energy boost, suggests Fair Oaks, California, aromatherapist Victoria Edwards.

For information on preparing and administering essential oils, including cautions about their use, see page 19. For information on purchasing essential oils, refer to the resource list on page 633.

AYURVEDA

To battle the fatigue that comes with or after illness, drink a mixture of almond milk and herbs once or twice a day, says Vasant Lad, B.A.M.S., M.A.Sc., director of the Ayurvedic Institute in Albuquerque, New Mexico. To make the mixture, soak ten almonds overnight in enough water to cover them. In the morning, peel off their skins, then put them in a blender with a cup of hot skim milk, a pinch each of ginger powder and cardamom and one teaspoon of date sugar (available in most health food stores). Blend and drink.

FATIGUE

HYDROTHERAPY

The cold mitten friction rub is a classic hydrotherapy remedy for fatigue, lethargy or general weakness, according to Agatha Thrash, M.D., a medical pathologist and co-founder and co-director of Uchee Pines Institute, a natural healing center in Seale, Alabama. Dip a small towel or washcloth into cold (50° to 60°F) water, curl one hand into a fist and wrap the towel or washcloth around it. Use your fist to rub your other arm in a vigorous circular motion, beginning with the fingers and finishing at the shoulder. Dip the cloth in cold water again and repeat the step. Your skin should be pink. Dry your arm with a towel using the same vigorous circular movement, then repeat the process on your other arm and on your legs, feet, chest and abdomen. Dr. Thrash says to perform this rub once or twice every day until you're free of fatigue, then use as needed.

IMAGERY

Imagine an energy machine suspended over your head. Give the machine any shape and color that suits you. This machine has a strong, thick wire that connects to the top of your head. You'll find an on/off switch on the wire just before it enters your head. When you feel comfortable, turn on the switch and feel the energy flow into your head and down through your body, says Dennis Gersten, M.D., a San Diego psychiatrist and publisher of *Atlantis*, a bimonthly imagery newsletter. He suggests practicing this imagery for five minutes twice a day.

MASSAGE

A vigorous ten-minute whole-body massage can give you a quick burst of energy, says Vincent Iuppo, N.D., massage therapist, naturopathic physician and director of the Morris Institute of Natural Therapeutics, a holistic health education center in Denville, New Jersey. Obviously, you can't reach every part of your body, but every little bit helps.

Start by lightly lubricating your hands with vegetable oil or massage oil. You can rub your legs and arms with the effleurage (page 570), tapotement (page 571) and vibration (page 571) strokes. Work from your feet to your hips. Then rub your abdomen and chest with gliding, circular strokes. Work each arm by running your hand vigorously from your wrist to your elbow, then from your elbow to your shoulder. Also take time to vigorously rub your shoulder and neck muscles.

REFLEXOLOGY

Working the following reflex points on your feet may help give you a little extra zip, says St. Petersburg, Florida, reflexologist Dwight Byers, author of *Better Health with Foot Reflexology*: diaphragm, whole spine and adrenal, pituitary and thyroid gland.

To help you locate these points, consult the foot reflex chart on page 592. For instructions on how to work the points, see "Your Reflexology Session" on page 110.

RELAXATION AND MEDITATION

Meditation is quite invigorating and can sweep aside any feelings of fatigue, even if it's practiced for just a few minutes a day, says Sundar Ramaswami, Ph.D., a clinical psychologist at the F. S. Dubois Community Mental Health Center in Stamford, Connecticut. To try a simple meditation technique, see page 117.

Begin meditating for 20 minutes twice a day, suggests Dr. Ramaswami. As you become more proficient and more aware of your body's sensations, he says, you may find you can meditate less and still get the same effect.

Deep breathing (see page 116), autogenics (see page 120) and progressive relaxation (see page 122) can also recharge you, according to Martha Davis, Ph.D., Elizabeth Robbins Eshelman and Matthew McKay, Ph.D., in *The Relaxation and Stress Reduction Workbook*.

SOUND THERAPY

Listening to upbeat music can be a great way to find some extra energy, writes Barbara Anne Scarantino in *Music Power: Creative Living through the Joys of Music*. Here are some suggested pieces: marching music by John Philip Sousa; ragtime music by Scott Joplin; *Graceland* by Paul Simon; *Best of the Beach Boys* by the Beach Boys; big band music by Glenn Miller, Benny Goodman, Duke Ellington and the Dorsey brothers; *Black Swan Pas De Deux* by Pyotr Ilich Tchaikovsky; and *Breezin'* by George Benson.

Scarantino warns against listening to too much pop and hard rock music, because it can make you more jittery than energized. Be sure to often vary what you listen to. You could try classical music one day, pop the next day and jazz the third.

Many of these selections are available at music stores. For mail-order information, refer to the resource list on page 642.

YOGA

Morning yoga practice will give you the extra zip you need to make it through tough days, says Alice Christensen, founder and executive director of the American Yoga Association. She recommends doing at least six yoga poses per day from the Daily Routine, which begins on page 606, including the standing sun (page 607), seated sun (page 616) and cobra (page 622). These, combined with 30 minutes of meditation (see page 153), will provide you with additional energy, Christensen says.

SEE ALSO Chronic Fatigue Syndrome; Drowsiness

FEVER

A fever can leave you hot and bothered—in more ways than one. Besides elevating body temperature to the point of discomfort or full-fledged pain, a fever often brings with it shivering, headaches, sweating, thirst, flushed skin and even rapid breathing. It can also include sore throat, body aches and coughing.

Actually, fever isn't a disease. It's a reaction to an infection or to certain medications. When you have a cold, for instance, your immune system tells the brain that it needs more body heat to attack the infectious cells, and body temperature rises. The natural remedies in this chapter—in conjunction with medical care and used with the approval of your doctor—may help relieve the discomfort of a fever, according to some health professionals.

SEE YOUR MEDICAL DOCTOR WHEN . . .

- Your fever is 103°F or higher.
- Your fever lasts longer than 72 hours.
- Your fever is accompanied by a stiff neck, a severe headache or severe back or abdominal pain, you're coughing up discolored phlegm or you have pain while urinating.
- You have a history of heart disease, diabetes or another chronic illness.

FEVER

AYURVEDA

Add ½ teaspoon of coriander, ½ teaspoon of cinnamon and ¼ teaspoon of ginger powder to a cup of hot water, steep for ten minutes, then drink without straining out the herbs, says Vasant Lad, B.A.M.S., M.A.Sc., director of the Ayurvedic Institute in Albuquerque, New Mexico. Dr. Lad says to drink ¼ cup of the hot tea every half-hour. The coriander is the active ingredient here, he explains. Also, he says, the remedy is tridoshic, meaning that it works equally well for vata, pitta and kapha constitutions. (For more information about the Ayurvedic doshas, see "All about Vata, Pitta and Kapha" on page 28.)

HERBAL THERAPY

Fevers can actually be beneficial, because "bacteria, parasites and viruses replicate more slowly at high temperatures," says Jane Guiltinan, N.D., a naturopathic physician and chief medical officer at the Natural Health Clinic of Bastyr University in Seattle. But when your temperature goes over 101°F and stays there for more than 24 hours, Dr. Guiltinan suggests drinking elder tea. She says to drink a cup or two every 15 to 20 minutes until you break into a sweat and your temperature starts going down. You can buy tea bags of elder at most health food stores, or you can make your own tea by steeping one teaspoon to one tablespoon of dried elder flowers (also available in most health food stores) in a cup of boiling water for 15 minutes, straining the mixture to remove the dried herb, then cooling the tea to a drinkable temperature.

HOMEOPATHY

If you develop a fever and sluggishness without other noticeable symptoms, such as headache, earache, cold, flu or stomachache, one of the first remedies to try is a 6C or 12C dose of Ferrum phosphoricum, says Mitchell Fleisher, M.D., a family practice physician and homeopath in Colleen, Virginia. "Sometimes one dose of Ferrum phosphoricum is enough to knock out the fever," he says. Take no more than four doses in 24 hours. If there is no improvement, Dr. Fleisher advises that you consult a medical doctor or homeopath.

Ferrum phosphoricum is available in many health food stores. To purchase homeopathic remedies by mail, refer to the resource list on page 637.

REFLEXOLOGY

Working the pituitary gland reflexes on both feet may help fight a fever, says St. Petersburg, Florida, reflexologist Dwight Byers, author of *Better Health with Foot Reflexology*.

To help you locate these points, consult the foot reflex chart on page 592. For instructions on how to work the points, see "Your Reflexology Session" on page110.

FIBROCYSTIC BREAST DISEASE

Y ou find a lump on your breast. That's all you need to know. After all, every woman realizes what that means, right?

Not necessarily. While any lump is cause for concern—and a trip to the doctor—it's not necessarily cancer. The term *fibrocystic breast disease* has been used to describe problems including mammary dysplasia, fibrocystic mastopathy, chronic cystic mastitis and other conditions that leave breasts painful, lumpy, swollen or tender. The natural remedies in this chapter—in conjunction with medical care and used with the approval of your doctor—may help prevent or relieve fibrocystic breast disease and its symptoms, according to some health professionals.

SEE YOUR MEDICAL DOCTOR WHEN . . .

- You find unusual lumps, swelling, bulging or dimpling in one or both breasts.
- Your breast pain is severe or lasts for more than two months.
- Your breasts are tender while you undergo hormone replacement therapy.

AYURVEDA

At night, apply a paste made from ½ teaspoon of yellow turmeric and 1 teaspoon of warm castor oil to the area of the breast where the cysts are, says Vasant Lad, B.A.M.S., M.A.Sc., director of the Ayurvedic Institute in Albuquerque, New Mexico. He adds this caution: Turmeric can stain skin and clothes, so cover the paste with something that you won't mind staining. Any discoloration should wash off your skin in about two weeks, he adds.

FOOD THERAPY

Food may not alleviate the pain of fibrocystic breast disease, but it can certainly intensify it. "Coffee is especially bad, not only because of the caffeine but also because of the oils in it," says Julian Whitaker, M.D., founder and president of the Whitaker Wellness Center in Newport Beach, California.

Cutting dietary fat can also reduce pain and inflammation, according to Dr. Whitaker. He points out that some women see improvement after switching to a very lean diet that gets no more than 20 percent of its calories from fat. He says the best way to lower fat is to reduce or eliminate fatty meats, oils and dairy products.

HERBAL THERAPY

In *Herbal Healing for Women*, Barre, Vermont, herbalist Rosemary Gladstar, author of several other herb books, offers this recipe for Immune Cleanser Tea, which she recommends as part of an overall health care program to treat fibrocystic breasts. You can find all of the ingredients—freshly dried herbs and powders—in most health food stores or by mail order (refer to the resource list on page 635).

Gladstar says to mix the ingredients in these proportions: one part yellow dock root, three parts dandelion root, two parts burdock root, one part ginger powder, one part dong quai, one part astragalus, one part licorice root, one part chaste berry and four parts pau d'arco. To make the tea, says Gladstar, use four to six tablespoons of this combination per quart of water. Simmer over low heat in a tightly covered pot for 20 minutes, then turn off the heat and let the herbs sit in the covered pot for another 20 minutes. Strain the tea so that no dried herb remains and let the tea cool to a drinkable temperature.

Gladstar suggests drinking three to four cups of the tea daily for five days, then going off it for two days. Continue this treatment for a maximum of three months, she says.

HYDROTHERAPY

Frequent water treatments can soothe tender, lumpy breasts, says Agatha Thrash, M.D., a medical pathologist and co-founder and co-director of Uchee Pines Institute, a natural healing center in Seale, Alabama. She suggests applying a hot, moist compress to each breast for three to five minutes every time you shower. Follow each hot application with a cool sponging, she says.

VITAMIN AND MINERAL THERAPY

"Some studies show that taking 800 international units of vitamin E each day might be helpful for some women," says JulianWhitaker, M.D., founder and president of the Whitaker Wellness Center in Newport Beach, California.

Other nutrients that have been found to help reduce breast tenderness, according to Dr. Whitaker, include vitamin A, the B-complex vitamins (thiamin, riboflavin, niacin, vitamin B_6, vitamin B_{12} and pantothenic acid), iodine and selenium. He says to look for a multivitamin/mineral supplement containing all of these nutrients.

FIBROMYALGIA

Some doctors say that fibromyalgia comes from using muscles too much, to the point where they are stressed or get injured. Others say it's the result of not using your muscles enough, another consequence of a sedentary lifestyle. Either way, this condition leaves muscles hurting so bad that the pain interferes with moving around and even sleeping.

Suspect fibromyalgia (which means pain in the fibrous muscle tissue) if you feel intense pain when you press on tender points in your neck, shoulders, chest, hips, back or buttocks or if you feel an all-over muscle pain that lasts three months or longer, especially if you're in your forties or older. The natural remedies in this chapter—in conjunction with medical care and used with the approval of your doctor—may help relieve some of the symptoms of fibromyalgia, according to some health professionals.

SEE YOUR MEDICAL DOCTOR WHEN . . .

- Your muscles in your neck, shoulders, chest, hips, back or buttocks are so tender that pressing them makes you jump with pain.
- Your muscle pain is accompanied by fever, sleeping problems or depression.
- You also have all-over achiness that has lasted longer than three months.

FOOD THERAPY

"Barley green can be helpful, because it acts as an anti-inflammatory agent when you have fibromyalgia," says Julian Whitaker, M.D., founder and president of the Whitaker Wellness Center in Newport Beach, California. "Try to have it once a day; just sprinkle it on your salad, or mix one to two tablespoons in water and drink it straight." Barley green is available in most health food stores.

YOGA

As part of your daily yoga routine, be sure to include poses that stretch and strengthen your joints, muscles and nerves, says Alice Christensen, founder and executive director of the American Yoga Association. These include the knee squeeze (page 612), spine twist (page 614), easy bridge (page 619) and cobra (page 622). Christensen says that these will help reduce the pain of muscle spasms by keeping you more flexible. *Note:* Do not do the easy bridge pose during the second half of pregnancy.

SEE ALSO Muscle Cramps and Pain

FLATULENCE

It may be the, er, butt of jokes in junior high school locker rooms, but flatulence is anything but funny when it's coming from you. (Of course, those on the receiving end are probably not laughing, either.)

Despite the embarrassment, breaking wind isn't worth getting all huffy about. We all do it, usually between 8 and 20 times a day. Flatulence means just that you have excessive gas in the stomach or intestine, which can result from being sedentary, swallowing air while chewing or having trouble digesting carbohydrates (although other foods can also produce gas, such as dairy products, sauerkraut and artificial sweeteners). Those on a high-fiber diet rich in fruits and vegetables are especially prone to flatulence.

What's bad about it, of course, is the odor, since trace amounts of methane gas are often released. The bottom line in this rump rumpus: Unless you are feeling pain with your flatulence, try to stop worrying and go with the flow, so to speak. But the natural remedies in this chapter, used with the approval of your doctor, may help relieve excessive flatulence, according to some health professionals.

SEE YOUR MEDICAL DOCTOR WHEN . . .

- Your flatulence is accompanied by stomach or abdominal pain for more than three days.
- You have an unexplained weight loss with the gas.
- Your pain is more severe than you've ever had before.

FLATULENCE

AROMATHERAPY

This remedy, from *Aromatherapy: Applications and Inhalations* by San Francisco herbalist Jeanne Rose, chairperson of the National Association for Holistic Aromatherapy, won't eliminate flatulence, but it will make you more pleasant to be around while the problem runs its course. Drink four ounces of water to which you've added a single drop of peppermint essential oil. Rose says that before long, your flatus will have the minty fragrance of toothpaste or breath mints!

For information on preparing and administering essential oils, including cautions about their use, see page 19. For information on purchasing essential oils, refer to the resource list on page 633.

AYURVEDA

A mixture of one teaspoon of grated fresh ginger pulp and one teaspoon of lime juice, taken immediately after eating, can prevent excess gas and lower abdominal pain, says Vasant Lad, B.A.M.S., M.A.Sc., director of the Ayurvedic Institute in Albuquerque, New Mexico.

FOOD THERAPY

Kombu, a sea vegetable that's available in most Asian grocery stores and some health food stores, can help neutralize foods that usually trigger flatulence, says Allan Magaziner, D.O., a nutritional medicine specialist and head of the Magaziner Medical Center in Cherry Hill, New Jersey. "Let's say you're boiling broccoli, a food that can cause flatulence in many people. Simply put a little strip of kombu in the pot while you're cooking. It helps neutralize the gas from the broccoli, so you avoid the flatulence afterward."

HOMEOPATHY

A 30C dose of Carbo vegetabilis, taken once or twice a day, may stop a sudden, acute attack of flatulence, particularly if it is accompanied by a lot of belching, says Judyth Reichenberg-Ullman, N.D., a naturopathic physician in Edmonds, Washington, and co-author of *The Patient's Guide to Homeopathic Medicine*. If your flatulence doesn't subside within 24 hours or two doses of the remedy, she says to consult your medical doctor or homeopath.

Carbo vegetabilis is available in many health food stores. To purchase homeopathic remedies by mail, refer to the resource list on page 637.

HYDROTHERAPY

Activated charcoal is great for relieving intestinal gas, according to Agatha Thrash, M.D., a medical pathologist and co-founder and co-director of Uchee Pines Institute, a natural healing center in Seale, Alabama. Her instructions: Put two to three tablespoons of activated charcoal powder in the bottom of a large glass and add a small amount of water (bottled may be best if you're traveling). Stir slowly with a long-handled spoon to keep the fine powder from flying everywhere, suggests Dr. Thrash. Fill the glass the rest of the way with water and drink through a straw. Dr. Thrash says to use this remedy whenever you have gas, drinking a glass of charcoal water every day until the problem clears. Activated charcoal is available in most health food stores and some pharmacies.

JUICE THERAPY

The licorice-flavored plant fennel has long been used to help relieve or expel gas, according to Michael Murray, N.D., a naturopathic physician and author of *The Complete Book of Juicing*. Since fresh fennel has a very strong flavor, Dr. Murray recommends juicing a few sprigs of the herb with apples, pears, carrots or celery and drinking eight ounces of the blend.

For information on juicing techniques, see page 93.

REFLEXOLOGY

Work the reflexes on your hands or feet for your intestine, stomach, liver, gallbladder and pancreas, says St. Petersburg, Florida, reflexologist Dwight Byers, author of *Better Health with Foot Reflexology*.

To help you locate these points, consult the hand and foot reflex charts beginning on page 582. For instructions on how to work the points, see "Your Reflexology Session" on page 110.

YOGA

You can relieve gas by trying the knee squeeze (page 612), says Stephen A. Nezezon, M.D., yoga teacher and staff physician at the Himalayan International Institute of Yoga Science and Philosophy in Honesdale, Pennsylvania. Practice this pose whenever needed. Dr. Nezezon also suggests chewing food consciously, concentrating on each bite, to slow down your eating and help digestion.

FLU

Not again! That deathbedlike fatigue. That brain-smashing headache. The feeling that you've been run over by a truck . . . or rather, General Motors.

It's flu season again. Time for vomiting, fever, sweats and shivers. Time for a few days of agony and more than a few curses over your failure to get a flu shot. Like colds and other viruses, the flu is spread from person to person, usually in the winter and early spring, and getting a vaccination is the best way to avoid it. The other way, unfortunately, is to avoid other people, especially indoors. Since the latter option usually isn't an option, the odds are good that the flu bug will bite you—at least on occasion. But the natural remedies in this chapter—in conjunction with medical care and used with the approval of your doctor—may help relieve the symptoms of the flu, according to some health professionals.

SEE YOUR MEDICAL DOCTOR WHEN . . .

- You want a flu shot, which you should get before flu season begins.
- You get the flu and are over age 65.
- You get the flu and experience hoarseness, pain in your chest or difficulty breathing.

AROMATHERAPY

When everyone around you seems to be coming down with the flu, mix a blend of essential oils to use in your diffuser, suggests John Steele, an aromatic consultant in Los Angeles. "Scenting a room with the right essences can stop the spread of airborne viruses," he explains.

In a five-milliliter bottle, says Steele, blend together three parts ravensare, one part naiouli or eucalyptus, one part lemon, one part rosewood and one part lavender. (Ravensare and naiouli have antiviral properties, according to Steele, while the other essential oils act as antiseptics and give the blend a wonderful aroma.) Add about 50 drops of this blend to your diffuser at a time.

For a steam inhalation, Steele suggests adding six to eight drops of this blend to a bowl of just-boiled water. Place a towel over your head and inhale. Repeat this treatment two or three times a day, if necessary, he says.

For chills, Steele suggests 3 drops of rosemary and 3 drops of ginger or black pepper essential oils added to your bath. Or, he says, make an energizing massage oil blend using 5 drops of ravensare and 15 drops of rosewood in ½ ounce of carrier oil such as olive or almond. Carrier oils are available in most health food stores.

For information on preparing and administering essential oils, including cautions about their use, see page 19. For information on purchasing essential oils, refer to the resource list on page 633.

AYURVEDA

At the first sign of the flu, switch to a bland diet, says Vasant Lad, B.A.M.S., M.A.Sc., director of the Ayurvedic Institute in Albuquerque, New Mexico. He especially recommends soft-cooked rice (rice that has a very soft, moist texture created by a longer cooking time with more water) with a pinch of cumin, ginger powder and turmeric for seasoning. The ginger and cumin heat up your body, so you can sweat out toxins, he explains. And, he says, turmeric has antibiotic and antiseptic qualities.

To ease the congestion that can accompany the flu, Dr. Lad suggests this formula: Mix just under ½ teaspoon each of sitopaladi powder (available from some Indian grocers and through mail order; refer to the resource list on page 634) and sudarshan (available from Ayurvedic practitioners), with ½ teaspoon of honey to sweeten. "Take a teaspoonful of this mixture every few hours," says Dr. Lad. "You'll be amazed at how quickly your symptoms disappear."

FOOD THERAPY

Feed your flu with fluids to replace what you lose through sweating and vomiting, suggests Julian Whitaker, M.D., founder and president of the Whitaker Wellness Center in Newport Beach, California. Besides water, which should be sipped regularly even when you don't feel thirsty, Dr. Whitaker recommends vitamin-rich beverages such as apple juice and vegetable juice, as well as soups. Once your stomach can handle it, stick with easy-to-digest, high-nutrient foods such as dry toast and bananas and rice, he says.

HERBAL THERAPY

To ward off the flu at the first hint of symptoms, take echinacea, an herb with powerful antiviral and immunity-boosting effects, says Barre, Vermont, herbalist Rosemary Gladstar, author of *Herbal Healing for Women* and other books about herbs. Echinacea is available in most health food stores in supplement form, as a tincture and as a tea, according to Gladstar; she advises following the dosage recommendations on the label of the product you choose.

Echinacea works best over a short period of time, she says, and isn't an effective immune strengthener when taken long term. She suggests using the herb for no more than a week.

HOMEOPATHY

Oscillococcinum, Flu Solution and other commerical combination remedies containing duck liver and heart extract are excellent flu fighters, says Mitchell Fleisher, M.D., a family practice physician and homeopath in Colleen, Virginia. "Combination flu remedies work for a lot of people, particularly if you take one in the first 4 to 12 hours after you start having symptoms," according to Dr. Fleisher. He says to follow the dosage recommendations on the label of the remedy you choose. If it's going to work, you should feel relief with a single dose, he adds.

If the flu persists, however, Dr. Fleisher says that you'll probably need a more specific remedy, such as a 12C or 30C dose of Eupatorium perfoliatum, which is good for a flu that causes aches and chills in your back and bones, fatigue, thirst and bad headaches. If you feel dizzy, drowsy and weak but momentarily better after urinating, he suggests trying a 12C or 30C dose of Gelsemium. Take up to four doses of one of these flu remedies in 24 hours. Then if you don't feel better, see your medical doctor or homeopath, says Dr. Fleisher.

All of these remedies are available in many health food stores. To purchase the remedies by mail, refer to the resource list on page 637.

HYDROTHERAPY

A hot bath followed by a cold mitten friction rub, two to four times a day, loosens congestion, improves circulation and strengthens the immune system, speeding healing from the flu. That advice is from Charles Thomas, Ph.D., co-author of *Hydrotherapy: Simple Treatments for Common Ailments* and a physical therapist at Desert Springs Therapy Center in Desert Hot Springs, California.

To do a cold mitten friction rub, follow these instructions from Agatha Thrash, M.D., a medical pathologist and co-founder and co-director of Uchee Pines Institute, a natural healing center in Seale, Alabama: Dip a small towel or washcloth into cold (50° to 60°F) water, curl one hand into a fist and wrap the cloth around it. Use your fist to rub your other arm in a vigorous circular motion, beginning with the fingers and finishing at the shoulder. Dip the cloth in the cold water again and repeat. Your skin should be pink. Dry your arm with a towel using the same vigorous circular movement, then repeat the process on your other arm and on your legs, feet, chest and abdomen.

JUICE THERAPY

Both apple and dark grape juices may be beneficial to those fighting the flu, says John Peterson, M.D., an Ayurvedic practitioner in Muncie, Indiana. Apple and dark grape juices have properties that work against congestion and runny nose, according to Dr. Peterson. And, he says, dark grape juice is rich in tannins, substances that have been shown to kill viruses under laboratory conditions.

Do not blend the juices, says Dr. Peterson, but you may dilute them if they are too sweet. He says to drink them at room temperature and at any time other than meals. He also suggests that pear, cranberry and pomegranate juices may be helpful.

For information on juicing techniques, see page 93.

REFLEXOLOGY

Pay special attention to the following reflexes on your hands or feet, says St. Petersburg, Florida, reflexologist Dwight Byers, author of *Better Health with Foot Reflexology*: chest and lung, diaphragm, intestine, lymphatic system and pituitary and adrenal gland.

To help you locate these points, consult the hand and foot reflex charts beginning on page 582. For instructions on how to work the points, see "Your Reflexology Session" on page 110.

FOOD ALLERGIES

It may be wheezing from wheat or a rash from radishes. But while food allergies are rare, affecting only 1 percent of the population and usually outgrown by age six, the foods that can trigger them aren't.

Cow's milk, eggs, peanuts, wheat and soybeans lead the list of eats that can cause swollen lips, throat or tongue, eczema, hives, vomiting, fainting, nausea, diarrhea and other reactions. But they're not alone. Even food additives such as yellow dye #5 and gum arabic can cause allergic reactions in some people, usually within a few minutes of consumption. Reactions range from minor to life-threatening, so see your doctor to pinpoint the cause and come up with a preventive strategy. But the natural remedies in this chapter—in conjunction with medical care and used with the approval of your doctor—may help relieve the symptoms of a food allergy, according to some health professionals.

FOOD ALLERGIES

SEE YOUR MEDICAL DOCTOR WHEN...

- You experience any of these symptoms within two hours of eating a certain food.

  Hives or another skin reaction
  Swelling, especially of the lips or face
  Vomiting or nausea
  A tight feeling in your chest
  Trouble breathing, whether from an asthmatic reaction or throat
    swelling
  Nasal congestion
  Diarrhea
  Cramping or feelings of faintness

AYURVEDA

What kinds of foods you're allergic to depends on your Ayurvedic dosha, says Vasant Lad, B.A.M.S., M.A.Sc., director of the Ayurvedic Institute in Albuquerque, New Mexico. Pitta people are allergic to hot, spicy foods, fermented foods, sour fruits, tomatoes, potatoes and eggplant, according to Dr. Lad. He says that kaphas develop allergies to dairy products and cold beverages. And, he says, vatas may have allergic reactions to hard-to-digest foods such as popcorn, beans and raw vegetables. No matter what your dosha, says Dr. Lad, the symptoms of food allergies include constipation, burping and hiccuping. (For more information about the Ayurvedic doshas, see "All about Vata, Pitta and Kapha" on page 28.)

To avoid adverse reactions to foods, "find out what your dosha is and follow the proper diet for that dosha," says Dr. Lad. He also offers the following remedies.

- For pitta allergies, Dr. Lad suggests eating cooked apple pulp (peel, core and mash the apples to make the pulp) with a pinch of cumin and one teaspoon of ghee, or clarified butter (for a recipe, see "How to Make Ghee" on page 26). Eat a small amount, about ½ cup, twice daily, at least an hour before or after a meal, he says.
- For kapha allergies, Dr. Lad suggests drinking licorice tea. To make the tea, he says to blend ½ teaspoon of licorice (which is available in most health food stores), ¼ teaspoon of cinnamon and ½ teaspoon of coriander, then steep the mixture in one cup of hot water for ten minutes. Don't strain out the herbs before drinking, he says. His suggested dosage: Sip about an ounce of the tea every half-hour for the first few hours, then for the next few hours, sip an ounce every hour. Continue as needed, he adds.

- For vata allergies, Dr. Lad recommends another variation of licorice tea: Mix ½ teaspoon of licorice, ½ teaspoon of honey and 1 teaspoon of ghee in a cup of hot water. As with the other tea, do not strain out the herbs before drinking. He says to sip an ounce of the tea every half-hour for the first two hours, then for the next few hours, sip an ounce every hour. Continue as needed, he adds.

One cautionary note from Dr. Lad: He says people with high blood pressure should not drink licorice tea. For them, Dr. Lad recommends cinnamon/clove tea as an alternative. His recipe: Steep ½ teaspoon of cinnamon and two or three cloves in a cup of boiling water for ten minutes. Sip an ounce of the tea every half-hour for the first two hours, then for the next few hours, sip an ounce every hour. Continue as needed, says Dr. Lad.

YOGA

Poor digestion may result in food allergies, especially as you get older, says Stephen A. Nezezon, M.D., yoga teacher and staff physician at the Himalayan International Institute of Yoga Science and Philosophy in Honesdale, Pennsylvania. To improve digestion, Dr. Nezezon suggests trying an exercise called *agni sara*, or "strengthening the fire."

Here are his instructions for performing the exercise: Stand with your feet about three feet apart, toes pointed slightly outward. Bend your knees slightly and place your right hand on your right thigh and your left hand on your left thigh. Your fingers should be pointing inward, toward the opposite leg. Bend your neck so that you're looking down at your stomach. Breathe out completely. Then suck in and lift your abdomen without taking a breath. Now pump your stomach muscles, pushing your abdomen in and out without breathing. Pump this way 10 to 15 times, then relax, stand up straight and breathe. Repeat the exercise three times per day.

Dr. Nezezon says not to do this exercise during menstruation or pregnancy, after surgery, if you are bleeding or if you have heart disease or high blood pressure.

SEE ALSO Allergies; Lactose Intolerance

FOOD CRAVINGS

I t's perfectly normal to feel hungry when you smell food cooking, see a delicious dish or feel the rumblings from down below. But when you start drowning with desire at the very thought of a particular food, you're no longer eating just for nourishment—at least not the kind that feeds your body.

Everyone knows what it's like to have food cravings and to succumb to them. And that's fine, as long as it doesn't occur on a routine basis. (One reason not to give in: Most of what we crave is high in sugar and fat.) But beyond that, a food craving can also be a symptom of a physical or an emotional problem. Those with diabetes often crave carbohydrates, for example. And sometimes food cravings are the result of anxiety or depression. The natural remedies in this chapter—in conjunction with medical care and used with the approval of your doctor—may help reduce food cravings, according to some health professionals.

SEE YOUR MEDICAL DOCTOR WHEN...

- Your food cravings dominate your thinking and you become so obsessed with satisfying your cravings that it interferes with your normal lifestyle.
- You think your cravings are a problem.

JUICE THERAPY

A craving for salty foods may be a symptom of adrenal exhaustion, especially in people who live fast-paced, stressful lives, says Cherie Calbom, M.S., a certified nutritionist in Kirkland, Washington, and co-author of *Juicing for Life*. In such cases, she recommends juices that she says are high in vitamin C (citrus, pepper and broccoli) and potassium (parsley, garlic, spinach and carrot). "Salt cravings can also be a symptom of serious conditions such as diabetes, high blood pressure and sickle cell anemia," says Calbom. "So anyone who is craving salt should really see a doctor for a complete physical."

For information on juicing techniques, see page 93.

RELAXATION AND MEDITATION

Meditation may be worth trying if you want to reduce your food cravings, says Roger Walsh, M.D., Ph.D., professor of psychiatry, philosophy and anthropology at the University of California, Irvine, California College of Medicine.

Cravings may be a substitute for a more meaningful spiritual experience, according to Dr. Walsh. Meditation may reduce those cravings by filling that void. To learn a simple meditation, see page 117. Practice this technique for 20 minutes once or twice a day, he suggests.

VITAMIN AND MINERAL THERAPY

The amino acid glutamine, which is sold in the vitamin and mineral section of most pharmacies and health food stores, can help you get over food cravings, says Julian Whitaker, M.D., founder and president of the Whitaker Wellness Center in Newport Beach, California. "Take 1,000 milligrams a day to avoid food cravings if you're prone to them."

FOOD POISONING

You fed your face, and now, hours later, your stomach is reacting. Badly. Uh-oh, this wasn't on the menu: nausea, vomiting, diarrhea, cramps and other below-the-belt discomfort that can last a day or two.

Usually, food poisoning is nothing serious—just the result of eating food or drinking water that has been contaminated with infectious bacteria. Within 24 to 48 hours of consuming the culprit, you'll get a reaction, which may also include sweating, itching or even a slight fever. Then it's over. If the bout goes on longer, see a doctor. But the natural remedies in this chapter—in conjunction with medical care and used with the approval of your doctor—may help relieve the symptoms of food poisoning, according to some health professionals.

SEE YOUR MEDICAL DOCTOR WHEN...

- Your condition doesn't improve after 24 to 48 hours.
- Your symptoms also include a high fever, worsening abdominal cramps, bloody diarrhea or the prolonged inability to hold down fluids.

FOOD THERAPY

"Eat bread when you have food poisoning," says Julian Whitaker, M.D., founder and president of the Whitaker Wellness Center in Newport Beach, California. "It has a tendency to soak up the poison for quicker relief." Dr.

FOOD POISONING

Whitaker says a few slices should do it, but he cautions not to top it with butter or jam, which could make you feel even sicker.

HOMEOPATHY

If you suspect that you have food poisoning and you feel anxious, restless and chilly and have simultaneous nausea, vomiting and diarrhea, try taking Arsenicum album in 6C or 12C potency every two to three hours until you feel better, says Mitchell Fleisher, M.D., a family practitioner and homeopath in Colleen, Virginia. If, however, you have similar symptoms but also have cold sweats and crave ice-cold beverages, Dr. Fleisher recommends trying a 6C or 12C dose of Veratrum album every two to three hours. If you feel bloated, sweaty and weak, develop flatulence and diarrhea and feel better after belching, he suggests taking a 6C or 12C dose of Carbo vegetabilis every two to three hours.

Arsenicum album, Veratrum album and Carbo vegetabilis are available in many health food stores. To purchase homeopathic remedies by mail, refer to the resource list on page 637.

HYDROTHERAPY

Activated charcoal is the remedy of choice for Agatha Thrash, M.D., a medical pathologist and co-founder and co-director of Uchee Pines Institute, a natural healing center in Seale, Alabama. "Start with ¼ cup of charcoal powder mixed with a glass of water," she suggests. "If you don't feel better in a half-hour, do it again." She says to continue this regimen until your symptoms subside.

Because charcoal powder is very fine, she suggests mixing it with a little water in the bottom of a tall glass to moisten it, then adding water a little at a time and stirring until the glass is full. You can find activated charcoal in most health food stores and some pharmacies.

FOOT ODOR

Maybe you do all of the right things to stay one step ahead of foot odor. You wash your feet regularly with warm, soapy water. You change shoes and socks daily (or even more). But those dogs still smell bad enough to make those around you want to roll over and play dead.

The problem with foot odor is more than skin-deep. Overactive sweat glands trigger the growth of bacteria and fungus, and they trigger that unforgettable odor (and the hasty exit of those around you). The natural remedies in this chapter, used with the approval of your doctor, may help prevent or relieve foot odor, according to some health professionals.

SEE YOUR MEDICAL DOCTOR WHEN...

• Your foot odor continues, despite all efforts to control it.

AROMATHERAPY

Try the following deodorizing foot wash, from *Aromatherapy: Applications and Inhalations* by San Francisco herbalist Jeanne Rose, chairperson of the National Association for Holistic Aromatherapy: Blend two ounces of water, ten drops of lemon essential oil and the juice of one lemon, then wipe your feet thoroughly.

For information on preparing and administering essential oils, including cautions about their use, see page 19. For information on purchasing essential oils, refer to the resource list on page 633.

FOOD THERAPY

Soak your feet in tea, suggests Jerome Z. Litt, M.D., assistant clinical professor of dermatology at Case Western Reserve University in Cleveland. He says that the tannic acid in tea eliminates the odor. Simply boil a few tea bags in a pint of water for 15 minutes, then pour the hot brew into a basin filled with two quarts of cool water. Dr. Litt recommends soaking for 30 minutes every day for a week.

HOMEOPATHY

In addition to washing your feet daily with antibacterial soap, try one of the following remedies in a 12C potency in the morning and evening until you see improvement, says Chris Meletis, N.D., a naturopathic physician and medicinary director at the National College of Naturopathic Medicine in Portland, Oregon. According to Dr. Meletis, Silicea may help if you have ice-cold, sweaty feet and pain from the instep through the sole of your foot and if your armpits and hands also have an offensive odor. If your symptoms are worse with warmth, and if you tend to have dry and rough skin in places, he suggests trying Graphites. Iodom can help, he says, if you have acrid, sweaty feet and if the symptoms are worse in warm rooms and better with walking around and when feet are aired.

All of these remedies are available in many health food stores. To purchase homeopathic remedies by mail, refer to the resource list on page 637.

SEE ALSO Sweating Excessively

FOOT PAIN

Ask anyone, and he'll probably admit to possessing three qualities: a great sense of humor, excellent driving ability and, at least occasionally, a certain amount of misery that's brought on by feet that burn, swell, sting, itch, ache or otherwise cause problems.

Foot pain is one of the most common health complaints, affecting nearly nine of every ten people. And often it's not related to any specific condition. Wearing properly fitting shoes can solve a lot of the problem. And the natural remedies in this chapter—in conjunction with medical care and used with the approval of your doctor—may also help prevent or relieve foot pain, according to some health professionals.

SEE YOUR MEDICAL DOCTOR WHEN...

- Your foot sore doesn't heal after one week.
- Your feet consistently feel either hot or cold or have increasing redness.
- You feel continual prickling or weakness or a change of sensation in your foot.

ACUPRESSURE

For pain in the big toe, press Lv 3, located on the top of the foot in the valley between the big toe and the second toe, advises Michael Reed Gach,

Ph.D., director of the Acupressure Institute in Berkeley, California, and author of *Acupressure's Potent Points*. He says to hold the point for one minute. To relieve foot cramps, press Sp 4 in the upper arch of the foot, one thumbwidth from the ball of the foot, says Dr. Gach. Press point Sp 4 for one minute. (For help in locating these points, refer to the illustrations beginning on page 564.)

AROMATHERAPY

To ease tired, aching feet, Greenwich, Connecticut, aromatherapist Judith Jackson, author of *Scentual Touch: A Personal Guide to Aromatherapy*, recommends a good foot soak: Add ten drops each of juniper and lavender essential oils to two quarts of warm water, then soak your feet for ten minutes.

For information on preparing and administering essential oils, including cautions about their use, see page 19. For information on purchasing essential oils, refer to the resource list on page 633.

HOMEOPATHY

If you have puffy feet that burn or sting, Andrew Lockie, M.D., in his book *The Family Guide to Homeopathy*, suggests taking a 6C dose of Apis three times a day. He says that a similar dose of Sulphur will help if you tend to feel hot most of the time and have burning feet that feel worse at night. If you have a burning sensation in your feet that feels worse when walking, Dr. Lockie recommends Graphite 6C three times a day. Take these remedies for up to three weeks, he says. If there is no improvement, see a medical doctor or homeopath.

Apis, Sulphur and Graphite are available in many health food stores. To purchase homeopathic remedies by mail, refer to the resource list on page 637.

MASSAGE

If your feet hurt because of overuse, a gentle sole massage can make them feel better, says Elliot Greene, past president of the American Massage Therapy Association. Sit in a comfortable chair and cross your left foot over your right leg. Lightly oil your fingers with vegetable oil or massage oil. With the tip of your thumb, glide up the middle of your sole from the back of the heel to the base of your toes. Repeat this on the right and left sides of your sole. This should take about two minutes per foot.

Then retrace all three lines—middle, right and left—pressing with the tip of your thumb. Do this until you reach the base of your toes. Then gently rub and squeeze your toes with your fingertips, paying special attention to the tips of your toes. Repeat with the other foot. You should spend about three to four minutes on each foot.

VITAMIN AND MINERAL THERAPY

If your feet are hurting because of bunions, you may get relief from a daily dose of 25,000 international units of vitamin A, says Julian Whitaker, M.D., founder and president of the Whitaker Wellness Center in Newport Beach, California. Discontinue use after one week if your symptoms don't improve, he says, since vitamin A can cause nerve damage when taken for extended periods.

SEE ALSO Calluses and Corns; Gout; Heel Spurs; Ingrown Toenails

FROSTBITE

When Jack Frost takes an innocent nip at our noses, we sing about it. But expect to cry the blues if those nips turn into big, sore frostbite on your fingers and toes, the result of spending time in the frigid outdoors.

Frostbite results when your body attempts to stay warm in the bitter cold. Trying to warm the vital inner organs, it cuts back on blood circulation to the extremities, especially the hands and feet. Without their share of 98.6°F blood, these parts can freeze, causing permanent damage. Skin that is frostbitten appears waxy and feels doughlike to the touch. The natural remedy in this chapter—in conjunction with medical care and used with the approval of your doctor—may help relieve the symptoms of frostbite, according to one health professional.

SEE YOUR MEDICAL DOCTOR WHEN . . .

- Your skin has ice crystals on it after exposure to the cold, the first sign of frostbite.
- Your pain continues for more than a few hours.
- Your skin is pale or white and doesn't respond to rewarming.
- You see dark blue or black areas under the skin.
- Your skin blisters.

GALLSTONES

HOMEOPATHY

"The most common homeopathic frostbite remedy is Agaricus. I've used it, and I've found it quite helpful," says Judyth Reichenberg-Ullman, N.D., a naturopathic physician in Edmonds, Washington, and co-author of *The Patient's Guide to Homeopathic Medicine*. She suggests taking a 30C dose once or twice a day to treat frostbite that causes red fingers or toes and itching or burning of the skin. If you don't notice any improvement in 48 hours, Dr. Reichenberg-Ullman says to discontinue use and see your medical doctor or homeopath.

Agaricus is available in many health food stores. To purchase homeopathic remedies by mail, refer to the resource list on page 637.

GALLSTONES

G et a "seed" of sand inside an oyster shell, and you can wind up with a pearl. When the same thing happens in your gallbladder, you can wind up with a gem of an ache.

Gallstones form when there's too much cholesterol in your bile. This excess forms tiny "seeds" that start out the size of a grain of sand but can grow to the size of a marble or even an egg. Pain in the upper abdomen or near the shoulder blades, along with vomiting and nausea, occurs when the stone gets stuck in the gallbladder's duct. The pain usually lasts a few hours, until the stone drops back into the gallbladder. If it stays stuck in the duct, a stone can block the flow of bile and cause damage to the liver, pancreas or gallbladder.

Women are three times more likely than men to develop gallstones, and stones seem to run in families. Being overweight and having high cholesterol or insulin levels are also risk factors. By age 60, nearly one in three people will have a gallstone. The natural remedies in this chapter—in conjunction with medical care and used with the approval of your doctor—may help prevent gallstones, according to some health professionals.

SEE YOUR MEDICAL DOCTOR WHEN...

- You are experiencing sharp, unexplained pain in your upper abdomen, between your shoulder blades or in your right shoulder that lasts more than 20 minutes.
- Your skin and the whites of your eyes turn yellow.

GALLSTONES

FOOD THERAPY

"It's easier to prevent gallstones than to treat them, and one of the best ways to prevent them is with a high-fiber diet," says Julian Whitaker, M.D., founder and president of the Whitaker Wellness Center in Newport Beach, California. To add more fiber to your diet, Dr. Whitaker suggests eating more beans and no fewer than five servings of fresh fruits and vegetables each day. He also says to add oat bran to recipes or sprinkle it on your cereal.

HYDROTHERAPY

Drinking plenty of water flushes the liver and dilutes the bile secretions that lead to gallstones, says Agatha Thrash, M.D., a medical pathologist and co-founder and co-director of Uchee Pines Institute, a natural healing center in Seale, Alabama. She suggests drinking 8 to 12 eight-ounce glasses of water a day.

JUICE THERAPY

"Green juices are great for preventing a recurrence in anyone who has had gallstones," says Elaine Gillaspie, N.D., a naturopathic physician in Portland, Oregon. Juices with spinach and parsley are rich in chlorophyll, a pigment that has a natural cleansing effect, according to Dr. Gillaspie. She suggests an eight-ounce blend of two ounces of green juice and two ounces of carrot juice, diluted with an equal amount of water. "Even one eight-ounce glass a day has a preventive effect," she says.

For information on juicing techniques, see page 93.

REFLEXOLOGY

To help relieve gallbladder problems, says New York City reflexologist Laura Norman, author of *Feet First: A Guide to Foot Reflexology*, try working these reflexes on your feet: solar plexus, diaphragm, thyroid and helper to thyroid, thoracic spine, liver and gallbladder.

To help you locate these points, consult the foot reflex chart on page 592. For instructions on how to work the points, see "Your Reflexology Session" on page 110.

VITAMIN AND MINERAL THERAPY

Use the food sensitivity diet (see "Food Sensitivity: How to Discover the 'Healthy' Foods That Can Cause Disease" on page 52) to eliminate any foods

that might have a role in causing gallstones, suggests David Edelberg, M.D., an internist and medical director of the American Holistic Center/Chicago. He also says people with gallstones may want to use the following nutritional regimen: 1,000 milligrams of vitamin C three times a day; 1,200 milligrams of lecithin twice a day; one tablespoon of flaxseed oil a day; and 1 gram of taurine twice a day. Lecithin, flaxseed oil and taurine are available in most health food stores.

GENITAL HERPES

L ove can hurt. Just ask anyone with genital herpes, also known as herpes simplex type 2. (Type 1 usually results in cold sores on the mouth and hands.) And the way it's passed isn't too complex: Have sexual intercourse with an infected person who is in the contagious stage—that is, with herpes sores on the body—and you might join the 500,000 people each year who get genital herpes, a condition that stays with you for life.

The virus may lie dormant for years, which is one reason why three of four people with genital herpes are unaware they have it. But during an outbreak, it doesn't exactly put you in the mood for sex. One or more open sores can appear on the genitals, creating a painful burning sensation. Not having sex with someone who's infected is how to avoid genital herpes, and the prescription drug acyclovir is the best way to control outbreaks. And the natural remedies in this chapter—in conjunction with medical care and used with the approval of your doctor—may help prevent outbreaks, relieve the symptoms of herpes lesions or speed their healing, according to some health professionals.

SEE YOUR MEDICAL DOCTOR WHEN . . .

- You notice a blister or sore that suddenly appears on your genitals, whether or not it is painful.
- Your itching or pain is so bad that you want medication for relief.

AROMATHERAPY

Apply a single drop of tea tree essential oil directly to herpes lesions once a day after showering, recommends San Francisco herbalist Jeanne Rose, chair-

GENITAL HERPES

person of the National Association for Holistic Aromatherapy and author of *Aromatherapy: Applications and Inhalations.* "Tea tree oil is gentle to the skin and helps any kind of external sore heal faster," says Rose.

For information on preparing and administering essential oils, including cautions about their use, see page 19. For information on purchasing essential oils, refer to the resource list on page 633.

FOOD THERAPY

"For some people, changing the diet to make it more alkaline can help prevent herpes outbreaks and help get over them more quickly," says Elson Haas, M.D., director of the Preventive Medical Center of Marin in San Rafael, California, and author of *Staying Healthy with Nutrition.* That means eating more fruits (with the exception of citrus fruits, which are too acidic), vegetables, sea vegetables such as kelp and seaweed, millet, seeds and herbs and less meats, fish, eggs, milk products, breads and baked goods, nuts and alcohol, according to Dr. Haas.

HERBAL THERAPY

Try a wash made from lemon balm, says Varro E. Tyler, Ph.D., professor of pharmacognosy at Purdue University in West Lafayette, Indiana. The fragrant leaves and flowering tops of the lemon balm plant have antiviral properties, he explains.

To make the wash, Dr. Tyler says you should pour ½ cup of boiling water over two to three teaspoons of finely cut leaves, available in most health food stores. Let it brew for 20 to 30 minutes, then strain it and saturate a clean cotton cloth with the solution. Dr. Tyler suggests applying the wash to herpes lesions three or four times a day.

VITAMIN AND MINERAL THERAPY

Use the food sensitivity diet (see "Food Sensitivity: How to Discover the 'Healthy' Foods That Can Cause Disease" on page 52) to eliminate any foods that may aggravate outbreaks of genital herpes, suggests David Edelberg, M.D., an internist and medical director of the American Holistic Center/Chicago. He also says people with genital herpes may want to use the following nutritional regimen to help control recurrences: 2,000 milligrams of vitamin C twice a day; one gram of citrus bioflavonoids a day; and 500 milligrams of lysine a day, increasing the amount to 3,000 milligrams during a flare-up. Citrus bioflavonoids are available in most health food stores.

GINGIVITIS

We spend the better part of our lives fighting cavities tooth and nail. Then when we hit our thirties and forties, we have to worry about another threat to our pearly whites: gum disease, or gingivitis. The problem can be caused by any number of the 300 or so different types of bacteria that take shelter in our mouths. Without proper brushing and flossing, some of these bacteria burrow into our gums, resulting in a plaque buildup known as gingivitis that causes gums to redden, swell and bleed easily. Although it's painless, gingivitis can lead to the more serious and more painful periodontitis as well as eventual tooth loss. The natural remedies in this chapter—in conjunction with medical care and used with your dentist's approval—may help control gingivitis, according to some health professionals.

SEE YOUR MEDICAL DOCTOR WHEN . . .

- You have bad breath that doesn't go away within 24 hours.
- Your teeth look longer, the result of gums shrinking away from your teeth.
- Your teeth are loose, fall out or break off near the gum line.
- You notice a change in your tooth alignment, the way your bite feels.
- Your dentures fit differently.
- Pus pockets form between your teeth and gums.
- Your gums are still swollen, sore or bleeding despite good oral hygiene.

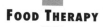

AROMATHERAPY

When gums look inflamed and irritated, add a drop of tea tree essential oil to your toothbrush, on top of the toothpaste, before brushing, says Fair Oaks, California, aromatherapist Victoria Edwards. This is also great preventive medicine, says Edwards. "Tea tree is a natural antiseptic and helps prevent gum disease before it starts."

For information on preparing and administering essential oils, including cautions about their use, see page 21. For information on purchasing essential oils, refer to the resource list on page 633.

FOOD THERAPY

"High intake of vitamin C has been shown to be as effective in controlling gingivitis as brushing and flossing," says Richard D. Fischer, D.D.S., a dentist in

Annandale, Virginia, and president of the International Academy of Oral Medicine and Toxicology. While that's not to say you shouldn't brush and floss, vitamin C makes gums less likely to bleed and promotes the healing process, says Dr. Fischer. And, he points out, it helps strengthen the gum tissue, making it less vulnerable to bacteria and other irritants. He recommends trying to eat at least five servings of fruits and vegetables each day, including vitamin C–rich broccoli, citrus fruits, peppers, strawberries and tomatoes. (For other food sources of vitamin C, see "Getting What You Need" on page 142.)

HERBAL THERAPY

Look for toothpastes and mouthwashes containing bloodroot, such as Viadent, says Varro E. Tyler, Ph.D., professor of pharmacognosy at Purdue University in West Lafayette, Indiana. Scientific studies show that bloodroot can help prevent the buildup of plaque and the development of gum disease.

HOMEOPATHY

If you think you have gingivitis, you may want to try one of the following 30C remedies two or three times a day until you see your dentist, says Chris Meletis, N.D., a naturopathic physician and medicinary director at the National College of Naturopathic Medicine in Portland, Oregon. If you have a persistent sour taste in your mouth, bleeding gums and bad breath, especially if the tip of your tongue feels like it is burning and your symptoms are worse with cold, Dr. Meletis suggests trying Calcarea carbonica. Carbo vegetabilis may help, he says, if you have retracted gums that bleed easily, especially after brushing at night. If your gums bleed and are spongy and swollen, Lachesis is the remedy to choose, he says.

All of these remedies are available in many health food stores. To purchase homeopathic remedies by mail, refer to the resource list on page 637.

VITAMIN AND MINERAL THERAPY

To help heal gingivitis, take 500 milligrams each of vitamin C and bioflavonoids each day, advises Richard D. Fischer, D.D.S., a dentist in Annandale, Virginia, and president of the International Academy of Oral Medicine and Toxicology.

GLAUCOMA

I t's called the sneak thief of sight because glaucoma has no obvious symptoms at first—it's painless, and there's no effect on vision. By the time you notice that your sight isn't what it used to be, glaucoma has done its damage.

Here's how it occurs: A normal eye is filled with fluid, and that fluid drains through tissue between the iris and cornea. With glaucoma, that drain backs up—no one knows why—and the fluid either flows out slowly or stops flowing. The backup builds pressure throughout the eye, damaging blood vessels that feed the retina and optic nerve. Without nutrients, the optic nerve begins to die, along with your vision. One of every seven legally blind people in America lost sight due to glaucoma. Once glaucoma is diagnosed through a regular eye exam, most people use medication to keep it from getting worse. The natural remedies in this chapter—in conjunction with medical care and used with the approval of your doctor—may help prevent glaucoma or slow its development, according to some health professionals.

SEE YOUR MEDICAL DOCTOR WHEN . . .

• You notice any vision loss, no matter how slight.

AYURVEDA

Glaucoma is a disorder of the kapha dosha, according to Vasant Lad, B.A.M.S., M.A.Sc., director of the Ayurvedic Institute in Albuquerque, New Mexico. (For more information on the Ayurvedic doshas, see "All about Vata, Pitta and Kapha" on page 28.) He says an Indian herb called punarnava helps minimize kapha accumulation and slowly reduces pressure on the affected eye. Punarnava is available in Indian pharmacies or by mail order (refer to the resource list on page 634).

To treat glaucoma in its early stages, Dr. Lad suggests making a tea by steeping one teaspoon of punarnava in one cup of hot water for two minutes. Strain the tea until there's no punarnava in the water, then drink the tea two or three times a day, he says. Dr. Lad also recommends abstaining from coffee, white sugar and dairy products.

This remedy is not a substitute for your eye doctor's care, says Dr. Lad. He says to be sure to consult your doctor before beginning this treatment.

GLAUCOMA

REFLEXOLOGY

Pay special attention to the eye, throat, neck, kidney and diaphragm reflexes on both feet, and make sure to thoroughly work all of the points on the sides and bottoms of your toes, too, says St. Petersburg, Florida, reflexologist Dwight Byers, author of *Better Health with Foot Reflexology*. (To work the toe points, use whichever technique you find most comfortable.)

To help you locate these points, consult the foot reflex chart on page 592. For instructions on how to work the points, see "Your Reflexology Session" on page 110.

SOUND THERAPY

For some people, listening to slow, relaxing music for 20 to 40 minutes each day might help reduce the eye pressure that marks glaucoma, says Janalea Hoffman, R.M.T., a composer and music therapist based in Kansas City, Missouri. Hoffman suggests her tapes *Musical Acupuncture* and *Musical Biofeedback*; for other selections, see "Sailing Away to Key Largo" on page 129. Many of these are available from music stores. For information on ordering the tapes, refer to the resource list on page 642.

VITAMIN AND MINERAL THERAPY

Take vitamin C, adds Jay Cohen, O.D., associate professor at the State University of New York College of Optometry in New York City. "Studies show that high doses help draw fluid out of the eye in some way," he says. "I advise my patients to take supplements of between 1,000 and 2,000 milligrams a day, amounts that would be difficult to get in foods alone."

SEE ALSO Vision Problems

GOUT

It's hard to put your best foot forward when your big toe has swollen as big as a beet and is just as red. But that's what occurs with this form of arthritis, once called the disease of kings because it usually resulted from too much of the good life.

These days, we know that even commoners can get gout if they produce too much of a chemical called uric acid or if their kidneys fail to flush away excess amounts through urination. The uric acid then forms into tiny crystals and eventually lodges in joints—the big toe is particularly vulnerable—causing a royal pain that leaves the affected area hot, swollen and extremely tender. The pain is especially bad at night and can wake you from a sound sleep, say doctors.

Gout tends to run in families, but it usually strikes middle-age men who are overweight, drink alcohol and eat a lot of organ meats, gravies and other foods rich in purines, a substance that causes excess uric acid. The natural remedies in this chapter—in conjunction with medical care and used with your doctor's approval—may help prevent gout attacks or relieve the symptoms of gout, according to some health professionals.

SEE YOUR MEDICAL DOCTOR WHEN . . .

- You have repeated gout attacks or they don't improve after three to four days.
- You suddenly lose a lot of weight.
- You suffer from dehydration, some symptoms of which are excessive thirst, dry lips and decreased urination.
- You've had diarrhea for 24 hours or more.
- You are prone to gout and also take medications such as salicylates, diuretics or some antibiotics or cancer drugs.
- You are prone to gout and frequently drink alcohol.

AROMATHERAPY

To ease the pain of gout, make a massage oil with one ounce of olive oil (available in most health food stores) and five drops of juniper oil, then massage into the joint several times a day, suggests San Francisco herbalist Jeanne Rose, chairperson of the National Association for Holistic Aromatherapy, in *Aromatherapy: Applications and Inhalations*.

To soothe gout pain in the feet, try a cool footbath spiked with juniper and rosemary essential oils, suggests Greenwich, Connecticut, aromatherapist Judith Jackson, author of *Scentual Touch: A Personal Guide to Aromatherapy*. She says to add ten drops of each oil to two quarts of cold water.

For information on preparing and administering essential oils, including cautions about their use, see page 19. For information on purchasing essential oils, refer to the resource list on page 633.

FOOD THERAPY

Eat more blueberries and cherries, because they're rich in substances that counteract purines, which cause gout, says Julian Whitaker, M.D., founder and president of the Whitaker Wellness Center in Newport Beach, California. He says that some gout patients report finding relief by eating from a handful to up to ½ pound of cherries each day. He also advises people with gout to avoid anchovies, asparagus, mushrooms and organ meats such as liver and kidney, since they're high in purines.

HOMEOPATHY

Gout often requires medical care, but you can use one of the following treatments until you see your medical doctor or homeopath or as a complementary treatment until you feel relief, says Chris Meletis, N.D., a naturopathic physician and medicinary director at the National College of Naturopathic Medicine in Portland, Oregon.

If you have red, hot, swollen joints that are worse with motion or from the lightest touch, Dr. Meletis says to try Belladonna 12C every couple of hours. He says Aconite 12C, taken every few hours, is the choice if you have an acutely painful and red joint. Colchicum 12C, taken every few hours, is very helpful when the swelling is in your big toe, which is red and tender, especially if you also feel irritated and weak, he says. For burning, itching and swelling in the gouty area, he suggests Urtica urens 12C, taken every few hours.

All of these remedies are available in many health food stores. To purchase homeopathic remedies by mail, refer to the resource list on page 637.

HYDROTHERAPY

Ice and cold water treatments are great first aid for painful gout attacks, says John Abruzzo, M.D., professor of medicine and director of the Rheumatology and Osteoporosis Center at Thomas Jefferson University Hospital in Philadelphia. Apply a cold, wet compress directly to the affected area for 20 minutes, or wrap an ice pack in a plastic bag and place it over a towel on the skin, suggests Dr. Abruzzo. "Never leave a cold treatment on for more than 20 minutes, though, or you could damage your skin," he cautions.

While cold treatments usually relieve the pain, see your doctor right away if a single application doesn't help. "Gout is comparatively easy to treat if it is recognized early enough. If you let it go for too long, it's much harder to get under control," says Dr. Abruzzo.

JUICE THERAPY

Juicing about four handfuls of pitted cherries with ½ cup of strawberries can help neutralize excess uric acid and may help prevent gout attacks, says Cherie Calbom, M.S., a certified nutritionist in Kirkland, Washington, and co-author of *Juicing for Life*. She says people prone to gout attacks should drink this juice every day as a preventive.

For information on juicing techniques, see page 93.

REFLEXOLOGY

Work the kidney reflexes on both feet, recommends St. Petersburg, Florida, reflexologist Dwight Byers, author of *Better Health with Foot Reflexology*.

To help you locate these points, consult the foot reflex chart on page 592. For instructions on how to work the points, see "Your Reflexology Session" on page 110.

SEE ALSO Arthritis; Foot Pain; Joint Pain

GRIEF

Lose a loved one, and you lose more than that person; you lose a part of yourself. Grief, the normal reaction to this and other deep losses, is the most draining of emotions, robbing you of both your energy and your brainpower day after dreaded day.

There are various stages of grief—shock, denial, protest and the most devastating, depression—although they don't occur in any particular order. Throughout these stages, it's not uncommon to have trouble concentrating or performing other thought processes. The natural remedies in this chapter—in conjunction with medical care and used with your doctor's approval—may help you deal with grief and speed your return to normal life, according to some health professionals.

GRIEF

- Your grief overwhelms you, interfering with your ability to perform normal, day-to-day activities.

AROMATHERAPY

The essential oil marjoram, a soothing, uplifting scent, is a traditional remedy for grief, says Fair Oaks, California, aromatherapist Victoria Edwards. She suggests applying a drop or two of the oil to a tissue or handkerchief and inhaling whenever you're in need of a little comfort.

For information on preparing and administering essential oils, including cautions about their use, see page 19. For information on purchasing essential oils, refer to the resource list on page 633.

FLOWER REMEDY/ESSENCE THERAPY

"Grief is a natural reaction to loss, whether it's the loss of a job, the death of a loved one or the end of a marriage," says Eve Campanelli, Ph.D., a holistic family practitioner in Beverly Hills, California. For those recovering from such a loss, Dr. Campanelli recommends the emergency stress relief formula, a blend of five essences used in times of crisis. "Place four drops of the formula under the tongue as often as needed, whenever the feeling of grief overwhelms you," she says. "Six to 12 times a day is common."

The emergency stress relief formula, sold under brand names such as Calming Essence, Rescue Remedy and Five-Flower Formula, is available in most health food stores and through mail order (refer to the resource list on page 635). For more information on preparing and administering the formula, see page 40.

FOOD THERAPY

"There's nothing scientific about it, but I would recommend consuming more ginseng during times of grief," says Julian Whitaker, M.D., founder and president of the Whitaker Wellness Center in Newport Beach, California. "It helps deal with stresses." Ginseng is available as a tea, a powder and capsules in most health food stores.

HOMEOPATHY

"If someone experiences the sudden loss of a loved one and is in a state of shock and grief, the remedy I usually recommend is one 30C dose of Ignatia," says Mitchell Fleisher, M.D., a family practice physician and homeopath in Colleen, Virginia.

Ignatia is available in many health food stores. To purchase homeopathic remedies by mail, refer to the resource list on page 637.

IMAGERY

Although it may be painful, picture the deceased person on the last day of his life. Then take time to speak to the image of that loved one. Say all of the things you wish you would have said before the person died, says Dennis Gersten, M.D., a San Diego psychiatrist and publisher of *Atlantis*, a bi-monthly imagery newsletter. If you're angry, sad or feeling confused, let the deceased person know that, too.

"The night my father died, I did that, and the effect it had on me was quite remarkable and healing," Dr. Gersten says.

RELAXATION AND MEDITATION

Progressive relaxation may elevate your mood and give your immune system a vital boost while you are coping with grief, according to researchers at the University of Pennsylvania School of Nursing in Philadelphia. To learn the technique for progressive relaxation, see page 122.

In a preliminary study of nine grieving widows whose husbands had died within the previous two months, the researchers found that the women who practiced progressive relaxation three or four times a day for four weeks had increases in their immune cell activity. That's important, because other studies have shown that people who are grieving are more susceptible to disease.

The immunity boost over such a short period and the corresponding reduction in stress show that relaxation holds real advantages, says Arlene Houldin, R.N., Ph.D., assistant professor of psychosocial oncology nursing at the University of Pennsylvania School of Nursing. In order to get the full benefit, practice progressive relaxation three or four times a day, 10 to 15 minutes per session.

YOGA

You may not feel much like exercising, but doing three yoga poses per day can help you deal with grief, according to Alice Christensen, founder and executive director of the American Yoga Association. She recommends the standing sun (page 607), knee squeeze (page 612) and seated sun (page 616) because they increase blood circulation, making it easier to overcome the physical effects of grief. She points out that people who are grieving can become sedentary, but a daily yoga routine can help keep you moving.

Meditation (see page 153) is also helpful, but don't be surprised if you break into tears in the middle of it. Christensen says you should let them flow freely, and eventually, the meditation will fall into a healing quiet.

SEE ALSO Depression

HAIR LOSS

If you're a typical adult, you have about 100,000 hairs on your head. And you're not willing to part with a single one of them.

Yet once your hair starts to thin, there's little Western medicine can do. Except in cases caused by radiation treatments, scalp infections or severe stress, hair loss in men and women is hereditary and permanent. Only one prescription product, minoxidil, has won approval as a hair loss cure. And it doesn't work for everyone, especially when there is actual baldness rather than thinning. The natural remedies in this chapter, used with the approval of your doctor, may help slow hair loss or increase hair growth, according to some health professionals.

SEE YOUR MEDICAL DOCTOR WHEN . . .

- Your hair loss is rapid.
- You experience hair loss after taking high doses of vitamins, such as vitamin A.
- Your hair loss accompanies other problems, such as hypothyroidism or malnutrition.

AROMATHERAPY

To stimulate the scalp, try a blend of bay and lavender essential oils, suggests Greenwich, Connecticut, aromatherapist Judith Jackson, author of *Scentual Touch: A Personal Guide to Aromatherapy.* She says to add six drops of each oil to four ounces of warm carrier oil (almond, soybean and sesame are popular carrier oils; all are sold in most health food stores). Massage the mixture into the scalp and allow it to absorb for 20 minutes, she says, then wash with your regular shampoo, to which you've added three drops of bay essential oil.

For information on preparing and administering essential oils, including cautions about their use, see page 19. For information on purchasing essential oils, refer to the resource list on page 633.

FOOD THERAPY

For women, thinning hair or hair loss can be a sign of a problem in the gastrointestinal tract, says Michael A. Klaper, M.D., a nutritional medicine specialist in Pompano Beach, Florida, and director of the Institute of Nutritional Education and Research, an organization based in Manhattan Beach, California, that teaches doctors about nutrition and its relationship to disease. "Occasionally, it's a sign of insufficient stomach acids or that she's not absorbing protein, zinc and other nutrients," he says. "If she takes acidophilus after meals for a month or so, that often helps." Dr. Klaper recommends nondairy powdered acidophilus, available in most health food stores. He says to take two tablets between meals (four to six tablets per day) for at least two months.

For men, Dr. Klaper says that a low-fat diet may help slow down the balding process. "On some level, male pattern baldness might be tied to increased testosterone levels during puberty, which are often the result of a high-fat diet or eating too many animal products," says Dr. Klaper. "If you look at Japan, male pattern baldness was almost unheard of prior to World War II. The Japanese diet is now far more fatty and Westernized, and Japanese men are going bald everywhere. It's clear that a high-fat, meat-based diet raises testosterone levels, and that may adversely affect hair follicles. I'm not sure eating low-fat foods will stop hair loss, but it might slow it down."

MASSAGE

Giving your scalp a three-minute massage each day may increase blood flow to your hair follicles and help hair growth, says John F. Romano, M.D., clinical assistant professor of dermatology at New York Hospital–Cornell Medical Center in New York City. He suggests using your fingertips to gently rub all over your scalp. Don't be too rough; vigorous pulling or brushing can actually pull hair out of your head.

HANGOVER

L et's skip the medical mumbo jumbo here. If every vein in your head is throbbing, your mouth tastes like a skunk died in it and you have vague recollections of dancing the fox-trot while wearing a lampshade last night, you probably have yourself a hangover. The natural remedies in this chapter, used with your doctor's approval, may help relieve the symptoms of a hangover, according to some health professionals.

SEE YOUR MEDICAL DOCTOR WHEN . . .

- You have severe headache pain that is still present the day after your hangover.
- You continue to feel nauseated or haven't regained your appetite after 48 hours.
- You feel disoriented despite abstaining from alcohol for two to three days.
- You have bouts of diarrhea that go on for more than three to four days.

ACUPRESSURE

To relieve the headache and gastrointestinal distress of a hangover, press point LI 4, located in the webbing between the thumb and index finger, close to the bone at the base of the index finger, says Michael Reed Gach, Ph.D., director of the Acupressure Institute in Berkeley, California, and author of *Acupressure's Potent Points*. (To help locate this point, refer to the illustration on page 565.) Hold this point with your thumb on top of the webbing and your index finger underneath, says Dr. Gach, then squeeze into the webbing, angling the pressure toward the bone that connects the index finger to the hand. He suggests stimulating the point for one minute, then repeating on your other hand. This is not recommended for pregnant women because it can cause uterine contractions, he says.

For a headache accompanied by sensitivity to light, Dr. Gach recommends the B 2 points, situated on the upper ridge of each eye socket close to the bridge of the nose. (To help locate these points, refer to the illustration on page 564.) He says to gently pinch the area with your thumb and index finger and press upward into the indentations of the eye sockets. Hold for two to three minutes while you concentrate on taking slow, deep breaths, he says.

AROMATHERAPY

In *Aromatherapy: Applications and Inhalations*, San Francisco herbalist Jeanne Rose, chairperson of the National Association for Holistic Aromatherapy, suggests an aromatic cocktail to ease hangover queasiness: Mix four ounces of water, the juice of half of a lemon and a drop or two of fennel essential oil, then drink it before breakfast.

For information on preparing and administering essential oils, including cautions about their use, see page 19. For information on purchasing essential oils, refer to the resource list on page 633.

AYURVEDA

For hangovers, stir one teaspoon of lime juice and a pinch of cumin into one cup of fresh orange juice and drink, says Vasant Lad, B.A.M.S., M.A.Sc., director of the Ayurvedic Institute in Albuquerque, New Mexico.

FOOD THERAPY

No matter how much you drink, have a few more before retiring—but this time, make it water. "The big problem with a hangover is dehydration, and you can make the morning after a little easier by drinking two or three large glasses of water before going to sleep," says Elson Haas, M.D., director of the Preventive Medical Center of Marin in San Rafael, California, and author of *Staying Healthy with Nutrition*. He also recommends replenishing your system the morning after with plenty of fruits rich in vitamin C, such as oranges, grapefruit, strawberries and guava, and foods rich in the B vitamins, including whole grains, fish and beans. "Vitamin C may help speed the alcohol out of the body, and the B vitamins are believed to do the same thing," he says. (For more food sources of vitamin C and the B vitamins, see "Getting What You Need" on page 142.)

HOMEOPATHY

Nux vomica is a homeopathic remedy for hangover that works for many people, says Mitchell Fleisher, M.D., a family practice physician and homeopath in Colleen, Virginia. He suggests taking one 6C or 12C tablet every three to four hours as needed until you begin to feel better.

Nux vomica is available in many health food stores. To purchase homeopathic remedies by mail, refer to the resource list on page 637.

IMAGERY

Picture yourself on a ship in a stormy sea. See huge waves tossing your ship wildly in every direction. Imagine the storm slowly subsiding. The giant waves become smoother and smoother until the boat bobs on the water, as if you were gently being rocked like a little baby. Now safely pull into port, says Dennis Gersten, M.D., a San Diego psychiatrist and publisher of *Atlantis*, a bimonthly imagery newsletter.

JUICE THERAPY

"Fresh juices are wonderful hangover medicine, since they flush out the system and rehydrate the body at the same time," says Eve Campanelli, Ph.D., a holistic family practitioner in Beverly Hills, California. She recommends a blend of 8 ounces of carrot juice, 1 ounce of beet juice, 4 ounces of celery juice and ½ to 1 ounce of parsley juice. "Drink one glass in the morning and a second glass later in the day," she suggests. "This will stimulate the liver and alleviate the diarrhea that severely dehydrated people often experience."

For information on juicing techniques, see page 93.

VITAMIN AND MINERAL THERAPY

"An easy way to get the nutrients that help treat a hangover is with a product called E-mergen-C, which is a ready-made mixture of the necessary B vitamins, vitamin C and minerals. It is very helpful for relief from hangovers," says Elson Haas, M.D., director of the Preventive Medical Center of Marin in San Rafael, California, and author of *Staying Healthy with Nutrition*. You can find E-mergen-C in drugstores and most health food stores. Follow the dosage recommendations on the label.

HEADACHE

Take one part tension, blended with a stiff neck, screaming children and expressway traffic. Mix well with a glass of red wine.
Voilà! Instant headache.

Headaches come in all sizes and shapes. Tension headaches are the most common. They start when muscles tighten in your head and neck, then press on blood vessels in your scalp. You may also get cluster headaches, which are extremely painful and isolated to one part of your head. Migraines are the granddaddy of headaches, can last for hours and hours and may be caused by anything from food reactions to changes in barometric pressure. The natural remedies in this chapter—in conjunction with medical care and used with your doctor's approval—may help prevent a headache or relieve its symptoms, according to some health professionals.

SEE YOUR MEDICAL DOCTOR WHEN . . .

- Your headaches are getting stronger and more frequent.
- You also notice numbness, blurred vision, memory loss or dizziness.
- You have a headache after a severe head injury.
- Your headaches are caused by exercise.
- Your headaches start disrupting your life—for example, you start missing work because of recurring headaches.

ACUPRESSURE

The Gates of Consciousness points, GB 20, can relieve tension headaches as well as neck pain, says Michael Reed Gach, Ph.D., director of the Acupressure Institute in Berkeley, California, and author of *Acupressure's Potent Points*. Dr. Gach says to use the thumbs of both hands to press the GB 20 points, which are situated two inches out from the middle of your neck, underneath the base of the skull. (To help locate these points, refer to the illustration on page 565.) He suggests sitting in a chair and bending over, with your elbows propped on a table or desk, to make holding these points most comfortable. Breathe deeply and press firmly for one to two minutes.

Point LI 4 is especially helpful for frontal headaches, according to Dr. Gach. He explains that the point lies in the webbing between the thumb and index finger, close to the bone at the base of the index finger. (To help locate this point, refer to the illustration on page 565.) Holding the point with your thumb on top of the webbing and your index finger underneath, angle the pressure toward the bone that connects the index finger to the hand, says Dr. Gach. Hold for one minute, then repeat on your other hand. This is not recommended for pregnant women, says Dr. Gach, because pressing the LI 4 points can cause uterine contractions.

AROMATHERAPY

The cool scent of peppermint can often relieve headache pain, says Los Angeles aromatherapist Michael Scholes, of Aromatherapy Seminars, an organization that trains professionals and others in the use of essential oils. He suggests adding a drop of peppermint essential oil to any unscented facial lotion and applying the lotion under the nose and behind the ears. Inhaling the fragrance of peppermint from the bottle can also take the edge off a headache, he says.

For information on preparing and administering essential oils, including cautions about their use, see page 19. For information on purchasing essential oils, refer to the resource list on page 633.

AYURVEDA

Throbbing, pulsating headaches that are aggravated by high altitude, that get worse when you move your body and that subside when you rest are vata headaches, according to Ayurvedic practitioners. They say these headaches are caused by constipation and an accumulation of toxins in the colon. (For more information on the doshas of Ayurveda, see "All about Vata, Pitta and Kapha" on page 28.)

Try a plain warm–water enema to relieve constipation, suggests Vasant Lad, B.A.M.S., M.A.Sc., director of the Ayurvedic Institute in Albuquerque, New Mexico. (See "How to Perform an Enema" on page 76 for instructions.) To relieve the pain of a vata headache, he suggests rubbing the scalp and the soles of the feet with sesame oil (available in most health food stores). "Massage the neck, shoulders and upper back with sesame oil, too, and then take a hot shower," he says.

Vata headaches are frequently accompanied by dehydration, says Dr. Lad. He suggests sipping a mixture of one tablespoon of sugar, ¼ teaspoon of salt, the juice of half of a lime and one pint of water.

Shooting, burning, piercing pitta headaches are worsened by bright light and associated with nausea, Dr. Lad says. Pain is often felt behind the eyes, and the headache may be accompanied by dizziness. These headaches are connected to stomach problems, he says.

Dr. Lad suggests this remedy for a pitta headache: Mix one teaspoon of sandalwood powder (available from Indian grocers or from Ayurvedic practitioners) with enough water to make a paste, then apply this sandalwood paste to your forehead and temples. Wash off the paste after it has become dry and crumbly. Then, he says, put a few drops of warm liquid ghee, or clarified butter (see "How to Make Ghee" on page 26 for a recipe), into the palm of your hand and sniff the drops into your nostrils. Sometimes pitta headaches can be relieved by eating something sweet, says Dr. Lad, who recommends tapioca pudding.

If your headaches tend to occur in winter and spring, generally strike in the morning and evening and get worse when you bend down, you're getting kapha headaches, according to Dr. Lad. Kapha headaches are usually accompanied by sinus congestion or colds, he says, and are symptoms of hay fever and other allergies. The pain is usually dull and deep-seated and makes you feel drowsy.

Here's Dr. Lad's remedy for kapha headaches: Mix ½ teaspoon of ginger powder, 1 teaspoon of cinnamon and a pinch of clove powder into a cup of boiling water, steep for a few minutes, strain to remove the powder and drink. Dr. Lad says you can also make a ginger paste by adding hot water to 1 teaspoon of ginger powder, then apply it to the bridge of your nose and over your cheekbones. He suggests putting it on when you have a headache and leaving it on until your symptoms are relieved.

Finally, Dr. Lad suggests this kapha headache remedy: Mix one tablespoon of warm water and at least ⅛ teaspoon of salt to make a thick solution, draw the solution into an eyedropper and squeeze three to five drops into each nostril. This will help unclog sinuses, he says.

FOOD THERAPY

Try having a cup of coffee, advises Fred Sheftell, M.D., co-founder and co-director of the New England Center for Headache in Stamford, Connecticut. He says that caffeine constricts blood vessels and is an ingredient in many pain relievers. In fact, studies show that having a cup of coffee or tea can boost the pain-relieving powers of aspirin and other such products by about one-third.

HERBAL THERAPY

For a headache caused by stress, try a soothing cup of this tea recommended by Mary Bove, L.M., N.D., a naturopathic physician and director of the Brattleboro Naturopathic Clinic in Vermont: Blend one part each of the dried herbs wintergreen, willowbark and meadowsweet (available in most health food stores). Pour boiling water over a teaspoon of this blend, steep for ten minutes, strain, let cool to a drinkable temperature and drink.

HOMEOPATHY

If you have an occasional mild headache, Andrew Lockie, M.D., recommends the following remedies in his book *The Family Guide to Homeopathy*. He suggests taking the remedy appropriate for your symptoms every 10 to 15 minutes for up to ten doses.

If the headache comes on suddenly, feels like a tight band is wrapped around your head and is worse in cold air and you feel apprehensive, Dr. Lockie says to try a 30C dose of Aconite. Take a 30C dose of Apis, he says, if your body feels bruised and tender and you have a stinging, stabbing or burning headache that feels worse in hot air. If you have a flushed face, dilated eyes and a throbbing headache that is worse in the hot sun, he recommends a 30C dose of Belladonna. And for a headache that feels like a nail is being driven into your skull, he says to take a 6C dose of Ignatia.

All of these remedies are available in many health food stores. To purchase the remedies by mail, refer to the resource list on page 637.

HYDROTHERAPY

Water treatments for headaches use a combination of heat and cold to draw blood away from the affected area. Try soaking your feet and ankles in a hot foot bath while applying an ice pack or a cold cloth to the forehead and temples, says Tori Hudson, N.D., a naturopathic physician and professor at the National College of Naturopathic Medicine in Portland, Oregon. When you use an ice pack, many experts suggest wrapping it in a plastic bag and placing it over a towel on the skin. Also, they advise limiting your cold treatment to 20 minutes, since prolonged exposure could damage the skin. This treatment is very effective for tension and sinus headaches and can be used as needed, says Dr. Hudson.

IMAGERY

Imagine that all of the muscles in your head and neck are like tightly coiled springs. Now imagine that all of those springs begin to loosen. As they do, the muscles become more relaxed, and your discomfort decreases, says Dennis Gersten, M.D., a San Diego psychiatrist and publisher of *Atlantis*, a bi-monthly imagery newsletter. He adds that if you do this for 30 seconds every hour on the hour, it will dramatically relax you and ease your headache.

HEADACHE

JUICE THERAPY

"The most common causes of headaches are constipation and liver malfunction," says Eve Campanelli, Ph.D., a holistic family practitioner in Beverly Hills, California. For those prone to headaches, Dr. Campanelli recommends twice-daily doses of apple-spinach juice for its gentle laxative qualities. "Mix one ounce of spinach juice into eight ounces of apple juice, and you'll never taste the spinach," she promises.

Once constipation has been cleared up, Dr. Campanelli advises getting the liver moving with a blend of 8 ounces of carrot juice, 1 ounce of beet juice, 4 ounces of celery juice and ½ to 1 ounce of parsley juice. "Drinking this juice once or twice a day helps the liver filter out toxins more effectively, resulting in fewer headaches," explains Dr. Campanelli. See your doctor if your headaches persist, she adds.

For information on juicing techniques, see page 93.

MASSAGE

Here's a fingertip massage from Elliot Greene, past president of the American Massage Therapy Association, that should help ease the pain of tension headaches.

Start by placing your fingertips on your scalp, with your left hand on the left side of your head and your right hand on the right side. Press down gently, and move the scalp back and forth about a half-inch. "Your fingers shouldn't slide across the skin," Greene says. "They should be moving the scalp itself." After a few seconds, move your fingertips farther back on the scalp and repeat. Do this until you have massaged the entire scalp from front to back. Make sure to massage the sides of your head above and around the ears.

Next, grasp a small amount of hair in one hand. Gently lift the hair away from your scalp and twist it slightly. This will stimulate the scalp, Greene says, and should help relieve tension. Repeat until you've covered the whole scalp.

Now use your fingertips to massage your temples and forehead. Make small circles as you massage. Do this for several minutes or until you feel the headache subsiding. You can also rub the back of your neck, especially at the base of the skull.

You can finish the massage with a shoulder rub. Use your right hand to grasp the muscle on your left shoulder and squeeze lightly for several seconds. Release and squeeze several times. Then switch sides, with your left hand grasping your right shoulder. Greene says you should breathe deeply and regularly during the entire massage, so you don't build up more tension.

In her book *Self-Massage*, Monika Struna recommends two other remedies for headache: the headache massage (page 574) and the towel trick for headaches (page 579).

REFLEXOLOGY

Reflexology's ability to relax the body makes it a perfect choice for treating headaches, say Kevin and Barbara Kunz, reflexology researchers in Santa Fe, New Mexico, and authors of *Hand and Foot Reflexology*. They suggest using the corresponding golf ball technique (page 588) to work the solar plexus, eye, ear and head points on your hands. They also say to work the face points on your hands and the lower back points on your feet.

To help you locate these points, consult the hand and foot reflex charts beginning on page 582. For instructions on how to work the points, see "Your Reflexology Session" on page 110.

RELAXATION AND MEDITATION

"We've had good success using stretch-based relaxation to help people who have tension headaches," says Charles Carlson, Ph.D., professor of psychology at the University of Kentucky in Lexington. See page 602 for one example of a stretch-based relaxation technique. Practice this sequence of exercises whenever you begin to feel a headache coming on.

For some people, other relaxation techniques, including deep breathing, meditation, autogenics, thermal biofeedback and progressive relaxation, are also effective, according to Dr. Carlson. For brief descriptions of each of these techniques, see page 113.

YOGA

A yoga exercise called the neck roll (page 627) can help, say Dr. Robin Monro, Dr. R. Nagarathna and Dr. H. R. Nagendra in their book *Yoga for Common Ailments*. They recommend doing this exercise three times per day to relieve headaches but caution not to do it if you have neck problems or neck pain.

SEE ALSO Migraines

HEARING PROBLEMS

In a world of blaring boom boxes, jarring jackhammers and screaming sirens, it's no wonder that hearing problems are on the rise.

Statistics show that one in 12 people suffers from some kind of hearing trouble. Hearing problems can range from hearing loss (caused by too much noise, an infection, a drug side effect, aging or other factors) to tinnitus, a constant ringing or buzzing in your ears.

Prevention is the best medicine for your ears. Stay away from loud noise when you can, especially when it's continuous, and wear ear protection when you can't. The natural remedies in this chapter—in conjunction with medical care and used with the approval of your doctor—may help prevent hearing loss, according to some health professionals.

SEE YOUR MEDICAL DOCTOR WHEN . . .

• You have sudden hearing loss or ringing in one or both ears.
• You have sharp pain in one or both ears.

FOOD THERAPY

A zinc deficiency could affect hearing, so get enough of it in your diet, says Michael A. Klaper, M.D., a nutritional medicine specialist in Pompano Beach, Florida, and director of the Institute of Nutritional Education and Research, an organization based in Manhattan Beach, California, that teaches doctors about nutrition and its relationship to disease.

He says that good sources of zinc are whole grains, fortified cereals and root vegetables. Other experts suggest oysters, crabmeat and other seafood as well as lean beef as good food sources of zinc.

Dr. Klaper adds that a high-fat diet might also cause hearing loss by blocking blood flow to the cochlea, the hearing mechanism in your inner ear. He suggests limiting the fat in your diet to less than 20 percent of your total calorie intake.

VITAMIN AND MINERAL THERAPY

Magnesium and zinc supplements can help restore stability to your inner ear, where some hearing problems begin, says Paul Yanick, Ph.D., a research scientist in Milford, Pennsylvania, who specializes in hearing problems. Some experts recommend that people with hearing loss take 30 milligrams of zinc and 400 milligrams of magnesium daily.

HEARTBURN

YOGA

Daily practice of an exercise called yawning (page 628) and a simple chant may help fight hearing loss, writes yoga teacher Rosalind Widdowson in her book *The Joy of Yoga*. The chant uses a mantra, a sound that is often used in yoga meditation. Widdowson's instructions: Sit in a comfortable chair and begin breathing deeply. As you exhale, repeat one of these phrases out loud: *ham* or *hrah*. Hold the last sound (either the *mmmm* in *ham* or the *ahhh* in *hrah*) and feel the vibrations. Widdowson suggests doing this for two to three minutes each day.

SEE ALSO Tinnitus

HEARTBURN

S ure you knew better. But how could you pass up the Nuclear Nachos plate at Harry's House of Jalapeños?
  Now your innards are fighting a five-alarm food fire, and ten straight glasses of water haven't doused the flames.

Hydrochloric acid is what puts the burn in heartburn. The discomfort you feel is caused by acid that has escaped from your stomach and into your throat. While your gut has a lining that protects it from the stuff, your esophagus gets no such help. The natural remedies in this chapter, used with the approval of your doctor, may help relieve heartburn, according to some health professionals.

SEE YOUR MEDICAL DOCTOR WHEN . . .

- You get heartburn frequently—every day or at least several times a week.
- You have what feels like heartburn along with vomiting, dizziness, chest pain, bloody or black stool or difficulty swallowing. If you have these symptoms, seek medical attention quickly.

ACUPRESSURE

You can get rid of heartburn by pressing CV 12, the Center of Power point, says Michael Reed Gach, Ph.D., director of the Acupressure Institute in Berkeley, California, and author of *Acupressure's Potent Points*. CV 12 is found near the center of the front of your body, halfway between the breastbone and the navel.

(For help in locating this point, refer to the illustration on page 564.) Dr. Gach says to press this point for no longer than two minutes and only when your stomach is fairly empty. This point should be touched gently if you are pregnant or have a hiatal hernia, he adds.

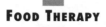

FOOD THERAPY

Think carbohydrates for dinner, says Michael A. Klaper, M.D., director of the Institute of Nutritional Education and Research, an organization based in Manhattan Beach, California, that teaches doctors about nutrition and its relationship to disease, and a nutritional medicine specialist in Pompano Beach, Florida. "When you dump a lot of protein into your stomach—like you do when you eat meat or fish—and then go to bed, you're going to have a lot of stomach acid churning around, which will create heartburn. What I suggest to people who have heartburn problems is to make dinner more of a carbohydrate-based meal centered around rice, beans, pastas and other nonmeat sources."

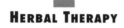

HERBAL THERAPY

For immediate relief of heartburn, make yourself a cup of ginger tea, says Mary Bove, L.M., N.D., a naturopathic physician and director of the Brattleboro Naturopathic Clinic in Vermont. Her instructions: Put ½ teaspoon of shredded fresh ginger in a cup of boiling water. Then let the ginger steep for about ten minutes, strain the tea so that no ginger remains, cool to a drinkable temperature and drink.

You can also try this tea, according to Dr. Bove: Add two teaspoons of anise seeds, fennel seeds or dill seeds to one cup of boiling water. Cover and steep for five to ten minutes, then strain, allow the tea to cool and drink a few teaspoons every few minutes.

HOMEOPATHY

If you have heartburn associated with heaviness after meals, excess gas and a bitter taste in your mouth, especially after large meals, try Nux vomica 30C every couple of hours until you feel better, says Chris Meletis, N.D., a naturopathic physician and medicinary director at the National College of Naturopathic Medicine in Portland, Oregon. If food feels stuck behind your breastbone, your tongue is coated and you crave starchy foods, which make the symptoms only worse, Dr. Meletis says to try Pulsatilla 30C every two hours. Natrum muriaticum 30C every two hours may offer relief if your heartburn is accompanied by nervousness, tension and pain in the upper abdomen, he says. If you tend to eat too fast and have gurgling and bloating after the meal, he suggests Zinc metallicum 30C every hour or two until you feel better.

All of these remedies are available in many health food stores. To purchase homeopathic remedies by mail, refer to the resource list on page 637.

HYDROTHERAPY

Activated charcoal provides quick relief from heartburn, says Agatha Thrash, M.D., a medical pathologist and co-founder and co-director of Uchee Pines Institute, a natural healing center in Seale, Alabama. She suggests mixing two tablespoons of activated charcoal powder with a little water in the bottom of a tall glass ("Stir gently, or the powder flies everywhere," she cautions). Continue stirring and adding water a little at a time until the glass is full, then drink it with a straw, suggests Dr. Thrash. Activated charcoal is available in most health food stores and some pharmacies.

REFLEXOLOGY

Work the diaphragm, gallbladder, pancreas and stomach reflexes on both feet, says St. Petersburg, Florida, reflexologist Dwight Byers, author of *Better Health with Foot Reflexology*. To help you locate these points, consult the foot reflex chart on page 592. For instructions on how to work the points, see "Your Reflexology Session" on page 110.

YOGA

To avoid heartburn, eat slowly and take a deep breath between bites, advises Stephen A. Nezezon, M.D., yoga teacher and staff physician at the Himalayan International Institute of Yoga Science and Philosophy in Honesdale, Pennsylvania. For instructions on deep breathing, see page 152.

SEE ALSO Indigestion

HEART DISEASE

Heart disease is serious business. The good news is that most of us are treating it that way. Death rates are declining as we learn to eat less fat, exercise more and quit smoking. And the natural remedies in this chapter—in conjunction with medical care and used with the approval of your doctor—may help prevent or reverse heart disease, according to some health professionals.

SEE YOUR MEDICAL DOCTOR WHEN . . .

- You feel uncomfortable pressure, fullness or squeezing in your chest that lasts for a few minutes or goes away and then returns.
- You feel pain spreading to your shoulders, neck or arms.
- You have chest discomfort along with light-headedness, fainting, nausea or shortness of breath.

AYURVEDA

Heart disease combines aspects of all three doshas, according to David Frawley, O.M.D., director of the American Institute of Vedic Studies in Santa Fe, New Mexico. (For more information on the Ayurvedic doshas, see "All about Vata, Pitta and Kapha" on page 28.) The angry, hard-driving type A behavior that seems to precipitate heart disease is a pitta characteristic, he explains, while poor circulation and atherosclerosis are vata problems. And the accumulation of cholesterol in the bloodstream is a kapha condition usually caused by eating too many rich, fatty foods, he says.

The primary Ayurvedic remedy for all three doshas is an herb called arjuna, says Dr. Frawley. The recommended dosage is 500 milligrams to one gram, two times a day, he says. Ayurvedic practitioners recommend arjuna to stimulate circulation, to strengthen the heart muscle, to stop bleeding and to promote healing after a heart attack. It is available by mail order (refer to the resource list on page 634).

Since heart disease is life-threatening, Ayurvedic practitioners suggest that you consult an M.D. before trying this or any other self-care remedy.

FOOD THERAPY

A low-fat, high-fiber diet not only can prevent heart disease but also can actually start you on the road to reversing it, says Michael A. Klaper, M.D., a nutritional medicine specialist in Pompano Beach, Florida, and director of the Institute of Nutritional Education and Research, an organization based in Manhattan Beach, California, that teaches doctors about nutrition and its relationship to disease. "That means eating little or no meats, dairy and processed foods, which are high in saturated fat, and more organically produced grains, legumes, fruits, vegetables and seeds, as fresh and as whole as possible."

IMAGERY

See yourself inside your bloodstream with a tiny scalpel. You are carefully removing the plaque that is attached to the inside of your blood vessels, says Elizabeth Ann Barrett, R.N., Ph.D., professor and coordinator of the Center for Nursing Research at Hunter College of the City University of New York in New York City. Keep doing this as you swim upstream toward your heart. Once you get there, see yourself easily swimming through the four chambers of your heart and out into the coronary arteries. Shine a blue healing light on the artery walls. See the walls relax and rejuvenate. Let go of all troubling emotions, which are the root of heart problems. Picture something troubling to your heart, such as anger or grief. Throw it over your left shoulder and let it go.

Dr. Barrett recommends that you practice this imagery three times a day: morning, afternoon and evening. Each session should last about ten minutes. Do this for 21 days, then discontinue the imagery for one week. She says to repeat this sequence for as long as needed.

REFLEXOLOGY

To relax and invigorate your heart muscle, focus on the heart, colon and pituitary gland reflexes on your feet, according to Rebecca Dioda, a reflexologist with the Morris Institute of Natural Therapeutics, a holistic health education center in Denville, New Jersey.

To help you locate these points, consult the foot reflex chart on page 592. For instructions on how to work the points, see "Your Reflexology Session" on page 110.

VITAMIN AND MINERAL THERAPY

Several vitamins and minerals have been found to reduce or even reverse symptoms of heart disease, says Richard Anderson, Ph.D., lead scientist for the Nutrient Requirements and Functions Laboratory at the U.S. Department of Agriculture Human Nutrition Research Center in Beltsville, Maryland. According to Dr. Anderson, scientific research shows that taking 400 micrograms of chromium daily can lower cholesterol and improve overall artery function.

Magnesium can also protect against heart disease, says Michael Janson, M.D., director of the Center for Preventive Medicine in Barnstable, Massachusetts, and an officer of the American College for Advancement in Medicine. He recommends a 400-milligram supplement each day.

The antioxidant vitamins can also help, according to Dr. Janson. He says many experts recommend taking daily supplements of 15 milligrams (25,000 international units) of beta-carotene, 1,000 to 5,000 milligrams of vitamin C, 400 to 800 international units of vitamin E and about 200 micrograms of selenium.

A person with heart disease may want to use the following vitamin, mineral and herbal regimen to help control or reverse the condition, says David Edelberg, M.D., an internist and medical director of the American Holistic Center/Chicago: magnesium/potassium aspartate capsules twice a day; 30 milligrams of coenzyme Q-10 three times a day; 1,000 milligrams of vitamin C three times a day; 400 international units of vitamin E twice a day; 200 micrograms of selenium a day; 50 milligrams of vitamin B$_6$ a day; 500 milligrams of carnitine three times a day; one capsule of the herb hawthorn berry three times a day; and one capsule of the herb *Ginkgo biloba* three times a day. Some manufacturers combine all of these dietary supplements into one capsule, according to Dr. Edelberg; these are available in most health food stores.

YOGA

Daily practice of the knee squeeze (page 612) can help your circulatory system by improving blood flow and making veins and arteries more elastic, according to Alice Christensen, founder and executive director of the American Yoga Association. Doing the complete breath exercise (see page 152) each day can also reduce stress, a major contributor to heart disease, Christensen says.

HEART PALPITATIONS

W hen it's working the way it should, your heart is a pretty boring organ. *Pa-pump. Pa-pump. Pa-pump.*

But what happens when things get a little crazy? What does it mean when your heart speeds up—pump-pump-pump-pump-pump—or misses a beat—pump-pump-pump-skip-pump?

It means you've had a heart palpitation. A palpitation is any heartbeat that's unusual enough to catch your attention, whether it's a rapid-fire series of beats, a fluttering beat or a misfire. The natural remedy in this chapter—in conjunction with medical care and used with the approval of your doctor—may help prevent heart palpitations, according to one health professional.

SEE YOUR MEDICAL DOCTOR WHEN . . .

- You have more than an occasional palpitation. Nearly everyone has a palpitation now and again. But if you feel a series of skipped beats, or if your heart seems to race for no reason, get medical attention immediately. That goes double if you feel dizziness or faintness along with the palpitation.

FOOD THERAPY

The cause of a heart palpitation could be as simple as having too much caffeine, says Michael A. Klaper, M.D., a nutritional medicine specialist in Pompano Beach, Florida, and director of the Institute of Nutritional Education and Research, an organization based in Manhattan Beach, California, that teaches doctors about nutrition and its relationship to disease. He suggests decreasing or even eliminating your intake of tea, cola, coffee and chocolate. "But a heart palpitation could also be an early warning sign of heart disease, thyroid disease, an anxiety attack or other serious problems," he says. "So it's smart to check with your doctor if they recur frequently or persist for more than a few seconds."

HEAT RASH

Acouple of laps around the walking path usually makes you feel great. So how come today you look like you just sprinted five miles through the Mojave Desert with a saguaro cactus strapped to your back?

Chances are you have a heat rash. Also known as prickly heat, these painful rashes occur when sweat gets stuck in your skin. Instead of flowing out from your pores, the sweat drains into your flesh, causing a bright red rash that feels like someone is sticking pins in it.

The natural remedies in this chapter, used with the approval of your doctor, may help prevent or relieve a heat rash, according to some health professionals.

SEE YOUR MEDICAL DOCTOR WHEN...

- You have a rash that's widely spread over your body.
- You experience fever and are fatigued.
- You get no relief in a cool environment.

FOOD THERAPY

"To get over heat rash more quickly, increase your intake of essential fatty acids," advises Julian Whitaker, M.D., founder and president of the Whitaker Wellness Center in Newport Beach, California. "Salmon and other cold water fish (such as herring and mackerel) are excellent sources of these fatty acids, as are flaxseed oil and dark green leafy vegetables such as spinach." Flaxseed oil is available in most health food stores.

HOMEOPATHY

To prevent heat rash, take a 30C dose of Sol three times a day for up to three weeks, writes Andrew Lockie, M.D., in his book *The Family Guide to Homeopathy*. If you do develop a rash, Dr. Lockie recommends trying a 30C dose of Apis as soon as the prickling or itching sensation starts. Take this remedy every two hours for up to ten doses, he says, and repeat this routine daily, if necessary.

Sol and Apis are available in many health food stores. To purchase homeopathic remedies by mail, refer to the resource list on page 637.

HYDROTHERAPY

Take an alkaline bath to soak away heat rash, suggests medical pathologist Agatha Thrash, M.D., co-founder and co-director of Uchee Pines Institute, a natural healing center in Seale, Alabama. Add one cup of baking soda to a tub filled with lukewarm water (94° to 98°F; you can use a regular thermometer to check) and soak for 30 to 60 minutes, using a cup to pour the water over any part of the body that isn't submerged in the bath. Pat dry.

SEE ALSO Rashes

HEEL SPURS

We already have 19 bones in each of our feet. So we don't need any more, especially when they come in the form of painful heel spurs. Spurs are knobs of unwanted bone that grow on the bottoms of your feet. They start when the main ligament that runs across your sole and connects to the heel gets irritated. Spurs are a common problem for runners and other folks who are hard on their feet. The natural remedies in this chapter—in conjunction with medical care and used with your doctor's approval—may help prevent or relieve the pain of heel spurs, according to some health professionals.

SEE YOUR MEDICAL DOCTOR WHEN...

- You have heel pain for more than five days.
- You experience calf pain in addition to heel pain.
- You are unable to walk.

HYDROTHERAPY

You can get relief from spur pain by using an ice pack, according to Terry Spilken, D.P.M., a podiatrist and adjunct faculty member at the New York College of Podiatric Medicine in New York City. He says to wrap an ice pack in a towel and apply it to the spur for ten minutes, then remove the pack for ten minutes before using it again. Do not apply the pack directly to the skin or leave it on for more than 20 minutes, since many experts say this can cause skin damage.

VITAMIN AND MINERAL THERAPY

Add more calcium and magnesium to your diet with supplements, says Julian Whitaker, M.D., founder and president of the Whitaker Wellness Center in Newport Beach, California. He suggests taking 1,000 milligrams of each daily at the first sign of heel spurs, continuing until symptoms improve. Calcium and magnesium will also help prevent or ease the pain of future heel spurs, he says.

SEE ALSO Foot Pain

HEMORRHOIDS

Hemorrhoids may be one of the most joked about medical problems, but they're also among the most common. At this very moment, nearly half of the men, women and children in the United States have hemorrhoids.

Rest assured none of them is laughing about it.

Hemorrhoids are varicose veins that form inside your rectum or around the opening of your anus. They're caused by increased pressure on the veins from sitting, being constipated or straining too hard to defecate. Hemorrhoids can be extremely painful or itchy and can rupture and bleed when they're irritated. The natural remedies in this chapter—in conjunction with medical care and used with the approval of your doctor—may help relieve the symptoms of hemorrhoids and prevent their recurrence, according to some health professionals.

SEE YOUR MEDICAL DOCTOR WHEN...

• You notice bleeding from your rectum.

AROMATHERAPY

Soothe painful hemorrhoids with a good soak, suggests Greenwich, Connecticut, aromatherapist Judith Jackson, author of *Scentual Touch: A Personal Guide to Aromatherapy*. She says to add 20 drops each of lavender and juniper essential oils to a hot, shallow bath, mixing the bathwater with your hand to make sure the oils are well-dispersed. Then soak for ten minutes, she says.

You can also treat hemorrhoids with a topical ointment after each bath or bowel movement, adds Jackson. She suggests trying two drops of lavender and one drop of geranium essential oils blended with one ounce of carrier oil. Carrier oils are available in most health food stores.

For information on preparing and administering essential oils, including cautions about their use, see page 19. For information on purchasing essential oils, refer to the resource list on page 633.

AYURVEDA

To relieve the itching and reduce the swelling from external hemorrhoids, Vasant Lad, B.A.M.S., M.A.Sc., director of the Ayurvedic Institute in Albuquerque, New Mexico, suggests applying a mixture of ½ teaspoon of turmeric and 1 teaspoon of ghee, or clarified butter, at bedtime for three nights in a row. (See "How to Make Ghee" on page 26 for a recipe.) Then stop for two nights, resume for three nights and continue with this pattern until the external hemorrhoids are cured, says Dr. Lad. Since turmeric can stain, be sure to wear a pair of old underwear to bed; any skin discoloration should wash off in about two weeks, he adds.

FOOD THERAPY

A high-fiber diet is the key to preventing or treating hemorrhoids, says Michael A. Klaper, M.D., a nutritional medicine specialist in Pompano Beach, Florida, and director of the Institute of Nutritional Education and Research, an organization based in Manhattan Beach, California, that teaches doctors about nutrition and its relationship to disease. Hard, constipated stool means you need to push harder to defecate, he explains, and when you push hard, your hemorrhoidal veins bulge and can become varicose, which is what hemorrhoids are—varicose veins. Fiber makes your stool soft, putting less pressure on the veins. Dr. Klaper suggests trying to consume at least 30 grams of fiber each day by eating at least five servings of fresh fruits and vegetables and more whole grains, beans and bran products.

HERBAL THERAPY

Saint-John's-wort can help relieve the itching and burning of hemmorhoids, says Barre, Vermont, herbalist Rosemary Gladstar, author of *Herbal Healing for Women* and several other books about herbs. Most health food stores carry salves made with this herb; Gladstar says to follow the directions on the label of the product you choose.

HEMORRHOIDS

Witch hazel, usually distilled in alcohol, helps, too, according to Gladstar. She says to moisten cotton cloths with witch hazel extract and apply the cloths as compresses, leaving them on for 15 to 20 minutes twice a day. Keep both the salve and the witch hazel extract in the refrigerator, Gladstar suggests; they'll retain their freshness and feel cool and soothing when you use them.

HOMEOPATHY

Take a 10- to 15-minute sitz bath in warm water twice a day, then apply Aesculus and Hamamelis ointment after each bath, says Maesimund Panos, M.D., a homeopathic physician in Tipp City, Ohio, and co-author with Jane Heimlich of *Homeopathic Medicine at Home*. (For instructions on using a sitz bath, see "Hydrotherapy at Home" on page 78.) Dr. Panos says that this ointment helps relieve pain and swelling and can speed healing. Taking two tablets of Aesculus 6X three or four times daily may also be helpful in speeding healing, she says.

These remedies are available in many health food stores. To purchase the remedies by mail, refer to the resource list on page 637.

HYDROTHERAPY

A compress soaked in strong, cold black tea is very soothing to hemorrhoids, says Agatha Thrash, M.D., a medical pathologist and co-founder and co-director of Uchee Pines Institute, a natural healing center in Seale, Alabama. She suggests holding the compress against the hemorrhoids for several minutes.

IMAGERY

In his book *Healing Visualizations*, New York City psychiatrist Gerald Epstein, M.D., suggests you close your eyes, breathe out three times and imagine that your hemorrhoids are puckering up like an old purse. Picture them shriveling and disappearing as the walls of the anus become pink and smooth. Dr. Epstein says to practice this imagery for one to two minutes of every waking hour, for up to 21 days, until the hemorrhoids fade.

JUICE THERAPY

Besides adding fiber to the diet, which softens the stool, a number of fruit juices contain substances that may help ease hemorrhoids, says Cherie Calbom, M.S., a certified nutritionist in Kirkland, Washington, and co-author of *Juicing for Life*. Dark-colored berries such as cherries, blackberries and blueberries contain anthocyanins and proanthocyanidins, pigments that, according to Calbom, tone and strengthen the walls of hemorrhoidal veins, which can minimize pain and swelling.

To maximize the therapeutic benefits of these pigments, Calbom suggests drinking four ounces of dark berry juice diluted with four ounces of apple juice at least once a day.

For information on juicing techniques, see page 93.

REFLEXOLOGY

Pay special attention to the diaphragm, adrenal gland, rectum, sigmoid colon and lower spine reflexes in both feet, suggests St. Petersburg, Florida, reflexologist Dwight Byers, author of *Better Health with Foot Reflexology*. To help you locate these points, consult the foot reflex chart on page 592. For instructions on how to work the points, see "Your Reflexology Session" on page 110.

HERNIA

It's another one of those manly things. No real man admits to being lost. No real man cries at the movies. And no matter how big the box, no matter how heavy the sofa, no real man asks for help on moving day.

Until he gets a hernia, that is.

A hernia occurs when a piece of your body slips through a wall of muscle and gets stuck. Men get hernias much more often than women do, and most of them are caused by heavy lifting. With these so-called inguinal hernias, a piece of intestine slides through the abdominal muscle into the groin or upper thigh area. See your doctor, since surgery is usually required to repair a hernia. The natural remedies in this chapter—in conjunction with medical care and used with your doctor's approval—may help relieve the pain of a hernia or prevent its recurrence, according to some health professionals.

SEE YOUR MEDICAL DOCTOR WHEN . . .

• You notice any bulge in your groin or upper thigh area.

FOOD THERAPY

A hernia can result from an abdominal muscle wall that is protein-deficient, says Elson Haas, M.D., director of the Preventive Medical Center of Marin in San Rafael, California, and author of *Staying Healthy with Nutrition*. He suggests eating more low-fat sources of protein, which include chicken breast, tuna, skim milk and 1 percent cottage cheese. While this therapy won't heal an existing condition, Dr. Haas says, it may help prevent future problems.

REFLEXOLOGY

Work the groin, colon and adrenal gland reflex points on both feet, says St. Petersburg, Florida, reflexologist Dwight Byers, author of *Better Health with Foot Reflexology*. To help you locate these points, consult the foot reflex chart on page 592. For instructions on how to work the points, see "Your Reflexology Session" on page 110.

HICCUPS

Hiccups remain one of life's great mysteries, right up there with Stonehenge, the pyramids and setting a digital wristwatch.

As far as anyone can tell, hiccups serve no biological purpose. They're just annoying little spasms in your diaphragm, the thin muscle below your lungs that helps with breathing. And while they're usually not serious, hiccups can sometimes hang around for minutes or even hours. The natural remedies in this chapter, used with your doctor's approval, may help you get rid of hiccups, according to some health professionals.

SEE YOUR MEDICAL DOCTOR WHEN...

- You have hiccups for several days or longer.
- You get repeated cases of hiccups.

ACUPRESSURE

A combination of acupressure and deep, relaxing breathing may be all that you need to get rid of hiccups, says Michael Reed Gach, Ph.D., director of the Acupressure Institute in Berkeley, California, and author of *Acupressure's Potent Points*. First, find the Sp 16 points, situated at the base of your rib cage, a half-inch in from each nipple line. (For help in locating these points, refer to the illustration on page 564.) Then with the fingertips of both hands, firmly hold the points on the left and right sides of the body, says Dr. Gach. Close your eyes and breathe deeply as you hold these points for several minutes, he adds.

HOMEOPATHY

If you have belching and violent, noisy hiccups, try a 6C dose of Cicuta every 15 minutes, up to six doses, writes Andrew Lockie, M.D., in *The Family Guide to Homeopathy*. Similar doses of the following remedies might also help, he says.

If your hiccups begin an hour or two after eating a large or rich meal and are accompanied by belching and retching, Dr. Lockie recommends Nux vomica. Ignatia is a good remedy, he says, if your hiccups occur soon after an emotional upset or eating, drinking or smoking. Persistent hiccups with a sore chest and retching may be relieved by Magnesia phosphoricum, he says. And if you feel feverish and chilled and cold drinks make your hiccups worse, he suggests trying Arsenicum.

All of these remedies are available in many health food stores. To purchase the remedies by mail, refer to the resource list on page 637.

IMAGERY

Close your eyes and picture a neon sign, like a theater marquee, with the word 'Think' blinking on and off. Concentrate on the sign and make it blink as intensely as possible, and your hiccups may vanish, says Dennis Gersten, M.D., a San Diego psychiatrist and publisher of *Atlantis*, a bi-monthly imagery newsletter, who first used this remedy when he was a child. "The technique has never failed me in my entire life," he says.

REFLEXOLOGY

Relax your diaphragm by working the diaphragm and stomach reflex areas on your feet, says St. Petersburg, Florida, reflexologist Dwight Byers, author of *Better Health with Foot Reflexology*. To help you locate these points, consult the foot reflex chart on page 592. For instructions on how to work the points, see "Your Reflexology Session" on page 110.

RELAXATION AND MEDITATION

Stop hiccups with deep breathing exercises, such as the one described on page 116, says Steven Fahrion, Ph.D., director of research at the Life Sciences Institute of Mind–Body Health in Topeka, Kansas.

HIGH BLOOD PRESSURE

Here's something that ought to get your heart pounding: By age 55, about 30 percent of White American men and 20 percent of White women have blood pressure readings above the recommended maximum of 140/90. Blacks are even worse off; about half of Black men and more than 40 percent of Black women have high blood pressure by the same age.

And if that's not scary enough, consider that nearly half of all people with high blood pressure don't even know it. There aren't many noticeable signs of the problem, but these folks are at much higher risk for heart attacks, kidney failure, hardened arteries, strokes and other problems.

Experts recommend having your blood pressure checked at least every other year. If your readings are high, follow your doctor's orders. The natural remedies in this chapter—in conjunction with medical care and used with your doctor's approval—may help prevent or lower high blood pressure, according to some health professionals.

SEE YOUR MEDICAL DOCTOR WHEN...

• You require a blood pressure reading. High blood pressure can cause strokes and heart attacks, but because there are so few symptoms, it is possible to have high blood pressure and not even know it. The American Heart Association suggests that you have your blood pressure checked at least every other year by your doctor or another qualified health professional. If your blood pressure is 140/90 or above, ask your doctor how often you should have it rechecked.

AROMATHERAPY

"Blue chamomile is great for people with high blood pressure," says Victoria Edwards, an aromatherapist in Fair Oaks, California. Carry the essential oil with you and inhale directly from the bottle whenever you feel flushed or agitated, suggests Edwards. She also recommends a daily massage using an everlast massage oil, which combines one drop of everlast (also called immortelle or helichrysum), two drops of blue chamomile and ten drops of lavender in one ounce of olive, almond, sunflower or another carrier oil. (Carrier oils are available in most health food stores.) Massage this blend into the area under the collarbone every day at bedtime, she says.

For information on preparing and administering essential oils, including cautions about their use, see page 19. For information on purchasing essential oils, refer to the resource list on page 633.

FOOD THERAPY

"It's important to increase your intake of potassium and magnesium, since the way to lower high blood pressure is to narrow the dietary ratios between sodium and potassium and between sodium and magnesium," says Julian Whitaker, M.D., founder and president of the Whitaker Wellness Center in Newport Beach, California. "And the best way to do that is to eat a lot of fresh fruits and vegetables, especially bananas, melons and dark green leafy vegetables." (For more food sources of potassium and magnesium, see "Getting What You Need" on page 142.)

One of the best ways to lower blood pressure is to eat more celery, which contains an oil that can lower blood pressure, adds registered pharmacist Earl Mindell, R.Ph., Ph.D., professor of nutrition at Pacific Western University in Los Angeles and author of *Earl Mindell's Food as Medicine* and other books on nutrition. Celery oil allows muscles that regulate blood pressure to dilate, says Dr. Mindell, and scientific studies show that rats who consumed the equivalent of four stalks of celery a day lowered their blood pressure an average of 13 percent.

HERBAL THERAPY

Eating up to three or four cloves of garlic every day may lower blood pressure, according to Varro E. Tyler, Ph.D., professor of pharmacognosy at Purdue University in West Lafayette, Indiana. If you'd rather not eat fresh cloves, try garlic supplements (they're available in many drugstores and most health food stores). Dr. Tyler recommends enteric-coated tablets such as Garlique for maximum absorption of allicin, the blood pressure–lowering ingredient in garlic. He says to follow the dosage recommendations on the label of the product you choose.

IMAGERY

To soothe your blood pressure, imagine going to your refrigerator and taking out three or four ice cubes, writes Gerald Epstein, M.D., a New York City psychiatrist and author of *Healing Visualizations*. Picture yourself slowly washing your head, face and neck with the ice. Feel the coolness seeping into every pore and entering your bloodstream in the brain. Envision an icy feeling tumbling down through your neck and trunk and into your fingers and toes. At that point, sense that your blood pressure is within a normal range.

Dr. Epstein suggests doing this imagery for three to five minutes three times a day or whenever you sense that your blood pressure is elevated.

JUICE THERAPY

"Celery juice has a mild diuretic effect, similar to many drugs that are prescribed for high blood pressure," says Elaine Gillaspie, N.D., a naturopathic physician in Portland, Oregon. She recommends an eight-ounce blend of one part celery juice, one part carrot juice and one part water, taken at least once a day. "This juice is highly nutritious and can be helpful for people with high blood pressure," says Dr. Gillaspie.

For information on juicing techniques, see page 93.

REFLEXOLOGY

Once you and your doctor have stabilized your blood pressure, you can help maintain normal levels by focusing on the following foot reflexes, says Rebecca Dioda, a reflexologist with the Morris Institute of Natural Therapeutics, a holistic health education center in Denville, New Jersey: solar plexus, to help control negative emotions; colon, to help your body eliminate toxins; urinary tract; heart; and lymphatic system. To help calm you down, she also suggests you do extra relaxation strokes.

To help you locate these points, consult the foot reflex chart on page 592. For instructions on how to work the points, including how to do the relaxation strokes, see "Your Reflexology Session" on page 110.

RELAXATION AND MEDITATION

Studies suggest that meditating for 20 minutes twice a day can help lower high blood pressure, says Sundar Ramaswami, Ph.D., a clinical psychologist at the F. S. Dubois Community Mental Health Center in Stamford, Connecticut. For an example of a meditation technique, see page 117.

SOUND THERAPY

Listening to relaxing music for 20 to 30 minutes each day can slow the heart rate and help lower blood pressure in some people, says Steven Halpern, Ph.D., composer, researcher and author of *Sound Health: The Music and Sounds That Make Us Whole*. To get started, turn on the music, then sit or lie comfortably, close your eyes and take a deep breath. Dr. Halpern suggests that you wear headphones to focus your attention and avoid distraction. He recommends, however, that you keep the speakers playing, so your body absorbs the sound energy. While the music plays, let your breath slow down and become steady. Listen not just to the notes but to the silence between the notes. Dr. Halpern says this will keep you from analyzing the music, which will allow it to relax you.

For suggested pieces to relax by, see "Sailing Away to Key Largo" on page 129. Many of those pieces are available in music stores. For mail-order information, refer to the resource list on page 642.

VITAMIN AND MINERAL THERAPY

Along with conventional therapy, the best ways to lower high blood pressure are to cut back on sugar, salt, caffeine and alcohol and to reduce or eliminate meats in your diet, says David Edelberg, M.D., an internist and medical director of the American Holistic Center/Chicago. He also says that people with high blood pressure may want to use the following vitamin, mineral and herbal regimen to help control the condition: 500 milligrams of calcium twice a day; 400 milligrams of magnesium twice a day; one tablespoon of flaxseed oil a day; 400 international units of vitamin E a day; 30 milligrams of coenzyme Q-10 three times a day; one hawthorn berry capsule three times a day; and one ginseng capsule twice a day. Flaxseed oil and coenzyme Q-10, hawthorn berry and ginseng supplements are available in most health food stores.

YOGA

Two yoga poses, the corpse (page 612) and the knee squeeze (page 612), are especially helpful with high blood pressure, according to Alice Christensen, founder and executive director of the American Yoga Association. These two poses help improve blood circulation and relieve tension, which is a major contributor to high blood pressure, she explains. An association study found that people with mild high blood pressure could lower it by doing these two poses every day, along with breathing exercises (see page 152) and meditation (see page 153). Christensen recommends meditating twice a day for 10 to 20 minutes each time. And she says to choose one or two other poses, in addition to the knee squeeze and corpse, for your daily yoga session. You can pick from the poses in the Daily Routine, which begins on page 606.

HIGH CHOLESTEROL

Many of us know our cholesterol counts as well as we know our phone numbers, and with good reason: High cholesterol is a risk factor for the heart attacks that kill more than a half-million Americans a year. Cholesterol itself isn't harmful. Produced in the liver, it's necessary for certain metabolic functions. But too much in the bloodstream leads to the formation of plaque, a sticky substance that accumulates in and blocks the arteries, which can lead to a heart attack.

Experts agree that a total cholesterol reading below 200 mg/dl (milligrams per deciliter of blood) is desirable. More important, though, is the ratio of HDL (high-density lipoprotein, the good cholesterol) to LDL (low-density lipoprotein, the harmful type that clogs your arteries). HDL helps remove LDL from your body. Exercise, not smoking and a high-fiber diet low in cholesterol and fat will improve your cholesterol count. And the natural remedies in this chapter—used in conjunction with medical care and with your doctor's approval—may help lower cholesterol, according to some health professionals.

SEE YOUR MEDICAL DOCTOR WHEN . . .

- You experience a sudden lapse in attention, paralysis, weakness or loss of consciousness, vision or the ability to speak.
- You experience chest pain or pressure, especially after exertion or emotional stress.
- You have cramping, pain or discomfort in your legs when you walk, especially if you are walking uphill or carrying heavy packages.

AYURVEDA

Cinnamon has blood-thinning properties that can help lower cholesterol levels, says Vasant Lad, B.A.M.S., M.A.Sc., director of the Ayurvedic Institute in Albuquerque, New Mexico. He suggests this tea: Mix 1 teaspoon of cinnamon and ¼ teaspoon of trikatu (a blend of ginger and two kinds of peppers) directly into a cup of hot water, then stir and steep for five minutes. Add a teaspoon of honey once the tea has cooled. Dr. Lad says to drink this beverage twice daily, once in the morning and once in the evening. Trikatu is available from Ayurvedic practitioners and in some health food stores; you can also purchase it by mail order (refer to the resource list on page 634).

FOOD THERAPY

Besides avoiding meats, dairy products and other foods that are high in dietary cholesterol and fat, another way to lower cholesterol is to eat more grapes, says Elson Haas, M.D., director of the Preventive Medical Center of Marin in San Rafael, California, and author of *Staying Healthy with Nutrition.* "There's a compound in grape skins and seeds that helps lower cholesterol." He says this is one reason why wine made from grapes has been shown to lower cholesterol. "In fact, grapeseed oil has been shown in several studies to help lower cholesterol better than other oils," he says. He says that his detoxification diet (see "Detoxing Your Ills" on page 48) can also help significantly lower cholesterol.

Garlic is another food that has been found to lower cholesterol, says Dr. Haas. And he points out that grapefruit, carrots and apples are rich in pectin, which reduces cholesterol levels by bonding with dietary fat and cholesterol and removing them from the body through the intestine before they are absorbed through your bloodstream.

HERBAL THERAPY

Scientific studies indicate that one clove of garlic or its equivalent, taken every day, is effective in reducing cholesterol levels, according to Varro E. Tyler, Ph.D., professor of pharmacognosy at Purdue University in West Lafayette, Indiana. He says that one way to get the equivalent is with garlic supplements, a processed form of the herb that is available in most health food stores (and in many drugstores, too). There are two advantages to these supplements, says Dr. Tyler. Allicin, the active ingredient in garlic, is best absorbed in supplemental form. And taking supplements allows you to bypass the bad breath that can be an unfortunate side effect of eating fresh garlic.

Dr. Tyler says the most effective form for a garlic supplement is enteric-coated capsules, which pass through the stomach and dissolve in the small intestine. But no matter which form you choose, he suggests following the dosage recommendations on the label.

IMAGERY

In *Rituals of Healing: Using Imagery for Health and Wellness,* Barbara Dossey, R.N., director of Holistic Nursing Consultants in Santa Fe, New Mexico, and her co-authors suggest that you imagine following a beam of light into one of your blood vessels. As you approach the wall of the vessel, notice the dome-shaped accumulation of sticky cholesterol that has collected over an old injury to the vessel. Now picture yourself gently peeling off layers of fatty material and handing them over to special cells that pass by. Like little garbage trucks, these cells haul the cholesterol to the intestine, where it begins its journey out of your body.

Next, travel over to your liver, where cholesterol is manufactured. Imagine talking to the supervisor of cholesterol production and suggesting that production quotas should be lower, so less cholesterol is made. He agrees and promises that your cholesterol will be maintained at a lower, healthy level.

Dossey recommends doing this exercise twice a day, 15 to 20 minutes each session.

REFLEXOLOGY

To help your body rid itself of cholesterol more efficiently, St. Petersburg, Florida, reflexologist Dwight Byers, author of *Better Health with Foot Reflexology*, says you should work the thyroid gland and liver reflexes on your hands or feet.

To help you locate these points, consult the hand and foot reflex charts beginning on page 582. For instructions on how to work the points, see "Your Reflexology Session" on page 110.

RELAXATION AND MEDITATION

Studies suggest that meditation can help reduce blood cholesterol levels, says Roger Walsh, M.D., Ph.D., professor of psychiatry, philosophy and anthropology at the University of California, Irvine, California College of Medicine. To try a simple meditation, see page 117. Practice this technique for 20 minutes once or twice a day, Dr. Walsh suggests.

VITAMIN AND MINERAL THERAPY

The first step in lowering cholesterol is to increase your intake of fiber and to eat more garlic, onions, oat bran and soy products, says David Edelberg, M.D., an internist and medical director of the American Holistic Center/Chicago. He also says that people with high cholesterol may want to use the following vitamin, mineral and herbal regimen to help control the condition: 100 milligrams of niacin twice a day; 200 micrograms of chromium twice a day; 400 milligrams of magnesium aspartate twice a day; 1,200 milligrams of lecithin three times a day; 500 milligrams of meta-sitosterol twice a day; one fish oil capsule three times a day; 2,000 milligrams of vitamin C twice a day; one garlic capsule three times a day; one ginseng capsule twice a day; and one guggulipid capsule twice a day. (Guggulipid is an Indian herb.) Lecithin, meta-sitosterol, fish oil, garlic and ginseng supplements are available in most health food stores. Guggulipid capsules can be purchased through mail order (refer to the resource list on page 643).

YOGA

Cholesterol can rise with your stress level, says Stephen A. Nezezon, M.D., yoga teacher and staff physician at the Himalayan International Institute of Yoga Science and Philosophy in Honesdale, Pennsylvania.

To lower stress, you can do a daily routine of breathing exercises, meditation and poses, says Alice Christensen, founder and executive director of the American Yoga Association.

The complete breath exercise (see page 152) can be done whenever you're feeling stress, whether it's at the office, in the car or at home, according to Christensen. She adds that daily meditation (see page 153) helps clear your mind and teaches you to relax at will.

And choose three or four yoga poses from the Daily Routine, which begins on page 606. Be sure to vary the poses from day to day to keep your interest high and strengthen different parts of your body, says Christensen. Dr. Nezezon adds that you should include at least one relaxation pose, such as the corpse (page 612), knee squeeze (page 612) or baby (page 618), in your daily yoga routine.

HYPERVENTILATION

Hyperventilation is proof that you can have too much of a good thing—even breathing.

When you feel extra tense or anxious, your body may react by breathing faster than normal. This can leave you feeling faint or light-headed. In some cases, hyperventilation can make your heart beat harder, cause pain in the stomach or leave you with a feeling of fullness in the throat.

First aid for hyperventilation is an old standby: Breathe into a paper bag. This helps adjust the mixture of carbon dioxide and oxygen in your system. The natural remedies in this chapter—in conjunction with medical care and used with your doctor's approval—may also help prevent or relieve hyperventilation, according to some health professionals.

SEE YOUR MEDICAL DOCTOR WHEN . . .

• You hyperventilate for the first time.

IMPOTENCE

FLOWER REMEDY/ESSENCE THERAPY

"Anyone who is hyperventilating needs to slow down both physically and emotionally," says Eve Campanelli, Ph.D., a holistic family practitioner in Beverly Hills, California. A few drops of the emergency stress relief formula (sold under brand names such as Calming Essence, Rescue Remedy and Five-Flower Formula) placed under the tongue will help restore emotional balance and make the person more receptive to other treatment, according to Dr. Campanelli.

The emergency stress relief formula is available in most health food stores and through mail order (refer to the resource list on page 635). For more information on preparing and administering the formula, see page 40.

YOGA

Learning deep breathing and practicing it regularly will help prevent bouts of hyperventilation, according to Stephen A. Nezezon, M.D., yoga teacher and staff physician at the Himalayan International Institute of Yoga Science and Philosophy in Honesdale, Pennsylvania. For instructions on deep breathing, see page 152.

IMPOTENCE

Forget the great myth of impotence. It's not all in your mind. An estimated 15 million American men are consistently unable to achieve or maintain erections, and 80 to 90 percent of the time, the cause is physical.

Egyptian researchers, for example, believe that wearing polyester underwear can cause a buildup of static electricity that may inhibit erections. But most often impotence is caused by something deadly serious: vascular disease. Clogged-up arteries, caused by a high-fat diet, lack of exercise or other reasons, can block the blood flow that causes erections. Impotence can also be a side effect of medication. The natural remedies in this chapter—in conjunction with medical care and used with your doctor's approval—may help prevent or relieve impotence, according to some health professionals.

SEE YOUR MEDICAL DOCTOR WHEN...

- You have diabetes or arteriosclerosis and aren't able to maintain an erection as frequently as usual.
- Your impotence is persistent or getting worse.

IMPOTENCE

ACUPRESSURE

"Acupressure on the Sea of Vitality points, B 23 and B 47, can fortify the body and, with repeated usage over a long period of time, can make a man stronger sexually," says Michael Reed Gach, Ph.D., director of the Acupressure Institute in Berkeley, California, and author of *Acupressure's Potent Points*. To find the B 47 points, measure four finger-widths away from the spine at waist level. The points are situated on the lower back on the left and right sides of the spine, in line with the navel. From B 47, you can move two finger-widths closer to the spine to find the B 23 points. (For help in locating these points, refer to the illustration on page 565.)

Dr. Gach says you can use your thumbs or fingers to work the points, pressing one or both B 47 points for one minute, then one or both B 23 points for one minute. He says to use this remedy three times daily. He adds that if you have a weak back, press these points lightly, and be sure not to press directly on the disks or vertebrae.

AROMATHERAPY

Jasmine is often inhaled for its aphrodisiac qualities, writes San Francisco herbalist Jeanne Rose, chairperson of the National Association for Holistic Aromatherapy, in her book *Aromatherapy: Applications and Inhalations*. Because the oil is expensive, Rose suggests using it in a candle diffuser to make it last longer. It can also be inhaled from a handkerchief or applied directly to the body, she says.

For information on preparing and administering essential oils, including cautions about their use, see page 19. For information on purchasing essential oils, refer to the resource list on page 633.

AYURVEDA

Here's a treatment regimen recommended by Vasant Lad, B.A.M.S., M.A.Sc., director of the Ayurvedic Institute in Albuquerque, New Mexico: Mix one cup of fresh grape juice with one teaspoon of fresh onion juice and one teaspoon of honey. Drink this mixture daily, one hour before going to bed, for 45 days. Dr. Lad says it will help increase sexual energy and sperm count.

Men with kapha constitutions should add a pinch of trikatu, says Dr. Lad. (For information on the doshas of Ayurveda, see "All about Vata, Pitta and Kapha" on page 28.) He explains that trikatu is an Indian herbal preparation combining dried ginger, black pepper and pippali, an Indian pepper. Trikatu and pippali are available from Ayurvedic practitioners and by mail order (refer to the resource list on page 634). You can also purchase trikatu in some health food stores.

FLOWER REMEDY/ESSENCE THERAPY

If a visit to your doctor has ruled out physical causes of impotence such as medication side effects and vascular disease, consider that your impotence may have an emotional cause, says Cynthia Mervis Watson, M.D., a family practice physician in Santa Monica, California, who specializes in homeopathic and herbal therapies. If a lack of sexual self-confidence is hampering you, Dr. Watson recommends the essence Pink Monkey Flower. If you're haunted by past episodes of impotence, the essence Sticky Monkey Flower may be helpful, she says.

"Impotence is always traumatic for a man, whether it's caused by physical or emotional factors," according to Dr. Watson. She says men receiving medical treatment for physically caused impotence can take the Bach flower remedy Star-of-Bethlehem, which will help them keep balanced emotionally.

Flower remedies/essences are available in some health food stores and through mail order (refer to the resource list on page 635). For information on preparing and administering flower remedies/essences, see page 37.

FOOD THERAPY

"You need to keep the arteries to the genitals open, and the way to do that is with a low-fat, low-cholesterol diet," says Michael A. Klaper, M.D., a nutritional medicine specialist in Pompano Beach, Florida, and director of the Institute of Nutritional Education and Research, an organization based in Manhattan Beach, California, that teaches doctors about nutrition and its relationship to disease. "The key to reversing impotence is to eat as you would to reverse heart disease." That means a diet centered around plenty of high-fiber fresh fruits and vegetables, legumes and other low-fat fare, says Dr. Klaper.

HERBAL THERAPY

Supplements of the herb ginkgo, found in most health food stores, can improve blood flow to the penile arteries and veins, which may help reverse impotence, says herbalist James Green, director of the California School of Herbal Studies in Forestville. He cautions that this herbal remedy isn't a quick fix; you'll need to take the supplements daily for six to eight weeks before you see results. Green says to follow the dosage recommendations on the product label.

HOMEOPATHY

After a thorough medical exam and diagnosis, try taking one of these 6C remedies two or three times a day until improvement occurs, says Chris Meletis,

N.D., a naturopathic physician and medicinary director at the National College of Naturopathic Medicine in Portland, Oregon. Agnus castus can be helpful for symptoms of a cold and relaxed penis and for lack of sexual desire, especially if accompanied by a fear of death and dilated pupils, says Dr. Meletis. If you are apprehensive and cannot have an erection, or if erections lead to premature emission, he recommends Lycopodium. Try Argentum nitricum, he says, if your erection fails when attempting intercourse, if intercourse is painful and if your symptoms are made worse at night, from warmth and when you eat sweets.

All of these remedies are available in many health food stores. To purchase the remedies by mail, refer to the resource list on page 637.

IMAGERY

Conquering impotence may be as simple as slaying an ogre, writes Gerald Epstein, M.D., a New York City psychiatrist and author of *Healing Visualizations*. Here's how: Imagine yourself descending into a valley. There you're confronted by a monster or an ogre. Fortunately, you have everything you need to defeat this beast. Fight the monster, and when you are triumphant and the monster is dead, skin it. Carry the skin with you and climb to the top of the valley. There you meet your loved one. Take her hand, walk with her to a tree and lie behind it. Picture the two of you surrounded by a cocoon of blue light and embrace.

Dr. Epstein suggests practicing this technique for five to seven minutes once a week, on the same morning each week, for three weeks.

REFLEXOLOGY

Pay special attention to the diaphragm reflex as well as to the spine, reproductive system and pituitary, parathyroid, thyroid and adrenal gland reflexes on your feet, says St. Petersburg, Florida, reflexologist Dwight Byers, author of *Better Health with Foot Reflexology*.

To help you locate these points, consult the foot reflex chart on page 592. For instructions on how to work the points, see "Your Reflexology Session" on page 110.

RELAXATION AND MEDITATION

Daily practice of thermal biofeedback can often help overcome impotence because it reduces anxiety and keeps your blood vessels open, says Steven Fahrion, Ph.D., director of research at the Life Sciences Institute of Mind-Body Health in Topeka, Kansas. To give this simple ten-minute technique a try, see page 121.

VITAMIN AND MINERAL THERAPY

"Vitamin A deficiency has been the cause of impotence in some men," says Elson Haas, M.D., director of the Preventive Medical Center of Marin in San Rafael, California, and author of *Staying Healthy with Nutrition*. Although vitamin A can be toxic in large doses, Dr. Haas says that most men can safely take between 10,000 and 25,000 international units daily without dangerous side effects. However, he recommends talking over possible supplementation with your doctor before beginning self-treatment.

YOGA

A yoga pose called the knee squeeze (page 612) may help against impotence, according to Alice Christensen, founder and executive director of the American Yoga Association. She recommends combining this exercise with two inverted yoga poses, the easy bridge (page 619) and the cobra (page 622), in a daily routine that should also include breathing exercises (see page 152) and meditation (see page 153). She also recommends several meditation breaks throughout the day of no more than five to ten minutes at a time.

INCONTINENCE

There are more serious conditions, more painful conditions and more noticeable conditions. But in most people's books, there are few conditions more embarrassing than urinary incontinence.

Simply put, incontinence is the inability to control your bladder.

Lots of things cause incontinence: urinary tract infections, aging, obesity, nerve damage, spinal cord injuries, prostate problems and more. The natural remedies in this chapter—in conjunction with medical care and used with your doctor's approval—may help control incontinence, according to some health professionals.

SEE YOUR MEDICAL DOCTOR WHEN . . .

- You urinate when you shouldn't or aren't trying to.
- You have no sensation that your bladder is full.

FOOD THERAPY

Sometimes overweight can cause incontinence, because fat around the abdomen pushes down on the bladder, says Michael A. Klaper, M.D., a nutritional medicine specialist in Pompano Beach, Florida, and director of the Institute of Nutritional Education and Research, an organization based in Manhattan Beach, California, that teaches doctors about nutrition and its relationship to disease.

"The answer is a low-fat diet and gentle exercise, because losing weight can help tremendously or even clear up the problem," he says. Eating more fresh fruits and vegetables is a great first step to losing weight, he says, since they're low in calories and fat yet very filling. He also recommends pastas, beans and rice—without fatty sauces or butter.

HOMEOPATHY

One remedy worth trying is Causticum, says Stephen Messer, N.D., dean of the National Center for Homeopathy's summer school and a naturopathic physician in Eugene, Oregon. He suggests taking a 6C dose after every episode of incontinence for three to four days. If that doesn't help, he advises that you seek medical care.

Causticum is available in many health food stores. To purchase homeopathic remedies by mail, refer to the resource list on page 637.

HYDROTHERAPY

"Many people with incontinence also experience bladder irritation, which aggravates the problem," says Agatha Thrash, M.D., a medical pathologist and co-founder and co-director of Uchee Pines Institute, a natural healing center in Seale, Alabama. "We find that drinking more water alleviates the irritation by diluting the irritants in the urine." Eight to ten eight-ounce glasses of water a day, plus Kegel exercises, often make a big difference in patients' ability to control urination, according to Dr. Thrash.

Kegel exercises are designed to strengthen the pubococcygeus muscles, a set of muscles that run from the pubic bone to the tailbone, according to Charles Kuntzleman, Ed.D., associate professor of kinesiology at the University of Michigan in Ann Arbor. These muscles help both men and women stop the flow of urine and squeeze off gas and permit women to tighten the vagina, he says.

To learn how to do Kegels, Dr. Kuntzleman suggests that the next time you are urinating, try to stop your flow when you are halfway finished without tensing the muscles in your legs, buttocks or abdomen. If you're able to stop the flow, you're using the right muscles, he explains. Once you've located them, he says, you can contract these muscles anytime, anywhere.

To control urinary incontinence, Dr. Kuntzleman recommends that you do Kegel exercises as often as possible during the day, slowly increasing the amount of time you hold the squeezing motion.

IMAGERY

In *Rituals of Healing: Using Imagery for Health and Wellness*, Barbara Dossey, R.N., director of Holistic Nursing Consultants in Santa Fe, New Mexico, and her co-authors recommend the following visualization exercise to help you overcome incontinence. Imagine that somewhere within you there is a brilliant glowing light that is penetrating and powerful. From this light, a beam shoots into your pelvic and bladder area that heals and calms your urinary tract.

Now imagine that the beam transforms into a tiny boat that journeys on a golden river from the kidneys to the bladder. In the bladder, the small boat of light drifts on a tiny inner lake. As you sail on, you notice the smooth layers of muscle tissue in the bladder. As the bladder fills, you see the muscles relax in response to increased pressure. When the time is right, watch the muscular bands that have been holding the urethra closed slowly relax. Feel the walls of the bladder contract to help empty the urine. Finally, picture the sphincter muscles closing after the last few drops have drained.

Dossey recommends practicing this imagery twice a day for 15 to 20 minutes each session.

REFLEXOLOGY

To help you with bladder control, New York City reflexologist Laura Norman, author of *Feet First: A Guide to Foot Reflexology*, recommends working these reflex points on your feet: solar plexus, diaphragm, chest, lung, bronchial tube, lower spine, bladder, kidney and adrenal gland. To help you locate these points, consult the foot reflex chart on page 592. For instructions on how to work the points, see "Your Reflexology Session" on page 110.

YOGA

A yoga exercise called the stomach lock can help strengthen muscles in the lower abdomen, increasing bladder control, says Alice Christensen, founder and executive director of the American Yoga Association. Her instructions for the exercise: Lie on your back and take a deep breath. Breathe out until the breath is completely gone, then pull in your buttock, groin and stomach muscles hard. Hold for a count of three, then release your muscles.

Christensen recommends doing this yoga exercise three times per session, two or three times per day. You should notice improvement in a couple of weeks, she says.

You should not practice this pose if you have high blood pressure, hiatal hernia, ulcers or heart disease, according to Stephen A. Nezezon, M.D., yoga teacher and staff physician at the Himalayan International Institute of Yoga Science and Philosophy in Honesdale, Pennsylvania. Dr. Nezezon also cautions that women should not practice stomach locks during menstruation or pregnancy.

INDIGESTION

You might as well have swallowed a cinder block. That mystery meat sandwich from the cafeteria is sitting in your stomach like a ten-pound hunk of marble, refusing to be digested, refusing to move along and leaving you with a bellyful of discomfort.

Lots of things can cause indigestion: eating too much too fast, eating spicy or fatty foods, even being tense, upset or emotional when you're eating. For whatever reason, your body occasionally has trouble breaking down the foods you eat, sometimes resulting in stomachaches, cramps, flatulence, nausea and other problems. The natural remedies in this chapter—in conjunction with medical care and used with the approval of your doctor—may help prevent or relieve indigestion, according to some health professionals.

SEE YOUR MEDICAL DOCTOR WHEN . . .

- You continue to feel pressure, fullness, squeezing or pain in your chest despite taking antacids.
- You develop other symptoms such as shortness of breath, sweating, nausea or vomiting, dizziness, fainting, general weakness or pain radiating from your chest into your back, jaw or arms.
- Your indigestion is accompanied by changes in the frequency or appearance of your bowel movements.

INDIGESTION

AROMATHERAPY

Massage an upset stomach with a blend of essential oils known to stimulate digestion, suggests Los Angeles aromatherapist Michael Scholes, of Aromatherapy Seminars, an organization that trains professionals and others in the use of essential oils. He says to add four drops each of peppermint, marjoram, coriander, fennel and basil essential oils to an ounce of olive or almond oil (both of these oils are available in most health food stores) and massage it gently into the abdomen.

For information on preparing and administering essential oils, including cautions about their use, see page 19. For information on purchasing essential oils, refer to the resource list on page 633.

AYURVEDA

According to Ayurvedic practitioners, bay leaf helps kindle *agni,* or gastric fire, one of the most vital elements of good digestion. To relieve indigestion, try steeping ½ teaspoon of crushed or ground bay leaf (available in most health food stores) in a cup of hot water for ten minutes, suggests Vasant Lad, B.A.M.S., M.A.Sc., director of the Ayurvedic Institute in Albuquerque, New Mexico. Strain the tea so that there's no bay leaf left in it, add a pinch of cardamom and drink the tea after eating.

You can also try chewing ½ teaspoon each of roasted fennel and cumin seeds after meals to aid digestion, he says. Or, he suggests, stir 1 teaspoon of lemon juice and ½ teaspoon of baking soda into a cup of cool water, then drink this mixture quickly whenever you're suffering from indigestion.

FOOD THERAPY

"There are two major forms of indigestion," says Michael A. Klaper, M.D., a nutritional medicine specialist in Pompano Beach, Florida, and director of the Institute of Nutritional Education and Research, an organization based in Manhattan Beach, California, that teaches doctors about nutrition and its relationship to disease. "One is in the upper tract: a stomach filled with acid, which is usually the result of plopping a lot of protein into the stomach and the stomach responding with a big gush of acid to digest it. For that kind of indigestion, it's a matter of not eating protein-rich foods too late in the day. So if you must have meat, have it for lunch, and stick with pasta for dinner.

"The other form of indigestion is due to swallowed air in the lower gastrointestinal tract, and that's often a matter of how fast you're eating. For that, the best thing is to slow down, chew each mouthful at least 10 to 15 times, avoid drinking with meals and minimize talking while eating," says Dr. Klaper.

INDIGESTION

HERBAL THERAPY

Traditional herbal remedies for indigestion include peppermint, ginger and chamomile teas, all of which you can find in tea bag form in most health food stores, says Varro E. Tyler, Ph.D., professor of pharmacognosy at Purdue University in West Lafayette, Indiana. He suggests drinking a cup of one of these teas after every meal.

HOMEOPATHY

If you have indigestion and have been eating lots of rich, fatty foods, try taking a 6C dose of Pulsatilla every 30 minutes until you begin to feel better, says Stephen Messer, N.D., dean of the National Center for Homeopathy's summer school and a naturopathic physician in Eugene, Oregon. If you have lots of abdominal gas, he says to try a 6C dose of Carbo vegetabilis every 30 to 60 minutes until you feel better.

Pulsatilla and Carbo vegetabilis are available in many health food stores. To purchase homeopathic remedies by mail, refer to the resource list on page 637.

HYDROTHERAPY

"I don't believe there is a gastric problem that doesn't respond to activated charcoal," says Agatha Thrash, M.D., a medical pathologist and co-founder and co-director of Uchee Pines Institute, a natural healing center in Seale, Alabama. To alleviate indigestion, mix two to three tablespoons of activated charcoal powder with a little water in the bottom of a tall glass. "Stir gently, or the powder flies everywhere," says Dr. Thrash. Continue stirring and adding water a little at a time until the glass is full, then drink it with a straw. Activated charcoal is available in most health food stores and some pharmacies.

IMAGERY

In *Rituals of Healing: Using Imagery for Health and Wellness*, Barbara Dossey, R.N., director of Holistic Nursing Consultants in Santa Fe, New Mexico, and her co-authors suggest that you envision a bright light beginning to glow within you. This light is powerful and penetrating. Imagine a beam spreading from this light that has a soft, healing color. The beam goes directly into your abdomen. Allow its healing color to fill your stomach with calm and quiet. Imagine the color slowly flowing out of your stomach and into your small intestine, like a tiny sailboat riding on smooth waves. Follow it down through your large intestine and into your rectum, gently healing and soothing your digestive tract as it goes.

Dossey recommends that you use this imagery twice a day, 15 to 20 minutes each time.

JUICE THERAPY

In *The Complete Book of Juicing*, naturopathic physician Michael Murray, N.D., recommends juicing a ¼-inch-thick slice of fresh ginger, half of a handful of fresh mint, one kiwifruit and one-fourth of a pineapple (both with skin, if your juicer can handle it). He says drinking this eight-ounce blend twice daily, in conjunction with proper medical treatment, should speed digestion, soothe the intestine and help eliminate gas.

For information on juicing techniques, see page 93.

REFLEXOLOGY

Use the corresponding golf ball technique (page 588) to work the stomach, colon and small intestine points on your hands, say Kevin and Barbara Kunz, reflexology researchers in Santa Fe, New Mexico, and authors of *Hand and Foot Reflexology*. They also suggest working the solar plexus points on both hands. To help you locate these points, consult the hand reflex chart on page 582. For instructions on how to work the points, see "Your Reflexology Session" on page 110.

RELAXATION AND MEDITATION

Thermal biofeedback can relieve indigestion by increasing blood flow to the gastronintestinal tract, says Steven Fahrion, Ph.D., director of research at the Life Sciences Institute of Mind-Body Health in Topeka, Kansas. Use the ten-minute technique described on page 121 whenever your digestive tract rebels.

SOUND THERAPY

Tension and stress may lead to indigestion, and relaxing music can help, says Janalea Hoffman, R.M.T., a composer and music therapist based in Kansas City, Missouri. For some people, music with a slow, steady beat calms the heart and other body parts, including the stomach, according to Hoffman. She says to try listening to relaxing music during meals and for 20 to 30 minutes after meals. Hoffman suggests her tape *Deep Daydreams*; for other pieces to relax by, see "Sailing Away to Key Largo" on page 129. Many of these recordings are available in music stores. For mail-order information, refer to the resource list on page 642.

YOGA

The knee squeeze (page 612) can help when you have indigestion, says Stephen A. Nezezon, M.D., yoga teacher and staff physician at the Himalayan International Institute of Yoga Science and Philosophy in Honesdale, Pennsylvania. He explains that this pose massages the large colon, easing constipation and improving digestion. It also reduces toxin buildup in the digestive tract, he adds.

SEE ALSO Heartburn

INFERTILITY

You've been trying for months, and still there's no baby on the way. You're beginning to wonder if you and your partner are infertile.

Most doctors won't even diagnose infertility until after a couple has tried to conceive for a year. They advise that women ages 35 and over seek medical help after six months, however, because of natural declines in a woman's fertility.

Male infertility is the problem about 35 percent of the time. This can include having too few sperm or sperm that are too weak to swim the distance to the fallopian tubes. Another 35 percent of infertility cases involve the female reproductive system, with problems such as blocked or damaged fallopian tubes and lack of ovulation. These conditions have many causes, including endometriosis, hormone deficiencies, infections, cysts and sexually transmitted diseases. In 30 percent of cases, there is a combination of problems, or the cause is unknown. The natural remedies in this chapter—in conjunction with medical care and used with the approval of your doctor—may help improve the possibility of conception, according to some health professionals.

SEE YOUR MEDICAL DOCTOR WHEN . . .

- You are a woman under age 35 and have been unable to conceive in a year of unprotected intercourse.
- You are a woman age 35 or over and have been unable to conceive after six months of unprotected intercourse.
- Your menstrual periods are scant or irregular and your cervical mucus doesn't change.

- Your medical history includes pelvic infections, endometriosis, polycystic ovary disease, abdominal or urinary tract surgery, excessively high fever or mumps or measles.
- You have used an intrauterine device.
- You or your partner has suffered from chlamydia.
- You are a woman and are producing milk or have male pattern hair growth on your breasts, upper lip or chin.

FLOWER REMEDY/ESSENCE THERAPY

"In ancient cultures, the pomegranate was a symbol of fertility," says Cynthia Mervis Watson, M.D., a family practice physician in Santa Monica, California, who specializes in homeopathy and herbal therapy. She recommends the essence Pomegranate to women who are trying to conceive. "It has a balancing effect on the female reproductive system and is also good for emotional issues surrounding sexuality and motherhood," says Dr. Watson.

Flower essences are available in some health food stores and through mail order (refer to the resource list on page 635). For information on preparing and administering flower essences, see page 37.

FOOD THERAPY

Eat more oysters, advises Julian Whitaker, M.D., founder and president of the Whitaker Wellness Center in Newport Beach, California. While there's no evidence that this much-ballyhooed "aphrodisiac" can increase libido, there is proof that the high zinc content of oysters may strengthen sperm count and motility, increasing chances for conception, according to Dr. Whitaker. He says you'll get nearly the entire Recommended Dietary Allowance of zinc from just one oyster. He suggests lean red meats and crab as other good sources of zinc.

"It's also good to eat more fruits and vegetables, which are high in vitamin C and other antioxidants," says Dr. Whitaker. "A lot of male infertility is due to oxidation, which can weaken or kill sperm."

For other food sources of zinc and vitamin C, see "Getting What You Need" on page 142.

HOMEOPATHY

Infertility should be treated on an individual basis by a homeopath or fertility specialist, write Andrew Lockie, M.D., and Nicola Geddes, M.D., in *The Women's Guide to Homeopathy*. But they add that there are several homeopathic remedies you can try while waiting for professional care. They suggest taking a 30C dose of one of the following remedies every 12 hours for up to seven days.

If you're a woman whose breasts feel tender, with pockets of hard swelling, and whose desire for sex is ebbing, try Conium, say Dr. Lockie and Dr. Geddes. They say that Lycopodium may help if you have a dry vagina and tenderness in your lower abdomen over the right ovary. If you feel weepy, chilly and irritable, have a lack of sexual desire and have irregular periods accompanied by a sensation that your womb is about to drop out of your vagina, they suggest trying Sepia. And if you've had a previous miscarriage before 12 weeks, try Sabina, they say.

All of these remedies are available in many health food stores. To purchase the remedies by mail, refer to the resource list on page 637.

IMAGERY

In his book *Healing Visualizations*, New York City psychiatrist Gerald Epstein, M.D., suggests this visualization to help women overcome infertility. Close your eyes, breathe out three times and imagine walking into a beautiful garden. There you find a tree and a stream of flowing water. Bathe in the water, allowing it to enter and clean all ova, or eggs. Then sit under the tree and enjoy the sunshine and blue sky reflecting through the leaves. Look up to your right and make a prayer for what you want. Do this quickly. Then ask your mate to join you in the garden. Lie down under the tree holding hands. Picture a blue light forming a dome over you. Now go out of the garden holding hands, cradling a child between you.

Do this imagery for two to three minutes once a day for seven days, beginning at the middle of your cycle.

REFLEXOLOGY

On your hands or feet, work the reflex points for the reproductive system, diaphragm, spine and pituitary, parathyroid, thyroid and adrenal glands, says St. Petersburg, Florida, reflexologist Dwight Byers, author of *Better Health with Foot Reflexology*.

To help you locate these points, consult the hand and foot reflex charts beginning on page 582. For instructions on how to work the points, see "Your Reflexology Session" on page 110.

VITAMIN AND MINERAL THERAPY

The antioxidants beta-carotene and vitamins C and E can increase sperm count (the number of sperm) and motility (the sperm's ability to swim into the egg), says Julian Whitaker, M.D., founder and president of the Whitaker Wellness Center in Newport Beach, California. In fact, he says, studies show that large doses of supplemental vitamin C can actually reverse some cases of male infertility. He recommends taking at least 1,000 milligrams of vitamin C each day, as well as 400 to 800 international units of vitamin E and 15 milligrams (25,000 international units) of beta-carotene.

And try taking 30 to 60 milligrams a day of zinc, which may also help increase sperm count, says Dr. Whitaker.

INGROWN TOENAILS

They don't call them toe*nails* for nothing. When one of them changes course and starts growing down into your toe, it feels like someone is driving a sharp tack right into your flesh.

Ingrown toenails happen mostly to the big toe on each foot. Sometimes a shoe that's too tight or an overzealous pedicure that leaves your toenail too short can cause the nail to grow into the flesh on the sides of your toe. This can be extremely painful and can become infected. Unfortunately, the tendency to develop ingrown toenails can be hereditary. The natural remedies in this chapter, used with the approval of your doctor, may help heal an ingrown toenail, according to some health professionals.

SEE YOUR MEDICAL DOCTOR WHEN ...

- You notice that the skin surrounding your toenail is red and swollen or discharging green or yellow fluid.
- You have diabetes.

HOMEOPATHY

At the first sign of discomfort from an ingrown toenail, soak your toe in five drops of Hypericum tincture and five drops of Calendula tincture diluted in ½ pint of warm water, write Andrew Lockie, M.D., and Nicola Geddes, M.D., in *The Women's Guide to Homeopathy*. After 15 to 30 minutes, they say, remove your toe from the water and gently wrap a small piece of soft linen around the side of the nail, slipping it between the skin over the top of the nail and the nail bed.

Dr. Lockie and Dr. Geddes also suggest taking one of these 6C remedies every

12 hours for two weeks. To strengthen nails that repeatedly ingrow, they say, try Magnetis polus australis. If your nails are quite brittle, they recommend Thuja. If there is no improvement in a month, see your medical doctor or homeopath.

All of these remedies are available in many health food stores. To purchase the remedies by mail, refer to the resource list on page 637.

HYDROTHERAPY

To help heal an ingrown toenail, soak your foot in hot, sudsy water for 20 minutes, suggests Agatha Thrash, M.D., a medical pathologist and co-founder and co-director of Uchee Pines Institute, a natural healing center in Seale, Alabama. Then, she says, cut off the corner of the nail (make sure it's square) and wrap your toe in a hot compress covered with a dry cloth, keeping it in place overnight.

In the morning, says Dr. Thrash, trim the toenail in a shallow U shape across the top, leaving it squared off in the corners. She suggests slipping a few fibers of cotton under the edge of the nail to stop it from digging into the flesh. Trim the ends of the cotton short to get them out of the way, so it can remain in place for several days or even weeks, she adds.

SEE ALSO Foot Pain

INHIBITED SEXUAL DESIRE

It used to be more, more, more. Now it's bore, bore, bore—or even chore, chore, chore. For whatever reason, sex has lost its appeal. The only thing you want to do in the bedroom these days is pull the covers over your head and hope your partner doesn't try to get frisky.

What's going on? Well, the problem could be inhibited sexual desire, defined by doctors as a lack of interest in sex or an inability to become sexually aroused. The possible causes vary greatly. Sometimes there's an obvious reason, such as a hormone deficiency or depression. But more often there's a hidden problem: excessive stress, trouble in your current relationship or past abuse. Counseling, alone or with your partner, often helps get your sex drive back. The natural remedies in this chapter—in conjunction with medical care and used with your doctor's approval—may also help reignite your sex drive, according to some health professionals.

- You notice a drop in your desire to have sex and are unable to discuss the matter with your mate.
- You lose interest in other activities that you once enjoyed greatly.

FLOWER REMEDY/ESSENCE THERAPY

The Bach remedy Crab Apple is often helpful, according to Susan Lange, O.M.D., of the Meridian Center for Personal and Environmental Health in Santa Monica, California. "Crab Apple is good for women who feel discomfort or shame about their sexuality or who simply feel 'dead' inside," she says. "Crab Apple can help get energy flowing again."

She also recommends the essence Sticky Monkey Flower, which helps balance sexual impulses. "This is good for women and men who feel either excessive sexual desire or none at all. It helps them achieve equilibrium," says Dr. Lange.

Flower remedies/essences are available in some health food stores and through mail order (refer to the resource list on page 635). For information on preparing and administering flower remedies/essences, see page 37.

FOOD THERAPY

Fava beans and soybeans are excellent sources of dopamine, which can enhance sex drive, says Julian Whitaker, M.D., founder and president of the Whitaker Wellness Center in Newport Beach, California. He recommends increasing your intake of these fiber-rich foods to improve your libido. *Note:* A very small number of people of Mediterranean descent may have a reaction to fava beans. If your skin and eyes turn yellow from jaundice within three days of eating fava beans, see your doctor.

Other lean foods may also do the trick, but in a different way, according to Dr. Whitaker. He explains that fatty foods can curb production of testosterone, the hormone that controls sex drive in both men and women. By cutting down on the fat in your diet, he says, you can increase testosterone production, improving sex drive.

HOMEOPATHY

Use a 30C dose of one of the following remedies once a day until improvement is noted, says Chris Meletis, N.D., a naturopathic physician and medicinary director at the National College of Naturopathic Medicine in Portland, Oregon. If you weep easily, are timid with a passive personality and do not tolerate heat well, Dr. Meletis recommends using Pulsatilla. Ignatia is a good remedy, he says, if your inhibition is due mainly to fear and anxiety, with symptoms that are worse in the morning and better while eating. If you have fear and anxiety, cannot relax and feel worse with music and heat and better in open, airy rooms and with pressure against your back, Natrum muriaticum may be helpful, he says.

All of these remedies are available in many health food stores. To purchase the remedies by mail, refer to the resource list on page 637.

IMAGERY

See yourself on a boat in the ocean with a crew composed entirely of the opposite sex, says Elizabeth Ann Barrett, R.N., Ph.D., professor and coordinator of the Center for Nursing Research at Hunter College of the City University of New York in New York City. Envision yourself lying on a massage table, facing down and wearing little or no clothing. Feel the warm sun on your bare skin as a gentle, cool breeze flows over you. A gorgeous man or woman approaches you and begins to give you a massage with what feel like velvet hands. As the massager rubs perfumed oils on your skin, you feel tingling sexual vibrations throughout your body. The massager leans over and whispers a beautiful sexual message in your ear that you have been waiting to hear all of your life. When you hear this message, open your eyes and keep this message for yourself.

Dr. Barrett suggests using this imagery every evening before bed, when you are as relaxed as possible. Continue the imagery for as long as the images and good feelings stay with you. If nothing happens with the imagery, says Dr. Barrett, let it go and try again the next night.

INSOMNIA

Think you're the only one who watches the late show, the later show, the latest show and the it's-so-late-it's-almost-early show?

Guess again, sleepyhead. An estimated 40 million Americans have chronic sleep disorders, and another 20 to 30 million have at least occasional problems catching some Zzzs. Women, especially those over age 40, seem to be more at risk for insomnia than men. The causes of insomnia are as numerous as the sheep you've probably tried to count, from caffeine to stress to working the graveyard shift. The natural remedies in this chapter—in conjunction with medical care and used with your doctor's approval—may help prevent or relieve insomnia, according to some health professionals.

ACUPRESSURE

Use the index and ring fingers of one hand to apply pressure to the indentation on the back of the head at the base of the skull for several minutes, suggests Jin Shin Jyutsu practitioner Priscilla Pitman, of Manchester, Massachusetts. (Jin Shin Jyutsu is a type of acupressure.) "Exhale first," she says, "then inhale, receiving a new breath as you guide your fingers to the spot. This area is among the 26 'safety energy locks' used in the art of Jin Shin Jyutsu. It marks the bridge between the spiritual and physical realms and helps release fears that may be keeping you awake." She adds that you can use this technique periodically throughout the day or when you can't fall asleep.

Pitman says you can also apply pressure to the fleshy pad of skin at the base of either thumb, switching hands as you feel is needed. This point can quiet the mind, according to Pitman. She suggests using this technique periodically throughout the day or as you fall asleep at night.

AROMATHERAPY

For occasional sleeplessness, add six to eight drops of lavender, marjoram or ylang-ylang essential oil to your bathwater before going to bed, suggests Los Angeles aromatic consultant John Steele. Or put four drops of lavender, marjoram, rum or chamomile essential oil on your pillow right before sleep, he says.

For information on preparing and administering essential oils, including cautions about their use, see page 19. For information on purchasing essential oils, refer to the resource list on page 633.

FLOWER REMEDY/ESSENCE THERAPY

"If you lie awake because of unwanted thoughts that go around and around in your head, the flower remedy White Chestnut can be effective," says Leslie J. Kaslof, an herbalist and author of *The Traditional Flower Remedies of Dr. Edward Bach.*

Kaslof cautions against expecting a quick response. "Flower remedies don't work in the same way that a chemical drug or a sleeping pill does. They work more gently and slowly and may not provide short-term relief," he notes. "But people with insomnia may often see improvement within a few weeks."

Flower remedies are available in some health food stores and through mail order (refer to the resource list on page 635). For information on preparing and administering flower remedies, see page 37.

HERBAL THERAPY

Herbal sleep formulas—in teas, tinctures and capsules—are available in most health food stores, says Varro E. Tyler, Ph.D., professor of pharmacognosy at Purdue University in West Lafayette, Indiana. For best results, he recommends choosing one that combines hops, valerian, chamomile, oats, passionflower and balm. He says to follow the directions on the product label for proper dosage.

Valerian, which reduces activity in the central nervous system, is the best-known herbal treatment for insomnia, and you could take that alone if the herbal formulas don't work, according to Dr. Tyler. Most health food stores carry valerian products; follow the dosage recommendations on the label, he says.

Hops, a digestive tonic and sedative, may also help you relax, says Dr. Tyler. He recommends purchasing dried hops flowers (available in most health food stores), putting them in a small muslin bag and placing the bag under your pillow.

HOMEOPATHY

For mild bouts of insomnia, try taking a 30C dose of one of the following remedies one hour before bedtime for ten consecutive nights, says Andrew Lockie, M.D., in *The Family Guide to Homeopathy*. He suggests repeating the dose if you wake and can't get back to sleep.

If you can't pop your mind out of gear because of some good or bad news, Dr. Lockie says to try Coffea. He recommends Pulsatilla if you feel restless when you first go to bed, alternate between being too hot and too cold and aren't thirsty and if your insomnia seems worse after eating rich foods. Ignatia is a good remedy, he says, if you yawn a lot but aren't able to drift off, you dread not being able to sleep or you have nightmares when you do fall asleep. If you're anxious, worried or restless, have ominous dreams about fire or danger and are wide awake between midnight and 2:00 A.M., Dr. Lockie says to try Arsenicum. Lycopodium may help if you talk and laugh in your sleep, are aware that you dream a lot and often wake about 4:00 A.M. and if your mind is usually very active at bedtime, he says.

All of these remedies are available in many health food stores. To purchase the remedies by mail, refer to the resource list on page 637.

INSOMNIA

HYDROTHERAPY

Brief cold water "treading" before bed may help you drop off, according to Agatha Thrash, M.D., a medical pathologist and co-founder and co-director of Uchee Pines Institute, a natural healing center in Seale, Alabama. To tread, fill the bathtub with enough water to cover your ankles. Holding on to a stable railing, march in place in the water for anywhere from five seconds to five minutes.

IMAGERY

Imagine a time when you had to stay awake when you really didn't want to, such as to study all night for a test. Picture yourself studying but struggling to stay awake. Finally, you just give in to the urge to sleep. It's a paradoxical imagery that seems to help some people fall asleep, says Dennis Gersten, M.D., a San Diego psychiatrist and publisher of *Atlantis*, a bimonthly imagery newsletter. He suggests practicing this imagery in bed, just before going to sleep.

MASSAGE

Slow, gentle massage of the neck and shoulders, done just before bedtime, can help you relax and get to sleep, says Vincent Iuppo, N.D., massage therapist, naturopathic physician and director of the Morris Institute of Natural Therapeutics, a holistic health education center in Denville, New Jersey.

Dr. Iuppo's instructions: Lubricate your hands with a small amount of vegetable oil or massage oil, then stroke your shoulders lightly. Rub your left shoulder with your right hand and your right shoulder with your left hand. Use gentle, gliding strokes. "You'll be able to tell what feels good for you," Dr. Iuppo says. Also rub the back of your neck, using the same gliding strokes. You can use your thumbs to make slow, small circles on the muscles in the back of your neck. Dr. Iuppo suggests taking about ten minutes for the entire massage.

REFLEXOLOGY

Working the diaphragm, ovary/testicle, pancreas and pituitary, parathyroid, thyroid and adrenal gland reflexes in both of your feet may help you rest easier, says St. Petersburg, Florida, reflexologist Dwight Byers, author of *Better Health with Foot Reflexology*. To help you locate these points, consult the foot reflex chart on page 592. For instructions on how to work the points, see "Your Reflexology Session" on page 110.

■
RELAXATION AND MEDITATION

For a swift voyage into dreamland, try progressive relaxation about 15 minutes before bedtime, suggests Julie Johnson, R.N., Ph.D., director of the School of Nursing at the University of Nevada at Reno. In a study of 176 men and women older than age 65 who had difficulty sleeping, Dr. Johnson found that progressive relaxation helped people fall asleep more quickly, sleep more soundly with fewer nighttime arousals and feel more satisfied with their night's rest.

"Progressive relaxation helps you relax, and as you relax, you tend to get drowsy," Dr. Johnson says. "No matter what your age, I think this technique can work for you." To try progressive relaxation, see page 122.

As an alternative, consider a quick ten-minute session of the thermal biofeedback technique described on page 121, says Steven Fahrion, Ph.D., director of research at the Life Sciences Institute of Mind-Body Health in Topeka, Kansas.

■
SOUND THERAPY

Listening to relaxing music shortly before going to bed can de-stress your body and help you get a good night's sleep, says Steven Halpern, Ph.D., composer, researcher and author of *Sound Health: The Music and Sounds That Make Us Whole.* To get started, turn on the music, then sit or lie comfortably, close your eyes and take a deep breath. Dr. Halpern suggests that you wear headphones to focus your attention and avoid distraction. He recommends, however, that you keep the speakers playing, so your body absorbs the sound energy. While the music plays, let your breath slow down and become steady. Listen not just to the notes but to the silence between the notes. Dr. Halpern says this will keep you from analyzing the music, which will allow it to relax you.

For suggested pieces to relax by, see "Sailing Away to Key Largo" on page 129. Many of these recordings are available in music stores. For mail-order information, refer to the resource list on page 642.

■
VITAMIN AND MINERAL THERAPY

Calcium, vitamin D and the B vitamins each play a role in the regulation of the nervous system, and each can help you sleep more soundly, says Richard Gerson, Ph.D., author of *The Right Vitamins.* His recommendation: daily intakes of between 800 and 1,400 milligrams of calcium and 400 international units of vitamin D, along with a B-complex supplement that contains the Recommended Dietary Allowances of the six important B vitamins (thiamin, riboflavin, niacin, vitamin B_6, vitamin B_{12} and pantothenic acid). For the Recommended Dietary Allowances, see "Getting What You Need" on page 142. He says to take this level of supplementation until insomnia is no longer a problem.

YOGA

A 30-minute meditation just before bedtime will encourage better sleep, says Alice Christensen, founder and executive director of the American Yoga Association. She suggests lying in bed to do the meditation, then rolling over and nodding off. You may even fall asleep during the meditation, she says. (Instructions for yoga meditation begin on page 153.)

If you should wake up during the night, Christensen suggests doing the yoga version of counting sheep: the complete breath (see page 152). As you breathe, she says, pay attention only to the sound of your breath. Don't hold your breath at any time; just let it flow in and out, says Christensen.

INTERCOURSE PAIN

Making love shouldn't hurt. So when sex with your mate becomes painful, it's time to take action.

Vaginal dryness is one of the most common causes of intercourse pain for women. The problem can become more pronounced as a woman approaches menopause, when secretions lessen because of a decline in hormones. The dryness, combined with a thinning vaginal lining, can make sex excruciating. Bladder infections can also cause pain for women, and herpes outbreaks can affect both men and women. The natural remedy in this chapter—in conjunction with medical care and used with your doctor's approval—may help relieve painful intercourse, according to one health professional.

SEE YOUR MEDICAL DOCTOR WHEN . . .

- You have so much pain that you and your partner can't enjoy sex.
- You feel a burning sensation during urination.
- You have severe pain deep within your pelvis.

FLOWER REMEDY/ESSENCE THERAPY

Pain during intercourse can signal emotional as well as physical problems, says Cynthia Mervis Watson, M.D., a family practice physician in Santa Monica, California, who specializes in homeopathy and herbal therapy. "Women who experience pain may be ashamed of their bodies or may feel that sex is dirty and contaminated," she explains. Men and women suffering from poor body images may benefit from the Bach flower remedy Crab Apple, according to Dr. Watson, while the California essence Easter Lily can help men and women with negative feelings about sex.

Flower remedies/essences are available in some health food stores and through mail order (refer to the resource list on page 635). For information on preparing and administering flower remedies/essences, see page 37.

IRRITABILITY

S ometimes life just piles up on you. Nothing's falling your way, nobody's giving you a break, your patience is completely shot, and Groucho Marx himself couldn't make you crack a smile.

Call it what you want. Cranky. Moody. Irritable. But when you're feeling this way, three words pretty much sum up how you feel: *Leave . . . me . . . alone.* The natural remedies in this chapter, used with your doctor's approval, may help prevent or relieve irritability, according to some health professionals.

SEE YOUR MEDICAL DOCTOR WHEN . . .

- Your irritability starts affecting your job performance and personal relationships.
- You have frequent or persistent headaches.
- Your irritability lasts for more than a week.
- You feel under constant pressure.

FLOWER REMEDY/ESSENCE THERAPY

For those who are easily annoyed and who quickly lose patience with others, the flower remedy Impatiens can be helpful, says Leslie J. Kaslof, an herbalist and author of *The Traditional Flower Remedies of Dr. Edward Bach.* Those who are irritated by and critical and judgmental of the idiosyncrasies of others can be helped by using the flower remedy Beech, he says.

Flower remedies are available in some health food stores and through mail order (refer to the resource list on page 635). For information on preparing and administering flower remedies, see page 37.

FOOD THERAPY

Fruits and vegetables are rich in complex carbohydrates, which increase serotonin, a brain chemical that produces an overall calming effect, says Julian Whitaker, M.D., founder and president of the Whitaker Wellness Center in Newport Beach, California. While it's always a good idea to eat plenty of produce, "when you're feeling irritable, it's especially important to eat more fruits and vegetables," he says.

HOMEOPATHY

If you demand attention and need to be comforted and your irritability worsens with noise and when you're spoken to, try Chamomile 30C in the morning and evening until symptoms lessen, says Chris Meletis, N.D., a naturopathic physician and medicinary director at the National College of Naturopathic Medicine in Portland, Oregon. Bryonia 30C twice a day may help, according to Dr. Meletis, if you have a tendency toward dry, parched lips and you are worse in the morning and when being touched. Nux vomica 30C in a similar dose can lessen your irritation if you also feel tense, have backaches and indigestion and feel worse when questioned, he says. If you have lots of anger and resentment, with vengeful tendencies, he suggests a similar dose of Staphysagria 30C.

You can find all of these remedies in many health food stores. To purchase the remedies by mail, refer to the resource list on page 637.

HYDROTHERAPY

The neutral bath has a balancing effect on anxious or irritable people, according to Charles Thomas, Ph.D., co-author of *Hydrotherapy: Simple Treatments for Common Ailments* and a physical therapist at Desert Springs Therapy Center in Desert Hot Springs, California. Fill your bathtub with water slightly cooler than body temperature, around 94° to 97°F, according to Dr. Thomas. Submerging as much of your body as possible, he says, stay in the bath for at least 30 minutes, adding water as needed to maintain the temperature of the bath. Dr. Thomas suggests trying this remedy whenever you feel irritable.

IMAGERY

Close your eyes and hear a silent cry from within. Feel this cry going out of you, says Elizabeth Ann Barrett, R.N., Ph.D., professor and coordinator of the Center for Nursing Research at Hunter College of the City University of New York in New York City.

"The idea behind this imagery is that there is an agony or crying inside you that isn't being expressed and that's why you're irritable. This can help you let go of that pain," Dr. Barrett says. She suggests doing this imagery once a day in the morning as needed. It might take practice, she says, so if you don't feel the cry the first time, try again the next day.

As an alternative, imagine that your nerves are a series of stretched rubber bands throughout your body. One by one, release the rubber bands. Envision yourself relaxing more and more as each rubber band is released, says Dr. Barrett. She recommends that you do this imagery twice a day, once in the morning and once in the evening, and let it continue until you feel relaxed. If needed, she adds, you can repeat this imagery at any time during the day.

RELAXATION AND MEDITATION

Meditation may help soothe irritability, says Sundar Ramaswami, Ph.D., a clinical psychologist at the F. S. Dubois Community Mental Health Center in Stamford, Connecticut. Meditation helps you become more aware of physical cues, such as increased muscle tension, that occur as you become irritable, according to Dr. Ramaswami. He says that learning to control those physical responses is the key to alleviating irritability.

To experiment with meditation, try the simple technique on page 117. Begin meditating for 20 minutes twice a day, suggests Dr. Ramaswami. As you become more proficient and more aware of your body's sensations and needs, he says, you may find you can meditate less and still get the same effect.

SOUND THERAPY

Think and hear green when you're feeling mean, says color-music therapist Mary Bassano in her book *Healing with Music and Color*. Bassano suggests taking a few minutes to imagine yourself swimming in a bubble of green light. While you do this, listen to one of these pieces of classical music, which Bassano says will help you calm down: *Melody in F* by Arthur Rubinstein, *Clair de Lune* by Claude Debussy or *Violin Concerto in E Minor* by Felix Mendelssohn. Or try these New Age recordings: *Fairy Ring* by Mike Rowland or *Pan Flute* by Za Mir. You should be able to find these recordings in music stores.

VITAMIN AND MINERAL THERAPY

A daily dose of an amino acid called gamma-aminobutyric acid, or GABA, can increase levels of the brain chemical serotonin, which has a calming effect and can help ease irritability, says Julian Whitaker, M.D., founder and director of the Whitaker Wellness Center in Newport Beach, California. You can buy GABA in supplement form in most health food stores. Follow the manufacturer's suggested dosage on the label.

YOGA

Take a rest break during the day, says Alice Christensen, founder and executive director of the American Yoga Association. She suggests scheduling a 10- to 15-minute break right on your calendar, then spending that time meditating. This will slow you down a little, she says, and help you deal with one of the root causes of irritability: the feeling that you can't produce fast enough to satisfy yourself. For more information about meditation, see page 153.

SEE ALSO Anger; Type A Personality

IRRITABLE BOWEL SYNDROME

Once, just once, you'd like your digestive system to work the way it's supposed to. But nothing's ever easy. Either you're constipated or you have diarrhea. You have terrible gas. And your stomach starts to ache after almost every meal.

If your doctor has ruled out other possible causes, you could have irritable bowel syndrome (IBS). Sometimes called spastic or nervous colon, it's the most common disorder among people with gastrointestinal problems. People with IBS have a difficult time staying regular and often complain of pain somewhere in the digestive system after eating. The good news is that IBS is not dangerous. The natural remedies in this chapter—in conjunction with medical care and used with your doctor's approval—may help prevent or relieve IBS, according to some health professionals.

SEE YOUR MEDICAL DOCTOR WHEN . . .

- Your bowel habits suddenly change.
- Your bowel habits change and you're suffering from abdominal pain or vomiting.

• Your pain is more severe than any you've had before.
• You have severe pain and a fever or bloody stool.
• You are losing weight without being on a diet.

AYURVEDA

Triphala, a gentle but powerful internal cleanser made from the Indian fruits amalaki, haritaki and bibhitaki, is the main Ayurvedic treatment for digestive and eliminative problems, says David Frawley, O.M.D., director of the American Institute of Vedic Studies in Santa Fe, New Mexico. Some health food stores sell triphala capsules or tablets; you can also purchase them in Indian pharmacies or by mail order (refer to the resource list on page 634). Dr. Frawley says to take one gram two times a day or to follow the directions on the label.

"It is a mild laxative, without side effects," says Dr. Frawley. "People who take triphala don't develop a laxative dependency. In fact, triphala helps restore the tone of the large intestine."

FLOWER REMEDY/ESSENCE THERAPY

People with IBS or colitis often have trouble expressing certain emotions, particularly anger, according to Eve Campanelli, Ph.D., a holistic family practitioner in Beverly Hills, California. Dr. Campanelli recommends a blend of three remedies: Cerato, to combat self-doubt, Gorse, for hopelessness, and Vervain, to quell anger.

Flower remedies are available in some health food stores and through mail order (refer to the resource list on page 635). For information on preparing and administering flower remedies, see page 37.

FOOD THERAPY

"Be nice to your colon, and your colon will be nice to you," says Michael A. Klaper, M.D., a nutritional medicine specialist in Pompano Beach, Florida, and director of the Institute of Nutritional Education and Research, an organization based in Manhattan Beach, California, that teaches doctors about nutrition and its relationship to disease.

"If you eat a lot of cooked protein, hydrogenated oils, concentrated sugars or other foods that are hard to digest, your colon can react—and not nicely," says Dr. Klaper. He advises that those with IBS avoid meats, dairy products, greasy snack foods, spicy fare and sweets. At the first sign of a flare-up and during the time the colon is inflamed, build your meals around easy-to-digest foods such as rice, sweet potatoes, well-steamed green and yellow vegetables and bananas, he suggests. Then after the bowel inflammation subsides, he says, you can start adding new foods to your daily diet, one at a time every 48 hours. This way, he explains, you can watch for any ill effects of the new foods.

HERBAL THERAPY

Peppermint is what herbalists call an antispasmodic, and it may help alleviate the bowel spasms that are often part of IBS, says Barre, Vermont, herbalist Rosemary Gladstar, author of *Herbal Healing for Women* and other books about herbs. She recommends peppermint oil, available in most health food stores. She says to take two or three drops of the oil, diluted in ¼ cup of warm water, three or four times a day.

RELAXATION AND MEDITATION

Progressive relaxation may reduce anxiety and help subdue the symptoms of IBS, says Edward B. Blanchard, Ph.D., a clinical psychologist at the Center for Stress and Anxiety Disorders at the State University of New York at Albany. In a small study of 16 people with IBS, for instance, Dr. Blanchard and his colleagues found that those who practiced progressive relaxation daily for a month were five times more likely to report improvement in their conditions than people who merely kept records of their symptoms. To try progressive relaxation, see page 122. Dr. Blanchard suggests practicing progressive relaxation for 15 to 20 minutes once each day for eight weeks. Then when the relaxation comes easily, use it whenever you feel stressed or anxious, he says.

VITAMIN AND MINERAL THERAPY

Use the food sensitivity diet (see "Food Sensitivity: How to Discover the 'Healthy' Foods That Can Cause Disease" on page 52) to eliminate any foods that might aggravate IBS, suggests David Edelberg, M.D., an internist and medical director of the American Holistic Center/Chicago. He also says to eliminate sugar and caffeine, which can contribute to episodes of irritable bowel. And he says that people with IBS may want to take 500 milligrams of glutamine three times a day and one peppermint oil capsule three to six times a day to help control the condition. These supplements are available in most health food stores; glutamine can also be purchased in most pharmacies.

YOGA

Stress often causes flare-ups of irritable bowel, says Stephen A. Nezezon, M.D., yoga teacher and staff physician at the Himalayan International Institute of Yoga Science and Philosophy in Honesdale, Pennsylvania. To lower stress, he suggests trying a daily routine of breathing exercises, meditation and poses.

Do the complete breath exercise (see page 152) whenever you're feeling stress, whether it's at the office, in the car or at home, suggests Alice Christensen, founder and executive director of the American Yoga Association. Daily meditation (see page 153) helps clear your mind and teaches you to relax at will, she says. And for the poses, choose three or four from the Daily Routine, which begins on page 606. Be sure to vary the poses from day to day to keep your interest high and to strengthen different parts of your body, according to Christensen. Dr. Nezezon says you should include at least one relaxation pose, such as the corpse (page 612), knee squeeze (page 612) or baby (page 618), in your daily yoga routine.

JEALOUSY

Everyone feels the pinch of jealousy now and again. Like when you think your boss is giving special treatment to the guy at the next desk. Or when your old flame shows up at the company Christmas party on the arm of some hard-bodied hunk from corporate sales.

While it's often harmless, jealousy can definitely get out of hand. Movies such as *Fatal Attraction* may be a bit overdramatic, but it's true that jealousy can harm relationships. The natural remedies in this chapter, used with the approval of your doctor, may help you deal more effectively with jealousy, according to some health professionals.

SEE YOUR MEDICAL DOCTOR WHEN . . .

- You notice that your attention is consumed by jealous thoughts to the point that your work and home life are suffering.
- You lose your ability to eat, sleep and concentrate.
- You find yourself unable to talk about your feelings.

FLOWER REMEDY/ ESSENCE THERAPY

"Holly is a great help to anyone suffering from jealousy or envy," says Eve Campanelli, Ph.D., a holistic family practitioner in Beverly Hills, California. She says it also helps even out other negative emotional states such as distrust and vengefulness.

Flower remedies are available in some health food stores and through mail order (refer to the resource list on page 635). For information on preparing and administering flower remedies, see page 37.

IMAGERY

Picture a box outside of yourself. Make it a good-size box, from material such as wood, metal or plastic, that will be big and strong enough to hold your emotions. Decorate it, if you wish. Now whenever jealousy arises within you, imagine that you throw that emotion into the box, says Dennis Gersten, M.D., a San Diego psychiatrist and publisher of *Atlantis*, a bi-monthly imagery newsletter. He suggests doing this imagery for 15 to 30 seconds whenever jealousy arises.

YOGA

Since yoga enhances your sense of ease and overall health, it can help turn aside feelings of jealousy, says Stephen A. Nezezon, M.D., yoga teacher and staff physician at the Himalayan International Institute of Yoga Science and Philosophy in Honesdale, Pennsylvania. He recommends a daily yoga routine of deep breathing (see page 152), meditation (see page 153) and three or four yoga poses (choose from the Daily Routine, which begins on page 606). Many yoga experts suggest varying the poses in your routine from day to day to keep your interest high and to strengthen different parts of your body.

JET LAG

Your plane has just landed in San Francisco, but your brain seems to have missed the connecting flight in Houston. And your body feels like it's spinning on a luggage carousel in Oklahoma City.

Jet lag will do that to you. Humans were not designed to travel such long distances in such short times. Flying long distances can mess up your body's circadian rhythms, which tell you when to sleep and when to wake up. Your body will figure things out by itself in a day or so, though you'll feel pretty sluggish until then. The natural remedies in this chapter, used with the approval of your doctor, may help prevent or relieve jet lag, according to some health professionals.

JET LAG

AROMATHERAPY

"Essential oils are so great for jet lag that some airlines have started giving aromatherapy kits to their first-class passengers," says Victoria Edwards, an aromatherapist in Fair Oaks, California. But there's a cheaper way to beat jet lag, according to Edwards: Travel coach and pick up the essential oils lavender, geranium and rosemary on your way to the airport.

While flying, Edwards says, put a drop or two of lavender on a wet washcloth and wipe your forehead and temples. "This eases flying jitters and gets rid of that keyed-up feeling," she explains. Once you're off the plane and settled in, banish exhaustion with a soothing bath. Edwards recommends adding 10 to 15 drops of geranium oil as the water is running. "Geranium is an adrenal stimulant and will help you get your second wind," she says. Finally, banish drowsiness by inhaling an invigorating scent such as rosemary. "Put a single drop on a tissue and inhale whenever you need an energy boost," Edwards suggests.

For information on preparing and administering essential oils, including cautions about their use, see page 19. For information on purchasing essential oils, refer to the resource list on page 633.

AYURVEDA

For jet lag, take one ginger capsule an hour before your flight takes off, says Vasant Lad, B.A.M.S., M.A.Sc., director of the Ayurvedic Institute in Albuquerque, New Mexico. You can take another capsule between flights, he says. Ginger capsules are available in most health food stores.

HOMEOPATHY

"One remedy for jet lag that people can try is Cocculus," says Stephen Messer, N.D., dean of the National Center for Homeopathy's summer school and a naturopathic physician in Eugene, Oregon. He suggests a 6C dose five to ten minutes before you board the airplane. Then after you arrive at your destination, continue taking it up to twice daily for two to three days to help you adjust to the new time zone, he says.

Cocculus is available in many health food stores. To purchase the remedy by mail, refer to the resource list on page 637.

HYDROTHERAPY

Drink plenty of water during the trip to prevent dehydration, which contributes to jet lag, says Agatha Thrash, M.D., a medical pathologist and co-founder and co-director of Uchee Pines Institute, a natural healing center in Seale, Alabama. She suggests drinking one eight-ounce glass of water for each hour you spend in the air.

RELAXATION AND MEDITATION

Deep breathing techniques are very helpful in fighting off jet lag, says Martin Shaffer, Ph.D., executive director of the Stress Management Institute in San Francisco and author of *Life after Stress*. During the first two days after your arrival, practice the slow, deep breathing technique described on page 116 for 15 minutes every four hours, he says.

YOGA

A session of deep breathing (page 152) and meditation (page 153) will help you overcome jet lag's effects, even while you're still on the plane, say Dr. Robin Monro, Dr. R. Nagarathna and Dr. H. R. Nagendra in their book *Yoga for Common Ailments*.

JOCK ITCH

Spend enough time at the gym, and you'll get the rippling biceps you've always dreamed about. But spend enough time in the locker room afterward, and you may also get a nightmare case of jock itch.

What puts the itch in jock itch? The same thing that puts the . . . uh, foot in athlete's foot: a fungus called trichophyton. This fungus loves warm, moist places such as a locker room—and your groin area. The fungus often spreads through towels that have not been properly cleaned. So consider packing your own towel instead of using the freebies at the gym. The natural remedy in this chapter, used with you doctor's approval, may help relieve jock itch, according to one health professional.

JOINT PAIN

SEE YOUR MEDICAL DOCTOR WHEN . . .

- Your itching has lasted for more than a week without relief.
- Your itching is accompanied by or causes severe redness, sores or oozing.
- Your itching precedes formation of a blister or sore.
- Your genitals are maddeningly itchy and the sensation seems to have spread to other parts of your body.

FOOD THERAPY

Garlic may help bring quicker relief because of its antifungal qualities, says Julian Whitaker, M.D., founder and president of the Whitaker Wellness Center in Newport Beach, California. "I'd advise eating as much raw garlic as possible at the first sign of jock itch. It's also a good idea to avoid yeast products such as breads, baked goods and alcohol, which may make some people more prone to getting jock itch."

But eating raw garlic can cause gastrointestinal upset, says registered pharmacist Earl Mindell, R.Ph., Ph.D., professor of nutrition at Pacific Western University in Los Angeles and author of *Earl Mindell's Food as Medicine* and other books on nutrition. If you find you have trouble tolerating raw garlic, Dr. Mindell suggests trying garlic supplements instead. Take one capsule with every meal, he says; they're available in most health food stores and in many drugstores.

JOINT PAIN

Yesterday you were Limber Larry, flexible as a willow tree. You weeded the garden, played hopscotch with the kids, then dashed off to the local alley for a few frames of bowling.

And this morning you're Rigid Roger, stiff as a two-by-four. Your ankles are aching, your knees are gnarly, and your shoulders are singing the blues. How can such simple activities cause such pain?

In a word, misuse. If you know that you don't have arthritis, bursitis or tendinitis, then maybe you're just asking too much of your joints. Perhaps you're not stretching enough before exercising. Over the long run, this kind of stress can cause inflammation and can break down cartilage, the natural shock absorbers in all of your joints. The natural remedies in this chapter—in conjunction with medical care and used with the approval of your doctor—may help relieve joint pain, according to some health professionals.

JOINT PAIN

ACUPRESSURE

For joint pain anywhere in the body, press both St 36 points, situated four finger-widths below each kneecap, in the indentation at the front of the shin-bone, says Michael Reed Gach, Ph.D., director of the Acupressure Institute in Berkeley, California, and author of *Acupressure's Potent Points*. He suggests holding these points for one minute three times daily. Pressing these points tones all of the muscles in the body, according to Dr. Gach, making it espe-cially helpful for relieving joint pain.

For joint pain and stiffness in your ankle, Dr. Gach says to press both GB 40 points, situated in the large hollow directly in front of each anklebone. Stimu-late these points for three to five minutes three times daily, he says.

The following pain-relieving points should be held for one minute three times daily any time you feel pain in the area indicated, according to Dr. Gach.

For knee joint pain, Dr. Gach recommends both Sp 9 points, located on the inside of each leg, just under the knee and below the head of the shinbone.

For wrist pain, press points P 7, located on the inside of each arm in the middle of the wrist crease, and TW 4, on the outside of each arm in the hollow at the center of the wrist crease, says Dr. Gach. These points can be stimulated simultaneously. So if you are experiencing pain in your left wrist, for example, Dr. Gach says to press the TW 4 point on your left wrist with your right thumb while stimulating the P 7 point on your left wrist with the fingers of your right hand. Then switch and apply pressure to the same points on your right wrist.

For shoulder pain, Dr. Gach says, hook your fingers into both TW 15 points, situated over the tops of your shoulders, midway between the base of the neck and the outer edges of the shoulders. Feel for the spots of greatest tension and press there, he explains. He also suggests using tennis balls to put pressure on these points. His instructions: Lie down with your knees bent. If you wish, put a pillow under your head for comfort. Reach behind your back and position the tennis balls on the points. Then cross your arms over your chest and breathe deeply.

For help in locating any of these acupressure points, refer to the illustrations beginning on page 564.

JOINT PAIN

FOOD THERAPY

Try the detoxification diet (see "Detoxing Your Ills" on page 48) to help correct the nutritional imbalance that could be triggering joint pain, suggests Elson Haas, M.D., director of the Preventive Medical Center of Marin in San Rafael, California, and author of *Staying Healthy with Nutrition*.

Or try eating vegetarian, says Neal Barnard, M.D., president of the Physicians Committee for Responsible Medicine in Washington, D.C., and author of *Food for Life* and other books on the healing aspects of food. Animal proteins have been found to trigger the joint pain associated with arthritis and other inflammatory diseases, he says.

HYDROTHERAPY

Simple hot or cold water treatments are easy ways to soothe joint pain, says John Abruzzo, M.D., professor of medicine and director of the Rheumatology and Osteoporosis Center at Thomas Jefferson University Hospital in Philadelphia. To relieve stiffness and dull, penetrating pain, he recommends a warm (not hot) compress applied directly to the affected area. For sharper, more intense pain, he says to try a cold compress or an ice pack wrapped in a plastic bag and placed over a towel on the skin. Hold in place for 10 to 20 minutes, he suggests, and repeat every four hours as needed. Don't apply a cold treatment for more than 20 minutes at a time, or you'll risk damaging your skin, he adds.

MASSAGE

Gently rub the muscles directly above and below the sore joint, says Vincent Iuppo, N.D., massage therapist, naturopathic physician and director of the Morris Institute of Natural Therapeutics, a holistic health education center in Denville, New Jersey. Use the friction technique (page 570) to massage for about ten minutes, and repeat daily until the pain has subsided. Do not rub directly on the affected joint.

REFLEXOLOGY

To help relieve pain in a joint, work the corresponding reflex points on your hands or feet, says St. Petersburg, Florida, reflexologist Dwight Byers, author of *Better Health with Foot Reflexology*. If you have knee pain, for example, he says to pay special attention to the knee reflex points.

To help you locate these points, consult the hand and foot reflex charts beginning on page 582. For instructions on how to work the points, see "Your Reflexology Session" on page 110.

KIDNEY STONES

VITAMIN AND MINERAL THERAPY

People with joint pain may get relief from the following daily nutrient intakes, says Richard Gerson, Ph.D., author of *The Right Vitamins*: 5,000 milligrams of vitamin C, 800 to 1,400 milligrams of calcium and a B-complex supplement containing the six important B vitamins (thiamin, riboflavin, niacin, vitamin B_6, vitamin B_{12} and pantothenic acid). He explains that vitamin C helps promote healing, calcium builds stronger bones and the B vitamins balance the nervous system, reducing pain.

SEE ALSO Arthritis; Gout

KIDNEY STONES

L et's take a minute to smash a couple of myths about kidney stones. For starters, they're not really stones at all. They're usually small, rough hunks of calcium that crystallize in your urine.

Second, kidney stones probably aren't caused by a diet too high in dairy products. Even though the stones are made from calcium, research shows that a diet high in calcium actually decreases your risk of forming them.

But one common belief about kidney stones is true: They can hurt like crazy. If a stone gets lodged in your urinary tract, you may feel extreme pain in your groin, lower back, inner thighs or genitals. If this happens, see your doctor immediately. Stubborn stones sometimes have to be surgically removed. The natural remedies in this chapter—in conjunction with medical care and used with your doctor's approval—may help prevent the recurrence of kidney stones, according to some health professionals.

SEE YOUR MEDICAL DOCTOR WHEN . . .

- You see blood in your urine.
- You experience sharp pain in your groin, lower back or testicles.

FOOD THERAPY

"Magnesium has been shown to prevent all types of kidney stones, so I'd recommend eating more foods rich in this mineral," says Julian Whitaker,

M.D., founder and president of the Whitaker Wellness Center in Newport Beach, California. "They include pumpkin seeds, tofu, wheat germ, seafood and dark green leafy vegetables such as spinach." (For other food sources of magnesium, see "Getting What You Need" on page 142.)

But the most important dietary therapy is to drink a lot of water, according to Dr. Whitaker. He says people who are prone to stones or who are recovering from them need at least ten eight-ounce glasses of water each day. Water helps decrease the concentration of stone-forming elements in the urine, he explains.

JUICE THERAPY

For those prone to kidney stones, cranberry is the juice of choice, says naturopathic physician Michael Murray, N.D., author of *The Complete Book of Juicing*. He explains that high levels of urinary calcium have been linked to kidney stones and that cranberry juice reduces the amount of calcium in your urine. He recommends two eight-ounce glasses daily as a preventive. Of course, if you develop kidney stones, see your physician immediately, he says.

For information on juicing techniques, see page 93.

REFLEXOLOGY

Work the kidney, bladder, diaphragm and parathyroid gland reflexes on the hands or feet, says St. Petersburg, Florida, reflexologist Dwight Byers, author of *Better Health with Foot Reflexology*. Also work the ureter points on your feet. To help you locate these points, consult the hand and foot reflex charts beginning on page 582. For instructions on how to work the points, see "Your Reflexology Session" on page 110.

VITAMIN AND MINERAL THERAPY

If you're prone to developing kidney stones, supplement your diet with 800 milligrams of magnesium and 100 milligrams of vitamin B6 each day, advises Julian Whitaker, M.D., founder and president of the Whitaker Wellness Center in Newport Beach, California. He says that these two nutrients have been found to prevent stones from recurring.

LACTOSE INTOLERANCE

You know it's good for you. So why does it make you feel so lousy? If drinking milk brings you hours of cramping, bloating and flatulence, you're probably suffering from lactose intolerance.

The intestinal fireworks are caused by a shortage of lactase, an enzyme produced in the intestinal walls that's necessary for breaking down lactose. While infants produce enough lactase to digest milk, those with inherited tendencies toward lactose intolerance begin to lose this ability in early childhood.

While lactose intolerance isn't dangerous, it can make it difficult to get enough calcium in your diet. Many adults who can't drink milk can digest cheeses and yogurt with no problem. Others find they can build up a tolerance by gradually increasing their intakes of dairy foods. The natural remedy in this chapter—in conjunction with medical care and used with your doctor's approval—may help relieve the symptoms of lactose intolerance, according to some health professionals.

SEE YOUR MEDICAL DOCTOR WHEN . . .

- Your flatulence is accompanied by stomach or abdominal pain for more than three days.
- You have severe abdominal cramping or severe diarrhea.

FOOD THERAPY

Some people find their symptoms disappear if they take their dairy products with meals, says Theodore M. Bayless, M.D., professor of medicine at Johns Hopkins Hospital in Baltimore. That's because one of the key factors in lactose intolerance is the rate at which the stomach empties. "If you can slow the stomach's emptying, you can reduce or prevent symptoms," adds Dennis Savaiano, Ph.D., a nutritionist and associate dean at the University of Minnesota College of Human Ecology in St. Paul. "And having a complete meal slows the rate at which your stomach empties." However, it's not advisable to load up on several dairy products at one meal.

You might also want to try fermented dairy products such as yogurt, buttermilk and hard cheeses. These foods don't carry the punch of regular milk for the lactose-intolerant. For instance, the organisms that make yogurt what it is also produce lactase to digest the lactose—which is why most lactose-intolerant people can eat yogurt with no problem, says Naresh Jain, M.D., a gastroen-terologist in Niagara Falls, New York.

But one cautionary note: Frozen yogurt will produce the same reaction as ice cream or ice milk. That's because once yogurt is frozen, it loses its "helpful" bacteria.

Buttermilk is also "pretty tolerable," adds Dr. Jain (and despite its name, it usually has less fat and cholesterol than 2 percent milk). And calcium-rich hard cheeses have less lactose than milk. "Swiss and extra-sharp Cheddar contain only trace amounts of lactose and are thus less likely to produce digestive upset," says Seymour Sabesin, M.D., a gastroenterologist and director of the Section of Digestive Diseases at Rush–St. Luke's–Presbyterian Medical Center in Chicago.

And some research suggests that cocoa may reduce symptoms of lactose in-tolerance—one reason why many lactose-intolerant people get no severe reac-tions when drinking chocolate milk. "I suspect that the cocoa helps slow stomach emptying, which reduces the rate at which lactose reaches the colon," says Dr. Savaiano. "If you must have milk, one of the easiest things to do is to make it chocolate milk." But use powdered cocoa, which has no fat, instead of chocolate syrup, which is high in fat.

SEE ALSO Allergies; Food Allergies

LARYNGITIS

Whether you got caught up in the excitement of rooting for your team or spent hours catching up with an old friend, there's a price to be paid for pushing your voice to the limit. An evening of aban-doned shouting, singing or even talking can leave your throat and larynx (also known as the voice box) sore and inflamed. You may wake up to find your voice has gone on strike, and no eleventh-hour concessions will get your sound system back on the job.

While laryngitis can also be caused by upper respiratory infections, flu, aller-gies and environmental irritants such as dust and smoke, in many cases it's an overuse injury. The natural remedies in this chapter, used with the approval of your doctor, may help relieve the symptoms of laryngitis, according to some health professionals.

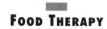

SEE YOUR MEDICAL DOCTOR WHEN . . .

- Your voice disappears all of a sudden, for no apparent reason.
- You lose your voice after a head or neck injury.
- You experience hoarseness for more than two weeks.

FOOD THERAPY

"Put some lemon juice and honey in a tablespoon with a pinch of cayenne pepper and suck on it," advises Elson Haas, M.D., director of the Preventive Medical Center of Marin in San Rafael, California, and author of *Staying Healthy with Nutrition*. He says the mixture helps coat your larynx, which can relieve laryngitis. There are no hard-and-fast rules about frequency: "Just as often as you deem necessary," suggests Dr. Haas.

HOMEOPATHY

If you suddenly develop laryngitis along with a bright red, dry throat but you don't want water or other fluids, try a 30C dose of Belladonna every two hours, says Chris Meletis, N.D., a naturopathic physician and medicinary director at the National College of Naturopathic Medicine in Portland, Oregon. If your condition persists for more than two days, or if you notice white spots on the back of your throat, see your medical doctor or homeopath.

Belladonna is available in many health food stores. To purchase homeopathic remedies by mail, refer to the resource list on page 637.

HYDROTHERAPY

Try steam inhalation (see "Hydrotherapy at Home" on page 78) and heating compresses to speed the healing of laryngitis, suggests Charles Thomas, Ph.D., co-author of *Hydrotherapy: Simple Treatments for Common Ailments* and a physical therapist at Desert Springs Therapy Center in Desert Hot Springs, California. To make a compress, you'll need a piece of old sheet that's long and wide enough to wrap around your throat and a same-size piece of wool flannel. Wring out the sheet in cold water and wrap it once around your throat; cover it with the dry flannel and secure it with a safety pin. As your body heat warms and dries the compress, circulation will increase.

Dr. Thomas suggests repeating the steam inhalation for five to ten minutes of every hour over the course of a day. By evening, he says, you should feel better. Change the compresses every six to eight hours, keeping the rest of your body warm with sweaters or blankets, until you're healed, he adds.

REFLEXOLOGY

Pay special attention to the throat, chest, lung, diaphragm and lymphatic system reflex points on both of your feet, says St. Petersburg, Florida, reflexologist Dwight Byers, author of *Better Health with Foot Reflexology*. He also suggests thoroughly working all of the points on the sides and bottoms of your toes, using whichever technique you find most comfortable.

To help you locate these points, consult the foot reflex chart on page 592. For instructions on how to work the points, see "Your Reflexology Session" on page 110.

VITAMIN AND MINERAL THERAPY

"People with laryngitis can get relief by sucking on zinc lozenges and taking up to 5,000 international units of vitamin A and 5,000 milligrams of vitamin C each day," says Elson Haas, M.D., director of the Preventive Medical Center of Marin in San Rafael, California, and author of *Staying Healthy with Nutrition*. He advises continuing these levels of supplementation until your symptoms clear up and never exceeding 100 milligrams of zinc each day.

SEE ALSO Sore Throat

LEG CRAMPS

If there's a more brutal way to wake up than a Monday morning alarm clock, this is it: a knot of pain grabbing your calf with the white-knuckle intensity of a clenched fist.

Nighttime cramps, known as recumbency cramps, usually occur during light sleep and are caused by spasmlike muscular contractions. Other leg cramps occur after exercise, especially if you're dehydrated, overheated or overtired.

Leg cramps usually aren't serious, but in rare cases, they can be symptoms of intermittent claudication, a form of atherosclerosis that causes inadequate blood supply to the legs. Minor cramps can often be prevented by drinking enough water and stretching before and after exercise. The remedies in this chapter—in conjunction with medical care and used with the approval of your doctor—may help prevent and relieve leg cramps, according to some health professionals.

SEE YOUR MEDICAL DOCTOR WHEN . . .

- You have frequent severe leg cramps that interfere with sleep.
- You have frequent leg cramps during or after exercise.

ACUPRESSURE

For a cramp in the calf, press point B 57, suggests Michael Reed Gach, Ph.D., director of the Acupressure Institute in Berkeley, California. Point B 57 is situated at the bottom of the calf muscle bulge—on the back of your leg in the center of the base of the calf muscle, midway between the crease behind the knee and the heel. (For help in locating the point, refer to the illustration on page 565.) Hold for one minute, says Dr. Gach.

AROMATHERAPY

"Lavender is the Swiss army knife of aromatic oils," says Los Angeles aromatic consultant John Steele. He packs the versatile oil on long road trips to treat "driver's leg," that painful cramp in the calf that comes from hours of braking and accelerating. To use, he suggests massaging four or five drops directly on the affected area. "It works every time," says Steele. Tarragon and chamomile essential oils are also effective for leg cramps, he says.

For information on preparing and administering essential oils, including cautions about their use, see page 19. For information on purchasing essential oils, refer to the resource list on page 633.

FOOD THERAPY

"Frequent leg cramps are often a sign of an electrolyte imbalance. I believe that part of the answer is to increase your intake of calcium and magnesium," says Michael A. Klaper, M.D., a nutritional medicine specialist in Pompano Beach, Florida, and director of the Institute of Nutritional Education and Research, an organization based in Manhattan Beach, California, that teaches doctors about nutrition and its relationship to disease. That means eating your vegetables, particularly dark green leafy ones such as broccoli and kale, which are good sources of both calcium and magnesium, and drinking calcium-fortified orange juice.

Other health professionals say that besides vegetables, good food sources of calcium include low-fat dairy products and sardines with bones. Good sources of magnesium include nuts, beans and whole grains.

Since some cramping may be caused by low potassium levels, eating foods rich in potassium may be the best thing for cramps, says Julian Whitaker, M.D., founder and president of the Whitaker Wellness Center in Newport Beach, California. The Daily Value for potassium is 3,500 milligrams. Foods high in it include bananas, orange juice, prune juice, broccoli, baked potatoes with the skin and red snapper.

For other food sources of calcium, magnesium and potassium, see "Getting What You Need" on page 142.

HOMEOPATHY

Gelsemium 6C is the remedy of choice if you have a burning sensation in your legs, feel better with movement and have fatigue after the slightest exercise, says Chris Meletis, N.D., a naturopathic physician and medicinary director at the National College of Naturopathic Medicine in Portland, Oregon. If you have twitching in your legs, with cramps localized in the calves and soles of your feet, Dr. Meletis says to try Cuprum metallicum 6C. He suggests a 6C dose of Veratrum album if the cramps are localized in your calves, you feel relief with massage and the pain is worse when walking, especially if your legs feel cold and look bluish. Take the remedy of choice two or three times a day until the cramps subside, he says.

All of these remedies are available in many health food stores. To purchase the remedies by mail, refer to the resource list on page 637.

MASSAGE

To relieve a cramp in your calf, sit on the floor or your bed and draw the cramped leg toward your chest, bending it at the knee. Now push your thumb gently into your calf, hold it and breathe normally until you feel the cramp relax, says Elaine Stillerman, L.M.T., a massage therapist in New York City.

You may also use the effleurage stroke (page 570) to work the calf for several minutes. Then place your hands on either side of the calf and roll the muscle from left to right, as if you were shaking it. Do this until the pain subsides. Stillerman warns that you shouldn't rub too hard on a cramp, because that may cause it to return.

VITAMIN AND MINERAL THERAPY

To prevent leg cramps that strike very quickly and unexpectedly—the so-called charley horse—take a daily supplement of 400 international units of vitamin E, suggests Charles Kuntzleman, Ed.D., associate professor of kinesiology at the University of Michigan in Ann Arbor. If this doesn't stop them, he says to add daily dosages of up to 1,000 milligrams of magnesium and 500 to 1,000 milligrams of calcium.

LYME DISEASE

YOGA

Yoga compression poses will increase blood circulation to your legs, relieving leg cramps, according to Alice Christensen, founder and executive director of the American Yoga Association. She suggests trying the knee squeeze (page 612), seated sun (page 616) and baby (page 618) whenever you have a cramp. You can also include these poses in your daily yoga routine as a preventive, she adds.

SEE ALSO Muscle Cramps and Pain

LYME DISEASE

Sure, Dorothy had to keep her wits about her in the forest, but at least lions, tigers and bears are beasts you can see. Today's hikers have their eyes peeled for ticks, the tiny carriers of Lyme disease.

Named for Old Lyme, Connecticut, the disease is caused by bacteria carried by ticks that are found mostly in the New England and mid-Atlantic regions as well as in Minnesota and Wisconsin.

Lyme disease is avoided if the tick is discovered and removed within 36 hours; if not, flulike symptoms such as chills, fever, a stiff neck and painful joints appear within a month. Many patients also develop a circular or oblong rash that looks reddish on light skin and resembles a bruise on dark skin.

When treated in its early stages, Lyme disease is about 95 percent curable. If you suspect Lyme disease, see your doctor for a diagnosis. The natural remedies in this chapter—in conjunction with medical care and used with the approval of your doctor—may help relieve the symptoms of Lyme disease, according to some health professionals.

SEE YOUR MEDICAL DOCTOR WHEN . . .

- You have a large bull's-eye rash that has a clear center and red circles of inflammation.
- You have flulike symptoms such as headache, fever, swollen glands and general fatigue.

■
FOOD THERAPY

The one-two punch that may help lessen the severity of Lyme disease is garlic and foods rich in vitamin C, says Julian Whitaker, M.D., founder and president of the Whitaker Wellness Center in Newport Beach, California. "Garlic is a generalized antibiotic, which may help you get over Lyme disease more quickly," explains Dr. Whitaker. And citrus fruits, strawberries, peppers and other foods rich in vitamin C can build immunity for quicker relief of the flulike symptoms of Lyme disease, he says. (For more food sources of vitamin C, see "Getting What You Need" on page 142.)

■
HYDROTHERAPY

Water treatments are useful for managing joint pain associated with Lyme disease, says John Abruzzo, M.D., professor of medicine and director of the Rheumatology and Osteoporosis Center at Thomas Jefferson University Hospital in Philadelphia. The best treatment depends on the type of pain. Hot applications relieve dull, penetrating pain, according to Dr. Abruzzo, while sharper, more intense pain responds better to cold.

You can apply a comfortably warm (not hot) compress directly to the affected area, according to Dr. Abruzzo, but an ice pack should be wrapped in a plastic bag and placed over a towel on the skin. He suggests holding the pack in place for 10 to 20 minutes; any longer, and you risk damaging your skin, he says. Repeat the hot or cold treatment every four hours until the pain subsides, he adds.

■
IMAGERY

Envision the Lyme spirochete, a coiled organism that causes the disease, as looking like a deer tick, a tiny, dark brown bug with a round body and eight legs. See it swimming in your bloodstream, says Elizabeth Ann Barrett, R.N., Ph.D., professor and coordinator of the Center for Nursing Research at Hunter College of the City University of New York in New York City. Now see yourself also swimming in your bloodstream, holding a candle. As you approach the Lyme disease spirochete, point the candle at the organism. Watch it shrivel up from the heat and die. Do this until all of the deer tick spirochetes are dead. Feel yourself recovering from the disease. Dr. Barrett suggests that you do this imagery once a day in the morning, taking as long as you need to complete it.

SEE ALSO Bites and Stings

MEMORY PROBLEMS

Maybe you forget appointments or constantly misplace things. Some consider such glitches a sign of old age, but the fact is that people of all ages can experience temporary memory shutdowns.

Experts agree that your memory is like a muscle; the less it is used, the more quickly it atrophies. If you do the same thing day in and day out—what is commonly known as being in a rut—your mind won't get the workout it needs to stay sharp, regardless of your age. The natural remedies in this chapter, used with the approval of your doctor, may help improve your memory, according to some health professionals.

SEE YOUR MEDICAL DOCTOR WHEN . . .

- You routinely have trouble remembering what month or year it is.
- You routinely become confused in familiar places and can't remember where you are.

ACUPRESSURE

Press the EX 2 points, says Michael Reed Gach, Ph.D., director of the Acupressure Institute in Berkeley, California, and author of *Acupressure's Potent Points*. According to Dr. Gach, EX 2, also called the Sun point, is an extra point that is not located directly on any of the meridians. Locate the EX 2 points in the depression of the temples, level with and a half-inch out from your eyebrows. (To help locate these points, refer to the illustration on page 567.) Try sitting in a chair, resting your elbows on a desk or table and pressing the heels of your hands on these points. Close your eyes, relax and breathe deeply as you press for at least one minute, suggests Dr. Gach. Do this several times a week, he says, but once a day is best.

AROMATHERAPY

Try using equal parts rosemary and geranium essential oils in your diffuser to stimulate the memory, suggests San Francisco herbalist Jeanne Rose, chairperson of the National Association for Holistic Aromatherapy and author of *Aromatherapy: Applications and Inhalations*. "Inhaled scents feed directly into the limbic system, the part of the brain that controls memory and learning," explains Rose. "Geranium has antidepressant properties, and rosemary is a general mental stimulant. When you combine them, they have a stronger effect."

For information on preparing and administering essential oils, including cautions about their use, see page 19. For information on purchasing essential oils, refer to the resource list on page 633.

AYURVEDA

Ayurvedic practitioners consider the spice saffron to be a nerve and heart tonic, a blood cleanser and a blood thinner. Because they think it has such broad-ranging effects, they use it to help relieve memory problems caused by circulatory disease.

To take saffron, boil a pinch of the spice along with ½ teaspoon of gotu kola powder in a cup of milk, says Vasant Lad, B.A.M.S., M.A.Sc., director of the Ayurvedic Institute in Albuquerque, New Mexico. (Gotu kola is an herb available in most health food stores.) Let the mixture cool a little, then drink. Dr. Lad suggests drinking this mixture once a day for a month and seeing if your memory improves. And, he says, as long as you don't have lactose intolerance or any other kind of sensitivity to dairy products, you can continue to drink this mixture for as long as you like.

FOOD THERAPY

Go for a low-fat diet, says Michael A. Klaper, M.D., a nutritional medicine specialist in Pompano Beach, Florida, and director of the Institute of Nutritional Education and Research, an organization based in Manhattan Beach, California, that teaches doctors about nutrition and its relationship to disease. "Many times, memory problems are caused by poor blood flow, and eating low-fat can help open up arteries and improve blood flow," Dr. Klaper explains. To reduce the fat in your diet, he suggests reducing or eliminating fatty cuts of beef, lamb and pork and replacing saturated fats such as butter with unsaturated oils such as flaxseed and safflower, which are available in most health food stores.

HERBAL THERAPY

The herb ginkgo may help reverse memory loss caused by poor circulation to the brain, says Varro E. Tyler, Ph.D., professor of pharmacognosy at Purdue University in West Lafayette, Indiana. According to Dr. Tyler, *Ginkgo biloba* is one of the oldest trees on the planet, and for thousands of years, Chinese herbalists have used its leaves—which increase blood flow to the brain and to other parts of the body—to treat cerebral and cardiovascular problems. Dr.

Tyler recommends ginkgo in supplement form, which you can find in most health food stores, and says to follow dosage recommendations on the label. He says you will need to take ginkgo for one to three months before you see any improvement in memory loss.

HOMEOPATHY

Try one of the following 12C remedies twice daily, says Chris Meletis, N.D., a naturopathic physician and medicinary director at the National College of Naturopathic Medicine in Portland, Oregon. If you have memory loss for recent events and general difficulty comprehending, Dr. Meletis says that Baryta carbonica can be helpful. He suggests Lycopodium for loss of memory due to anxiety, associated with a fussy, agitated and worrisome state. Argentum nitricum can help a generally weak memory, he says. And he suggests trying Anacardium if you have impaired memory that seems worse after a hot bath and better after eating.

These remedies can be taken for up to 30 days, according to Dr. Meletis. If your memory doesn't improve in that time, see your medical doctor or homeopath.

All of these remedies are available in many health food stores. To purchase the remedies by mail, refer to the resource list on page 637.

IMAGERY

Imagine taking an oxygen tank into your brain. Spray your brain cells with a blast of oxygen. Now recall something that you'd like to forget, says Elizabeth Ann Barrett, R.N., Ph.D., professor and coordinator of the Center for Nursing Research at Hunter College of the City University of New York in New York City.

As people get older, there may be certain issues or memories they don't want to face or deal with, so they block those out, according to Dr. Barrett. Unfortunately, by doing that, they also suppress a lot of other memories they'd like to keep. So recalling something you'd like to forget may help you rekindle fond memories as well, she explains.

Dr. Barrett recommends using this imagery once a day in the morning. It may take up to ten minutes to complete, she says, but stop after ten minutes if nothing happens. Practice the imagery for 21 days, stop for 7 days, then repeat the cycle, she suggests.

SOUND THERAPY

Listening to music can improve your concentration and help you remember what you've learned, suggests Don G. Campbell, director of the Institute for

Music, Health and Education in Boulder, Colorado, and author of *Music: Physician for Times to Come*. His suggestions: Mozart's C Major Piano Concerto, performed by Elvira Madigan; *December* by George Winston; *Sunsinger* by Paul Winter; *Relax with the Classics*, andante version, from the Lind Institute; and Campbell's *Crystal Meditations* and *Angels* (side 2). Most of these can be found in music stores. For mail-order information, refer to the resource list on page 642.

VITAMIN AND MINERAL THERAPY

Studies show that beta-carotene can help improve some aspects of memory and word fluency and recall, especially in people over age 60, says James G. Penland, Ph.D., a research psychologist at the U.S. Department of Agriculture Human Nutrition Research Center in Grand Forks, North Dakota. Some experts recommend daily supplements of 15 milligrams (25,000 international units).

YOGA

Daily meditation helps with memory, says Stephen A. Nezezon, M.D., yoga teacher and staff physician at the Himalayan International Institute of Yoga Science and Philosophy in Honesdale, Pennsylvania. For instructions on meditation, see page 153.

Dr. Nezezon also suggests this daily concentration exercise (improving concentration is an aspect of traditional yoga practice): Sit quietly in a comfortable position and start silently counting backward from 50. As your concentration improves, you can move the starting count higher, to 100, 200 or even 500. Dr. Nezezon says that this exercise will improve your concentration and help you remember things better.

MENOPAUSE PROBLEMS

I t used to be called the change of life, and for many women, the name is an accurate one. Menopause isn't just the end of a woman's childbearing years, it's the beginning of a new stage.

Most women experience menopause in their forties or fifties. Like puberty and pregnancy, menopause is packed with physical and psychological changes caused by shifts in a woman's hormonal makeup. These changes may cause night sweats, vaginal dryness and hot flashes. Menstruation becomes irregular and finally stops. For some women, this process take as little as six months; others have symptoms for three years or longer. The natural remedies in this chapter—in conjunction with medical care and with your doctor's approval—may help lessen the severity of the symptoms of menopause, according to some health professionals.

SEE YOUR MEDICAL DOCTOR WHEN . . .

- Your hot flashes are so severe or frequent that they result in fatigue, depression or mood swings or interrupt your sleep.
- You are on hormone replacement therapy and your bleeding is not on the cycle your doctor told you to expect.
- You experience bleeding after your menstrual cycle has ceased for six months or longer.

AROMATHERAPY

Clary sage essential oil, used in a home diffuser, may help ease hot flashes, says San Francisco herbalist Jeanne Rose, chairperson of the National Association for Holistic Aromatherapy and author of *Aromatherapy: Applications and Inhalations*. For portable relief, she suggests carrying a handkerchief scented with a drop of clary sage and inhaling whenever you feel a flush coming on. Keep the hankie in a plastic bag, so the smell doesn't dissipate.

For information on preparing and administering essential oils, including cautions about their use, see page 19. For information on purchasing essential oils, refer to the resource list on page 633.

AYURVEDA

For hot flashes, David Frawley, O.M.D., director of the American Institute of Vedic Studies in Santa Fe, New Mexico, recommends swallowing a teaspoon or two of aloe vera gel before meals and before going to bed at night. "It's very cooling to the whole system," he says. Be sure to purchase the aloe vera gel that is intended for internal use; ask your Ayurvedic practitioner or herbalist to recommend a brand that won't have a laxative side effect. It's available in most health food stores.

FLOWER REMEDY/ESSENCE THERAPY

"For most women, the emotional issues surrounding menopause are at least as difficult as the physical symptoms," says Eve Campanelli, Ph.D., a holistic family practitioner in Beverly Hills, California. She recommends the remedy Walnut. "Menopausal women are entering a new phase of their lives, and Walnut helps them achieve emotional balance during the transition," says Dr. Campanelli.

For women prone to hot flashes, Susan Lange, O.M.D., of the Meridian Center for Personal and Environmental Health in Santa Monica, California, suggests the flower essence Aloe Vera. "It has a soothing, cooling effect and can be very helpful for mental and emotional burnout," says Dr. Lange.

Flower remedies/essences are available in some health food stores and through mail order (refer to the resource list on page 635). For information on preparing and administering flower remedies/essences, see page 37.

FOOD THERAPY

Eat a low-fat vegetarian diet, suggests Michael A. Klaper, M.D., a nutritional medicine specialist in Pompano Beach, Florida, and director of the Institute of Nutritional Education and Research, an organization based in Manhattan Beach, California, that teaches doctors about nutrition and its relationship to disease. "Vegan women (vegans eat no animal products, including dairy) tend to breeze through menopause, while those who eat the typical meat-laden, high-fat American diet often have worse problems," he says. "A high-fat diet produces high estrogen levels, and when you go through menopause, there's a big drop in these hormone levels, setting off a tremendous number of hot flashes. But a low-fat vegetarian-based diet seems to keep natural hormone levels steady and less likely to cause problems."

HERBAL THERAPY

Scientific studies conducted in Europe show that the herb black cohosh may be effective at relieving menopausal symptoms, according to Varro E. Tyler, Ph.D., professor of pharmacognosy at Purdue University in West Lafayette, Indiana. In one study, he says, a group of menopausal women had fewer hot flashes and felt less nervous tension after they began taking the herb.

Dr. Tyler says you can find black cohosh in most health food stores, where it's usually sold as an extract. He says to follow the dosage recommendations on the label and, because there are no studies of the herb's effects when it's taken for years at a time, to not take the herb continuously for more than six months. Instead, he suggests taking it for six months, stopping for about a month and then resuming treatment again, staying on this regimen for as long as your menopausal symptoms persist.

Homeopathy

In his book *The Family Guide to Homeopathy*, Andrew Lockie, M.D., suggests taking one of the following 30C remedies every 12 hours for up to seven days to cope with menopause.

If you feel unusually talkative and dizzy and have a headache when you wake, a tight feeling around your belly, hot flashes and an usually heavy menstrual flow, Dr. Lockie says to try Lachesis. He suggests Sepia if you feel irritable, chilly and tearful and have a backache, periods of sweating, hot flashes and an usually heavy menstrual flow. Amyl nitrosum is a good remedy for hot flashes that develop suddenly, he says.

Pulsatilla is the remedy of choice if you have hot flashes, hemorrhoids and varicose veins, prefer open air to stuffy rooms and are often weepy and chilled, says Dr. Lockie. He recommends Sulphuric acidum if you feel fatigued and your hot flashes seem worse in the evening or after exercise. To calm hot flashes that are worse at about 3:00 A.M. and are accompanied by loss of appetite, backaches, heart palpitations and nervousness, take Kali carbonicum, he says.

All of these remedies are available in many health food stores. To purchase the remedies by mail, refer to the resource list on page 637.

Hydrotherapy

For minimizing hot flashes, Tori Hudson, N.D., a naturopathic physician and professor at the National College of Naturopathic Medicine in Portland, Oregon, recommends beginning each day with a neutral bath in water just slightly cooler than body temperature. "The neutral bath improves vasodilation, which might help release the heat of a hot flash," says Dr. Hudson. "Some women prevent hot flashes entirely by taking a coolish bath every morning. It's wonderful for easing the tension and anxiety some women experience during menopause." Soak for about 20 minutes, Dr. Hudson suggests, adding water as needed to maintain the temperature of the bath.

A daily perineal wash may reduce vaginal dryness, says Agatha Thrash,

M.D., a medical pathologist and co-founder and co-director of Uchee Pines Institute, a natural healing center in Seale, Alabama. After urinating or having a bowel movement, rinse the area around the vagina with a quart of plain water while you're still sitting on the toilet, suggests Dr. Thrash. Use a squirt bottle or a square container and pour from one corner. Hold the container in one hand and use the other hand to open the folds a bit. Women prone to urinary tract infections or yeast infections should add one to two tablespoons of apple cider vinegar per quart of water, says Dr. Thrash.

JUICE THERAPY

"Hot flashes often flare up when women drink wine or coffee, which acidifies the blood and strains the liver," says Eve Campanelli, Ph.D., a holistic family practitioner in Beverly Hills, California. "One way to avoid this acidification is to cut down on these beverages and to drink more fresh vegetable juices, which counteract the effect by alkalinizing the system." She recommends a liver-stimulating blend of 8 ounces of carrot juice, 1 ounce of beet juice, 4 ounces of celery juice and ½ to 1 ounce of parsley juice. Drinking an eight-ounce glass of this juice blend in the morning and the remainder in the afternoon can prevent or reduce hot flashes, says Dr. Campanelli.

For information on juicing techniques, see page 93.

REFLEXOLOGY

You may help control hot flashes by working the diaphragm, reproductive system and pituitary, thyroid and adrenal gland reflexes on your feet, says St. Petersburg, Florida, reflexologist Dwight Byers, author of *Better Health with Foot Reflexology*.

To help you locate these points, consult the foot reflex chart on page 592. For instructions on how to work the points, see "Your Reflexology Session" on page 110.

RELAXATION AND MEDITATION

Slow, deep breathing may reduce the number and severity of hot flashes by calming the central nervous system, says Robert R. Freedman, Ph.D., professor of psychiatry, obstetrics and gynecology and director of behavioral medicine at Wayne State University School of Medicine in Detroit. Practice deep breathing twice a day for 15 minutes at a time as a preventive measure, or use it as an on-the-spot treatment when you feel a flash coming on, Dr. Freedman says. To learn a deep breathing technique, see page 116.

VITAMIN AND MINERAL THERAPY

You may be able to reduce the severity of menopausal symptoms with the following vitamin and mineral regimen, says Elson Haas, M.D., director of the Preventive Medical Center of Marin in San Rafael, California, and author of *Staying Healthy with Nutrition*: 300 to 500 milligrams of magnesium, 500 to 1,000 milligrams of calcium, 800 international units of vitamin E (400 international units twice a day) and a multivitamin/mineral supplement that contains at least 100 percent of the six important B vitamins (thiamin, riboflavin, niacin, vitamin B_6, vitamin B_{12} and pantothenic acid). "It's also a good idea to take evening primrose oil supplements as well, according to the manufacturer's specifications," he adds. These supplements are available in most health food stores.

MENSTRUAL PROBLEMS

It comes once a month, like the phone bill and the mortgage payment—and for some women, it's about as welcome. For them, the menstrual period can be an endurance contest. While their more fortunate sisters barely notice their periods or get by with the occasional mild cramp, others suffer with headaches, heavy bleeding and cramps severe enough to cause them to miss work or school. Add up all of the days a woman has her period, month after month, year after year, and you'll find that she spends a lot of time menstruating. The natural remedies in this chapter, used with your doctor's approval, may help relieve the symptoms of menstruation, according to some health professionals.

SEE YOUR MEDICAL DOCTOR WHEN . . .

- You are an adult and you experience severe menstrual cramps for the first time or start passing clots for the first time.
- You are on birth control pills and have severe cramps.
- You experience nausea, headaches, diarrhea and vomiting as well as cramps.
- You have severe cramps and very heavy bleeding for more than one day.
- Your cramps interfere with normal activity and aren't relieved by aspirin or ibuprofen.
- You experience heavy bleeding and feel weak and light-headed during your period or you bleed between periods.
- You have a heavy menstrual flow and your periods are more than 45 days apart.

ACUPRESSURE

Retreat to a quiet, comfortable room so you can get the most out of these cramp-relieving acupressure points, says Michael Reed Gach, Ph.D., director of the Acupressure Institute in Berkeley, California, and author of *Acupressure's Potent Points*. He suggests pressing points Sp 12 and Sp 13, which are situated in the pelvic area, in the middle of the crease where the leg joins the trunk of the body. Sp 12 is slightly lower and a little more toward center than Sp 13. (For help in locating these points, refer to the illustration on page 564.) Dr. Gach says you can stimulate all of these points at one time by positioning your left fist over points Sp 12 and Sp 13 on your left side and your right fist over the points on your right side. Lie on your stomach with your fists in place, using the weight of your body to apply gentle pressure. Find a comfortable position and relax for at least two minutes, says Dr. Gach.

AYURVEDA

To ease menstrual problems, take one tablespoon of aloe vera gel with one pinch of black pepper, suggests Vasant Lad, B.A.M.S., M.A.Sc., director of the Ayurvedic Institute in Albuquerque, New Mexico. He says to start taking this mixture after every meal one week before your period begins. You should continue taking it during your period if you have cramps, he adds, one dose every half-hour until your symptoms are relieved.

Aloe vera gel is available in most health food stores. Be sure to purchase the kind that's intended for internal use; ask your Ayurvedic practitioner or herbalist to recommend a brand that won't have a laxative side effect.

FLOWER REMEDY/ESSENCE THERAPY

"In some women, very painful periods are the result of anxiety about their sexuality," says Cynthia Mervis Watson, M.D., a family practice physician in Santa Monica, California, who specializes in homeopathy and herbal therapy. To these women, Dr. Watson recommends the California flower essence Pomegranate.

"Pomegranate balances the female organs and helps women accept their sexuality, which can make a huge difference in their experience of menstruation," says Dr. Watson. This essence is also helpful for women with premenstrual syndrome, she says. These remedies should be taken every day, not just when you're menstruating.

Flower essences are available in some health food stores and through mail order (refer to the resource list on page 635). For information on preparing and administering flower essences, see page 37.

HERBAL THERAPY

Drink cramp bark tea for painful menstrual cramps, says Barre, Vermont, herbalist Rosemary Gladstar, author of *Herbal Healing for Women* and other books about herbs. To make the tea, Gladstar says, place four tablespoons of cramp bark, one tablespoon of pennyroyal and one to two teaspoons of freshly grated ginger in a pot and add a quart of cold water. Slowly bring the water to a simmer. Cover the pot and allow it to simmer for 2 to 3 minutes. Then remove it from the heat, steep for 30 minutes and strain. Drink ¼ cup every 15 minutes until cramping stops, says Gladstar. Cramp bark and pennyroyal are available in most health food stores.

HOMEOPATHY

Occasional menstrual pain can be relieved with a few doses of one of the following homeopathic remedies, according to Maesimund Panos, M.D., a homeopathic physician in Tipp City, Ohio, and co-author with Jane Heimlich of *Homeopathic Medicine at Home*. If you double up with pain or can relieve your cramps by pressing a book or pillow into your belly, Dr. Panos says to try Colocynthis 6X. She suggests Magnesia phosphorica 6X if placing a heating pad or warm water bottle on your belly relieves your pain. If you produce bright red blood during your period and your menstrual pain comes and goes, but when it strikes, it feels as if your uterus were trying to push its way out of your body, give Belladonna 6X a try, she says. If you feel impatient and snappy, she recommends Chamomilla 6X.

Take the remedy of choice every 15 minutes for up to four doses, then wait two hours, says Dr. Panos. If you don't feel any improvement, she advises repeating the doses.

All of these remedies are available in many health food stores. To purchase the remedies by mail, refer to the resource list on page 637.

HYDROTHERAPY

"Hydrotherapy is very effective for relieving menstrual cramps," says Tori Hudson, N.D., a naturopathic physician and professor at the National College of Naturopathic Medicine in Portland, Oregon. "Most cramps are caused by muscle contractions in the pelvic area. A hot pack on the abdomen for 5 to 30 minutes relaxes the muscles and makes you feel better fast."

In some women, cramps are caused by congestion of blood in the pelvis, says Dr. Hudson. In such cases, she recommends applying an ice pack to the lower abdomen for 5 to 30 minutes while sitting in a hot bath. She says this draws blood to the extremities, away from the pelvis, and does a super job of taking away the pain. She advises patients to try both treatments to see which works better for them.

JUICE THERAPY

To ease menstrual cramps, try this blend of apple, celery and fennel juices, suggests naturopathic physician Michael Murray, N.D., in *The Complete Book of Juicing*: Juice two apples, two celery ribs and one small bulb of fennel. According to Dr. Murray, both celery and fennel are rich in phytoestrogens, which mimic the effects of the female hormone estrogen and may reduce menstrual discomfort. He recommends two eight-ounce glasses of this juice every day, along with proper medical treatment.

Women who suffer cramps may also benefit from drinking fresh pineapple juice, according to Cherie Calbom, M.S., a certified nutritionist in Kirkland, Washington, and co-author of *Juicing for Life*. "Pineapples are rich in the enzyme bromelain, which is believed to be a muscle relaxant," says Calbom.

For information on juicing techniques, see page 93.

MASSAGE

The following two massages can help relieve menstrual cramps, according to Elaine Stillerman, L.M.T., a New York City massage therapist. First, lie on your back with your legs bent. Press your palms gently over the pubic area. Then begin to make small circles with your fingertips, going in a clockwise direction over the uterus. Continue for three to five minutes.

Next, lie on your side, with a pillow under your neck and one between your knees. Reach behind your back, and with the palm of your hand, massage the sacrum, the triangle-shaped bone at the base of your spine, in a clockwise direction. Spiral out from the sacrum in a clockwise manner until you have massaged the entire lower back. Continue for five to seven minutes.

REFLEXOLOGY

To help relieve cramps and other menstrual problems, focus on these reflex points on your hands or feet: reproductive system, pancreas, thyroid and pituitary gland, spine and lymphatic system, says Rebecca Dioda, a reflexologist with the Morris Institute of Natural Therapeutics, a holistic health education center in Denville, New Jersey. She says this will help relax key points in your body and ease menstrual symptoms.

To help you locate these points, consult the hand and foot reflex charts beginning on page 582. For instructions on how to work the points, see "Your Reflexology Session" on page 110.

MIGRAINES

It may start as a dull ache that gradually worsens or come on like gang-busters and stay that way for hours or days. About 16 million Americans suffer from migraines, severe headaches often accompanied by nausea and vomiting. A migraine can stop you dead in your tracks and lead you to wonder if your head is a body part you could manage just as well without.

Migraines are caused by a number of different factors, from skipping meals to eating certain foods such as cheeses and chocolate. Alcohol, caffeine and food additives can also trigger migraines. And migraines can be a side effect of certain prescription drugs, including oral contraceptives and some high blood pressure medications. Ask your doctor whether your medication might be to blame. The natural remedies in this chapter—in conjunction with medical care and used with the approval of your doctor—may help prevent migraines or reduce their severity, according to some health professionals.

SEE YOUR MEDICAL DOCTOR WHEN . . .

- You experience fever, convulsions or confusion in addition to a headache.
- Your headache is accompanied by weakness or loss of sensation over half of your body.
- You have a sharp pain in your ear or anywhere on your face or head.
- You have a headache after a severe head injury.

ACUPRESSURE

The Gates of Consciousness points, GB 20, can relieve migraine headaches as well as neck pain, says Michael Reed Gach, Ph.D., director of the Acupressure Institute in Berkeley, California, and author of *Acupressure's Potent Points*. Dr. Gach says to use the thumbs of both hands to press the GB 20 points, which are situated two inches out from the middle of your neck, underneath the base of the skull. (To help locate these points, refer to the illustration on page 565.) He suggests sitting in a chair and bending over, with your elbows propped on a table or desk, to make holding these points most comfortable. Breathe deeply and press firmly for one to two minutes.

AROMATHERAPY

To ease the pain of a migraine, surround yourself with the healing aroma of the essential oil rosemary, says Victoria Edwards, an aromatherapist in Fair

Oaks, California. If you're at home, says Edwards, massage your face and neck with a solution of ten drops of rosemary essential oil per ounce of carrier oil, which is available in most health food stores, and use a few drops of rosemary in a diffuser or an aroma lamp to create a soothing atmosphere. If you're on the road, she suggests applying a drop or two to a tissue and inhaling. "Rosemary, especially rosemary verbenon, also has a balancing effect on the liver and gallbladder, which tend to be sluggish in people who get migraines," says Edwards.

For information on preparing and administering essential oils, including cautions about their use, see page 19. For information on purchasing essential oils, refer to the resource list on page 633.

FLOWER REMEDY/ESSENCE THERAPY

"People prone to migraines often have a hard time dealing with anger," says Eve Campanelli, Ph.D., a holistic family practitioner in Beverly Hills, California. Such people may benefit from the Bach remedy Gentian, which helps balance out the hopelessness and frustration that can lead to migraines.

Flower remedies are available in some health food stores and through mail order (refer to the resource list on page 635). For information on preparing and administering flower remedies, see page 37.

FOOD THERAPY

"A lot of migraines are food-related," says Michael A. Klaper, M.D., a nutritional medicine specialist in Pompano Beach, Florida, and director of the Institute of Nutritional Education and Research, an organization based in Manhattan Beach, California, that teaches doctors about nutrition and its relationship to disease. "In my experience, dairy products are the biggest trigger, followed by poultry, including eggs. Then come chocolate, wheat products and beef. You'll know your trigger by noticing when you get a migraine. If you have a big glass of milk and get a migraine within an hour, it's likely dairy that's causing it."

His solution: "Try to stick with a vegetarian-based diet without food additives such as monosodium glutamate, artificial sweeteners and food colorings. If you get rid of all of the trigger foods, processed foods and synthetic additives, you can often end migraines." Dr. Klaper recommends avoiding red wine, tea, unrefined cider and other beverages that contain tannin, another major trigger. Also, he says, try to eat foods high in magnesium content, such as spinach and other dark green leafy vegetables, whole grains, cashews and soybeans. Magnesium relaxes muscles in the walls of blood vessels, including those running to the brain, which may help prevent migraines, says Dr. Klaper. (For other food sources of magnesium, see "Getting What You Need" on page 142.)

HERBAL THERAPY

Scientific studies show that the herb feverfew can reduce the frequency and severity of migraine headaches, says Varro E. Tyler, Ph.D., professor of pharmacognosy at Purdue University in West Lafayette, Indiana. That's because parthenolide, the plant's active ingredient, inhibits the brain chemicals that dilate blood vessels and cause a migraine, he explains.

Feverfew will work effectively only if you take it every day—not just when you get a migraine—and only if you take enough of it, according to Dr. Tyler. This is because feverfew functions mainly a preventive, so it won't help much once you already have a migraine, he explains. The recommended dosage is a daily supplement of 125 milligrams, he says, and the supplement must contain at least 0.2 percent parthenolide. Check the labels on feverfew products to make sure the product you choose contains parthenolide and follow the dosage recommendations on the label, he adds. Feverfew supplements are available in most health food stores.

HYDROTHERAPY

Contrast showers can sometimes head off a migraine, suggests Agatha Thrash, M.D., a medical pathologist and co-founder and co-director of Uchee Pines Institute, a natural healing center in Seale, Alabama. She suggests a brief hot shower followed by a slightly longer cold shower every morning and any time during the day that you feel a migraine coming on. Place your entire body, including your head, under the hot water until the skin reddens. Switch to cold water and stay under until you start shivering.

When migraines don't respond to any other treatment, a hot enema can provide temporary pain relief, says Dr. Thrash. Enemas work on what is called the gate theory of pain control, she says. "Immediately after an enema, there are so many impulses traveling up to the brain that pain impulses are temporarily crowded out." In many cases, an enema provides relief long enough to help you fall asleep, she says. For instructions, see "How to Perform an Enema" on page 76.

IMAGERY

Imagine there is a control room in your mind that regulates all of your bodily functions. Find the valve that regulates blood flow to your right hand and open up that valve. Feel the sensation of blood rushing out of your head and into your right hand. As the blood travels down your right arm, notice how the pain of your migraine diminishes, says Dennis Gersten, M.D., a San

Diego psychiatrist and publisher of *Atlantis*, a bi-monthly imagery newsletter. He recommends practicing this imagery for six to ten minutes twice a day.

JUICE THERAPY

Celery juice is rich in coumarins, substances that have a soothing effect on the vascular system and that may benefit those prone to migraines, says naturopathic physician Michael Murray, N.D., author of *The Complete Book of Juicing*. Fresh celery juice may be drunk alone or combined with other vegetable juices, such as carrot, cucumber, parsley and spinach. Dr. Murray says to drink an eight-ounce glass of the juice twice a day as a preventive, in conjunction with proper medical treatment.

For information on juicing techniques, see page 93.

RELAXATION AND MEDITATION

Thermal biofeedback can help redirect blood flow out of dilated blood vessels in the scalp and ease migraine pain, says Steven Fahrion, Ph.D., director of research at the Life Sciences Institute of Mind-Body Health in Topeka, Kansas. To learn more about this simple ten-minute technique, see page 121.

SEE ALSO Headache

MOOD SWINGS

It doesn't take much to change your moods: a song on the radio, the color of the walls, your spouse's voice telling you good night. Your moods are legendary among friends and family, who've seen them shift faster than an Indy 500 driver.

In women, mood swings are often related to hormonal fluctuations and may occur before the monthly period, during and right after pregnancy and during menopause. But female hormones aren't the only culprits: Men, too, can go into funks—over a cloudy sky, a spouse's offhand comment or just a stressful day at work. The natural remedies in this chapter, used with the approval of your doctor, may help control mood swings, according to some health professionals.

FLOWER REMEDY/ESSENCE THERAPY

"Chamomile is a classic remedy for a moody personality," says Patricia Kaminski, co-director of the Flower Essence Society, a Nevada City, California, organization that studies and promotes the use of flower remedies/essences.

For the generally stable person who finds himself pouting like a child when things don't go his way, Kaminski recommends the remedy Chicory. "Self-centeredness isn't something we outgrow, so this can be helpful for both adults and children," says Kaminski.

Flower remedies/essences are available in some health food stores and through mail order (refer to the resource list on page 635). For information on preparing and administering flower remedies/essences, see page 37.

FOOD THERAPY

"When people have an overgrowth of yeast in their intestines, they can have a lot of emotional shifts, because certain substances are released into their blood that affect their psyches," says Elson Haas, M.D., director of the Preventive Medical Center of Marin in San Rafael, California, and author of *Staying Healthy with Nutrition*. Other people develop emotional reactions to certain foods, such as refined sugar, he says. If you're prone to mood swings, he recommends limiting your intake of yeast-producing foods such as vinegar and baked goods as well as of refined sugar, caffeine and alcohol.

"Mood swings can also be caused by foods that typically cause allergic reactions in people—things such as milk products and wheat," says Dr. Haas. "So if you notice mood swings after consuming these foods, you might have a food allergy and should avoid them."

HYDROTHERAPY

The neutral bath is a classic water treatment for emotional ups and downs, says Tori Hudson, N.D., a naturopathic physician and professor at the National College of Naturopathic Medicine in Portland, Oregon. The next time you need to chill out, fill your tub with water just slightly cooler than body temperature. It should feel like a hot bath that's beginning to get a little chilly, says

Dr. Hudson. Soak for 20 minutes, adding water as needed to maintain the temperature of the bath.

JUICE THERAPY

"Mood swings are often caused by problems in the pancreas," says Eve Campanelli, Ph.D., a holistic family practitioner in Beverly Hills, California. "Carrot juice contains natural insulin and stabilizes the pancreas." Many people may be able to control mood swings by minimizing the amount of sugar in their diets and by drinking two glasses of fresh carrot juice a day, according to Dr. Campanelli. Because carrot juice is quite sweet, she recommends diluting four ounces of the juice with an equal amount of water for each glass.

For information on juicing techniques, see page 93.

SOUND THERAPY

Mood swings often arise because of stress, anger or anxiety, says Janalea Hoffman, R.M.T., a composer and music therapist based in Kansas City, Missouri. Some people find relief from shifting moods by listening to relaxing music with a slow, steady beat, which slows your heart rate and calms your mind, she says. Try listening to this type of music for about 30 minutes a day. She suggests her tapes *Musical Hypnosis* and *Deep Daydreams*; for other selections, see "Sailing Away to Key Largo" on page 129. Many of these pieces are available in music stores. For mail-order information, refer to the resource list on page 642.

Here's another idea: If you live near the ocean, try sitting on or near the beach for a half-hour or so each day. Ocean waves crash the shore at a steady rhythm that helps calm you down, Hoffman says. "That's why people feel so good at the ocean," she says. "It's a constant sound, a relaxing sound. And people really respond to the rhythm."

If you can't get near the ocean, Hoffman suggests buying or making a tape recording of ocean waves. "It's probably not quite as good as the real thing, but the rhythm will still be the same," she says. You can find these tapes in many music stores. But, she adds, the sound of real waves is better than synthesized waves.

YOGA

Mood swings may mean that you've lost balance in your life, says Alice Christensen, founder and executive director of the American Yoga Association. To bring things back in line, Christensen suggests these yoga poses that stress balance: standing sun (page 607), tree (page 608) and dancer (page 609). Make them part of your daily yoga routine, Christensen says.

MOTION SICKNESS

I t's Detroit's favorite image for selling sports cars: the slick red convertible on a scenic, winding mountain road. "Take them for a spin in the country in this baby," the ads seem to say, "and your friends will be green with envy."

But subject some people to this kind of souped-up Sunday drive, and they might turn green for a different reason: motion sickness.

Whether you travel by car or plane, elevator or roller coaster, motion sickness can make your journey unpleasant. Caused by a disturbance in the inner ear, motion sickness can be aggravated by hunger, anxiety or unpleasant odors such as tobacco smoke. Staying calm and keeping your vehicle well-ventilated can help stop the world (and your stomach) from spinning. The natural remedies in this chapter—in conjunction with medical care and used with your doctor's approval—may help prevent or relieve motion sickness, according to some health professionals.

SEE YOUR MEDICAL DOCTOR WHEN . . .

- You have severe symptoms of dizziness that interfere with walking or even sitting up.
- You have severe nausea and/or vomiting.
- You have a change in hearing and ringing or fullness in the ear.
- You have ear pain, discharge or bleeding.

ACUPRESSURE

For motion sickness, firmly press points P 5 and P 6, which are near your wrists, says Michael Reed Gach, Ph.D., director of the Acupressure Institute in Berkeley, California, and author of *Acupressure's Potent Points*. To find P 5, place your right thumb on the inside of your left forearm, three finger-widths from the center of your wrist crease. Breathing deeply, apply firm pressure with your thumb for one minute, suggests Dr. Gach. Then move your thumb about half of a finger-width closer to the wrist crease to point P 6. Dr. Gach says to apply pressure for one more minute, then repeat the procedure on your right forearm.

For help in locating these points, refer to the illustration on page 564.

FLOWER REMEDY/ESSENCE THERAPY

The flower remedy Scleranthus can help motion sickness, says Leslie J. Kaslof, herbalist and author of *The Traditional Flower Remedies of Dr. Edward Bach*. He suggests placing two to four drops under the tongue and holding them in your mouth for a moment before swallowing. He also says you can apply the remedy topically, putting it on the temples and inside the belly button.

Flower remedies are available in some health food stores and through mail order (refer to the resource list on page 635). For information on preparing and administering flower remedies, see page 37.

HERBAL THERAPY

A scientific study from Britain says that ginger is more effective than Dramamine, an over-the-counter drug, in stopping motion sickness, says Varro E. Tyler, Ph.D., professor of pharmacognosy at Purdue University in West Lafayette, Indiana. You can buy candied ginger in Asian food markets and chew on it while traveling, according to Dr. Tyler. Or, he suggests, buy ginger supplements (they're available in most health food stores), then take two 500-milligram capsules about an hour before embarking on your trip and one or two more capsules every four hours while you're traveling.

HOMEOPATHY

If you feel like your surroundings are spinning, feel nauseated from motion in a car or boat and feel better when you close your eyes, try a 6C or 12C dose of Cocculus, says Mitchell Fleisher, M.D., a family practice physician and homeopath in Colleen, Virginia. Taking Cocculus 30 to 60 minutes prior to your trip may also be a good preventive measure if it has relieved your motion sickness in the past, he says.

Another option for motion sickness is a 30C dose of Tabacum, says Judyth Reichenberg-Ullman, N.D., a naturopathic physician in Edmonds, Washington, and co-author of *The Patient's Guide to Homeopathic Medicine*. She recommends using Tabacum if you feel better in the open air with your eyes closed.

If you don't know which remedy—Cocculus or Tabacum—is best for you, Dr. Reichenberg-Ullman says to carry both with you on your trip and take them one at a time. "Try one, and if it works, great. If it doesn't, then you have the option of trying the next one," she says. "You'll know within 30 minutes of taking it if one of these remedies is going to work."

Cocculus and Tabacum are available in many health food stores. To purchase the remedies by mail, refer to the resource list on page 637.

JUICE THERAPY

Scientific studies have shown that ginger works better than commercial motion sickness products such as Dramamine, says naturopathic physician Michael

Murray, N.D., in *The Complete Book of Juicing*. Those prone to motion sickness may be able to head off nausea by sipping Dr. Murray's Ginger Hopper juice blend about an hour before a trip. To prepare, juice a slice of fresh ginger (about ¼ inch thick) with an apple and four carrots.

For information on juicing techniques, see page 93.

REFLEXOLOGY

To help prevent motion sickness, or to help control it once it has started, work the diaphragm, pituitary gland, ear, neck and spine reflexes on your hands or feet, says St. Petersburg, Florida, reflexologist Dwight Byers, author of *Better Health with Foot Reflexology*.

To help you locate these points, consult the hand and foot reflex charts beginning on page 582. For instructions on how to work the points, see "Your Reflexology Session" on page 110.

SEE ALSO Nausea and Vomiting

MUSCLE CRAMPS AND PAIN

M uscles are the foot soldiers of the human body. Some, such as the heart, are independent. But more than 600 others bend and stretch to accommodate our every whim.

Only when we've forced them to do something ridiculous do muscles make their presence known, often in the form of muscle cramps, which are painful, spasmodic muscular contractions. Cramps often mean you've spent too long in an unnatural position: sitting in a cramped car for several hours or sleeping in a position fit for a circus contortionist. Muscle pain can mean you've pushed your body too far, whether in a vigorous game of touch football or by attacking the weeds in your garden like a Tasmanian devil. The natural remedies in this chapter—in conjunction with medical care and used with your doctor's approval—may help prevent or relieve muscle cramps, according to some health professionals.

SEE YOUR MEDICAL DOCTOR WHEN . . .

• You have cramps several times in one day or cramps that "lock" for several minutes.

- Your muscle pain is accompanied by a fever or tender areas in the neck, shoulders, back, chest, hips and buttocks.
- You have a muscle spasm in your back or neck that causes weakness, numbness or tingling.
- You have a muscle spasm that doesn't improve within three days.

ACUPRESSURE

Press point GV 26, situated on your face above your upper lip, two-thirds of the way to the nose, says Michael Reed Gach, Ph.D., director of the Acupressure Institute in Berkeley, California, and author of *Acupressure's Potent Points*. (For help in locating this point, refer to the illustration on page 564.) "You can stimulate this point with your knuckle or your thumb," says Dr. Gach. "You can also press firmly between your thumb and index finger to relieve aches and pains." Hold this point until the cramp releases, he says.

AROMATHERAPY

For a fragrant massage oil to relieve your aching muscles, Los Angeles aromatic consultant John Steele suggests a blend of anti-inflammatory blue chamomile, analgesic birch, stimulating rosemary and soothing lavender essential oils. To prepare, says Steele, add three drops of blue chamomile, three drops of birch, three drops of rosemary (or coriander), eight drops of lavender and three drops of ginger (or black pepper) to ½ ounce of a carrier oil such as olive, almond, grapeseed or avocado. (Carrier oils are available in most health food stores.) Massage into the affected area after a warm bath, says Steele.

For information on preparing and administering essential oils, including cautions about their use, see page 19. For information on purchasing essential oils, refer to the resource list on page 633.

AYURVEDA

To stop muscle spasms, soak your feet for 10 to 20 minutes in a large pot of hot water with a homemade tea bag of black or brown mustard seeds (two teaspoons of seeds tied up in some cotton or cheesecloth) immersed in it, says Vasant Lad, B.A.M.S., M.A.Sc., director of the Ayurvedic Institute in Albuquerque, New Mexico. Mustard seeds are available in most health food stores.

FOOD THERAPY

Eat your vegetables raw, since cooking them depletes their potassium, magnesium and calcium, the three nutrients most important in preventing and treating muscle cramps and pain, says Julian Whitaker, M.D., founder and president of the Whitaker Wellness Center in Newport Beach, California. "Eating foods rich in potassium and magnesium is the best thing for muscle cramps," he says. (For good sources of each of these nutrients, see "Getting What You Need" on page 142.)

HERBAL THERAPY

For massaging out muscle tension, Mary Bove, L.M., N.D., a naturopathic physician and director of the Brattleboro Naturopathic Clinic in Vermont, recommends this herbal massage oil. Start with one cup of extra-virgin olive oil or almond oil (available in most health food stores). Pour the oil into a bottle or jar and add the following herbs in tincture form: 1 ounce of cramp bark, ½ ounce of lobelia and ¼ ounce of willowbark or wintergreen. (If you don't have wintergreen tincture, Dr. Bove says to substitute 30 drops of wintergreen oil.) These ingredients are also available in most health food stores and through mail order (for mail-order information, refer to the resource list on page 635).

HOMEOPATHY

Rubbing Arnica ointment, cream, gel or oil into a sore muscle, then applying a warm washcloth, three or four times a day can help relieve cramping and pain, says Mitchell Fleisher, M.D., a family practice physician and homeopath in Colleen, Virginia. He says that taking a 12C or 30C tablet of Arnica two or three times a day until the pain and soreness are relieved may also help.

These remedies are available in many health food stores. To purchase the remedies by mail, refer to the resource list on page 637.

HYDROTHERAPY

A frozen bandage is great for minor sprains, minor sports injuries and spasms that do not respond to heat, says Agatha Thrash, M.D., a medical pathologist and co-founder and co-director of Uchee Pines Institute, a natural healing center in Seale, Alabama. Dip a hand towel in very cold water, squeeze it out, place it in a plastic bag and store it in the freezer over a piece of cardboard, so the towel freezes flat. To use, remove the plastic and lay the bandage over the affected area. The rigid bandage will quickly become soft as it's warmed by your body heat. Replace with a fresh bandage when the towel feels warm. Dr. Thrash recommends 20-minute sessions of this treatment two to four times a day for a week or until symptoms subside.

MUSCLE CRAMPS AND PAIN

IMAGERY

Close your eyes, breathe out three times and imagine your muscle encased in a block of ice, writes New York City psychiatrist Gerald Epstein, M.D., in his book *Healing Visualizations*. Picture the ice melting, and as it melts, feel the muscle relax. After the ice has completely melted, open your eyes, and the muscle spasm or cramp should be gone.

Dr. Epstein suggests doing this imagery for 2 to 3 minutes as needed every 15 to 30 minutes until the pain subsides.

MASSAGE

Using the effleurage stroke (page 570), run your fingertips very lightly up and down the length of the affected muscle, says Vincent Iuppo, N.D., naturopathic physician, massage therapist and director of the Morris Institute of Natural Therapeutics, a holistic health education center in Denville, New Jersey. Make sure the strokes are gentle, as if you were running a feather duster over the muscle. Continue until the pain or cramp has subsided.

RELAXATION AND MEDITATION

Whenever muscle cramps put a crimp in your day, reduce them with the stretch-based relaxation technique described on page 602, says Charles Carlson, Ph.D., professor of psychology at the University of Kentucky in Lexington.

SEE ALSO Fibromyalgia; Leg Cramps

NAUSEA AND VOMITING

Every once in a while, what goes down must come up. Whether the cause is flu, food poisoning, motion sickness or morning sickness, vomiting and nausea (which is feeling as though you might vomit) are natural reactions to stomach irritation. Be aware, though, that nausea can signal a heart attack and can be a symptom of some types of cancer as well as of kidney and liver disorders. The natural remedies in this chapter—in conjunction with medical care and used with your doctor's approval—-may help relieve nausea or prevent vomiting, according to some health professionals.

SEE YOUR MEDICAL DOCTOR WHEN . . .

- You feel frequent nausea for more than two days.
- You're pregnant and you can't eat or drink because your nausea is so severe.
- You vomit periodically for more than 24 hours.
- You have nausea and you're suffering from sudden, severe pain in the chest or abdomen.
- You vomit blood or a substance that looks like coffee grounds.
- You're elderly and your nausca is accompanied by fever.

ACUPRESSURE

Press points P 5 and P 6 on the insides of your forearms, says Michael Reed Gach, Ph.D., director of the Acupressure Institute in Berkeley, California, and author of *Acupressure's Potent Points*. For P 5, place your right thumb on the inside of your left forearm, three finger-widths from the center of your wrist crease. Breathing deeply, apply firm pressure with your thumb for one minute, suggests Dr. Gach. For P 6, move your thumb about half of a finger-width closer to the wrist crease. Dr. Gach says to apply pressure for one more minute, then repeat the procedure on your right forearm.

For help in locating these points, refer to the illustration on page 564.

AROMATHERAPY

Peppermint is a traditional cure for nausea and vomiting, according to San Francisco herbalist Jeanne Rose, chairperson of the National Association for Holistic Aromatherapy and author of *Aromatherapy: Applications and Inhalations*. She suggests adding a single drop of the essential oil to a sugar cube and sucking slowly until the cube is completely melted. An eight-ounce glass of water spiked with two drops of the essential oil has a similar effect, she says.

For information on preparing and administering essential oils, including cautions about their use, see page 19. For information on purchasing essential oils, refer to the resource list on page 633.

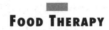

Ayurveda

Relieve nausea with two pinches of cardamom and ½ teaspoon of honey mixed into ½ cup of plain yogurt, says Vasant Lad, B.A.M.S., M.A.Sc., director of the Ayurvedic Institute in Albuquerque, New Mexico. Or, suggests Dr. Lad, you could try stirring a pinch each of nutmeg and cardamom into ½ cup of warm milk and slowly sipping this beverage. And he offers a third option: a tea made from 1 teaspoon of cumin seeds and a pinch of ground nutmeg steeped in 1 cup of boiling water for ten minutes. Strain the tea to remove the seeds, then drink it.

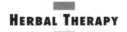

Food Therapy

The best foods to eat when you feel nauseated are low-fat, plain foods, such as dry soda crackers, says Robert M. Stern, Ph.D., a researcher on motion sickness and nausea for NASA and professor of psychology at Pennsylvania State University in University Park. He explains that high-fat foods take hours to digest, but lighter foods can ease stomach pain and are digested easily. Be careful not to overdo it, he says; a few crackers may ease your pain, but too many will make it worse.

When you're vomiting, Dr. Stern says, don't eat anything for at least one hour, since it will take your stomach that long to settle. Then, he suggests, have small portions of bread, broth or other bland foods, or drink soda that has gone flat.

Herbal Therapy

For mild nausea, drink ginger tea, says Varro E. Tyler, Ph.D., professor of pharmacognosy at Purdue University in West Lafayette, Indiana. To make the tea, slice a piece of fresh ginger and put a few shavings or slivers of it in a tea ball. Pour a cup of boiling water over it, steep for ten minutes, then allow it to cool before drinking.

When nausea is more intense, Dr. Tyler suggests trying a stronger dose of ginger, available in gelatin capsules of 500 milligrams in most health food stores. Take one or two capsules every four hours, or follow label instructions for dosage, he says.

HOMEOPATHY

If you feel nauseated and don't know why, the first thing to try is a dose of Ipecacuanha 6X every 15 minutes until you begin to feel better—but take no more than four doses, says Maesimund Panos, M.D., a homeopathic physician in Tipp City, Ohio, and co-author with Jane Heimlich of *Homeopathic Medicine at Home*.

Ipecacuanha is available in many health food stores. To purchase the remedy by mail, refer to the resource list on page 637.

HYDROTHERAPY

For anyone in gastric distress, Agatha Thrash, M.D., a medical pathologist and co-founder and co-director of Uchee Pines Institute, a natural healing center in Seale, Alabama, recommends this water-and-charcoal cocktail: Put two to three tablespoons of activated charcoal powder in the bottom of a large glass and add a small amount of water (bottled may be best if you're traveling). Stir slowly with a long-handled spoon to keep the fine powder from flying everywhere, suggests Dr. Thrash. Fill the glass the rest of the way with water and drink with a straw. Available in most health food stores and some pharmacies, activated charcoal doesn't taste very good, she says, but it's cheap, effective and safe for everyone.

IMAGERY

Picture your nausea as having any size, shape or color. Then transform it into a liquid that flows down one of your legs, out the bottom of your foot, across the room and out your front door. Watch it as it continues down your street and disappears miles away, says Dennis Gersten, M.D., a San Diego psychiatrist and publisher of *Atlantis*, a bi-monthly imagery newsletter. If you do that, your nausea may vanish within minutes.

JUICE THERAPY

Ginger is a well-known traditional remedy for gastric problems, says naturopathic physician Michael Murray, N.D., in *The Complete Book of Juicing*. That's because ginger is a carminative, a natural substance that helps eliminate gas and soothes the gastrointestinal tract, according to Dr. Murray. To ease nausea, he recommends a juice blend of a slice of fresh ginger (about ¼ inch thick), an apple and four carrots.

For information on juicing techniques, see page 93.

REFLEXOLOGY

Pay special attention to the following reflex points on your hands or feet, says New York City reflexologist Laura Norman, author of *Feet First: A Guide to Foot Reflexology*: solar plexus, diaphragm, chest, lung, esophagus, stomach, liver, gallbladder and thyroid, pituitary and adrenal gland.

To help you locate these points, consult the hand and foot reflex charts beginning on page 582. For instructions on how to work the points, see "Your Reflexology Session" on page 110.

NECK PAIN

Whether it's from sleeping in a contorted position or hunching over a computer screen all day, that stiff, achy feeling is truly a pain in the neck.

While a muscular injury or ruptured disk can cause neck pain, a less obvious cause is poor posture. Take a look in the mirror; if your shoulders are hunched over and your neck is bent forward, the weight of your head—about 18 pounds—isn't properly balanced over your shoulders, the way nature intended it. The muscles and ligaments in your neck do their best to compensate, but they aren't happy with the situation, and they're letting you know about it. The natural remedies in this chapter—in conjunction with medical care and used with your doctor's approval—may help relieve neck pain, according to some health professionals.

SEE YOUR MEDICAL DOCTOR WHEN . . .

- You have recurring neck pain or pain that lasts for more than three days.
- You have neck pain after a fall or an accident.
- Your neck pain runs down your arms or legs.

ACUPRESSURE

To get rid of neck pain, press the GB 20 points, which are two inches out from the middle of your neck, underneath the base of the skull, says Michael Reed Gach, Ph.D., director of the Acupressure Institute in Berkeley, California, and author of *Acupressure's Potent Points*. (For help in locating these points, refer to the illustration on page 565.) He says to close your eyes and press both GB 20 points for at least one minute, using the thumbs of both hands. To make holding these points most comfortable, Dr. Gach suggests sitting in a chair and bending over, with your elbows propped on a table or desk.

HYDROTHERAPY

Relieve neck pain with an ice massage, suggests Charles Thomas, Ph.D., co-author of *Hydrotherapy: Simple Treatments for Common Ailments* and a physical therapist at Desert Springs Therapy Center in Desert Hot Springs, California. His instructions: Freeze water in a plastic cup, remove the ice, and after rubbing your neck with your hand to prime the area, use the ice cube to rub your neck for 5 to 15 minutes. (Wear a glove or mitt to protect your hand from the cold.)

IMAGERY

Picture your neck pain as a ball that has a particular size, shape, color and texture. It may be as small as a marble or as large as a basketball. Allow the ball to grow larger and larger. As it does, the pain may momentarily increase. Now let the ball shrink smaller than its original size, but don't let it disappear. As the intensity of the pain changes, allow the ball to change color, too. Now imagine that the ball turns into a liquid that flows down your arm, drips on the floor and reforms into a ball. Now kick or throw the ball out into space. Watch it disappear. Most of your pain should be gone, says Dennis Gersten, M.D., a San Diego psychiatrist and publisher of *Atlantis*, a bi-monthly imagery newsletter. He suggests doing this imagery for ten minutes twice a day and whenever the pain flares up.

MASSAGE

Two exercises with a rolled-up towel can help you relieve tension and pain in your neck, writes Monika Struna in *Self-Massage*. For instructions, see the towel tricks for neck pain on page 580.

REFLEXOLOGY

Work the following reflex points on your feet, suggests New York City reflexologist Laura Norman, author of *Feet First: A Guide to Foot Relexology*: adrenal gland, solar plexus, diaphragm, shoulder, neck and spine, with special emphasis on the cervical spine. Also work all of the points on the tops and bottoms of the toes, using whichever technique you find most comfortable.

To help you locate these points, consult the foot reflex chart on page 592. For instructions on how to work the points, see "Your Reflexology Session" on page 110.

RELAXATION AND MEDITATION

Studies have shown that stretch-based relaxation techniques are an excellent way to reduce neck pain, says Charles Carlson, Ph.D., professor of psychology at the University of Kentucky in Lexington. See the illustrations on page 602 to learn one such technique. Dr. Carlson suggests using it whenever your neck begins to feel sore. It is also a good preventive measure if you practice it for 20 minutes twice a day, he adds.

NIGHT BLINDNESS

You used to do just fine anytime. Now evening strolls and moonlight drives have lost their appeal because it's harder to see after an oncoming car passes.

Often associated with aging, night blindness can be caused by a shortage of rhodopsin, a pigment found in the retina that allows nervous impulses to travel from the eyes to the brain. Rhodopsin is found in vitamin A, so problems with night vision may mean that you're not getting enough of this nutrient.

But because night blindness can also be caused by glaucoma or inadequate blood circulation to the eyes, you should see your doctor any time you notice a change in your night vision. The natural remedies in this chapter—in conjunction with medical care and used with the approval of your doctor—may help improve your night vision, according to some health professionals.

SEE YOUR MEDICAL DOCTOR WHEN . . .

- You notice a change in your night vision.
- You have trouble driving at night.
- You don't see the stars in the sky that others do.

FOOD THERAPY

Night blindness can be caused by a deficiency of vitamin A, so eat more yellow-orange vegetables such as carrots, pumpkin and squash, says Julian

Whitaker, M.D., founder and president of the Whitaker Wellness Center in Newport Beach, California. "Dark green leafy vegetables such as spinach are also good." (For more food sources of vitamin A, see "Getting What You Need" on page 142.)

JUICE THERAPY

Bilberries, a type of blueberry available in Europe, are a popular folk remedy for poor night vision, according to naturopathic physician Michael Murray, N.D., author of *The Complete Book of Juicing*. Believing it would improve their night vision, British Royal Air Force pilots prepared for nocturnal flights by eating bilberry preserves.

More recently, studies have shown that extracts of the common American blueberry can also improve night vision, according to Dr. Murray. For maximum therapeutic effect, he suggests drinking at least 16 ounces of fresh blueberry juice a day, alone or mixed with other fresh juices such as pear or pineapple for added taste and variety.

For information on juicing techniques, see page 93.

SEE ALSO Vision Problems

NIGHTMARES

Children have bogeymen. Adults have career failure, sickness and death, not to mention the latest horror story from the evening news.

No matter what your age, life supplies you with plenty of material for nightmares. Besides being unpleasant, nightmares also cut into your shut-eye time, and as modern life becomes more and more complicated, you need all of the rest you can get. The natural remedies in this chapter, used with your doctor's approval, may help prevent nightmares or decrease their incidence, according to some health professionals.

SEE YOUR MEDICAL DOCTOR WHEN . . .

- Your nightmares are so disturbing or persistent that they keep you from falling asleep or getting enough sleep.

NIGHTMARES

AYURVEDA

"If you dream about falling from heights, your nightmares are a sign of increased vata dosha, stemming from unresolved fears and anxieties," says Vasant Lad, B.A.M.S., M.A.Sc., director of the Ayurvedic Institute in Albuquerque, New Mexico. (For more information on the Ayurvedic doshas, see "All about Vata, Pitta and Kapha" on page 28.) He suggests eating early in the evening, avoiding carbonated beverages and drinking a cup of warm milk with a pinch of nutmeg before retiring.

Pitta nightmares are often violent, such as a house on fire. Heartburn, acid indigestion and other kinds of stomach upset can cause such dreams, Dr. Lad says. He recommends taking a mixture of warm water and ½ teaspoon each of the Indian herbal powders shatavari and brahmi every day after lunch and dinner. If your pitta nightmares are accompanied by fever and sweating, Dr. Lad says to take ½ teaspoon of the herbal preparation sudarshan churna two or three times daily.

Drowning dreams are a sign of excess kapha in the lungs and lymphatic tissue, Dr. Lad says. To stop these dreams, he recommends this mixture of powdered herbs: Add a pinch of pippali to ½ teaspoon each of punarnava and licorice, and mix with 1 teaspoon of honey. He says to eat this preparation at breakfast, lunch and dinner.

All of these herbs are available through Ayurvedic practitioners or by mail order (refer to the resource list on page 634). Punarnava is also available in Indian pharmacies; licorice can be purchased in most health food stores.

FLOWER REMEDY/ESSENCE THERAPY

Daily use of the flower remedy Rockrose at bedtime can be very helpful for people prone to nightmares, according to Leslie J. Kaslof, an herbalist and author of *The Traditional Flower Remedies of Dr. Edward Bach*. Rockrose is available in some health food stores and through mail order (refer to the resource list on page 635).

For occasional nightmares, Eve Campanelli, Ph.D., a holistic family practitioner in Beverly Hills, California, recommends the emergency stress relief formula (sold under brand names such as Calming Essence, Rescue Remedy and Five-Flower Formula). "I have seen children who had horrible nightmares after losing their homes in the earthquakes," says Dr. Campanelli. "I told their parents to give them a few drops of Rescue Remedy at bedtime, and the children slept peacefully all night." The emergency stress relief formula is available in most health food stores and through mail order (refer to the resource list on page 635).

For more information on preparing and administering flower remedies, see page 37.

FOOD THERAPY

Eat light at night, says Julian Whitaker, M.D., founder and president of the Whitaker Wellness Center in Newport Beach, California. "Heavy food at night is thought to cause nightmares in some people, so if you're prone, try to eat light for dinner." That means fewer protein-rich meats and more pastas and other high-carbohydrate meals, which are more easily digested, he says.

HOMEOPATHY

If you have nightmares about dying, hunger or problems at work and are depressed when you wake, try a 30C dose of Aurum, according to Andrew Lockie, M.D., in *The Family Guide to Homeopathy*. If you have disturbing dreams about fire or danger and have difficulty sleeping between midnight and 2:00 A.M., Dr. Lockie suggests a 30C dose of Arsenicum. Take these remedies one hour before going to bed for ten consecutive nights, he says. If your nightmares persist, see your medical doctor or homeopath.

Aurum and Arsenicum are available in many health food stores. To purchase the remedies by mail, refer to the resource list on page 637.

IMAGERY

If a nightmare wakes you, sit up in bed and turn on the light. Close your eyes, and as you do, imagine yourself surrounded by a warm, loving white light, say Elizabeth Ann Barrett, R.N., Ph.D., professor and coordinator of the Center for Nursing Research at Hunter College of the City University of New York in New York City. This light can't be penetrated by anything negative or harmful. See the light expand around you until it is three times your size. Know that the light loves you just the way you are and will allow nothing to hurt you. Open your eyes and turn out the light in the room, all the while keeping yourself embraced in the white light. Get comfortable in bed and close your eyes. Now let the nurturing white light fill the room. As you begin to drift off to sleep, sense that you have become a part of this loving light and that you are totally protected.

OILY HAIR AND SKIN

You thought you'd left this problem in high school. But unlike vocabulary lists, algebra and cafeteria pizza, oily hair and skin have followed you into adulthood. The results? Limp hair caused by oil clinging to it and flattening it out, and shiny spots on your face where oil collects.

The problem starts in your sebaceous glands, which lie just below the surface of the skin. In some people, these glands produce an excess of oil, which flows through pores and onto your hair and skin. Oily hair and skin are usually hereditary conditions, say experts. The natural remedies in this chapter, used with your doctor's approval, may help prevent or treat oily hair and skin, according to some health professionals.

SEE YOUR MEDICAL DOCTOR WHEN . . .

- Your extremely oily hair is accompanied by acne, excessive hairiness or, in women, hair loss.

AROMATHERAPY

The best way to regulate oily skin may be to add more oil to it—essential oil, that is, according to Los Angeles aromatic consultant John Steele. "Essential oils don't have the greasy consistency we associate with the word *oil*," he explains. "They're very light and quickly absorbed into the skin." For a purifying facial oil that's light enough for oily skin, Steele says to add two drops of lemongrass essential oil to ½ ounce of carrier oil such as apricot or hazelnut (available in most health food stores) and apply to the face after every cleansing. "Lemongrass has antibacterial properties and does a wonderful job of degreasing the skin and regulating overactive sebaceous glands," says Steele. Do not use more than two drops of this essential oil, he cautions, as it can irritate sensitive skin.

Essential oils can also be used to care for oily hair, says San Francisco herbalist Jeanne Rose, chairperson of the National Center for Holistic Aromatherapy, in *Aromatherapy: Applications and Inhalations*. To boost the cleaning power of your regular shampoo, she recommends adding eight drops of rose geranium essential oil and eight drops of lemongrass essential oil to an eight-ounce bottle.

For information on preparing and administering essential oils, including cautions about their use, see page 19. For information on purchasing essential oils, refer to the resource list on page 633.

OILY HAIR AND SKIN

FOOD THERAPY

De-grease your diet, says Michael A. Klaper, M.D., a nutritional medicine specialist in Pompano Beach, Florida, and director of the Institute of Nutritional Education and Research, an organization based in Manhattan Beach, California, that teaches doctors about nutrition and its relationship to disease. "Oily hair and skin sometimes are the result of eating too many fats in your diet—things such as doughnuts and potato chips. The heavy fats in these foods work their way into the skin oils, contributing to overly oily skin and acne. If it leaves a grease spot on a paper towel, avoid it."

HOMEOPATHY

Personal treatment by a medical doctor or homeopath may be necessary to control oily hair and skin, but try these 6C remedies first, writes Andrew Lockie, M.D., author of *The Family Guide to Homeopathy*. He says to take one of these remedies every 12 hours. If you notice no improvement in a month, see your medical doctor or homeopath.

If you have greasy hair, Dr. Lockie suggests trying Bryonia first. If that doesn't work, he says you may need to try a more specific remedy such as Mercurius, which helps people who have oily hair, a sweaty, tight sensation in the scalp, excessive saliva and intolerance of heat and cold. If you have oily, thinning hair, particularly after an extended period of stress or grief, try Phosphoricum acidum, he says.

If you have oily, shiny skin that is worse on hairy parts of your body and you feel constipated, Dr. Lockie recommends Natrum muriaticum. Mercurius is a good remedy for a trembling person who has sticky perspiration, increased saliva production and an unpleasant oily film on his face that is worse in cold and hot weather, he says.

All of these remedies are available in many health food stores. To purchase the remedies by mail, refer to the resource list on page 637.

OSTEOPOROSIS

Here are a couple of bone-chilling facts: Half of all American women over age 50 will suffer a fracture caused by osteoporosis sometime in their lives. And lest you think osteoporosis is a sexist disease, one in five sufferers is male.

Osteoporosis causes bones to thin, making them more likely to break when stressed. Most women with osteoporosis are past menopause. Though doctors don't know why, the drop in estrogen levels that occurs with menopause appears to speed the loss of bone mass.

Lifestyle can play a role in bone loss, too. People who consume too little calcium or too much caffeine and salt are at higher risk, along with people who smoke, don't exercise or are constantly dieting. The natural remedies in this chapter—in conjunction with medical care and used with the approval of your doctor—may help prevent or slow osteoporosis, according to some health professionals.

SEE YOUR MEDICAL DOCTOR WHEN . . .

- You notice a change in your height, which you should measure at least every two years.

AYURVEDA

To help prevent osteoporosis, eat a handful of sesame seeds every morning, says Vasant Lad, B.A.M.S., M.A.Sc., director of the Ayurvedic Institute in Albuquerque, New Mexico. He also suggests drinking calcium-rich almond milk twice a day, before breakfast and before bedtime. He says you can make your own almond milk by soaking ten almonds in a cup of warm water for ten minutes, peeling them and mixing them in a blender with one cup of cow's milk, goat's milk or soya milk, adding a pinch each of cardamom, ginger powder and saffron for flavor. Goat's milk and soya milk are available in most health food stores.

FOOD THERAPY

"Osteoporosis is a disease of calcium loss, not deficiency," says Michael A. Klaper, M.D., a nutritional medicine specialist in Pompano Beach, Florida, and director of the Institute of Nutritional Education and Research, an organization based in Manhattan Beach, California, that teaches doctors about nutrition and its relationship to disease. "You need to avoid things that make your kidneys excrete excess calcium, which is a steady drain upon your body's calcium stores." These foods include animal proteins such as meats, poultry and fish as well as refined sugars, alcohol, salt, tobacco and caffeine, found in coffee, black tea, cola and chocolate, he says.

Go for food sources that are rich in calcium, such as dark green leafy vegetables, low-fat dairy products and sardines with bones, says Richard Gerson, Ph.D., author of *The Right Vitamins*. (For more food sources of calcium, see "Getting What You Need" on page 142.)

JUICE THERAPY

It can be a challenge to get enough calcium in your diet, says naturopathic physician Michael Murray, N.D., in *The Complete Book of Juicing*. He offers this nondairy alternative: Juice three kale leaves, two collard leaves and a handful of parsley, followed by three carrots, one apple and half of a green pepper. According to Dr. Murray, this cocktail contains about 212 milligrams of calcium and 102 milligrams of magnesium, both essential for building bone mass.

For information on juicing techniques, see page 93.

VITAMIN AND MINERAL THERAPY

A person with osteoporosis may want to use the following daily regimen of supplements to help control the condition, says David Edelberg, M.D., an internist and medical director of the American Holistic Center/Chicago: 1,200 milligrams of calcium; 800 milligrams of magnesium; 10 milligrams of zinc; 1 milligram of copper; 1,000 milligrams of vitamin C; 200 international units of vitamin D; 50 milligrams of vitamin B_6; 1 milligram of folic acid; 1 milligram of silicon; 0.5 milligram of boron; and 5 milligrams of manganese. Some manufacturers combine all of these supplements in one capsule, according to Dr. Edelberg; these can be purchased in most health food stores.

YOGA

Standing poses such as the mountain (page 606) and the tree (page 608) can help your leg bones stay strong, says Stephen A. Nezezon, M.D., yoga teacher and staff physician at the Himalayan International Institute of Yoga Science and Philosophy in Honesdale, Pennsylvania. Try to do at least one of these exercises each day. (Dr. Nezezon cautions that the elderly and people with advanced osteoporosis should not try the tree pose.)

OVERWEIGHT

A slice of cheesecake here. A bag of potato chips there. They don't seem like much. But those sneaky calories can add up to one of the most common health problems: being overweight.

Sometimes people gain weight for medical reasons. Diseases of the endocrine system or problems with metabolism can cause you to store more fat. But most of us pack on the pounds the old-fashioned way: by eating too much and exercising too little.

Being overweight can contribute to a number of health problems, including high blood pressure, heart disease, diabetes, back and joint pain and the increased tendency to contract infectious diseases. But losing weight can help you fight these and other conditions such as osteoarthritis. The natural remedies in this chapter, used with the approval of your doctor, may help you prevent weight gain or lose weight, according to some health professionals.

SEE YOUR MEDICAL DOCTOR WHEN . . .

- You gain weight suddenly, especially after you start taking a new medication.
- You notice that you are urinating more at night or you have a history of chest pain or heart problems.
- You gain weight and also develop insomnia or feel either weak or depressed.

FOOD THERAPY

Eat more fiber, suggests Rosemary Newman, R.N., Ph.D., a registered dietitian and professor of foods and nutrition at Montana State University in Bozeman who has studied fiber and its relationship to cholesterol since the early 1980s. Dietary fiber fills you up, so you eat less, she says. Besides that, she adds, high-fiber foods tend to be very low in calories and fat, so they're great for any weight loss plan.

Dr. Newman advises aiming for no less than 25 grams of fiber a day. (Most women get only 11, and men, 18.) She says that good sources of fiber include fruits, vegetables and whole grains in breads and cereals. Soluble fiber, which acts to lower cholesterol, is found in barley, oats and legumes such as dried beans, she says.

IMAGERY

In his book *Healing Visualizations*, New York City psychiatrist Gerald Epstein, M.D., suggests the following weight loss imagery. Picture yourself in a mirror, seeing a vision of a thinner you. Now envision yourself entering the mirror and merging with the image. Notice the sensations you feel. Now come out of the mirror and stand in front of it again. Push the image out of the mirror and to the right with your right hand.

Each time you sit down to eat, take one to two minutes to conjure the image of your thinner self. Draw a picture of it if you'd like, and hang it where you can see it or carry it with you. This image will reinforce your resolve to lose weight.

RELAXATION AND MEDITATION

In *Meditating to Attain a Healthy Body Weight*, Lawrence LeShan, Ph.D., suggests choosing a word such as "hungry," "diet," "thin," "fat" or the name of your favorite binge food (such as "chocolate" or "Oreos") as a mantra, a word to repeat over and over again. He says to focus your mind on that word until an association forms. So if you choose the word "hungry," for example, the first association that pops into your mind might be "full." Think about the connection between the two words for five or six seconds, says Dr. LeShan, but do not try to make emotional sense of the connection or to gain any deeper insights. Real insights can be explored after the meditation, he explains. Then return to your mantra and wait for the next association. Dr. LeShan suggests doing this for 15 minutes a day, five times a week, for at least six weeks. It may help you understand and control your eating habits.

SOUND THERAPY

Playing slow, soft music during meals will encourage you to eat slower—and maybe to eat less, says Maria Simonson, Sc.D., Ph.D., professor emeritus and director of the Health, Weight and Stress Clinic at the Johns Hopkins Medical Institutions in Baltimore. The music will help you take smaller bites, she says. And as an added bonus, you'll enjoy the smell and the taste of the food more, because you're eating slower, she says.

YOGA

Yoga's gentle exercises are perfect to get you started on losing weight, especially if you have been inactive for a long time, says Alice Christensen, founder and executive director of the American Yoga Association. She recommends a simple daily routine of deep breathing, meditation and three or four yoga poses. Deep breathing (see page 152) will improve your strength, concentration and willpower, making it easier to stick to a weight management program, according to Christensen, while meditation (see page 153) will help you keep a positive self-image. You can choose three or four yoga poses from the Daily Routine, which begins on page 606.

PANIC ATTACKS

Y ou're out there living your day to the fullest—walking in the sunshine, reading a great novel, cooking a special dinner—and suddenly, you're stricken by irrational and intense terror. Nothing in the outside world has changed, but your heart is racing, you're having trouble breathing and you feel a sense of impending doom.

Panic attacks such as this are common and could be a sign of panic disorder, an anxiety-related condition that affects as much as 5 percent of the population. Panic attacks are also marked by dizziness, shaking, fainting and fear of dying or of losing your mind. They are often linked to agoraphobia, an intense fear of open spaces. Overcoming panic attacks may require medical care. The natural remedies in this chapter—in conjunction with medical care and used with the approval of your doctor—may help prevent panic attacks or reduce their severity, according to some health professionals.

SEE YOUR MEDICAL DOCTOR WHEN . . .

- You have episodes marked by rapid heartbeat, shortness of breath, severe anxiety and a feeling of impending doom.
- You find yourself avoiding situations, places or people in order to not feel anxious.

AROMATHERAPY

"Lavender is very calming in times of emotional or psychological distress," says Los Angeles aromatic consultant John Steele. He suggests inhaling directly from the bottle or scenting a handkerchief with three or four drops of lavender essential oil. Inhale slowly and deeply whenever panic strikes, he says.

For information on preparing and administering essential oils, including cautions about their use, see page 19. For information on purchasing essential oils, refer to the resource list on page 633.

FLOWER REMEDY/ESSENCE THERAPY

Anyone prone to panic attacks should keep a bottle of the emergency stress relief formula on hand, says Eve Campanelli, Ph.D., a holistic family practitioner in Beverly Hills, California. "Place three or four drops of the formula under the tongue as soon as you feel an attack coming on," she recommends. "The effect is subtle, but it's a very safe, effective way to restore emotional balance."

The emergency stress relief formula, sold under brand names such as Calming Essence, Rescue Remedy and Five-Flower Formula, is available in most health food stores and through mail order (refer to the resource list on page 635). For information on preparing and administering the formula, see page 40.

FOOD THERAPY

"Try to eat more whole grains, rice and millet," advises Allan Magaziner, D.O., a nutritional medicine specialist and head of the Magaziner Medical Center in Cherry Hill, New Jersey. "These foods are good sources of B vitamins, which have an overall calming effect and keep the nervous system healthy." (For other food sources of the B vitamins, see "Getting What You Need" on page 142.) And, he adds, there's another bonus: These foods are unprocessed. "It's best to stay away from foods with artificial colorings, additives and sugar, because they can make panic attacks worse," he says.

HOMEOPATHY

"If someone experiences panic and shock following a traumatic event such as an earthquake, a car accident or seeing another person injured or killed, you might try giving him one 30C dose of Aconite. That will often calm a person down," says Mitchell Fleisher, M.D., a family practice physician and homeopath in Colleen, Virginia.

Aconite is available in many health food stores. To purchase the remedy by mail, refer to the resource list on page 637.

IMAGERY

To subdue panic, close your eyes, breathe out very slowly three times and imagine that you are in a closed coffin wrapped like a mummy, writes New York City psychiatrist Gerald Epstein, M.D., in his book *Healing Visualizations*. Accept your feelings and stay with them for a long moment. Then push open the coffin, step out and unwrap your bandages. Make the bandages into a ball and throw the ball into a dark cloud, which has formed overhead. Watch the ball go into the center of the cloud and break it up. Allow the rain to wash over you, and realize that your panic is gone. Before you open your eyes, visualize the landscape around you.

Dr. Epstein suggests doing this for three minutes every one to two hours until the panic ebbs.

RELAXATION AND MEDITATION

Panic attacks can be helped by various forms of relaxation training, says Martin Shaffer, Ph.D., executive director of the Stress Management Institute in San Francisco and author of *Life after Stress*. It's a matter of finding the one that works best for you. Ask your therapist for help or see page 113 for a brief description of each of these techniques and how to use them.

YOGA

Fifteen to 20 minutes of daily meditation (see page 153) will give you the strength and courage to beat panic attacks, says Alice Christensen, founder and executive director of the American Yoga Association. Meditation calms and focuses your mind, she says, helping you to overcome the fear and feelings of helplessness that can trigger an attack.

In addition to meditation, Christensen suggests a daily routine of at least six yoga poses. She says to include those that require a complete breath movement, such as the standing sun (page 607), windmill (page 610) and seated sun (page 616). This will help make you physically strong and more able to cope with stress, she explains. Choose your poses from the Daily Routine, which begins on page 606, and be sure to vary the poses from day to day. This will keep your interest high and strengthen different parts of your body, according to Christensen.

SEE ALSO Anxiety; Phobias

PASSIVE SMOKING

Y ou? Smoke? Of course not. Never did, never will. But that doesn't mean you're free of all of the health dangers that tobacco smoke can pose. Because every time you sit in the living room with Aunt Madge and her ultra slims or in a restaurant next to Joe Schmoe and his menthols, you're a passive smoker, breathing in their hazardous secondhand smoke.

The link between passive smoking and lung cancer becomes clearer every day. For example, studies show that children and teens are at greater risk of developing lung cancer sometime in their lives if they grow up in homes with smokers. The smartest thing to do, of course, is avoid secondhand smoke. But that's not always possible. The natural remedies in this chapter, used with the approval of your doctor, may help lessen the damaging effects of secondhand smoke, according to some health professionals.

SEE YOUR MEDICAL DOCTOR WHEN . . .

- You are troubled by a persistent cough, especially if it is accompanied by thick yellow or blood-tinged sputum.
- You are troubled by wheezing, asthmalike problems or shortness of breath.

FOOD THERAPY

Just as research shows that eating more antioxidant-rich foods can help smokers by reducing at least some of the damage caused by cigarettes, it can also benefit the people around them, says Julian Whitaker, M.D., founder and president of the Whitaker Wellness Center in Newport Beach, California. He says that people who are regularly exposed to secondhand smoke should consume more foods high in beta-carotene (carrots, squash, yams, sweet potatoes and other yellow-orange vegetables) as well as foods rich in vitamin C (citrus fruits, peppers and broccoli) and vitamin E (wheat germ and nuts). For other food sources of vitamin C and vitamin E, see "Getting What You Need" on page 142.

VITAMIN AND MINERAL THERAPY

"If you're around someone who smokes heavily, you need high doses of vitamin C to offset the oxidative damage done by the secondhand smoke," says Michael Janson, M.D., director of the Center for Preventive Medicine in Barnstable, Massachusetts, and an officer of the American College for Advancement in Medicine. He recommends taking a minimum of 3,000 milligrams of vitamin C a day.

YOGA

After being exposed to secondhand smoke, you can remove bad air from your lungs with a breathing exercise called *kapalabhati*, says Stephen A. Nezezon, M.D., yoga teacher and staff physician at the Himalayan International Institute of Yoga Science and Philosophy in Honesdale, Pennsylvania. His instructions: Sit upright in a chair or on the floor, with your legs in a comfortable position. Practice a few minutes of the complete breath exercise (see page 152) to make sure you're breathing with the aid of your diaphragm. To start kapalabhati, breathe out forcefully, using your stomach muscles and diaphragm. Then relax the muscles and allow air to gently flow into your lungs; the inhalation should be comfortably deep. Repeat this seven to ten times, then return to normal breathing.

PHLEBITIS

Phlebitis is the ultimate pain in the vein. It's a condition marked by inflammation of the blood vessels, usually in the legs. When phlebitis strikes veins near the surface of the skin, it hurts like crazy but generally isn't dangerous. But when the inflammation occurs deep within the leg, it can be serious; if left untreated, an infection may develop. On rare occasions, a clot can form, break free and lodge in a dangerous spot such as your head or lungs.

Overweight people are more likely to develop phlebitis, as are women who have just given birth and people who have suffered injury to a leg or who have had recent surgery. Anyone with recurring phlebitis should be under a doctor's care. The natural remedies in this chapter—in conjunction with medical care and used with your doctor's approval—may help prevent phlebitis or ease its symptoms, according to some health professionals.

SEE YOUR MEDICAL DOCTOR WHEN...

- You have pain in one leg, along with redness, swelling, itching, tenderness or a cordlike formation under your skin.
- Your symptoms don't clear up in a week and are accompanied by a fever.

FOOD THERAPY

"Citrus fruits are rich in vitamin C and bioflavonoids, which are very helpful in building blood vessel walls, and that can help those with phlebitis," says Julian Whitaker, M.D., founder and president of the Whitaker Wellness Center in Newport Beach, California. He recommends eating several servings of oranges, grapefruit and strawberries each day for both prevention and treatment. (For other food sources of vitamin C, see "Getting What You Need" on page 142.)

REFLEXOLOGY

Work the adrenal gland, colon and liver reflex points on the hands or feet, says St. Petersburg, Florida, reflexologist Dwight Byers, author of *Better Health with Foot Reflexology*.

To help you locate these points, consult the hand and foot reflex charts beginning on page 582. For instructions on how to work the points, see "Your Reflexology Session" on page 110.

PHOBIAS

It started off small enough: You got stung by a bee while pruning the petunias. But the next time you saw a bee, you ran inside, locked the door and dove under the kitchen table. Then the very thought of bees made you shake. You stopped putting honey in your tea for fear that somehow—hey, you never know—there could be a bee inside the jar.

Sounds like a phobia. It's an unrealistic fear of something, a fear that you know is not rational. Phobias can progress to the point where they interfere with daily life. Common phobias include fear of animals, insects, lightning, water, heights and closed-in places such as elevators. Fortunately, 90 percent of phobias respond well to therapy such as relaxation and gradual exposure to the thing a person fears. The natural remedy in this chapter—in conjunction with professional care and used with the approval of your doctor—may help you overcome a phobia, according to one health professional.

SEE YOUR MEDICAL DOCTOR WHEN . . .

• You develop an unrealistic fear of something and this fear begins to interfere with the normal course of your life.

FLOWER REMEDY/ ESSENCE THERAPY

The flower remedy Mimulus is helpful for people trying to overcome specific fears, such as fear of the dark or fear of flying, says Leslie J. Kaslof, an herbalist and author of *The Traditional Flower Remedies of Dr. Edward Bach.*

Flower remedies are available in some health food stores and through mail order (refer to the resource list on page 635). For information on preparing and administering flower remedies, see page 37.

SEE ALSO Anxiety; Panic Attacks

POOR BODY IMAGE

Sure, people say you're attractive. Nice features and all that. But when you stare into the bathroom mirror, you see someone entirely different—someone who just doesn't measure up in the looks or weight department. Chances are you're suffering from poor body image. We become aware of our bodies in childhood and pay more attention to our appearance as we grow up. But sometimes our vision becomes distorted. We think we're fat when we're not; we think we're ugly when we're not; we think our noses are too big when they're not. Sometimes it takes professional counseling to change the way we look at our bodies. And the natural remedies in this chapter, used with your doctor's approval, may help improve body image, according to some health professionals.

SEE YOUR MEDICAL DOCTOR WHEN . . .

- You experience an unintended weight loss or gain of over 25 pounds in a six-month period.
- You routinely go on eating binges.
- You vomit or use laxatives specifically to lose weight.
- Your concerns about your body image and weight dominate your thoughts or interfere with other aspects of your life.

FLOWER REMEDY/ ESSENCE THERAPY

"Many people have grown up with low self-esteem and poor body image. The media feed this by giving us unrealistic expectations. Or perhaps we were taught that sex is dirty, and we have difficulty understanding or feeling comfortable with our sexual desires," says Cynthia Mervis Watson, M.D., a family practice physician in Santa Monica, California, who specializes in homeopathy and herbal therapy. For those who have trouble accepting their physical selves, Dr. Watson recommends the Bach flower remedy Crab Apple. For people whose negative body images stem from conflicting feelings about their sexuality, she recommends the California essence Easter Lily.

Flower remedies/essences are available in some health food stores and through mail order (refer to the resource list on page 635). For information on preparing and administering flower remedies/essences, see page 37.

IMAGERY

"Imagine looking at a statue of yourself, a statue that is the perfect, All-American ideal for your sex," says Dennis Gersten, M.D., a San Diego psychiatrist and publisher of *Atlantis*, a bi-monthly imagery newsletter. "Walk around this statue of yourself. Notice that it has all of the right dimensions, all of the right curves, even the perfect smile. Touch it, feel it. What is the statue made from? Stone, bronze, wood, glass or even flesh? Talk to the figure and ask it how it feels about itself. How do you feel about this perfect statue?

"Now imagine that inside this statue is a being who is unwillingly confined within this mold and who longs to escape. Get ready to liberate him. Take a big strong object, such as a hammer or an ax, and shatter the statue. Rejoice as the inner being emerges, as he dances, sings and flies free of the shackles of this mold." Dr. Gersten suggests practicing this imagery for 10 to 20 minutes twice a day.

RELAXATION AND MEDITATION

A few moments of meditation each day may help you improve body image and self-esteem, says Sundar Ramaswami, Ph.D., a clinical psychologist at the F. S. Dubois Community Mental Health Center in Stamford, Connecticut. For an example of a simple meditation technique, see page 117. Begin meditating for 20 minutes twice a day, suggests Dr. Ramaswami. As you become more proficient at meditation, you may find you can meditate less and still get the same effect.

POSTNASAL DRIP

It's like Chinese water torture inside your sinuses. Drip. Drip. Drip. The constant drainage of mucus from your nose into the back of your throat can be infuriatingly annoying—and it can also be a sign of allergies, sinus infection or other problems.

Actually, your sinuses drain mucus down your throat all of the time. It's just that you don't notice it unless there's an unusually heavy flow or the mucus become thicker than normal. The natural remedies in this chapter, used with your doctor's approval, may help prevent or ease postnasal drip, according to some health professionals.

SEE YOUR MEDICAL DOCTOR WHEN . . .

- Your postnasal drip is thick and colored and persists for seven days or more.
- You have a fever and facial pain along with postnasal drip or are coughing up mucus from deep in your chest.
- Your chronic postnasal drip leads to sore throats, hoarseness or repeated throat clearing.

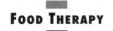

FOOD THERAPY

"Get the dairy out of your diet," advises Michael A. Klaper, M.D., a nutritional medicine specialist in Pompano Beach, Florida, and director of the Institute of Nutritional Education and Research, an organization based in Manhattan Beach, California, that teaches doctors about nutrition and its relationship to disease. Milk, cheeses and other dairy foods tend to promote mucus production, which can trigger or aggravate postnasal drip, according to Dr. Klaper.

JUICE THERAPY

People with postnasal drip may benefit from drinking apple or dark grape juice, says John Peterson, M.D., an Ayurvedic practitioner in Muncie, Indiana. He suggests drinking one eight-ounce glass every day, preferably before a meal. If the juice seems too strong, it can be diluted with water, he says. Cranberry juice can also be helpful, he adds.

For information on juicing techniques, see page 93.

YOGA

To ease postnasal drip, try a *neti*, a yogic nasal wash, suggests Stephen A. Nezezon, M.D., yoga teacher and staff physician at the Himalayan International Institute of Yoga Science and Philosophy in Honesdale, Pennsylvania. The wash can help reduce excess sinus flow, he says.

His instructions: Start by filling a four-ounce paper cup halfway with warm water and then add ½ teaspoon of salt. Put a small crease in the lip of the cup so that it forms a spout. Slightly tilt your head back and to the left. Then slowly pour the water into your right nostril. The water will flow out of your left nostril or down the back of your throat if your left nostril is clogged. Spit out the water if it goes down your throat, or wipe the water from your face with a hand towel if it flows out of your left nostril. Fill the cup again, then repeat the procedure on the other side, pouring the water into your left nostril and tilting your head back and to the right so that the water flows out of your right nostril.

Dr. Nezezon suggests using this treatment daily to relieve postnasal drip and to keep the sinuses clear and healthy.

SEE ALSO Sinus Problems

POST-TRAUMATIC STRESS SYNDROME

Some things are just too horrible to forget. A brutal battle, a natural disaster, a personal tragedy—all can haunt you for decades, and all can lead to post-traumatic stress syndrome.

The Vietnam War brought the syndrome to the nation's consciousness. Soldiers unable to deal with the ravages of war brought their emotional baggage home, where it severely altered their lives. People with post-traumatic stress syndrome suffer many of these symptoms: angry outbursts, depression, overreaction to seemingly small matters, feelings of alienation, nightmares and flashbacks, insomnia and abuse of alcohol and other drugs.

Women who are raped and people who witness terrifying events can develop post-traumatic stress syndrome months or years later. Those with the syndrome usually need counseling and other help. The natural remedies in this chapter—in conjunction with professional care and used with your doctor's approval—may help ease post-traumatic stress syndrome, according to some health professionals.

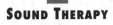

SEE YOUR MEDICAL DOCTOR WHEN . . .

- Your symptoms begin to interfere with your work or family life.
- You begin to use alcohol excessively or to abuse other drugs.

SOUND THERAPY

To ease anxiety related to post-traumatic stress syndrome, try listening to relaxing music for at least 20 to 30 minutes each day, says Steven Halpern, Ph.D., composer, researcher and author of *Sound Health: The Music and Sounds That Make Us Whole.*

To get started, turn on the music, then sit or lie comfortably, close your eyes and take a deep breath. Dr. Halpern suggests that you wear headphones to focus your full attention and to avoid distraction. He recommends, however, that you keep the speakers playing, so your body absorbs the sound energy. While the music plays, let your breathing slow down and become steady. Listen not just to the notes but to the silence between the notes. Dr. Halpern says this will keep you from analyzing the music, which will allow it to relax you.

For suggested pieces to relax by, see "Sailing Away to Key Largo" on page 129. Many of those pieces are available in music stores. For mail-order information, refer to the resource list on page 642.

YOGA

Stress reduction is an essential part of recovery from post-traumatic stress syndrome, says Stephen A. Nezezon, M.D., yoga teacher and staff physician at the Himalayan International Institute of Yoga Science and Philosophy in Honesdale, Pennsylvania. To lower stress, he says, you can try a daily routine of breathing exercises, meditation and yoga poses.

Do the complete breath exercise (see page 152) whenever you're feeling stressed, suggests Alice Christensen, founder and executive director of the American Yoga Association. Meditation (see page 153) helps clear your mind and teaches you to relax, she says. For the poses, select three or four from the Daily Routine, which begins on page 606. Christensen recommends varying the poses daily to keep your interest high and to strengthen different parts of your body. Dr. Nezezon says you should include at least one relaxation pose, such as the corpse (page 612), knee squeeze (page 612) or baby (page 618), in your daily yoga routine.

Dr. Nezezon also recommends doing the alternate nostril breath each day as a way of helping you regain emotional balance. For instruction in this breathing technique, see page 623.

POSTURE PROBLEMS

As babies, we just can't wait to stand up straight. But after a few decades, some of us start to sag a little. Osteoporosis, slumping in chairs and hunching over desks can put a painful pinch in perfect posture.

There's no real definition of "good" posture. Basically, if you can stand naturally straight without making your muscles rigid and can sit with your back comfortably straight, you're doing fine. But if the natural curves in your spine become exaggerated, all sorts of problems can crop up: back and neck pain, headaches, hip pain, fatigue, cramped internal organs and restricted blood flow and breathing, which can contribute to stress and feelings of helplessness. The natural remedy in this chapter, used with your doctor's approval, may help improve posture, according to one health professional.

SEE YOUR MEDICAL DOCTOR WHEN . . .

- You are unable to stand straight for a few moments, even with your best effort.
- You notice that your posture is getting worse over a period of two months.
- You have posture problems and are experiencing back pain.

YOGA

To help improve posture, you need to stretch the spine and the tendons at the backs of your legs, says Alice Christensen, founder and executive director of the American Yoga Association. Two poses, the standing sun (page 607) and the boat (page 621), are especially good for this type of stretch, according to Christensen; she suggests including them, along with two or three other poses from the Daily Routine, which begins on page 606, in your daily yoga session. (Practice the half boat pose, shown on page 620, for about one week before moving on to the boat pose.)

PREGNANCY PROBLEMS

Pregnancy brings many welcome changes—you'll no doubt revel in the joys of impending motherhood. But be aware that pregnant women may also face a battery of problems, from minor to serious.

One of the most dangerous is preeclampsia, a combination of high blood pressure, swelling and weight gain that affects 5 to 7 percent of pregnant women and can threaten the health of mother and baby.

Pregnancy can cause all sorts of other annoyances that are not as critical, including nausea and vomiting, backaches, swelling of the legs, feet, ankles and hands, stretch marks, hemorrhoids, even minor gum disease. (Did you know that pregnancy can even temporarily change the curve of your eyes, making contact lenses difficult to wear?) Pregnant women should have regular checkups with their doctors. The natural remedies in this chapter—in conjunction with medical care and used with the approval of your doctor—may help relieve pregnancy problems, according to some health professionals.

SEE YOUR MEDICAL DOCTOR WHEN . . .

- You experience sudden swelling anywhere on your body.
- You feel dehydrated or you are not urinating.
- You are losing weight.
- You can't keep anything down, including water and/or juice, over a period of 24 hours.
- Your gums bleed and there is also swelling, puffiness, soreness or persistent bad breath despite regular dental hygiene.
- You feel decreased fetal movement or a different pattern of movement than before.
- You begin to have visual disturbances such as double vision or you have persistent headaches.

AROMATHERAPY

To prevent or minimize stretch marks, Fair Oaks, California, aromatherapist Victoria Edwards swears by this fragrant, nourishing oil: Add 20 drops of mandarin orange and 5 drops of jasmine essential oils to four ounces of cocoa butter, unscented lotion or massage oil. "I tell women to start using it in the fourth month, or as soon as their skin begins to stretch," says Edwards. Apply daily after a bath or shower, while the skin is still damp, to the breasts, belly and wherever else your skin has stretched, she says.

For information on preparing and administering essential oils, including cautions about their use, see page 19. For information on purchasing essential oils, refer to the resource list on page 633.

FLOWER REMEDY/ESSENCE THERAPY

"Pregnancy is full of physical and emotional changes that can be difficult for a woman," says Eve Campanelli, Ph.D., a holistic family practitioner in Beverly Hills, California. "Walnut can help her achieve and maintain emotional balance as she adjusts to her new role as a mother." Walnut is available in some health food stores and through mail order (refer to the resource list on page 635).

The emergency stress relief formula can also ease the discomfort of pregnancy and childbirth, says Leslie J. Kaslof, an herbalist and author of *The Traditional Flower Remedies of Dr. Edward Bach.* "My wife used the formula during pregnancy, and she felt much calmer and more relaxed," according to Kaslof. During the birth, she took the remedy orally, says Kaslof, and he applied it in cream form to her temples and forehead, which also had a calming effect.

The emergency stress relief formula is sold under brand names such as Calming Essence, Rescue Remedy and Five-Flower Formula. It's available in most health food stores and through mail order (refer to the resource list on page 635).

Note: Since all flower remedy concentrates contain some alcohol as a preservative, pregnant women should consult a health professional before using them, says Kaslof.

For more information on preparing and administering flower remedies, see page 37.

HERBAL THERAPY

Red raspberry leaf tea tones the uterine muscles, says Barre, Vermont, herbalist Rosemary Gladstar, author of *Herbal Healing for Women* and other books about herbs. It is also rich in iron, she says, and makes a pleasant-tasting, all-purpose tea to drink daily during pregnancy. Drink ginger tea with a little honey and lemon to ease morning sickness symptoms, she advises. Chamomile tea aids digestion, she says, and its calming effects will help you relax. For ease of use, try these teas in tea bag form, she adds. All of them are available in most health food stores.

HOMEOPATHY

If you have morning sickness and even the thought of food makes you feel ill, try a dose of Colchicum autumnale 6X, says Maesimund Panos, M.D., a homeopathic physician in Tipp City, Ohio, and co-author with Jane Heimlich of *Homeopathic Medicine at Home*. If you crave cold water but vomit as soon as the water warms in your stomach, Dr. Panos suggests a dose of Phosphorus 6X. If you vomit first thing in the morning but feel better after eating, Nux vomica 6X may relieve your morning sickness, she says. If you have nausea with no other symptoms, she says to try a dose of Natrum phosphoricum 6X.

For each of these remedies, Dr. Panos suggests taking a dose every 15 minutes until your nausea begins to diminish. She adds this caution: Do not exceed four doses in a day of any of these remedies without consulting your homeopath.

All of these remedies are available in many health food stores. To purchase the remedies by mail, refer to the resource list on page 637.

HYDROTHERAPY

The alternating foot bath is an effective way to relieve swelling in the feet and legs, says Tori Hudson, N.D., a naturopathic physician and professor at the National College of Naturopathic Medicine in Portland, Oregon. Fill one bucket or plastic wastebasket with enough comfortably hot water (about 104°F; use a regular oral thermometer to check the temperature) to cover your legs up to the knees. Fill another container with the same amount of cold water. Soak your feet and legs in the hot water for about three minutes, then immerse them in the cold water for about 30 seconds. Dr. Hudson suggests repeating this cycle three to six times every day. The treatment functions like a pump to improve circulation. "The heat brings blood to the area, and the cold sends it away," says Dr. Hudson. "This is why you should always finish with cold water. The last thing you want is for blood to pool in the feet and legs." People with serious circulatory problems should check with their doctors before using this treatment.

Water treatments can also ease the nausea and vomiting common in pregnancy, says Dr. Hudson. She suggests applying a warm compress (a towel dipped in comfortably hot water and wrung out is fine) to the entire midriff area, from armpits to hips. Leave the compress in place for 20 minutes while holding a hot water bottle to the abdomen. Dr. Hudson recommends doing the treatment about a half-hour before each meal.

Finally, to ease backaches and improve tone in the abdominal area, she suggests an alternating hot and cold shower on the lower pelvis (below the belly) and lower back. "Sixty seconds of hot water to 30 seconds cold is the most comfortable," she says. "Alternate three times and finish with cold." Repeat this treatment twice a day, morning and evening, she says.

"Pregnant women should avoid excessive heat or steam," cautions Dr. Hudson. "Don't even think about going into a hot tub or sauna." High temperatures may harm the fetus.

IMAGERY

When you feel stress building or are suffering through a bout of morning sickness, try this imagery technique, says Barbara L. Rees, R.N., Ph.D., an imagery expert and professor of nursing at the University of New Mexico College of Nursing in Albuquerque.

Imagine yourself looking out into deep space. Count backward from five. By the time you get to one, you will be surrounded by deep space. Focus your attention on your breathing. Take a deep breath and let it out slowly, then breathe easily and gently. As you breathe, see and feel your chest filling with pure, clear light, power and love. As you let out your breath, imagine all of the tension flowing out of you. As you breathe in, feel yourself becoming more relaxed and increasingly filled with light, power and love. Imagine going through your day joyfully and peacefully, feeling very well and full of light, power and love. Count again from one to five, and as you count, gradually bring yourself back. When you reach five, slowly open your eyes.

Dr. Rees suggests practicing this imagery exercise once a day, preferably in the morning and in the same place every day. During the imagery, you may feel as though your arms, legs and body are heavy or numb. This is normal, according to Dr. Rees. Leave the imagery slowly, and try to maintain the sensations of wellness, she adds.

JUICE THERAPY

Ginger relaxes the intestinal tract and is very effective against morning sickness, writes naturopathic physician Michael Murray, N.D., in *The Complete Book of Juicing*. He suggests juicing a thin slice of fresh ginger (about ¼ inch thick) and half of a handful of fresh mint with one kiwifruit and one-fourth of a fresh pineapple.

For information on juicing techniques, see page 93.

MASSAGE

A three-part massage on the breasts can help relieve soreness and engorgement, says Elaine Stillerman, L.M.T., a New York City massage therapist and author of *Mother Massage: A Handbook for Relieving the Discomforts of Pregnancy*. Rub a small amount of massage oil or cream between your hands to warm it. Then rub either one or both breasts. Make large circles around the outside of each breast, but avoid directly touching your nipple or areola. Do this for several minutes. Now massage one breast at a time, using the fingertips of one hand to make small circles around the outside of the breast. After several minutes, repeat the same stroke on the other breast. For the third part, place both hands flat on either side of the areola, with your thumbs pointing toward your head and your fingers pointing toward your waist. Then slowly slide your hands away from the areola until you reach the edge of the breast. Be sure to avoid direct massage to the sensitive areola region. Turn your hands slightly to cover a different portion of the breast, and repeat. Do this for one to two minutes, then massage the other breast.

PREMATURE EJACULATION

In sex, as in life, every man would like to last a little longer. But how fast is too fast for an orgasm? And what can you do if lovemaking loses its appeal because of premature ejaculation?

First of all, let's define premature ejaculation. Most men ejaculate faster than you might think—usually one to six minutes after beginning intercourse. But about 15 to 20 percent of men have trouble delaying ejaculation that long; some ejaculate before penetrating a woman's vagina.

Physical problems such as prostatitis and urinary tract infections can cause premature ejaculation. But experts say it more often has a psychological basis. The natural remedies in this chapter—in conjunction with medical care and used with your doctor's approval—may help prevent premature ejaculation, according to some health professionals.

SEE YOUR MEDICAL DOCTOR WHEN . . .

- You consistently ejaculate immediately after, or even before, starting sexual intercourse.

FLOWER REMEDY/ESSENCE THERAPY

Men prone to premature ejaculation may benefit from regular use of the California flower essence Hibiscus, suggests Santa Monica, California, family practice physician Cynthia Mervis Watson, M.D., who specializes in homeopathy and herbal therapy. "Tension and lack of emotional connection are often underlying reasons why a man has sexual problems. Hibiscus helps him relax and restores warmth to the sexual relationship," says Dr. Watson.

Flower essences are available in some health food stores and through mail order (refer to the resource list on page 635). For information on preparing and administering flower essences, see page 37.

HOMEOPATHY

If you have a strong sexual desire but avoid intercourse, and if you ejaculate either early or not at all, try Graphites 12C two to four times a day until you improve, suggests Chris Meletis, N.D., a naturopathic physician and medicinary director at the National College of Naturopathic Medicine in Portland, Oregon. He says that a similar dose of Nux vomica 12C may help if your symptoms include irritability, anger and intolerance of your own and others' imperfections, especially if you are very busy and have lots of worries. If you experience premature ejaculation and have itchy genitals, which may be cold and relaxed (a limp penis and sagging scrotum), Dr. Meletis recommends Sulfur 12C two to four times a day. Lycopodium 12C in a similar dose may be helpful if your symptoms are worse in the evening and with heat and better with cold, he says.

All of these remedies are available in many health food stores. To purchase the remedies by mail, refer to the resource list on page 637.

IMAGERY

"Picture yourself performing onstage. Who's watching this performance? Your mother? Your father? Your minister? Whoever it is, tell that person to go away," says Dennis Gersten, M.D., a San Diego psychiatrist and publisher of *Atlantis*, a bi-monthly imagery newsletter. "Now get off the stage and follow a trail out into the countryside until you come to a haystack in a barn. Picture it as the most down-to-earth place you can imagine. Now imagine you and your lover having a grand old time. Fill in all of the details yourself." Dr. Gersten suggests using this imagery for 10 to 20 minutes twice a day.

PREMENSTRUAL SYNDROME

Most women know the feelings: breast tenderness, acne, weight gain, bloating, mood swings, food cravings, headaches, nausea, diarrhea and constipation. They're the telltale symptoms of premenstrual syndrome, or PMS.

Experts still aren't sure exactly what causes PMS. Some research shows that it's related to hormonal changes that occur during a woman's menstrual cycle. The symptoms may arise during ovulation or just before menses, or they may appear, disappear and reappear during the same cycle. For about one in 20 women, the combination is so bad that it creates a general depression that affects the daily course of their lives. The natural remedies in this chapter—in conjunction with medical care and used with the approval of your doctor—may help ease premenstrual symptoms, according to some health professionals.

SEE YOUR MEDICAL DOCTOR WHEN . . .

- Your symptoms of PMS become so strong that they interfere with daily life.
- You show signs of depression that occur regularly during your menstrual cycle, including food cravings, crying, insomnia, emotional withdrawal and mood swings.

ACUPRESSURE

To relieve tension and bloating, press points Sp 12 and Sp 13 in the pelvic area, says Michael Reed Gach, Ph.D., director of the Acupressure Institute in Berkeley, California, and author of *Acupressure's Potent Points*. Both points are located in the middle of the crease where the leg joins the trunk of the body. Sp 12 is slightly lower and a little more toward the center than Sp 13. (To help locate these points, refer to the illustration on page 564.) Dr. Gach says you can stimulate all of these points at one time by positioning your left fist over points Sp 12 and Sp 13 on your left side and your right fist over the points on your right side. Lie on your stomach with both fists in place, using the weight of your body to apply gentle pressure. Find a comfortable position and relax for at least two minutes, suggests Dr. Gach.

He also recommends pressing Sp 4, which is located in the upper arch of each foot, one thumb-width from the ball of the foot. (For help in locating these points, refer to the illustration on page 566.) He says to firmly press one Sp 4 point with your thumb for one minute, then switch feet and press the other Sp 4 point.

FLOWER REMEDY/ESSENCE THERAPY

Women who suffer severe PMS symptoms often have deep anxieties about their sexuality, says Cynthia Mervis Watson, M.D., a family practice physician in Santa Monica, California, who specializes in homeopathy and herbal therapy. She recommends taking the California flower essence Pomegranate throughout the months to balance the female organs and encourage a healthy acceptance of reproductive processes. Over time, this may improve premenstrual symptoms, according to Dr. Watson.

Flower essences are available in some health food stores and through mail order (refer to the resource list on page 635). For information on preparing and administering flower essences, see page 37.

FOOD THERAPY

"PMS is improved with a low-fat diet," says Michael A. Klaper, M.D., a nutritional medicine specialist in Pompano Beach, Florida, and director of the Institute of Nutritional Education and Research, an organization based in Manhattan Beach, California, that teaches doctors about nutrition and its relationship to disease. High-fat foods, especially animal fats, increase symptoms and pain, so he advises that you cut down—or cut out—beef, lamb and pork. And he says to replace butter with polyunsaturated omega-3 oils such as flaxseed, canola, walnut and pumpkin seed, which are available in most health food stores.

A woman with PMS may want to try Progest HP cream, which is made from wild yam, says David Edelberg, M.D., an internist and medical director of the American Holistic Center/Chicago. To use the cream, apply ¼ to ½ teaspoonful over your hips, stomach, buttocks or thighs three times each day from the time you ovulate to the end of your period. He also suggests reducing dairy products and eliminating caffeine, sugar and alcohol. And he says that a woman with premenstrual symptoms may want to use the following regimen of dietary supplements: 400 international units of vitamin E twice a day; 50 milligrams of pyridoxine twice a day; 50 milligrams of B-complex vitamins a day; 400 milligrams of magnesium twice a day; and one capsule of evening primrose oil twice a day. Pyridoxine and evening primrose oil capsules are available in most health food stores.

HERBAL THERAPY

To prevent or reduce premenstrual symptoms, Barre, Vermont, herbalist Rosemary Gladstar, author of *Herbal Healing for Women* and other books about herbs, recommends a daily regimen of fish oil, flaxseed oil, evening primrose oil or black currant seed oil. These oils are high in gamma-linolenic acid, which helps relieve PMS symptoms, especially breast tenderness, she says. She suggests taking 500 milligrams of any one of these oils three times a day (every day, not just when you're experiencing symptoms) or following the dosage recommendations on the product's label. The oils are available in most health food stores.

HOMEOPATHY

Although PMS is usually treated on a personal, case-by-case basis by homeopaths, you might want to try one of the following 30C remedies before seeking professional help, writes Andrew Lockie, M.D., in his book *The Family Guide to Homeopathy*. He suggests taking the remedy for the symptoms that most closely match yours every 12 hours for up to three days, beginning 24 hours before PMS usually starts in your cycle.

If your breasts are tender and your symptoms are worse in the morning, try Lachesis, says Dr. Lockie. He recommends Calcarea if you crave eggs and sweets, have cold sweats and swollen and painful breasts and feel clumsy or tired. He says Nux vomica will help if you feel irritable, chilly and constipated, urinate frequently and crave sweet or fatty foods. If you are disinterested in sex, crave sweet or salty foods and feel irritable, weepy, chilly and emotionally detached, he says to try Sepia.

All of these remedies are available in many health food stores. To purchase the remedies by mail, refer to the resource list on page 637.

HYDROTHERAPY

Water treatments can ease a variety of premenstrual symptoms, according to Tori Hudson, N.D., a naturopathic physician and professor at the National College of Naturopathic Medicine in Portland, Oregon. To alleviate premenstrual headaches, Dr. Hudson recommends soaking your feet and ankles in a hot foot bath for 30 minutes while applying a cold cloth to the forehead and temples. "This treatment directs blood away from the head, which is good for the congestive headaches some women get before their periods," says Dr. Hudson.

For premenstrual mood swings, Dr. Hudson recommends a neutral bath, an extended tub soak in water just slightly cooler than body temperature. (It's the temperature at which you start to feel chilly when a hot bath cools off, says Dr. Hudson.) She recommends soaking for about 20 minutes first thing in the morning, before bed or whenever you're feeling particularly frazzled, adding water as needed to maintain the temperature of the bath.

PREMENSTRUAL SYNDROME

IMAGERY

To help relieve bloating associated with PMS, try this imagery suggested by New York City psychiatrist Gerald Epstein, M.D., in his book *Healing Visualizations*. Close your eyes and breathe out three times. Picture yourself in a desert. Cover your body with sand and let the sun bake it into your skin. Sense the sand soaking up excessive water from your body and the sun drying up the sand. Open your eyes.

Dr. Epstein suggests that you begin doing this imagery at the first sign of premenstrual symptoms. Repeat three or four times a day, one to two minutes at a time, until the end of your menstrual cycle.

JUICE THERAPY

Beta-carotene and magnesium may help reduce PMS symptoms, says Cherie Calbom, M.S., a certified nutritionist in Kirkland, Washington, and co-author of *Juicing for Life*. She recommends increasing your beta-carotene intake during the week before your period by drinking a juice blend of five to seven carrots (for beta-carotene) and a handful of parsley (for magnesium) every day.

If you experience premenstrual bloating due to water retention, try drinking fresh grape or watermelon juice once a day. "These are natural diuretics," says Calbom.

For information on juicing techniques, see page 93.

REFLEXOLOGY

To help control hormone balance, relieve stress and help you relax, work the diaphragm and pituitary, thyroid and adrenal gland reflex points on your hands or feet, suggests St. Petersburg, Florida, reflexologist Dwight Byers, author of *Better Health with Foot Reflexology*.

To help you locate these points, consult the hand and foot reflex charts beginning on page 582. For instructions on how to work the points, see "Your Reflexology Session" on page 110.

RELAXATION AND MEDITATION

Meditating for 20 minutes twice a day triggers deep muscle relaxation, which may lessen the pain of PMS, says Sundar Ramaswami, Ph.D., a clinical psychologist at the F. S. Dubois Community Mental Health Center in Stamford, Connecticut. For information on how to meditate, see page 117.

VITAMIN AND MINERAL THERAPY

"The key treatments are vitamin B₆, evening primrose oil, calcium and magnesium," says Elson Haas, M.D., director of the Preventive Medical Center of Marin in San Rafael, California, and author of *Staying Healthy with Nutrition*. He suggests taking 50 milligrams of vitamin B_6 twice a day, along with the Recommended Dietary Allowances (RDAs) for calcium and magnesium, starting seven to ten days before your period and continuing until your period begins. (The RDAs for these nutrients are listed in "Getting What You Need" on page 142.) For evening primrose oil, Dr. Haas says to follow the manufacturer's recommendations on the package; these supplements are available in most health food stores.

YOGA

A pose called the butterfly (page 624) can help relieve PMS symptoms, say Dr. Robin Monro, Dr. R. Nagarathna and Dr. H. R. Nagendra in their book *Yoga for Common Ailments*. They recommend including this pose in your daily yoga routine whenever you're experiencing symptoms.

PROSTATE PROBLEMS

The prostate is a small gland that encircles the neck of the bladder and the tube that carries urine from the bladder. Found only in men, the prostate adds fluid to sperm just before ejaculation.

It's also responsible for a lot of discomfort. In about 60 percent of men over age 50, the prostate becomes enlarged—sometimes as big as an orange—and restricts the flow of urine. The condition is painless but can be frustrating to live with.

Prostate cancer is another major concern. More than 30 percent of men over age 50 may already have it, but it's a very slow-growing form of cancer that won't cause immediate health problems for most of them. Still, doctors recommend a yearly rectal exam for all men over 40. The natural remedies in this chapter—in conjunction with medical care and used with the approval of your doctor—may help prevent a prostate problem or lessen its symptoms, according to some health professionals.

PROSTATE PROBLEMS

SEE YOUR MEDICAL DOCTOR WHEN . . .

- You experience painful urination, coupled with lower back pain, fever and pelvic pain.
- You frequently feel the urge to urinate but can't get a stream started.
- Your urine stream is weak.
- You repeatedly urinate two or three times a night.
- You finish urinating but your bladder still feels full.

AYURVEDA

First, see a medical professional to find out what's causing the problem, says Vasant Lad, B.A.M.S., M.A.Sc., director of the Ayurvedic Institute in Albuquerque, New Mexico. If the cause is benign, the following remedy can be useful for self-treatment, according to Dr. Lad: Mix equal amounts of punarnava, gokshura and shilajit, which are herbal powders available in Indian pharmacies or by mail order (refer to the resource list on page 634). Dr. Lad says to take ¼ teaspoon of this mixture twice daily, either dry or mixed with a little warm water.

Or buy horsetail, ginseng or hibiscus tea, Dr. Lad says (these teas are available in most health food stores). Drink any one or more of these teas daily, as frequently as you wish.

FOOD THERAPY

"Eat more pumpkin seeds, sunflower seeds and other foods high in zinc," advises Allan Magaziner, D.O., a nutritional medicine specialist and head of the Magaziner Medical Center in Cherry Hill, New Jersey. "Zinc has been shown to have a beneficial effect in shrinking an enlarged prostate." (For other food sources of zinc, see "Getting What You Need" on page 142.)

HYDROTHERAPY

A hot sitz bath may be beneficial for prostate inflammation, according to Agatha Thrash, M.D., a medical pathologist and co-founder and co-director of Uchee Pines Institute, a natural healing center in Seale, Alabama. Fill a tub with enough comfortably hot water to cover the navel, then sit down and soak for 20 to 45 minutes. Follow with a cold bath or shower. Dr. Thrash suggests using this treatment once a day for 30 days or until symptoms subside.

PROSTATE PROBLEMS

IMAGERY

This imagery exercise from *Healing Visualizations* by New York City psychiatrist Gerald Epstein, M.D., may help you corral an enlarged prostate. Close your eyes, breathe out three times and imagine entering your body through any opening you choose. Find your prostate and examine it from every angle. Next, envision putting a thin golden net around the gland. This net has a drawstring that you can tighten. Cinch the drawstring so that the net is wrapped snugly around the prostate. As you do this, picture the prostate shrinking to its normal size. Then imagine using your other hand to massage your prostate. Sense that urine can now flow evenly and smoothly.

Dr. Epstein says to practice this imagery twice a day, three to five minutes a session, for six cycles of 21 days on and 7 days off.

REFLEXOLOGY

Focus on the prostate reflex as well as on the endocrine gland reflexes (pituitary, parathyroid, thyroid and adrenal glands and pancreas) on your hands or feet, according to Rebecca Dioda, a reflexologist with the Morris Institute of Natural Therapeutics, a holistic health education center in Denville, New Jersey. A reflexology session helps relax the entire body, and paying special attention to the prostate reflex may help the body heal itself, she says.

To help you locate these points, consult the hand and foot reflex charts beginning on page 582. For instructions on how to work the points, see "Your Reflexology Session" on page 110.

VITAMIN AND MINERAL THERAPY

"Take a 15- to 30-milligram supplement of zinc each day," says Allan Magaziner, D.O., a nutritional medicine specialist and head of the Magaziner Medical Center in Cherry Hill, New Jersey. "It's also good to get more essential fatty acids, such as those in flaxseed oil, which help prevent inflammation and swelling of the prostate." Dr. Magaziner recommends taking up to two teaspoons of flaxseed oil a day; if it's in capsule form, he says to follow the dosage recommendations on the label (about three capsules equals one teaspoon of the liquid). Both forms of flaxseed oil are available in most health food stores.

A person with prostate problems may want to use the following vitamin, mineral and herbal regimen to help control or reverse the disease, suggests David Edelberg, M.D., an internist and medical director of the American Holistic Center/Chicago: 400 international units of vitamin E a day; 30 milligrams of zinc twice a day; 1 milligram of copper twice a day; one tablespoon of flaxseed oil a day; and 160 milligrams of saw palmetto twice a day. Saw palmetto is also available in most health food stores.

YOGA

Make two poses—the knee squeeze (page 612) and the seated sun (page 616)—part of your daily yoga routine, says Alice Christensen, founder and executive director of the American Yoga Association. She explains that these poses can increase circulation to your groin and ease prostate troubles. She recommends practicing the two poses, along with a yoga exercise called the stomach lock, every day.

To do the stomach lock, says Christensen, lie on your back and take a deep breath. Breathe out until the breath is completely gone, then pull in hard on your buttocks, groin and stomach muscles. Hold for a count of three, then release your muscles. Christensen suggests doing this two or three times per day, three times per session, to help prevent prostate problems. You can also use the exercise as needed when problems flare up, she adds.

You should not practice this pose if you have high blood pressure, hiatal hernia, ulcers or heart disease, according to Stephen A. Nezezon, M.D., yoga teacher and staff physician at the Himalayan International Institute of Yoga Science and Philosophy in Honesdale, Pennsylvania.

PSORIASIS

Psoriasis isn't a hidden problem. When it flares up, red, scaly sores form on your elbows, knees, scalp, chest and back, itching like crazy and defying all attempts to make them go away.

Psoriasis is skin growth gone bananas. Your average skin cell grows, matures and sheds in about a month, leaving room for new skin. But when you have psoriasis, some cells grow about seven times faster than normal. Your body has a hard time shedding them off because they develop so quickly. The result is the telltale crusty lesions.

No one is sure what causes psoriasis. Doctors know that it doesn't spread from person to person, though it does run in families. There's no known cure for psoriasis. But the natural remedies in this chapter—in conjunction with medical care and used with your doctor's approval—may help lessen the severity of psoriasis, according to some health professionals.

SEE YOUR MEDICAL DOCTOR WHEN . . .

- You notice flaking skin that itches intensely.
- Your flaking skin becomes red or infected or resembles fish scales.
- Your home treatment for the flaking skin fails to help after three weeks.

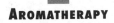

AROMATHERAPY

The gentle oil German chamomile is great for soothing inflamed, sensitive skin, says Fair Oaks, California, aromatherapist Victoria Edwards. She recommends a ten-minute soak in warm (not hot) water spiked with five drops of German chamomile. After the bath, says Edwards, apply a nourishing oil made from one drop of German chamomile per one ounce of carrier oil. (Carrier oils are available in most health food stores.)

For information on preparing and administering essential oils, including cautions about their use, see page 19. For information on purchasing essential oils, refer to the resource list on page 633.

FOOD THERAPY

Salmon, mackerel and other fish rich in omega-3 fatty acids have long been touted as a way to help ease psoriasis. But if you prefer your main course to be a land animal, take another look at turkey. "In one study, people who ate a lot of turkey showed marked improvement, but the researchers weren't sure whether it was something in the turkey itself or the fact that people were forgoing other meats that are higher in saturated fat," says registered pharmacist Earl Mindell, R.Ph., Ph.D., author of *Earl Mindell's Food as Medicine* and other books on nutrition and professor of nutrition at Pacific Western University in Los Angeles.

Dr. Mindell adds that celery, parsley, lettuce, limes and lemons may also help you rid your skin of those nasty blotches, since these foods contain psoralens, compounds that make the skin more sensitive to light (and, as a result, can reduce psoriasis lesions). In fact, synthetic psoralens, which can be applied on the skin or taken orally, are often used to treat psoriasis.

HOMEOPATHY

Psoriasis should be treated on an individual basis by a medical doctor or homeopath. But while waiting for professional care, you can try one of the following 6C remedies four times daily for up to 14 days, writes Andrew Lockie, M.D., in *The Family Guide to Homeopathy*.

For psoriasis that is aggravated by cold and is worse in the winter, try Petroleum, according to Dr. Lockie. If you have patches of extremely scaly skin that are worsened by heat, he recommends Kali arsenicosum. Graphites will help, he says, if the skin behind your ears is affected and secretes honey-colored pus. If you feel chilly and mentally restless but physically exhausted and your psoriasis feels burning hot, he says to try Arsenicum.

A 30C dose of Sulphur taken orally four times a day for up to 14 days may soothe your symptoms if you often feel overheated and you have dry, scaly, itchy patches of skin that are worse after bathing, says Dr. Lockie.

All of these remedies are available in many health food stores. To purchase the remedies by mail, refer to the resource list on page 637.

HYDROTHERAPY

A warm bath with salt may benefit psoriasis, according to Agatha Thrash, M.D., a medical pathologist and co-founder and co-director of Uchee Pines Institute, a natural healing center in Seale, Alabama. Use a pound or more of table salt, mineral salts or sea salts (available in most health food stores) per tub of warm water. Dr. Thrash suggests keeping the bath brief—10 to 30 minutes—and always finishing with a short cold shower. Use this treatment once or twice a day for a month, she adds.

IMAGERY

Close your eyes, breathe out three times and see, sense and feel yourself naked, suggests New York City psychiatrist Gerald Epstein, M.D., in his book *Healing Visualizations*. Now imagine you are sitting at the North Pole with a golden ice pick. Take the ice pick and remove all of the white scales on your body until you see healthy skin. After you have done that, dive into the cold Arctic water, washing your skin thoroughly. When you emerge from the water, picture an icy film of Arctic water covering your entire body. Scoop a glob of golden whale oil from a jar and smear it all over your ice-coated body. Put on a royal purple robe and see yourself as a healthy person free of scales.

Dr. Epstein says to practice this imagery for three minutes a day for 21 days, then take 7 days off. Repeat for one to two minutes a day for another 21 days, followed by another 7 days off. Then do it for up to one minute a day for 21 days. If there is no improvement at that point, consult your doctor.

JUICE THERAPY

"Many people with psoriasis have congestion in the bowels and liver," says Cherie Calbom, M.S., a certified nutritionist in Kirkland, Washington, and co-author of *Juicing for Life*. "A high-fiber diet will absorb toxins in the gut, and beet juice is wonderful to help detoxify the liver." Because beets have a strong flavor, she suggests blending beet juice with carrot juice and lemon. "One beet to four carrots (add one-fourth of a lemon to improve the flavor) is an ideal proportion," according to Calbom. She recommends drinking one glass of the juice every day.

For information on juicing techniques, see page 93.

REFLEXOLOGY

Work the kidney points on the bottoms of both feet, say Kevin and Barbara Kunz, reflexology researchers in Santa Fe, New Mexico, and authors of *Hand and Foot Reflexology*. They also suggest working these points on your hands: kidney, brain, uterus/prostate, ovary/testicle, pancreas and pituitary and thyroid gland.

To help you locate these points, consult the hand and foot reflex charts beginning on page 582. For instructions on how to work the points, see "Your Reflexology Session" on page 110.

VITAMIN AND MINERAL THERAPY

"Take one teaspoon of flaxseed oil each day, along with 400 international units of vitamin A and a zinc supplement ranging from 15 to 30 milligrams," says Michael A. Klaper, M.D., a nutritional medicine specialist in Pompano Beach, Florida, and director of the Institute of Nutritional Education and Research, an organization based in Manhattan Beach, California, that teaches doctors about nutrition and its relationship to disease. Flaxseed oil has been shown to improve a number of skin conditions, including psoriasis, according to Dr. Klaper. Flaxseed oil is available in liquid and capsule form in most health food stores. If you choose the capsules, Dr. Klaper says to follow the dosage recommendations on the label (generally, about three capsules equals one teaspoon of the liquid).

YOGA

Psoriasis can worsen during periods of stress, says Stephen A. Nezezon, M.D., yoga teacher and staff physician at the Himalayan International Institute of Yoga Science and Philosophy in Honesdale, Pennsylvania. To lower stress, Dr. Nezezon recommends a daily routine of breathing exercises, meditation and yoga poses.

Do the complete breath exercise (see page 152) whenever you're feeling stressed out, suggests Alice Christensen, founder and executive director of the American Yoga Association. Meditation (see page 153) helps clear your mind and teaches you to relax at will, she says. And for the poses, choose three or four from the Daily Routine, which begins on page 606. Christensen suggests varying the poses daily to keep your interest high and to strengthen different parts of your body. Dr. Nezezon says you should include at least one relaxation pose, such as the corpse (page 612), knee squeeze (page 612) or baby (page 618), in your daily yoga routine.

SEE ALSO Dermatitis and Eczema

RASHES

Arash can leave you scratching your head as well as your skin, and with good reason. From sunscreens to detergents, poisonous plants to cosmetics, there seems to be no end to the number of substances that can trigger a rash.

And apparently, there's no end to the hassles that a rash can cause. Whether red and itchy, wet and oozing, dry and flaky, hot and bumpy or cold and clammy, rashes have one thing in common: They're aggravating. From obvious culprits such as poison ivy and razor burn to that mysterious reaction to eating the "wrong" food or to wearing clothing made with an allergy-causing chemical, a rash is your skin's way of telling your body that something is not right. The natural remedies in this chapter, used with your doctor's approval, may help soothe or heal a rash, according to some health professionals.

SEE YOUR MEDICAL DOCTOR WHEN...

- Your rash develops when you feel sick or run a fever or after you take any medication.
- Your rash stings or burns, turns raw or blisters.
- You develop a bull's-eye rash after being bitten by a tick—even months later.
- Your household includes more than one person with the same type of rash.
- You have small black or purplish dots on most of your skin and have a bad headache or feel lethargic.

AYURVEDA

For hot, itchy skin rashes, mix one teaspoon of ghee, or clarified butter, with a pinch of black pepper and take this mixture twice a day until your symptoms clear, says Vasant Lad, B.A.M.S., M.A.Sc., director of the Ayurvedic Institute in Albuquerque, New Mexico. (For a recipe for ghee, see "How to Make Ghee" on page 26.)

To soothe hives and the nausea that can accompany an allergic rash, Dr. Lad suggests steeping 1 teaspoon of coriander, ½ teaspoon of cumin and 1 teaspoon of raw sugar in one cup of hot milk. Drink this mixture once or twice a day until your symptoms are gone, he says.

HERBAL THERAPY

Try dried chamomile to make a soothing wash for poison ivy, poison oak or poison sumac rashes, says Varro E. Tyler, Ph.D., professor of pharmacognosy at Purdue University in West Lafayette, Indiana. He says to steep two tablespoons of dried chamomile (available in most health food stores) in two cups of boiling water for about ten minutes. Let it cool, dip a washcloth in the wash and spread it on the rash. You can use this remedy as often as you like, he says.

HYDROTHERAPY

An oatmeal bath helps soothe and heal irritated skin, says Agatha Thrash, M.D., a medical pathologist and co-founder and co-director of Uchee Pines Institute, a natural healing center in Seale, Alabama. Using your blender, grind a cup of rolled oats into a fine powder and add it to a hot bath. Soak for 20 to 30 minutes, then pat the skin dry. Dr. Thrash recommends using this treatment once or twice a day for one to two weeks or until symptoms subside.

JUICE THERAPY

Both apple and dark grape juices may be beneficial to those with reddish skin rashes, says John Peterson, M.D., an Ayurvedic practitioner in Muncie, Indiana. These sweet juices are used to "cool" many skin problems, according to Dr. Peterson. He recommends drinking the juices at about room temperature and apart from meals. If the juices seem too strong, he says, they can be diluted with water. He adds that papaya and pineapple juices may also be beneficial.

For information on juicing techniques, see page 93.

VITAMIN AND MINERAL THERAPY

Many rashes respond to increased intakes of zinc and vitamins A and C, nutrients that repair and build skin tissue, says Elson Haas, M.D., director of the Preventive Medical Center of Marin in San Rafael, California, and author of

Staying Healthy with Nutrition. He recommends 5,000 international units of vitamin A a day, along with 5,000 milligrams of vitamin C and up to 30 milligrams of zinc. He says to continue these levels of supplementation until the rash clears up.

SEE ALSO Heat Rash; Lyme Disease

RAYNAUD'S DISEASE

You can understand when Jack Frost does his nipping in the dead of winter. In fact, you almost expect it. But when you're reaching for a Labor Day beer or sitting in air-conditioning to beat the July 4th heat? That's a sign of Raynaud's disease, which leaves hands and feet cold, painful and numb at the slightest change in temperature, such as opening a refrigerator door or walking into an air-conditioned room. Caused by a loss of blood circulation to the outer extremities, Raynaud's does more than cause pain. Fingers and toes turn white or bluish as they get colder. When they warm again, they become red and may throb with pain for hours.

Experts say that Raynaud's may result from overactive blood vessels, disorders of connective tissue or even emotional upset. Wearing gloves and heavy socks and sticking extremities in warm water can help. And the natural remedies in this chapter—in conjunction with medical care and used with your doctor's approval—may help ease the symptoms of Raynaud's disease, according to some health professionals.

SEE YOUR MEDICAL DOCTOR WHEN . . .

• Your fingers feel weaker or your sense of touch seems compromised.
• You think your condition is getting worse.

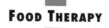

FOOD THERAPY

"Cayenne pepper helps with circulation," says registered pharmacist Earl Mindell, R.Ph., Ph.D., author of *Earl Mindell's Food as Medicine* and other books on nutrition and professor of nutrition at Pacific Western University in Los Angeles. He suggests sprinkling it on foods or mixing it (or another chili pepper powder) in a glass of water and drinking up.

HOMEOPATHY

Although most cases of Raynaud's disease are treated by homeopaths on an individual basis, you could try one of these 6C remedies suggested by Andrew Lockie, M.D., in his book *The Family Guide to Homeopathy*. He says to take the remedy of your choice every 30 minutes until your symptoms subside. Do not take more than ten doses of any of these remedies, he adds.

If your body feels cold except for a burning sensation in the fingers or toes that is worsened by heat, take Secale, according to Dr. Lockie. He says that Carbo vegetabilis is a good treatment when your skin is icy cold and mottled and your natural color returns after fanning. If your skin appears bluish purple, particularly after sleep, he says to try Lachesis. If heat or letting your arms or legs hang down makes the symptoms worse, he recommends Pulsatilla. For pale skin that flushes easily and is improved when you apply cold, try Ferrum phosphoricum, he says. If your hands are icy cold, your feet are swollen and you have restless legs, he suggests Cactus.

All of these remedies are available in many health food stores. To purchase the remedies by mail, refer to the resource list on page 637.

RELAXATION AND MEDITATION

Autogenics and thermal biofeedback may improve your circulation and take the chilling bite out of Raynaud's disease, says Steven Fahrion, Ph.D., director of research at the Life Sciences Institute of Mind-Body Health in Topeka, Kansas. To learn how to do autogenics, see page 120; for more on thermal biofeedback, see page 121.

VITAMIN AND MINERAL THERAPY

Take vitamin E to improve blood flow, says registered pharmacist Earl Mindell, R.Ph., Ph.D., author of *Earl Mindell's Food as Medicine* and other books on nutrition and professor of nutrition at Pacific Western University in Los Angeles. He recommends a daily supplement of between 100 and 400 international units.

REPETITIVE STRAIN INJURY AND CARPAL TUNNEL SYNDROME

The computer age has revolutionized nearly every facet of modern life, from paying taxes to making hotel reservations to finding a book at the library. It has also brought us repetitive strain injury, a disabling pain of the neck, shoulders, wrists or hands that commonly affects those who spend their days typing on computers.

Repetitive strain injury is caused by overuse of tendons, resulting in pain, swelling and pressure on nearby nerves. The best-known form of repetitive strain injury is carpal tunnel syndrome, a debilitating pain in the wrist caused by pressure on the median nerve where it passes through the bony carpal tunnel in the wrist.

Common symptoms of repetitive strain injury include persistent tingling, pain or numbness in the wrists, hands or forearms. Some people also experience swelling in the hands or start dropping things because they have trouble controlling their fingers. If you're experiencing any of these symptoms, see your doctor for an evaluation, since early intervention can keep this condition from worsening. The natural remedies in this chapter—in conjunction with medical care and used with your doctor's approval—may help those with repetitive strain injury or carpal tunnel syndrome, according to some health professionals.

SEE YOUR MEDICAL DOCTOR WHEN...

- Your hands, wrists or forearms become numb or tingly while you're performing repetitive tasks.
- You have pain in the neck, shoulders, wrists or hands that limits your usual activities.
- Your hands are swollen and painful.

ACUPRESSURE

While sitting comfortably, press points P 7, located on the inside of each arm in the middle of the wrist crease, and TW 4, on the outside of the arm in the hollow at the center of the wrist crease, says Michael Reed Gach, Ph.D., director of the Acupressure Institute in Berkeley, California, and author of *Acupressure's Potent Points*. (To help locate these points, refer to the illustrations beginning on page 564.) You can work the two points simultaneously, says Dr. Gach, by placing your left thumb on the TW 4 point of your right wrist and your left fingers on the P 7 point of your right wrist. He recommends pressing these points for a few minutes, then switching sides. Repeat this treatment throughout the day, he adds.

You can also use a shiatsu technique to press points in a line on your forearm, from the wrist to the elbow, according to Dr. Gach. He says to use all of your fingers to press up the outside of your forearm and your thumb to exert complementary pressure on the inside of your forearm. Press into the muscles on both sides of the bone structure, starting about three inches up from the wrist crease. "Squeeze for ten seconds and release. Then slide up a half-inch, squeeze and hold again for ten seconds. Repeat by half-inches all the way up to the elbow. Do this exercise on both arms whenever you think of it, as frequently as possible throughout the day," says Dr. Gach.

HOMEOPATHY

If you have stiff and painful joints that are hot and swollen and that feel worse with motion, take a 30C dose of Bryonia once a day or a 12C dose twice a day until you begin to feel better, says Cynthia Mervis Watson, M.D., a family practice physician in Santa Monica, California, specializing in homeopathy and herbal therapy. She says a similar dose of Rhus toxicodendron will relieve painful joints accompanied by stiffness in the neck and the small of the back that is worse in cold weather and better on warm, dry days or after exercise.

A 30C dose of Cimicifuga, taken once a day until you feel better, is a good remedy for symptoms such as an uneasy, restless feeling and achy muscles that are worse in the cold and in the morning, says Dr. Watson. She suggests a similar dose of Ruta graveolens if you have a tendon injury or ganglion cysts along with pain and stiffness, especially in cold and wet weather.

All of these remedies are available in many health food stores. To purchase the remedies by mail, refer to the resource list on page 637.

HYDROTHERAPY

Try nightly water treatments for carpal tunnel syndrome, suggests Agatha Thrash, M.D., a medical pathologist and co-founder and co-director of Uchee Pines Institute, a natural healing center in Seale, Alabama. She says to soak the hand and wrist in warm to hot water for 12 to 15 minutes, moving the fingers to increase circulation. Finish with a splash of cold water.

"The repetitive strain injuries of musicians and office workers are usually treated better with ice water than with heat," says Dr. Thrash. She has found that some people respond better to a 12- to 15-minute ice water soak done nightly. She says to put ice cubes in enough cold water to submerge the hand and arm to just above the elbow.

RELAXATION AND MEDITATION

Progressive relaxation is a terrific way to relieve hand and wrist tension, says Glenda L. Key, P.T., a physical therapist in Minneapolis who uses the technique to cope with her own carpal tunnel syndrome.

"The wrist is an area that you very easily tense up unconsciously. I find that progressive relaxation is one of the best ways to relax that area," Key says. To give progressive relaxation a try, see page 122. For the best results, practice this technique before starting work and then after every break.

VITAMIN AND MINERAL THERAPY

"Research shows that taking 50 milligrams of vitamin B_6 every day can help those with carpal tunnel syndrome," says Alan Gaby, M.D., a physician specializing in preventive and nutritional medicine in Baltimore and president of the American Holistic Medical Association. In fact, he says, research indicates that people who are deficient in B vitamins are more likely to develop the problem than those who aren't.

RESTLESS LEGS SYNDROME

After you've been running all day, the last thing you want your gams to do is the cha-cha—especially while you're trying to sleep. But that's what happens to people who suffer from restless legs syndrome, which causes an irresistible urge to thrash about, usually within 30 minutes after going to bed.

What makes legs restless? It's usually an impulse to relieve the tickling, prickling or burning discomfort triggered by this syndrome. Doctors aren't sure what causes these sensations, but some suspect that it's due to an abnormality in brain chemistry that affects nerve signals to the limbs. Others believe that caffeine or nicotine may play a role or that it may be related to anxiety, fatigue, iron deficiency anemia or stress. It tends to run in families, and pregnant women are the most likely candidates. (The problem usually disappears after delivery.) The natural remedies in this chapter—in conjunction with medical care and used with the approval of your doctor—may help ease restless legs syndrome, according to some health professionals.

SEE YOUR MEDICAL DOCTOR WHEN . . .

- Your legs feel tingly or numb or jerk suddenly and often, with a crawling sensation under the skin.
- Your leg discomfort seriously interferes with your sleep.

FOOD THERAPY

"There have been medical studies advising people with restless legs to increase their intakes of folate, which is found in dark green leafy vegetables," says Allan Magaziner, D.O., a nutritional medicine specialist and head of the Magaziner Medical Center in Cherry Hill, New Jersey. (For other food sources of folate, see "Getting What You Need" on page 142.)

HOMEOPATHY

If you have weakness, twitching and jerking in your legs and you are always moving them, try Tarentula hispanica 12C three times a day until improvement is noted, says Chris Meletis, N.D., a naturopathic physician and medicinary director at the National College of Naturopathic Medicine in Portland, Oregon. For legs that are restless at night, he says that Causticum 12C in a similar dose may be helpful. Zinc metallicum 12C three times a day is the remedy of choice if your legs are worse in the evening and your feet are continuously moving, according to Dr. Meletis.

All of these remedies are available in many health food stores. To purchase the remedies by mail, refer to the resource list on page 637.

JUICE THERAPY

Restless legs syndrome is sometimes caused by a folate deficiency, writes Cherie Calbom, M.S., a certified nutritionist in Kirkland, Washington, in *Juicing for Life*. In such cases, a daily dose of asparagus, spinach or kale juice, all rich sources of the nutrient folate, may be enough to keep your legs still at night. Calbom recommends mixing four ounces of one of the folate-rich juices with an equal amount of carrot juice and drinking the blend daily.

For information on juicing techniques, see page 93.

MASSAGE

If you can reach your calf muscles with your hands, you may be able to relieve restless legs with massage, says Elliot Greene, past president of the American Massage Therapy Association. Begin by placing the palm of your left hand on the largest part of your right calf. Your fingers should be pointing toward your heel. Then grab the muscle firmly in your hand and pull it away from your leg as far as is comfortable. Squeeze the muscle gently several times, then release the muscle. Repeat this for about five minutes, then switch to your left calf, using your right hand to do the massage.

If your thighs feel restless, Greene says to try stroking and grasping them gently with both hands. Start at the knees and pull your hands toward your hips. Use the effleurage (page 570) and petrissage (page 570) strokes. Do this for three to five minutes on each leg.

YOGA

Yoga exercises that improve circulation to your lower body are a great way to handle restless legs, according to Alice Christensen, founder and executive director of the American Yoga Association. She says that two useful poses are the knee squeeze (page 612) and the spine twist (page 614). Make them part of your daily yoga routine.

ROSACEA

It may come in handy when you're making like Santa Claus, but this chronic skin condition usually leaves you anything but jolly. Rosacea causes the nose and cheeks to suddenly turn beet red, often after eating spicy foods, drinking alcohol or a hot beverage or being out in hot weather.

While its cause is unknown, rosacea affects about 5 percent of the population, most often women between ages 30 and 40. It can cause permanent redness of the skin, sometimes with tiny pustules that resemble acne. In men, it can lead to a reddened, bulbous nose, à la W. C. Fields. Generally, a lengthy antibiotic treatment can suppress symptoms. The natural remedies in this chapter—in conjunction with medical care and used with the approval of your doctor—may help those with rosacea, according to some health professionals.

ROSACEA

• Your nose and cheeks are persistently red.
• You also have acnelike bumps on affected areas.

FOOD THERAPY

"Don't drink alcohol, because it makes rosacea worse," says Allan Magaziner, D.O., a nutritional medicine specialist and head of the Magaziner Medical Center in Cherry Hill, New Jersey. He explains that alcohol causes blood vessels in the skin to dilate, making rosacea much more noticeable. For the same reason, he says, it's also wise to avoid hot beverages and hot or spicy foods. Instead, Dr. Magaziner suggests that you try eating more dark green vegetables such as broccoli, kale, asparagus and spinach. He points out that these foods are high in vitamins A and C, beta-carotene and bioflavonoids, which can improve rosacea by strengthening capillaries and boosting the immune system. (For other food sources of vitamin A and vitamin C, see "Getting What You Need" on page 142.)

JUICE THERAPY

Both apple and dark grape juices may be beneficial to those suffering from rosacea, says John Peterson, M.D., an Ayurvedic practitioner in Muncie, Indiana. Drink the juices at room temperature and at a time other than mealtime, he advises. And, he says, you can dilute the juices with water if they taste too strong.

For information on juicing techniques, see page 93.

SCARRING

Usually, the only purpose of a scar is to forever remind you of an incident that you'd rather forget—an injury, illness, vaccination or surgery.

But these often unsightly marks don't have to be permanently etched in skin. Often you can help scars fade faster or even avoid them by treating your skin right during the healing process. Don't pick at a wound while it's healing, since that can increase your chances of developing a scar. And protect new scars from the sun's ultraviolet rays with sunscreen. Scars have less pigment than the rest of your skin, so they're especially vulnerable to sunburn and prolonged redness, making them even more prominent. The natural remedies in this chapter, used with your doctor's approval, may help minimize scarring, according to some health professionals.

SEE YOUR MEDICAL DOCTOR WHEN . . .

- Your wound continues to be inflamed or discolored or produces pus after several days.
- Your wound increases in size or severity.
- You have a cut or gash that doesn't heal within a month.

AROMATHERAPY

While treating her daughter's chickenpox scars, Victoria Edwards, an aromatherapist in Fair Oaks, California, discovered the skin-saving power of rose hip seed oil. Her recipe calls for one ounce of rose hip seed, one drop of rose and two drops of everlast (also known as immortelle or helichrysum) essential oils. Edwards says to store the mixture in a dark glass bottle and apply it to scars once a day after bathing. "It's a little expensive because of the rose oil, but there's simply nothing better for minimizing scarring," she says. She also recommends it for preventing keloids, which are enlarged, elevated scars that sometimes result from cuts, burns and surgical incisions.

For information on preparing and administering essential oils, including cautions about their use, see page 19. For information on purchasing essential oils, refer to the resource list on page 633.

AYURVEDA

To keep scar tissue from forming, David Frawley, O.M.D., director of the American Institute of Vedic Studies in Santa Fe, New Mexico, recommends this remedy for the week immediately following surgery: Blend ¼ teaspoon of turmeric, ¼ teaspoon of myrrh and a pinch of saffron (it's for flavor, so it's optional) with a little warm water or honey, then take this twice a day. You can get myrrh in most health food stores or through mail order (refer to the resource list on page 634).

HERBAL THERAPY

Calendula's bright orange flowers help reduce inflammation and promote the healing of wounds, says Varro E. Tyler, Ph.D., professor of pharmacognosy at Purdue University in West Lafayette, Indiana. Look for calendula gel or cream (available in most health food stores), he says, and follow the label directions for application.

HOMEOPATHY

A 1X or 10 percent ointment made from Thiosinaminum, which is oil of mustard seed, is an effective remedy for painful scarring if it is applied two or three times a day for several weeks, says Mitchell Fleisher, M.D., a family practice physician and homeopath in Colleen, Virginia. Although it is usually not available, some homeopathic pharmacies will prepare the ointment for you if you request it. For homeopathic pharmacies with mail-order services, see the resource list on page 637.

MASSAGE

A technique called rolling can help you loosen and break down stiff scar tissue, suggests Elliot Greene, past president of the American Massage Therapy Association. Do this only on well-healed scars, he cautions. Start at one end of the scar and pinch it gently between your forefinger and thumb. Moving lengthwise, continuously roll the scar between your fingers as you work your way to the other end of the scar. Work a fresh scar for one to two minutes. If the scar is older, work it for three to four minutes. Stop if you feel discomfort or tenderness. Once you are finished, you can rub on some vitamin E oil to soften your skin. (You can either buy the oil, which is available in most health food stores, or break open a capsule of vitamin E.) Greene recommends doing this once a day unless you notice redness or soreness. If you develop these symptoms, he says, stop until they subside.

SCIATICA

The largest nerve in your body can be quite unnerving, causing one massive pain in your buttocks—literally. Sciatica is a pain in the sciatic nerve that radiates from the buttocks down the back of the leg to the knee or even to the big toe. Often one side of the hip feels worse than the other.

Sciatica can result when the nerve is pinched from sitting on a hard stool, wearing a tight belt or even carrying a wallet in your back pocket. It's usually treated with a series of supervised exercises by a physical therapist. The natural remedies in this chapter—in conjunction with medical care and used with the approval of your doctor—may help prevent or ease sciatica, according to some health professionals.

SEE YOUR MEDICAL DOCTOR WHEN...

- You feel unexplained pain, weakness or numbness in your buttocks, in one side of your hip or in the back of your leg.
- You experience a loss of bowel or bladder control.

FOOD THERAPY

"I don't know why it works, but studies show that some people with sciatica have gotten relief by consuming large amounts of potassium," says Julian Whitaker, M.D., founder and president of the Whitaker Wellness Center in Newport Beach, California. "I'd advise eating as many potassium-rich foods as possible—things such as bananas, oranges and potatoes." (For more food sources of potassium, see "Getting What You Need" on page 142.)

HYDROTHERAPY

A shallow bath provides effective relief of sciatica pain, suggests Agatha Thrash, M.D., a medical pathologist and co-founder and co-director of Uchee Pines Institute, a natural healing center in Seale, Alabama. Fill your bathtub with enough warm water, about body temperature, to cover you up to the waist, then soak for 20 minutes to two hours. Finish each bath with a shower that starts out with lukewarm water and ends with cool. If the pain is too intense to sit in a tub, Dr. Thrash recommends a hot shower. Stay in it for 20 minutes or so, holding the water in the tub, since it warms up the venous blood returning from the feet.

MASSAGE

Here is a massage for sciatica from Elaine Stillerman, L.M.T., a massage therapist in New York City: First, sit comfortably in a chair, on a bed or on a padded surface on the floor. Support your lower back with pillows or cushions. Rub massage cream between your hands, and with open palms, use effleurage (page 570) to stroke from behind the knee to the hip for two to three minutes. Second, massage from the hip down to the back of the knee, moving your fingertips back and forth to apply friction. Follow the course of the sciatic nerve as you go down your leg, rubbing across the nerve. Do this three times, followed by three effleurage strokes. Third, using a loose fist to apply tapotement (page 571), gently tap on the back of the thigh from the hip to the knee and back again. Continue doing this for 10 to 30 seconds. Finish the sequence with three effleurage strokes.

If any of these strokes feels particularly comfortable, Stillerman suggests repeating it several times before continuing with the sequence. When you are finished, she says, rub an ice cube or put a cloth-covered ice pack on the painful area to soothe the nerve. You can do this massage every day, she adds. Besides helping to relieve existing pain, the massage may also prevent sciatica flare-ups, she explains.

Do not do this massage if the sciatic nerve is inflamed, according to Stillerman. She also cautions that pregnant women should use extremely gentle pressure when they do tapotement; too much pressure could stimulate the saphenous nerve, which leads into the pelvic area, causing uterine contractions.

REFLEXOLOGY

Work the sciatic nerve and shoulder reflex points on the bottoms of your feet, says St. Petersburg, Florida, reflexologist Dwight Byers, author of *Better Health with Foot Reflexology*. He also suggests working the hip/sciatic nerve points near your ankles.

To help you locate these points, consult the foot reflex chart on page 592. For instructions on how to work the points, see "Your Reflexology Session" on page 110.

YOGA

If your doctor says your sciatica is caused by a herniated or severely bulging disk, you may need surgery, says Mary Pullig Schatz, M.D., physician, yoga teacher and author of *Back Care Basics*. But if the problem is diagnosed as a slightly bulging disk or a tight piriformis muscle, Dr. Schatz says that daily practice of the following yoga stretches may be the best remedy: the easy bridge pose (page 619), the leg up, leg out exercise (page 626) and the piriformis stretch (page 627). These exercises may also serve as good preventive maintenance against sciatica pain, says Dr. Schatz. *Note:* Do not do the easy bridge pose during the second half of pregnancy.

Daily practice of the baby pose (page 618) may also help relieve or prevent sciatica flare-ups, notes Stephen A. Nezezon, M.D., yoga teacher and staff physician at the Himalayan International Institute of Yoga Science and Philosophy in Honesdale, Pennsylvania.

SEE ALSO Backache

SHINGLES

I t's *baaaack*! Just when you thought that childhood bout of chickenpox would never irritate your epidermis again, it has returned with a vengeance. There's the same maddening itch that you had as a child, those unsightly dots—as well as severe burning and a blistering rash.

Shingles is caused by the same virus (herpes zoster) as chickenpox, and it can lie dormant for decades. It reappears when the immune system is weakened by age, disease or unmanaged stress. You'll need to see your doctor to determine if you have shingles. The natural remedies in this chapter—in conjunction with medical care and used with the approval of your doctor—may help ease shingles, according to some health professionals.

SEE YOUR MEDICAL DOCTOR WHEN . . .

- Your skin is itchy, burning or blistering or has poxlike marks, especially near your eyes.
- Your pain is more than you can stand.

FOOD THERAPY

Although a diet rich in cayenne pepper may not prevent shingles, it can bring quicker relief from pain, says Allan Magaziner, D.O., a nutritional medicine specialist and head of the Magaziner Medical Center in Cherry Hill, New Jersey. In fact, he points out, the medication that's usually prescribed for shingles pain, Zostrix, is made from capsaicin, a derivative of hot peppers that indirectly helps prevent pain messages from reaching the brain.

HOMEOPATHY

"The best homeopathic remedy for shingles is Ranunculus bulbosus, especially when the shingles are on the trunk of the body," says Stephen Messer, N.D., dean of the National Center for Homeopathy's summer school and a naturopathic physician in Eugene, Oregon. He recommends taking a 6C dose up to four times a day as needed for pain. You should notice improvement within a couple of days, Dr. Messer says. If not, see your medical doctor or homeopath.

Ranunculus bulbosus is available in many health food stores. To purchase it by mail, refer to the resource list on page 637.

REFLEXOLOGY

Try working the diaphragm, spine, ovary/testicle, pancreas and pituitary, parathyroid, thyroid and adrenal gland reflex points on your hands or feet, suggests St. Petersburg, Florida, reflexologist Dwight Byers, author of *Better Health with Foot Reflexology*.

To help you locate these points, consult the hand and foot reflex charts beginning on page 582. For instructions on how to work the points, see "Your Reflexology Session" on page 110.

VITAMIN AND MINERAL THERAPY

A person with shingles may want to use the following supplemental regimen to help control the condition, suggests David Edelberg, M.D., an internist and medical director of the American Holistic Center/Chicago: 2,000 milligrams of vitamin C twice a day; 400 international units of vitamin E twice a day; and one gram of citrus bioflavonoids twice a day. Citrus bioflavonoids are available in most health food stores.

YOGA

Reduce stress, and you'll probably reduce the incidence—and possibly lessen the severity—of shingles, says Stephen A. Nezezon, M.D., yoga teacher and staff physician at the Himalayan International Institute of Yoga Science and Philosophy in Honesdale, Pennsylvania. To lower stress, Dr. Nezezon suggests trying a daily routine of breathing exercises, meditation and yoga poses.

Do the complete breath exercise (see page 152) whenever you're stressed, suggests Alice Christensen, founder and executive director of the American Yoga Association. Meditation (see page 153) helps clear your mind and teaches you to relax whenever you want to, she says. And for the poses, choose three or four from the Daily Routine, which begins on page 606. Christensen suggests varying the poses daily to keep your interest high and to strengthen different parts of your body. Dr. Nezezon says you should include at least one relaxation pose, such as the corpse (page 612), knee squeeze (page 612) or baby (page 618), in your daily yoga routine.

SHINSPLINTS

J ust do it," says the commercial. So you did. And now you've really done it, earning agony in the process.

Shinsplints are those sharp pains in the bones and tissue of the lower legs that may be caused by overuse when working out or running. This irritation of the tissue surrounding the shin muscles commonly occurs after exercising too much too soon, running on hard surfaces, not warming up enough or wearing inadequate footwear. Prevention is the key here. The natural remedies in this chapter, used with the approval of your doctor, may help ease the pain of shinsplints, according to some health professionals.

SEE YOUR MEDICAL DOCTOR WHEN...

- Your leg pain lasts for more than three days.
- Your pain is accompanied by a bluish skin discoloration, ulceration or tender lumps below the skin.
- Your pain recurs with only mild activity.

HOMEOPATHY

To ease the pain of shinsplints, try taking a 6C dose of Ruta graveolens three times a day until the discomfort begins to subside, says Stephen Messer, N.D., dean of the National Center for Homeopathy's summer school and a naturopathic physician in Eugene, Oregon.

Ruta graveolens is available in many health food stores. To purchase it by mail, refer to the resource list on page 637.

MASSAGE

Use the friction stroke (page 570) along the muscles in your calf and along the front of your shin, says Vincent Iuppo, N.D., naturopathic physician, massage therapist and director of the Morris Institute of Natural Therapeutics, a holistic health education center in Denville, New Jersey. Work each leg for about 15 minutes, then finish with a few minutes of the effleurage stroke (page 570). You should do this massage every day until the pain subsides.

SHYNESS

It may be appealing in song, but once the music stops, shyness is nothing to sing about. This social anxiety can be so severe that its sufferers may have trouble speaking, remembering names and even making decisions in front of other people.

What causes it? Experts say it's usually the result of traumatizing events in childhood that zap self-esteem. Heredity may also play a role. Serious shyness may require professional help. The natural remedies in this chapter, used with the approval of your doctor, may help you overcome shyness, according to some health professionals.

SEE YOUR MEDICAL DOCTOR WHEN . . .

- Your shyness is so overwhelming that it interferes with being able to function as you'd like.

FLOWER REMEDY/ESSENCE THERAPY

For shyness arising from low self-esteem, the flower essence Buttercup is most helpful, says Patricia Kaminski, co-director of the Flower Essence Society, a Nevada City, California, organization that studies and promotes the therapeutic use of flower remedies/essences.

"Shyness can also be caused by a deep-seated sense of shame that comes from past abuse," she adds. "This kind of person is terrified of self-revelation and has difficulty trusting." Such people benefit from the essence Pink Monkey Flower, according to Kaminski.

Flower essences are available in some health food stores and through mail order (refer to the resource list on page 635). For information on preparing and administering flower essences, see page 37.

HOMEOPATHY

Try a 30C dose of any of these remedies once a day until you feel improvement, says Chris Meletis, N.D., a naturopathic physician and medicinary director at the National College of Naturopathic Medicine in Portland, Oregon. Pulsatilla is an especially good remedy for shy, timid, agreeable individuals who are eager to please, according to Dr. Meletis. If you are solitary, want to be alone to cry, feel awkward in social settings and are prone to arguing about trivial things, he suggests trying Natrum muriaticum. Argentum nitricum can be helpful, he says, if you are impulsive and fearful of many things and want things hurried along.

All of these remedies are available in many health food stores. To purchase the remedies by mail, refer to the resource list on page 637.

SINUS PROBLEMS

Take a deep breath, and you may inhale hundreds of irritants that can result in clogged sinuses. Among them are pollen, cigarette smoke, dust, cold germs and exhaust fumes from cars, trucks, buses and lawn mowers. And when sinuses are clogged, the mucus they produce often can't drain properly. Fluid builds up, causing pressure and pain—along with any number of problems, from bad breath and stuffy nose to toothache and infection. The natural remedies in this chapter—in conjunction with medical care and used with your doctor's approval—may help ease sinus pain, according to some health professionals.

SEE YOUR MEDICAL DOCTOR WHEN...

- Your sinus pain doesn't improve after taking over-the-counter medication for three to five days.
- You also have a fever, cough or headache that has lasted longer than one day.
- You develop swollen eyelids and swelling along the sides of your nose.
- You have green or yellowish discharge.
- You have blurred or double vision.

SINUS PROBLEMS

ACUPRESSURE

To help get rid of sinus pressure and pain, gently press both LI 20 points for a couple of minutes, says Michael Reed Gach, Ph.D., director of the Acupressure Institute in Berkeley, California, and author of *Acupressure's Potent Points*. There is one point on each side of your nose, found near your nostrils. (For help in locating these points, refer to the illustration on page 567.) You can press them simultaneously by using the index and middle fingers of one hand, says Dr. Gach.

AYURVEDA

A sinus problem is caused by an excess of kapha dosha, according to Vasant Lad, B.A.M.S., M.A.Sc., director of the Ayurvedic Institute in Albuquerque, New Mexico. (For more information on the Ayurvedic doshas, see "All about Vata, Pitta and Kapha" on page 28.) He suggests the following remedy for severe and painful bouts of sinus congestion. The remedy is rather unpleasant, says Dr. Lad, but it works—fast.

"Use a garlic press to squeeze fresh garlic juice, then put the juice into an eyedropper," he says. "Put a few drops into your nostrils and keep your head back so that the juice stays inside your nose for about five minutes." Then, says Dr. Lad, sit up and let the garlic juice drain out onto a handkerchief or a tissue. He says your sinuses should be quite clear. Use this remedy no more than once a day when needed for sinus congestion, according to Dr. Lad; during a severe sinus attack, he says it may be repeated up to three times a day—morning, afternoon and evening.

For less severe sinus problems, a lukewarm saltwater solution may help restore easy breathing, according to Dr. Lad. To make the solution, he says to mix ½ teaspoon of salt in ½ cup of warm water. Then, he says, hold the salt water in the palm of your hand and sniff a bit into each nostril to help drain the sinuses. He suggests using this remedy as needed, up to three times an hour, to clear sinuses.

You can also sniff a pinch of ginger powder into the nostrils to help relieve the pain of swollen sinuses, says David Frawley, O.M.D., director of the American Institute of Vedic Studies in Santa Fe, New Mexico. He says to do this whenever you have sinus congestion. Do not use this remedy if you develop or are prone to bloody noses, he cautions.

To prevent sinus problems from developing, Dr. Lad recommends keeping your nostrils moisturized. "Using an eyedropper, put five drops of warm ghee in each nostril," he says. "Do this at least once a day, either once in the morning or once in the evening, and the ghee will moisturize your sinuses." Dr. Frawley says you can use either ghee or sesame oil for this purpose. For a recipe for ghee, or clarified butter, see "How to Make Ghee" on page 26. (Sesame oil is available in most health food stores.)

SINUS PROBLEMS

FOOD THERAPY

Barley green, which can be used in juices or simply sprinkled on salads as a topping, helps some people with sinus problems, says Julian Whitaker, M.D., founder and president of the Whitaker Wellness Center in Newport Beach, California. Barley green is available in most health food stores.

Some sinus problems are caused by a nutritional imbalance, adds Elson Haas, M.D., director of the Preventive Medical Center of Marin in San Rafael, California, and author of *Staying Healthy with Nutrition*. To restore the balance, he recommends following his three-week detoxification diet (see "Detoxing Your Ills" on page 48).

HYDROTHERAPY

A hot water bottle is a simple, effective way to relieve sinus pain, says Agatha Thrash, M.D., a medical pathologist and co-founder and co-director of Uchee Pines Institute, a natural healing center in Seale, Alabama. Fill about half of the bottle with hot (never boiling) water, wrap it in a towel and hold it against your nose and forehead until the pain subsides.

JUICE THERAPY

Both apple and dark grape juices may be beneficial to those with sinus problems, says John Peterson, M.D., an Ayurvedic practitioner in Muncie, Indiana. He recommends drinking the juice at room temperature and apart from meals. You can dilute either juice with water if it seems too strong, he adds.

For information on juicing techniques, see page 93.

REFLEXOLOGY

Using the corresponding golf ball technique (page 588) is a perfect way to work the adrenal gland, sinus, head and face reflex points on both hands, say Kevin and Barbara Kunz, reflexology researchers in Santa Fe, New Mexico, and authors of *Hand and Foot Reflexology*.

To help you locate these points, consult the hand reflex chart on page 582. For instructions on how to work the points, see "Your Reflexology Session" on page 110.

VITAMIN AND MINERAL THERAPY

Use the food sensitivity diet (see "Food Sensitivity: How to Discover the 'Healthy' Foods That Can Cause Disease" on page 52) to eliminate any foods

that might have a role in causing sinus problems, says David Edelberg, M.D., an internist and medical director of the American Holistic Center/Chicago. He also says to use steam inhalation (see "Hydrotherapy at Home" on page 78), with eucalyptus oil added to the water. And he says a person with sinus problems may want to try the following regimen of dietary supplements to help relieve symptoms: 2,000 milligrams of vitamin C twice a day; 400 international units of vitamin E twice a day; and 500 milligrams of n–acetylcysteine twice a day. Both eucalyptus oil and n–acetylcysteine are available in most health food stores.

YOGA

You can help both prevent and treat sinus problems if you do a yoga nasal wash, called *neti*, once a day, says Stephen A. Nezezon, M.D., yoga teacher and staff physician at the Himalayan International Institute of Yoga Science and Philosophy in Honesdale, Pennsylvania. Start by filling a four-ounce paper cup halfway with warm water, then add ½ teaspoon of salt. Put a small crease in the lip of the cup so that it forms a spout. Slightly tilt your head back and to the left. Then slowly pour the water into your right nostril. The water will flow out of your left nostril or down the back of your throat if your left nostril is clogged. Spit out the water if it goes down your throat, or wipe the water from your face with a hand towel if it flows out of your left nostril. Fill the cup again, then repeat the procedure on the other side, pouring the water into your left nostril and tilting your head to the right so that the water flows out of your right nostril.

SEE ALSO Postnasal Drip

SLEEP APNEA

For the one in ten Americans with sleep apnea, there's no such thing as sound sleep. Just ask their bedmates. The snarfing, gurgling and harrumphing are enough to rattle the walls as well as the nerves.

We're not talking just snoring here. During serious cases of sleep apnea, the throat relaxes and actually closes during sleep, which stops breathing for anywhere from ten seconds to up to three minutes. The gruff snoring sound occurs when the sleeper gasps for air and resumes breathing. A thorough examination of your sleeping habits can determine if you have sleep apnea, which usually afflicts overweight middle-age men. The natural remedy in this chapter—in conjunction with medical care and used with the approval of your doctor—may help relieve sleep apnea, according to one health professional.

SEE YOUR MEDICAL DOCTOR WHEN . . .

- Your spouse notices that your loud snoring is interrupted by pauses in breathing of ten seconds or more, perhaps followed by gruff snorts or gasps for air.
- You snore and also have high blood pressure, leg swelling, memory lapses, trouble concentrating or problems getting or maintaining erections.
- You also complain of frequent daytime sleepiness or fall asleep during the day.

FLOWER REMEDY/ESSENCE THERAPY

To treat sleep apnea, Eve Campanelli, Ph.D., a holistic family practitioner in Beverly Hills, California, has used the flower remedy Vervain. "Vervain is a very calming essence that is indicated for people with strong feelings about everything," says Dr. Campanelli. "This personality type seems to be associated with sleep apnea, and when these people use Vervain, it seems to help them solve problems in all areas of their lives, including sleeping problems."

Flower remedies are available in some health food stores and through mail order (refer to the resource list on page 635). For information on preparing and administering flower remedies, see page 37.

SMOKING

You've heard it all before. How smoking can kill you. How it annoys those around you. How being addicted to that smoldering stick of tobacco burns a hole in your bank account faster than a California brushfire. About the only thing you don't know about America's vilest vice is a surefire way to quit once and for all.

Sorry, but that's one question that isn't easily answered, at least not by the 50 million Americans who continue to smoke despite all they have to lose. Nicotine, the active ingredient in tobacco, is as addictive as heroin. But just because quitting is hard doesn't mean it can't be done. The natural remedies in this chapter—in conjunction with professional help and used with your doctor's approval—may help you quit smoking, according to some health professionals.

SEE YOUR MEDICAL DOCTOR WHEN . . .

• You want to quit and previous efforts haven't worked.

AROMATHERAPY

To help you ride out a cigarette craving, Fair Oaks, California, aromatherapist Victoria Edwards suggests mixing three essential oils—three parts lemon, two parts geranium and one part everlast (also known as immortelle or helichrysum)—in a small bottle that you keep in your pocket, briefcase or purse. Whenever a craving hits, she says, inhale directly from this bottle. "Lemon is a detoxifying agent, and geranium helps balance the adrenal system," explains Edwards. "Everlast is a powerful cellular rejuvenator and will help your body heal the damage smoking has done." This blend is also good when used in a diffuser, says Edwards.

For information on preparing and administering essential oils, including cautions about their use, see page 19. For information on purchasing essential oils, refer to the resource list on page 633.

AYURVEDA

To help you quit smoking or cut down on your habit, try chewing on small pieces of dried pineapple (about ½ teaspoon's worth) mixed with ½ teaspoon of honey, suggests Vasant Lad, B.A.M.S., M.A.Sc., director of the Ayurvedic

Institute in Albuquerque, New Mexico. He says to use this remedy whenever you desire a cigarette.

FOOD THERAPY

Load up on citrus fruits and other foods rich in vitamin C, suggests John Pinto, Ph.D., associate professor of biochemistry at Cornell University Medical College and director of the nutrition research laboratory at Memorial Sloan-Kettering Cancer Center, both in New York City. "There is no doubt that smokers can benefit from extra vitamin C, since it protects against the oxidative damage caused by smoking," he says. "You can get this extra vitamin C through foods if you eat plenty of fresh fruits and vegetables." He recommends having well over the Recommended Dietary Allowance for vitamin C, which is 60 milligrams, the amount you'd find in one orange. (For more food sources of vitamin C, see "Getting What You Need" on page 142.)

If you're trying to quit smoking cold turkey, drink a lot of orange juice, adds Thomas Cooper, D.D.S., professor of oral health sciences at the University of Kentucky in Lexington and an expert on nicotine dependency. But if you're quitting with the aid of a nicotine patch, you should avoid orange juice, says Dr. Cooper. Here's his explanation: By making your urine more acidic, the juice will clear your body of nicotine faster. But the purpose of the patch is to keep some nicotine in your body as you try to wean yourself off the weed.

HYDROTHERAPY

The body wrap, or wet sheet pack, can help detoxify your system if you're trying to quit, according to Charles Thomas, Ph.D., co-author of *Hydrotherapy: Simple Treatments for Common Ailments* and a physical therapist at Desert Springs Therapy Center in Desert Hot Springs, California. This treatment can be done at home but will probably require help from a partner.

After warming up with a hot shower, lie down on a bed with your entire body wrapped in a sheet wrung out in cold water. Then wrap yourself in one or more wool blankets. While the pack feels cool at first, your body heat will gradually dry the sheet, and you will begin to sweat. Leave the wrap in place for one to two hours after you start perspiring. Dr. Thomas suggests using this treatment once a day until you no longer feel as intense a craving for cigarettes.

IMAGERY

See yourself smoking. While you're doing it, do you perceive yourself as a smoker? In your mind, continue to see yourself smoking, but say to yourself

"At this time, I have the habit of smoking, but I am not a smoker," says Dennis Gersten, M.D., a San Diego psychiatrist and publisher of *Atlantis*, a bi-monthly imagery newsletter. That will help you adjust and maintain your self-image as you begin to make the transition from smoker to nonsmoker.

Now picture something that is good for you that you desire tremendously. It could be health, better looks or more control of your life. Focus on your desire. See yourself as an incredibly healthy, beautiful or self-reliant nonsmoker. Let that image overpower any desire that you have to smoke. Dr. Gersten recommends using this imagery for 10 to 20 minutes twice a day.

In addition, before you do this imagery, it may help to write down how and when you smoke, Dr. Gersten says. So if you light up after dinner, for example, jot down each step of the process, including getting up from the table, finding a match, grabbing your pack of cigarettes, tapping it on the kitchen counter, pulling out one cigarette, putting it in your mouth and lighting it. Doing that will help you understand and break the rituals of your habit, an important step in your effort to quit.

RELAXATION AND MEDITATION

Meditation techniques can help you overcome your urge to smoke, says Sundar Ramaswami, Ph.D., a clinical psychologist at F. S. Dubois Community Mental Health Center in Stamford, Connecticut.

"Studies have shown that many smokers use tobacco to help them reduce anxiety and tension. If you meditate, your mind learns another way to counteract that anxiety, so you may become less reliant on cigarettes," says Dr. Ramaswami, a practitioner of meditation for more than 20 years.

To try a simple meditation technique, see page 117. Meditate for 20 minutes twice a day or for a few minutes whenever you feel the urge to smoke, suggests Dr. Ramaswami.

VITAMIN AND MINERAL THERAPY

"Studies show that smokers who take extra vitamin C in supplement form get some extra protection from the harmful effects of smoking," says Judith S. Stern, R.D., Sc.D., professor of nutrition and internal medicine at the University of California, Davis. "Still, I wouldn't recommend that smokers depend on this. The extra protection isn't going to mean much compared with the overall damage that you're doing to your body from smoking."

SORE THROAT

I t's a special kind of torture that everyone from opera stars to off-key shower warblers dreads. Yet the raw, burning sensation of a sore throat is an extremely common symptom that usually means you have an inflammation somewhere between the back of your tongue and your voice box.

Often it is the first sign of a cold, the flu or a viral or bacterial infection such as strep throat or mononucleosis. In other cases, that tickle in your throat can be caused by dry indoor air, allergies or exposure to smoke, chemicals or pollution. In most cases, a sore throat will subside on its own in a few days. The natural remedies in this chapter, used with the approval of your doctor, may help lessen the symptoms of a sore throat and speed its healing, according to some health professionals.

SEE YOUR MEDICAL DOCTOR WHEN . . .

- The pain lasts for more than two to three days.
- You also have a fever of 101°F or higher, difficulty swallowing, swollen glands in your neck or white patches on your tonsils or in the area where your tonsils used to be.
- You also have a reddish, sandpaper-like rash on your trunk.
- You have a history of rheumatic fever.
- You have been exposed to either strep throat or mononucleosis or there is a community outbreak.
- You get sore throats frequently but haven't been to the doctor.

AROMATHERAPY

To speed the healing of a sore throat, Los Angeles aromatic consultant John Steele recommends applying a thin film of carrier oil externally over the throat area. Canola, sunflower, grapeseed and safflower are popular choices and are available in most health food stores. Apply seven drops of sandalwood essential oil over the carrier oil and rub gently into the skin, suggests Steele. "This treatment is soothing and smells wonderful, and the carrier oil prevents skin irritation," he explains. Or, he says, add two drops of tea tree, ginger, sandalwood or geranium essential oil to ½ ounce of warm water and gargle. Any of these essential oils can be taken with a spoonful of honey to coat the throat, says Steele.

For information on preparing and administering essential oils, including cautions about their use, see page 19. For information on purchasing essential oils, refer to the resource list on page 633.

SORE THROAT

AYURVEDA

Stir ½ teaspoon of salt and 1 teaspoon of turmeric into a cup of hot water, and gargle with this mixture before going to bed, says Vasant Lad, B.A.M.S., M.A.Sc., director of the Ayurvedic Institute in Albuquerque, New Mexico. If your sore throat doesn't go away within a few days, see a doctor, he adds.

FOOD THERAPY

Allicin, the compound that puts the pungent odor in garlic, has antibiotic and antifungal properties that can heal many types of sore throat, says registered pharmacist Earl Mindell, R.Ph., Ph.D., professor of nutrition at Pacific Western University in Los Angeles and author of *Earl Mindell's Food as Medicine* and other books on nutrition. Take two or more cloves, crushed or whole, at the first sign of a sore throat and continue eating two cloves a day until your symptoms clear up, he says.

Raw garlic is the most effective, says Dr. Mindell, but it can cause gastrointestinal upset. He suggests baking and stir-frying as other ways of getting garlic into your diet. Or, he says, take garlic supplements for all of the benefits with none of the digestive upset. Garlic supplements are available in most health food stores and many drugstores; Dr. Mindell recommends taking three capsules twice a day with meals until your symptoms clear up.

HERBAL THERAPY

Try gargling with goldenseal tea, says Varro E. Tyler, Ph.D., professor of pharmacognosy at Purdue University in West Lafayette, Indiana. To make the tea, Dr. Tyler says to pour boiling water over one to two teaspoons of the dried herb, which you can buy in most health food stores. Steep for ten minutes, strain to remove the herb and cool before using as a mouthwash, he says.

Sage is another good choice for a sore throat, according to Dr. Tyler. He says to chop two teaspoons of fresh leaves (available in most health food stores), then pour boiling water over them and steep for ten minutes. Strain the tea to remove the leaves and cool before using as a mouthwash, he says.

Dr. Tyler suggests that you repeat the gargles as necessary for a maximum of two to three days.

HOMEOPATHY

To treat a bright red sore throat that develops suddenly on the right side of the throat, is sore to the touch and is accompanied by high fever and thirst, take a 6C or 12C dose of Belladonna and consult your doctor, says Mitchell Fleisher,

M.D., a family practice physician and homeopath in Colleen, Virginia.

If you feel irritable and the soreness begins on the right side and then moves to the left, and if your throat feels better after you drink warm beverages, Dr. Fleisher suggests a 6C or 12C dose of Lycopodium. If the soreness begins on the left side and moves to the right and is worse when you swallow saliva but better when you eat, he says to try a 6C or 12C dose of Lachesis. Take one of these remedies up to four times daily, says Dr. Fleisher, and if your throat doesn't feel better within 48 hours, see your medical doctor or homeopath.

All of these remedies are available in many health food stores. To purchase the remedies by mail, refer to the resource list on page 637.

HYDROTHERAPY

"Charcoal has been shown to adhere to certain pathogenic germs that cause sore throats," says Agatha Thrash, M.D., a medical pathologist and co-founder and co-director of Uchee Pines Institute, a natural healing center in Seale, Alabama. Using activated charcoal powder (available in most health food stores and some drugstores) and cold water, make a paste thick enough to roll into a ball. Suck on the ball as long as it lasts to heal a sore throat fast, suggests Dr. Thrash.

JUICE THERAPY

Ginger and pineapple both contain natural anti-inflammatory agents that can speed the healing of a sore throat, according to Cherie Calbom, M.S., a certified nutritionist in Kirkland, Washington, and co-author of *Juicing for Life*. She suggests juicing three pineapple rings together with a ¼-inch-thick slice of fresh ginger for a delicious healing cocktail.

For information on juicing techniques, see page 93.

REFLEXOLOGY

Work the throat reflex points on your feet, say Kevin and Barbara Kunz, reflexology researchers in Santa Fe, New Mexico, and authors of *Hand and Foot Reflexology*. They also suggest using the corresponding golf ball technique (page 588) to work the adrenal gland and throat points on both hands.

To help you locate these points, consult the hand and foot reflex charts beginning on page 582. For instructions on how to work the points, see "Your Reflexology Session" on page 110.

VITAMIN AND MINERAL THERAPY

Whether caused by a virus, pollutants or just misusing your voice, a sore throat usually means that a more acute infection will follow. Vitamin C can help prevent infection and speed up the healing process, says Richard Gerson, Ph.D., author of *The Right Vitamins*. He says you can safely take up to 10,000 milligrams a day of vitamin C at the first sign of a problem, provided you drink plenty of water to flush away excess amounts of the nutrient.

SEE ALSO Laryngitis

SPRAINS

You've been down the basement steps so many times that you can do it in the dark. Or so you think. Now where is that bottom step? Oops. Stumble, bumble, tumble. There goes your ankle.

In fact, 85 percent of ankle injuries are sprains. A sprain occurs when a sudden impact—stepping off a curb the wrong way or tripping and landing on your hands—damages ligaments, the tough elastic bands that help hold a joint such as the ankle or wrist together.

A sprain can cause painful swelling of the joint and muscle spasms. Elevating the joint, wrapping it in an elastic bandage, applying ice to reduce swelling and resting the injured area are among the first things that most experts recommend you do. The natural remedies in this chapter—in conjunction with medical care and used with your doctor's approval—may help ease the pain and swelling of a sprain and speed healing, according to some health professionals.

SEE YOUR MEDICAL DOCTOR WHEN . . .

- You're unable to move or put weight on the injured joint.
- Your injured joint appears to be misshapen.
- Your pain spreads to other parts of the limb.
- Your pain and swelling persist for more than two to three days.

SPRAINS

ACUPRESSURE

For an ankle sprain, press point GB 40, situated in the large hollow directly in front of the outer anklebone, says Michael Reed Gach, Ph.D., director of the Acupressure Institute in Berkeley, California, and author of *Acupressure's Potent Points*. (To help locate the point, refer to the illustration on page 566.) He says to hold the point on the injured ankle for two minutes: For the first minute, alternate between light and firm pressure, and for the second minute, hold the point with a very light touch. Dr. Gach recommends using this remedy at least twice a day to help heal a sprain. To strengthen your ankle and prevent future injury, press one or both GB 40 points daily, he adds.

AYURVEDA

Salt can relieve the swelling that comes with a sprain, says Vasant Lad, B.A.M.S., M.A.Sc., director of the Ayurvedic Institute in Albuquerque, New Mexico. He suggests making a paste of one part salt and two parts turmeric, mixed with enough water to get the right consistency. Apply this paste to the injured area once a day, he says, letting it set for 20 minutes to an hour. He advises covering the paste with cotton flannel or muslin to keep it from rubbing off and to protect your clothing, since turmeric stains. Any skin discoloration from the turmeric should wash off in about two weeks, he adds.

FOOD THERAPY

Foods high in vitamin C help mend collagen, the supportive protein in skin, bones, tendons and cartilage that can become damaged in a sprain, says Julian Whitaker, M.D., founder and president of the Whitaker Wellness Center in Newport Beach, California. For faster relief, Dr. Whitaker recommends eating more vitamin C–rich foods such as oranges, grapefruit, strawberries and peppers. (For other food sources of vitamin C, see "Getting What You Need" on page 142.)

HERBAL THERAPY

The dried flower heads of the arnica plant contain chemical compounds that help heal sprains and relieve muscle pain, according to Varro E. Tyler, Ph.D., professor of pharmacognosy at Purdue University in West Lafayette, Indiana. Look for arnica tincture, cream or ointment in most health food stores. Apply directly to the injured area as recommended on the label.

HOMEOPATHY

In the first 24 hours after a sprain, take a dose of Arnica 6C to help the pain subside, says Stephen Messer, N.D., dean of the National Center for Homeopathy's summer school and a naturopathic physician in Eugene, Oregon. If that doesn't seem to help and your sprain is less painful if you keep the joint moving rather than immobilized, Dr. Messer suggests trying a dose of Rhus toxicodendron 6C. If neither of these remedies works, he says to try a dose of Ruta graveolens 6C. Take any of these remedies as needed, but no more than every two hours, he says.

All of these remedies are available in many health food stores. To purchase the remedies by mail, refer to the resource list on page 637.

HYDROTHERAPY

A frozen bandage is a great way to ease the pain and swelling, says Agatha Thrash, M.D., a medical pathologist and co-founder and co-director of Uchee Pines Institute, a natural healing center in Seale, Alabama. Dip a hand towel in very cold water, squeeze it out, place it in a plastic bag and store it in the freezer over a piece of cardboard, so the towel freezes flat. To use, remove the plastic and lay the bandage over the sprain. The rigid bandage will quickly become soft as it's warmed by your body heat. Replace with a fresh bandage when the towel feels warm. Dr. Thrash recommends 20-minute sessions of this treatment two to four times a day for a week or until symptoms subside.

MASSAGE

You can reduce swelling in a sprained joint with a rake massage, says Elliot Greene, past president of the American Massage Therapy Association. Start by placing your hands on either side of the sprained joint. If the joint is on the arm, you'll be able to use only one hand—the one on the other arm. Spread your fingers about a half-inch apart. Place the fingertips on the part of the joint that is farthest from the heart. If you're working on your knee, for example, place the fingertips just below the knee, closest to your ankle.

Now pull the fingertips over the joint, applying light pressure. "It's just like you were running a rake lightly across the joint," Greene says. When you go past the top of the joint a few inches, lift your hands and place them back at the starting point. You can do this massage for about five minutes at a time, several times a day, until the sprain has healed. But be sure to wait 24 to 48 hours after the sprain has occurred before you start using this massage.

![]

REFLEXOLOGY

To deal with a sprain, work the reflex points on the hands or feet that correspond to the injured area, says St. Petersburg, Florida, reflexologist Dwight Byers, author of *Better Health with Foot Reflexology*. If you have a sprained knee, for example, try working the knee reflex points on your feet, he says.

To help you locate these points, consult the hand and foot reflex charts beginning on page 582. For instructions on how to work the points, see "Your Reflexology Session" on page 110.

STOMACHACHE

After leftover pizza for breakfast, tacos for lunch and Cajun-style chicken for dinner, it's no wonder there's a brawl going on inside your belly.

Eating too much too quickly and consuming lots of rich, spicy or fatty foods are common causes of stomachaches. But the heartburn, cramping, nausea, flatulence and other symptoms typically associated with an upset tummy could also be caused by excessive stress, an irregular eating schedule, food poisoning or a flu bug. If the ache persists or recurs, it could be sign of appendicitis, an ulcer or gallstones, so see your doctor. The natural remedies in this chapter, used with your doctor's approval, may help ease a stomachache, according to some health professionals.

SEE YOUR MEDICAL DOCTOR WHEN . . .

- You experience sudden severe abdominal pain.
- Your pain persists for more than 24 hours.
- You have vomiting, fever or excessive nausea.
- You also have rectal bleeding or weight loss.

ACUPRESSURE

Press both Sp 16 points, situated below the edge of the rib cage, a half-inch in from each nipple line, says Michael Reed Gach, Ph.D., director of the Acupressure Institute in Berkeley, California, and author of *Acupressure's Potent Points*. (For help in locating these points, refer to the illustration on page 564.) "These are instinctual spots to press," Dr. Gach explains. "You're pressing these points when you bend over and hold your stomach." He suggests holding the points for one minute while breathing deeply.

AROMATHERAPY

The essential oil peppermint is great for easing gastric discomfort, says Los Angeles aromatherapist Michael Scholes, of Aromatherapy Seminars, an organization that trains professionals and others in the use of essential oils. "Peppermint oil was used for years to flavor after-dinner mints, because it's a very effective digestive," says Scholes. But, he cautions, most of today's peppermint candies do not contain the essential oil and probably wouldn't help your stomachache. He suggests sucking on a sugar cube flavored with a single drop of peppermint oil whenever your stomach feels a bit queasy.

For information on preparing and administering essential oils, including cautions about their use, see page 19. For information on purchasing essential oils, refer to the resource list on page 633.

FLOWER REMEDY/ESSENCE THERAPY

"People who get stomachaches respond really well to Crab Apple, which is a cleansing remedy," says Eve Campanelli, Ph.D., a holistic family practitioner in Beverly Hills, California. "It works especially well on stomachaches caused by bad food or a parasitic or yeast overload."

Flower remedies are available in some health food stores and through mail order (refer to the resource list on page 635). For information on preparing and administering flower remedies, see page 37.

FOOD THERAPY

"Cut a piece of ginger and suck on it," advises Allan Magaziner, D.O., a nutritional medicine specialist and head of the Magaziner Medical Center in Cherry Hill, New Jersey. He says that ginger helps calm activity in the stomach. A cup of ginger tea can also help, he adds. Ginger tea is available in tea bag form in most health food stores.

HERBAL THERAPY

Peppermint and chamomile are two traditional herbal remedies for stomachache, according to Mary Bove, L.M., N.D., a naturopathic physician and director of the Brattleboro Naturopathic Clinic in Vermont. She says both work gently to soothe an upset stomach, stop stomach spasms and reduce gas.

She recommends that you drink three to four cups of peppermint or chamomile tea daily to treat minor digestive problems. You can also sip a cup of either of these teas after meals to aid digestion, she adds. Peppermint and chamomile teas are available in tea bag form in most health food stores.

HYDROTHERAPY

"I don't believe there is a gastric problem that doesn't respond to activated charcoal," says Agatha Thrash, M.D., a medical pathologist and co-founder and co-director of Uchee Pines Institute, a natural healing center in Seale, Alabama. For quick relief of stomachache, mix two to three tablespoons of activated charcoal powder (available in most health food stores and some pharmacies) with a little water in the bottom of a tall glass. "Stir gently, or the powder flies everywhere," she says. Continue stirring and adding water a little at a time until the glass is full, then drink it with a straw.

IMAGERY

Imagery can be a powerful weapon against stomachache, according to Barbara Dossey, R.N., director of Holistic Nursing Consultants in Santa Fe, New Mexico, and co-author of *Rituals of Healing: Using Imagery for Health and Wellness*. Picture a bright light that is powerful and penetrating glowing within you. Now picture a beam that has a soft, healing color spreading from this light. Allow this beam's healing color to fill your stomach with calm and quiet. Now imagine the color slowly flowing out of your stomach and into your small intestine like a tiny sailboat riding on smooth waves. Follow it down through your large intestine and into your rectum, gently healing and soothing your digestive tract as it goes. Dossey recommends that you use this imagery for 15 to 20 minutes twice a day.

JUICE THERAPY

In *The Complete Book of Juicing*, naturopathic physician Michael Murray, N.D., suggests an apple juice cocktail flavored with ginger, mint and fennel. All three are potent carminatives, natural substances that help dispel gas and facilitate digestion, according to Dr. Murray. To prepare, juice a ¼-inch-thick slice of fresh ginger wrapped in half of a handful of mint leaves, followed by half of a small fennel bulb and two sliced apples.

For information on juicing techniques, see page 93.

STRESS

Y ou wake up late, dive into the shower, scramble into your clothes, grab a stale muffin from the kitchen, dash out to the car, roar out of the driveway and drive smack into the middle of a massive traffic jam. At the office, your boss and two impatient clients wait for you.

Welcome to the world of stress, an inescapable reality of modern life that has been linked to many disorders ranging from allergies to asthma, from stomach problems to heart disease. In fact, some physicians estimate that at least 80 percent of their patients have stress-related symptoms. The natural remedies in this chapter, used with your doctor's approval, may help ease stress, according to some health professionals.

SEE YOUR MEDICAL DOCTOR WHEN...

- You have uncontrollable anger and you don't know why.
- You have insomnia.
- You have difficulty sustaining relationships.
- You have persistent feelings of guilt.
- You consistently rehash incidents in your mind.

AROMATHERAPY

To melt away stress at the end of the day and ease the transition between work and home, aromatherapist Victoria Edwards, of Fair Oaks, California, recommends clary sage and lavender, two essential oils that relax. "If you have a long commute, put a drop or two of the oil on a tissue or napkin and let it heat up in the sun on your dashboard," says Edwards. "The heat diffuses the fragrance and helps you unwind. It's like the old after-work martini, but without the alcohol."

For information on preparing and administering essential oils, including cautions about their use, see page 19. For information on purchasing essential oils, refer to the resource list on page 633.

FLOWER REMEDY/ESSENCE THERAPY

"So much of the stress in our lives comes from adjusting to change," says Eve Campanelli, Ph.D., a holistic family practitioner in Beverly Hills, California. For anyone whose life has been turned upside down by a major lifestyle change (a move, a career change or a new baby, for example), Dr. Campanelli recommends daily doses of the flower remedy Walnut.

Flower remedies are available in some health food stores and through mail order (refer to the resource list on page 635). For information on preparing and administering flower remedies, see page 37.

HERBAL THERAPY

Siberian ginseng tones the nervous system and increases your resistance to stress, says Mary Bove, L.M., N.D., a naturopathic physician and director of the Brattleboro Naturopathic Clinic in Vermont. She suggests taking this herb in either capsule or tincture form, following the dosage recommendations on the label. Siberian ginseng supplements are available in most health food stores.

IMAGERY

Imagine that you are a feather floating in the air. You become more and more relaxed as you drift downward toward the ground. You finally glide to the ground, gently and softly touching down. As you're lying there, all stress has left your body, and you feel totally and completely relaxed, says Dennis Gersten, M.D., a psychiatrist and publisher of *Atlantis*, a bi-monthly imagery newsletter. He recommends using this imagery for two to five minutes three times a day.

If you're stressed out from work, Dr. Gersten says to try this imagery as you leave your job at the end of the day: Imagine that your stress is liquefying and running out of your body so that with each step, you leave on the ground a colored footprint or impression that represents your stress. As you walk farther away from your job, the footprints begin to fade, and any stress that you felt when you left work diminishes.

MASSAGE

Stress results in tense neck and shoulder muscles, leading to stiffness, headaches and even more stress, says Dan Bienenfeld, certified Hellerwork practitioner, massage therapist and director of the Los Angeles Healing Arts Center. You can stop the cycle with a 15-minute Hellerwork self-massage (page 575). Do the massage every day, even if you're not feeling stressed, Bienenfeld says. "That way, you can stop the knotted muscles before they even start," he says.

REFLEXOLOGY

An overall reflexology session, touching all of the major points of the hands and feet, will help relax you and ward off stress, says St. Petersburg, Florida, reflexologist Dwight Byers, author of *Better Health with Foot Reflexology*. To deal with extra tension, Byers suggests paying special attention to the diaphragm, the spine and the pituitary, parathyroid, thyroid and adrenal gland reflexes.

To help you locate these points, consult the hand and foot reflex charts beginning on page 582. For instructions on how to work the points, see "Your Reflexology Session" on page 110.

RELAXATION AND MEDITATION

Any of the relaxation and meditation techniques, such as mindfulness meditation, autogenics, progressive relaxation and stretching, will relieve stress, according to Steven Fahrion, Ph.D., director of research at the Life Sciences Institute of Mind-Body Health in Topeka, Kansas. It's a matter of finding the one that works best for you. See page 113 for a brief description of each of these techniques and how to do them.

SOUND THERAPY

To wash away stress, try taking a 20-minute "sound bath," says Steven Halpern, Ph.D., composer, researcher and author of *Sound Health: The Music and Sounds That Make Us Whole*. Put some relaxing music on your stereo, then lie in a comfortable position on a couch or on the floor near the speakers. For a deeper experience, you can wear headphones to focus your attention and to avoid distraction. Dr. Halpern says you should bend your knees slightly and support your neck by placing a folded towel underneath it.

As the music plays, Dr. Halpern says, allow it to wash over you, rinsing off the stress from the day. Focus on your breathing, letting it deepen, slow and become regular. Concentrate on the silence between the notes in the music; this keeps you from analyzing the music and makes relaxation more complete.

Here are some suggested pieces of music: *Seapeace* by Georgia Kelly; *Spectrum Suite, Inner Peace* and *Comfort Zone*, all by Dr. Halpern; and any recording of Gregorian chants. For mail-order information, refer to the resource list on page 642.

Dr. Halpern also says that listening to the sounds of nature—ocean waves or the calm of a deep forest, for instance—can reduce stress. Try taking a 15- to 20-minute walk if you're near the seashore or a quiet patch of woods. If not, you can buy tapes of these sounds in many music stores. For mail-order information, refer to the resource list on page 642.

For another stress-reducing experience, try the simple toning exercise described in "Hum Yourself to Health" on page 125. The sound of your own voice can bring a tremendous feeling of relaxation that can cut stress in just a few minutes, says Don G. Campbell, director of the Institute for Music, Health and Education in Boulder, Colorado, and author of *Music: Physician for Times to Come*.

VITAMIN AND MINERAL THERAPY

To help offset some of the damage caused by stress, try these daily supplements, says Alan Gaby, M.D., a physician specializing in preventive and nutritional medicine in Baltimore and president of the American Holistic Medical Association: 200 to 400 milligrams of magnesium, 10 to 100 milligrams of B-complex vitamins and 500 to 3,000 milligrams of vitamin C. "The magnesium blocks the damaging effects of excess adrenaline," says Dr. Gaby. "It's not exactly clear how the B-complex vitamins and vitamin C protect the body, but animal studies show that the physical damage caused by stress is minimized with these vitamins."

YOGA

Yoga really shines here, according to Alice Christensen, founder and executive director of the American Yoga Association. If you want a portable stress buster, Christensen recommends the complete breath exercise (see page 152), which you can do at your desk, in the car or anywhere else when you start to feel stressed out. Meditation (see page 153) helps calm your mind, she says, teaching you to relax at will and giving you a quick mental vacation whenever you need one. And daily practice of three or four yoga poses, chosen from the Daily Routine, which begins on page 606, will help ease knotted muscles, according to Christensen. She suggests varying the poses daily to keep your interest high and to strengthen different parts of your body.

SEE ALSO Burnout

STUTTERING

O ne in 100 adults has difficulty with stuttering, but no one really knows what causes it.

Stuttering is common among young children, but half of the children who stutter beyond age five will continue to do it as adults. It also tends to run in families and is more prevalent among males, twins and left-handed people. If stuttering begins in adulthood, it could be a sign of a neurological disorder or a head injury.

Some researchers suspect that stuttering is habit forming and that stress has a major role in its onset. When a child is learning to speak, or when an adult has to talk in a tense situation, stress increases tension on the vocal cords. As the person struggles to speak, words sputter out of his mouth as if he were trying to start a reluctant car engine on a cold winter morning. Keeping the vocal chords open and relaxed can help control stuttering, experts say. Speech therapy can benefit, too. The natural remedies in this chapter, used with your doctor's approval, may help stop you from stuttering, according to some health professionals.

SEE YOUR MEDICAL DOCTOR WHEN . . .

- You suddenly develop a stutter for the first time as an adult.
- Your periods of stuttering begin to occur more often or talking seems to require more effort or sounds strained.

FLOWER REMEDY/ESSENCE THERAPY

Flower essences can help alleviate the underlying anxiety associated with stuttering, says Patricia Kaminski, co-director of the Flower Essence Society, a Nevada City, California, organization that studies and promotes the therapeutic use of flower remedies/essences. For stuttering that arises from overexcitement and "information overload" (when the mouth can't keep up with the flow of thought), Kaminski recommends the California essence Cosmos. For people who have no problem speaking to friends and acquaintances but stutter when speaking in public, Trumpet Vine may help, she says.

Flower essences are available in some health food stores and through mail order (refer to the resource list on page 635). For information on preparing and administering flower essences, see page 37.

HOMEOPATHY

To help stop stuttering or stammering, try one of the following 6C or 12C remedies once a day for a month, says Chris Meletis, N.D., a naturopathic physician and medicinary director at the National College of Naturopathic Medicine in Portland, Oregon. If one remedy doesn't work, he says to try another one the following month.

Stramonium is the remedy of choice if you are imaginative, red-faced and excitable and your speech is irregular and erratic, according to Dr. Meletis. If you are nervous and tense with a ticlike movement, and if your symptoms are worse when you're excited, he says Agaricus may help. He suggests Cuprum metallicum if you are prone to spasms in general and have spasmodic and labored speech that gets worse when you're frightened. General stuttering or stammering is often helped by Arsenicum, he says.

All of these remedies are available in many health food stores. To purchase the remedies by mail, refer to the resource list on page 637.

SUBSTANCE ABUSE

Whether you're talking about drugs, tobacco or alcohol, substance abuse can take control of your life and send it spiraling downward. The misuse of alcohol, cigarettes and legal and illegal drugs is the main cause of premature death and preventable illness in the United States, according to the American Psychiatric Association. Some people—particularly those from families with histories of drug and alcohol problems—seem to be more susceptible than others to substance abuse. If you suspect that you have a problem, seek professional treatment. The natural remedies in this chapter—in conjunction with professional care and used with your doctor's approval—may help you overcome substance abuse, according to some health professionals.

SEE YOUR MEDICAL DOCTOR WHEN . . .

- You drink or use drugs after a confrontation, an argument or another emotional trauma.
- You find yourself developing a tolerance to drugs or alcohol.
- You have blackout spells when you can't remember what you did while drinking or using drugs.

- You have withdrawal symptoms such as trembling, diarrhea, cramps, vomiting and confusion.
- You find that using drugs or alcohol has become the focal point of your life, more important to you than your family or career.

AROMATHERAPY

The essential oil everlast (also known as helichrysum or immortelle) encourages cellular regeneration and helps the body repair the damage done by drugs or alcohol, says Fair Oaks, California, aromatherapist Victoria Edwards. According to Edwards, everlast is a key ingredient in the following blend of essential oils, developed to help those in recovery combat cravings for drugs or alcohol: Mix three parts lemon (to detoxify), two parts geranium (to balance the adrenal system) and one part everlast essential oils. Edwards suggests storing the mixture in a bottle small enough to fit in your pocket or purse. "You can inhale directly from this bottle whenever you have a craving," she says. She adds that the blend can also be used in a diffuser.

For information on preparing and administering essential oils, including cautions about their use, see page 19. For information on purchasing essential oils, refer to the resource list on page 633.

FLOWER REMEDY/ESSENCE THERAPY

"For most people, overcoming addiction is a very frightening experience," says Eve Campanelli, Ph.D., a holistic family practitioner in Beverly Hills, California. She recommends taking the Bach remedy Rockrose three or four times a day to alleviate these fears. People recovering from addictions who are prone to anxiety attacks should also take the emergency stress relief formula whenever feelings of panic arise, says Dr. Campanelli.

Flower remedies, including the emergency stress relief formula, are available in some health food stores and through mail order (refer to the resource list on page 635). The formula is sold under brand names such as Calming Essence, Rescue Remedy and Five-Flower Formula. For information on preparing and administering flower remedies, see page 37.

FOOD THERAPY

"It's especially important to eat more citrus fruits and vegetables, which are rich in antioxidant vitamins. Those who abuse substances are more prone to tissue damage, and antioxidant vitamins can help offset some of that damage," says Allan Magaziner, D.O., a nutritional medicine specialist and head of the Magaziner

Medical Center in Cherry Hill, New Jersey. He also advises people who abuse alcohol to consume foods rich in magnesium and vitamin B_6. "Drinking alcohol depletes magnesium and B vitamins, especially B_6," he says. Foods high in magnesium include nuts, tofu, spinach and wheat germ; beans, whole grains and dark green leafy vegetables are among the foods rich in vitamin B_6. (For other food sources of these nutrients, see "Getting What You Need" on page 142.)

IMAGERY

Imagine there is a hole in the ground that you throw all of your alcohol and drugs into; they fall to the center of the earth and are burned. Then imagine that the same thing happens to the rest of the alcohol and drugs in the world, says Dennis Gersten, M.D., a San Diego psychiatrist and publisher of *Atlantis*, a bi-monthly imagery newsletter. There are now no drugs or alcohol in your world. How do you feel about that? Scared? Relieved? Joyous? Allow yourself to experience any emotion that pops into your head without judging it.

Next, imagine that there is a giant switchboard in your mind that regulates all of your cravings and desires. Find the wires that spark your addiction. Unplug those wires, so you won't crave drugs or alcohol. Dr. Gersten suggests practicing this imagery for 10 to 20 minutes twice a day.

REFLEXOLOGY

You can help your body deal with the toxic effects of substance abuse by working the pituitary, parathyroid and adrenal gland, pancreas, diaphragm, liver and kidney reflex points on your hands or feet, says St. Petersburg, Florida, reflexologist Dwight Byers, author of *Better Health with Foot Reflexology*.

To help you locate these points, consult the hand and foot reflex charts beginning on page 582. For instructions on how to work the points, see "Your Reflexology Session" on page 110.

RELAXATION AND MEDITATION

Studies have found that meditation reduces the use of illegal drugs and the misuse of legal drugs such as tranquilizers and painkillers, says Roger Walsh, M.D., Ph.D., professor of psychiatry, philosophy and anthropology at the University of California, Irvine, California College of Medicine. "People find the meditative experience satisfying in and of itself, and this can reduce the spiritual or inner lack that was driving them toward drug use."

To give meditation a try, see page 117. Do it for 20 minutes once or twice a day, Dr. Walsh suggests.

SUNBURN

VITAMIN AND MINERAL THERAPY

Those who abuse alcohol may be damaging the mucus lining of their intestines, says John Pinto, Ph.D., director of the nutrition research laboratory at Memorial Sloan-Kettering Cancer Center and associate professor of biochemistry at Cornell University Medical College, both in New York City. "Because of this, they could benefit from certain vitamins—thiamin, riboflavin, niacin and B$_6$," according to Dr. Pinto. He says that supplements may be preferable, because the nutrients in foods aren't absorbed as efficiently in the bodies of people who abuse alcohol. You can get all of these vitamins in most multivitamin/mineral supplements, he adds. For Recommended Dietary Allowances, see "Getting What You Need" on page 142.

SUNBURN

You paddled to the middle of the lake, cast a fishing line and promptly fell asleep. Two hours later, you could star in *Invasion of the Lobster People from Outer Space.*

Sunburns hurt, and the damage they inflict on your skin is long lasting and dangerous. The redness of a sunburn is caused by clogged and swollen capillaries that supply blood to the skin. Severe burns, caused by the ultraviolet rays in sunlight, can damage blood vessels and destroy elastic fibers in the skin, causing it to sag and wrinkle. Excessive sun exposure can also lead to skin cancer, the most common of all cancers.

Prevention is your best bet. Do outdoor activities before 10:00 A.M. or after 2:00 P.M., when the ultraviolet rays are less intense. And remember to wear a sunscreen with an SPF (sun protection factor) of 15 or higher. The natural remedies in this chapter, used with your doctor's approval, may help soothe a sunburn, according to some health professionals.

SEE YOUR MEDICAL DOCTOR WHEN . . .

- You have nausea, chills or fever.
- You feel fatigued or faint.
- You have extensive patches of blistered, purple or discolored skin.
- You have intense itching.

SUNBURN

AROMATHERAPY

A cool aromatic bath is a wonderful way to soothe sunburned skin, says Greenwich, Connecticut, aromatherapist Judith Jackson, author of *Scentual Touch: A Personal Guide to Aromatherapy*. Add 20 drops each of lavender and chamomile essential oils to a tubful of cool water and soak for ten minutes, suggests Jackson.

For information on preparing and administering essential oils, including cautions about their use, see page 19. For information on purchasing essential oils, refer to the resource list on page 633.

FOOD THERAPY

The fat content of milk is soothing, so milk makes a great compress for sunburn pain, says John F. Romano, M.D., clinical assistant professor of dermatology at New York Hospital–Cornell Medical Center in New York City. His instructions: Dip some gauze in whole milk and apply it to sunburned areas for about 20 minutes, repeating this process every two to four hours. Be sure to wash off the milk to avoid having your skin smell sour.

For healing, eat more foods rich in vitamin C, which speeds the healing process for burns, says Julian Whitaker, M.D., founder and president of the Whitaker Wellness Center in Newport Beach, California. (For food sources of vitamin C, see "Getting What You Need" on page 142.)

HERBAL THERAPY

Keep an aloe vera plant in your house, and when you have a sunburn, break open a leaf and apply the clear gel inside directly to your tender skin, says Tori Hudson, N.D., a naturopathic physician and professor at the National College of Naturopathic Medicine in Portland, Oregon. Apply as often as needed for relief, says Dr. Hudson. Or for convenience, she says to use the aloe vera sunburn products available in most drugstores and health food stores. Just be sure that the product you're buying contains more aloe vera gel than water, she says.

HOMEOPATHY

For a mild sunburn, put 20 drops of Calendula tincture in four ounces of water and bathe the skin with it until the pain goes away, says Mitchell Fleisher, M.D., a family practice physician and homeopath in Colleen, Virginia. If the skin is itchy, prickly and stinging, Dr. Fleisher suggests using a mixture of 20 drops of Urtica urens tincture and four ounces of water to bathe the skin. He says you can also take a 6C or 12C dose of Calendula or Urtica urens every two to three hours as needed. If the skin is swollen and bothered by heat and feels better with an application of cold, he says to try taking a 12C or 30C dose of Apis every two to three hours.

All of these remedies are available in many health food stores. To purchase the remedies by mail, refer to the resource list on page 637.

HYDROTHERAPY

A baking soda bath is great for soothing a sunburn, according to Agatha Thrash, M.D., a medical pathologist and co-founder and co-director of Uchee Pines Institute, a natural healing center in Seale, Alabama. Add one cup of baking soda to a tub filled with lukewarm (94° to 98°F) water and soak for 30 minutes to an hour, using a cup to pour the water over any part of the body that isn't submerged in the bath. Pat dry.

VITAMIN AND MINERAL THERAPY

After a sunburn, taking these supplements for a few days can speed healing, says Julian Whitaker, M.D., founder and president of the Whitaker Wellness Center in Newport Beach, California: 1,000 milligrams of vitamin C, 400 international units of vitamin E and 15 milligrams (25,000 international units) of beta-carotene. "It's also a good idea to get more essential fatty acids, such as those in flaxseed oil," suggests Dr. Whitaker. Take one to two tablespoons of the liquid form, he says, or follow the manufacturer's label for the suggested dose if you are taking capsules (about three capsules equals one teaspoon of the liquid). Flaxseed oil is available in most health food stores.

SEE ALSO Burns

SURGICAL PREPARATION AND RECOVERY

Whether it's your first operation or your fifth, whether you're having a cyst removed or a heart bypass, surgery is scary.

But you might be able to relieve your fears, speed your recovery and lessen your pain after surgery if you heed the old Boy Scout motto and be prepared, experts say. If you're among the estimated 23 million Americans who undergo surgery each year, carefully follow your doctor's directions before the operation. And the natural remedies in this chapter—in conjunction with medical care and used with your doctor's approval—may help you prepare for and recover from surgery, according to some health professionals.

SEE YOUR MEDICAL DOCTOR WHEN . . .

- You experience nausea, constipation or diarrhea after surgery.
- You have increased bleeding or pain after release from the hospital.

FLOWER REMEDY/ESSENCE THERAPY

The emergency stress relief formula is very helpful in preparing fearful patients for surgery, according to Eve Campanelli, Ph.D., a holistic family practitioner in Beverly Hills, California. Begin treatment a week or two before the surgery, she suggests, taking four drops of the formula under the tongue four times a day.

The emergency stress relief formula, sold under brand names such as Calming Essence, Rescue Remedy and Five-Flower Formula, is available in most health food stores and through mail order (refer to the resource list on page 635). For more information on preparing and administering the formula, see page 40.

HOMEOPATHY

If possible, begin taking Arnica 30C three times a day a couple of days before your surgery to reduce swelling and soreness after the operation, says Stephen Messer, N.D., dean of the National Center for Homeopathy's summer school and a naturopathic physician in Eugene, Oregon. To speed your healing, he suggests taking one 200C dose of Arnica as soon as possible after surgery.

Arnica is available in many health food stores. To purchase it by mail, refer to the resource list on page 637.

Imagery

The night before your operation, imagine getting ready for your surgery. Picture that you are given medicine to relax you. Then imagine going into the operating room, where a skilled surgeon, anesthesiologist and nursing staff are waiting for you. As the general anesthetic is given to you, you peacefully fall asleep. Picture your surgery proceeding easily without problems. There is little bleeding, and you are sewn back up. The operation is a great success, says Dennis Gersten, M.D., a San Diego psychiatrist and publisher of *Atlantis*, a bi-monthly imagery newsletter. Then imagine that you are in the recovery room, slowly becoming more alert. You may feel some discomfort, but you are re-laxed and able to handle it easily, Dr. Gersten says. Repeat this imagery on the day of your surgery just before you leave your room for the operation.

After surgery, says Dr. Gersten, picture your pain. Give it a size, shape, color and texture. Transform your pain into a liquid and allow it to roll out of your hand or foot, drip onto the floor and flow out of the room into space.

Relaxation and Meditation

Stretch-based relaxation techniques may help relieve muscle tension and calm your body as you prepare for surgery, says Charles Carlson, Ph.D., pro-fessor of psychology at the University of Kentucky in Lexington. See page 602 for one such technique. Dr. Carlson suggests using this sequence of stretches at least once a day before surgery or whenever you feel tense.

For recovery, consider autogenics. "Autogenics is a good technique for a person who is recovering from surgery," says Martin Shaffer, Ph.D., executive director of the Stress Management Institute in San Francisco and author of *Life after Stress*. "I tell people to practice it for five minutes every hour the first day after surgery, every other hour the next day, every three hours the third day, every four hours the fourth day and then once a day until they feel well again." To learn how to do autogenics, see page 120.

SWEATING EXCESSIVELY

S ome days it seems like your sweat glands produce enough perspiration to fill the Hoover Dam.

The average person has about three million sweat glands that release fluids to help keep the body cool. Almost all sweating is triggered by activity, heat, humidity, stress or anxiety. It is a side effect of puberty, menopause and other times of hormonal upheaval. Spicy foods, alcohol and smoking can also stimulate your body to sweat more.

In most cases, people who sweat excessively have genetic predispositions to it. But profuse sweating could also be a sign of infection, heart disease, an overactive thyroid or tuberculosis. The natural remedies in this chapter, used with your doctor's approval, may help you control excess sweating, according to some health professionals.

SEE YOUR MEDICAL DOCTOR WHEN . . .

- Your sweat continually soaks and soils your clothes and shoes or trickles down your skin even when the room is cold.
- Your sweating adversely affects your career or personal life.
- You also experience persistent or recurrent fever, dizziness or rapid heartbeat.
- Your sweat has a color, crystallizes on the skin or causes skin irritation.

HOMEOPATHY

Excessive sweating can be controlled by taking one of the following 6C remedies four times a day for up to two weeks, writes Andrew Lockie, M.D., in his book *The Family Guide to Homeopathy*. Dr. Lockie recommends Acidum hydrofluoricum if your sweat is sour smelling and worse on your head and if cold weather and walking relieve it. For a thin person who tends to have sweaty, unpleasant-smelling feet, he suggests Silicea. And he says that Calcarea is a good remedy for an overweight person who is cold and clammy and has sour-smelling sweat that pours off his head at night.

All of these remedies are available in many health food stores. To purchase the remedies by mail, refer to the resource list on page 637.

IMAGERY

Picture yourself standing at the base of a mountain. There is a cool wind blowing off of it. Imagine that it's the perfect atmosphere in which to have your skin cool and dry, and if you are sweaty, the breeze will dry you off, says Dennis Gersten, M.D., a San Diego psychiatrist and publisher of *Atlantis*, a bi-monthly imagery newsletter. He recommends that you use this imagery for 10 to 20 minutes twice a day, depending on the severity of your problem.

SEE ALSO Foot Odor

TEMPOROMANDIBULAR JOINT DISORDER

If you think pronouncing "temporomandibular joint disorder" is tough on your jaws, try living with it. This ailment, also called TMD, is best known for the pain it causes in your jaw joint.

As many as one in three Americans is said to suffer from TMD, but the pain can go well beyond the jaw, affecting the temples, back teeth, cheeks, throat and the area behind the eyes. It even causes earaches and headaches.

And TMD may mean more than pain: It can cause a clicking or popping sound when the jaw moves as well as a stiff neck, stuffy nose and ringing in the ears. It's usually caused by improper alignment of the teeth, arthritis or trauma such as whiplash or a punch to the jaw. The natural remedies in this chapter—in conjunction with medical care and used with your doctor's approval—may help reduce the symptoms of TMD, according to some health professionals.

SEE YOUR MEDICAL DOCTOR WHEN . . .

- You have trouble opening your mouth more than two inches.
- Your efforts at yawning, chewing or talking result in jaw pain.
- You also feel pain in your neck, shoulders or ears.

ACUPRESSURE

To relieve the jaw aches and pains of TMD, press both St 6 points near the jaw area, recommends Michael Reed Gach, Ph.D., director of the Acupressure Institute in Berkeley, California, and author of *Acupressure's Potent Points*. Find the points by clenching your back teeth together. Feel for the muscles that bulge between the upper and lower jaw, near the jaw area. (To help locate these points, refer to the illustration on page 567.) Press these points with your middle fingers for one minute, two or three times daily, to train your jaw muscles, says Dr. Gach.

MASSAGE

To help ease the painful muscle tension in the jaw area that can accompany TMD, you can use a simple technique to massage your jaw muscles, suggests Elliot Greene, past president of the American Massage Therapy Association. The first set of muscles is located at the back of your jaw away from your chin. To find them, clench your teeth. Feel for the muscles with your fingers—left fingers on the left side of your jaw, right fingers on the right side. Once you have found them, unclench your teeth and rub the muscles with small, firm circular strokes until you feel the tension release. You can also press into the muscles with your fingertips and hold for 10 to 15 seconds.

To find the second set of muscles, clench your teeth again and feel on your scalp in front of the tops of your ears. Unclench your teeth, and rub or press the muscles.

Greene recommends doing this massage for about ten minutes once a day. For acute pain, you can repeat it two or three times a day, he says.

RELAXATION AND MEDITATION

Practicing stretch-based relaxation twice a day may help reduce symptoms of TMD, says Charles Carlson, Ph.D., professor of psychology at the University of Kentucky in Lexington. Relaxation slows the part of the nervous system that is responsible for regulating muscle tension and heart and breathing rates in response to stress, Dr. Carlson explains. That slowdown reduces a person's sensitivity to pain caused by TMD. See page 602 for one stretch-based relaxation technique.

SEE ALSO Tooth Grinding

TINNITUS

Buzzing, swishing, hissing, whirring, chirping, ringing. If you're hearing those noises *inside* your ears, you have tinnitus. It won't cause deafness, but it can impair hearing. It's usually caused by a head injury, an infection, a disease or exposure to loud sounds such as gunshots and explosions. The natural remedies in this chapter—in conjunction with medical care and used with the approval of your doctor—may help relieve tinnitus, according to some health professionals.

SEE YOUR MEDICAL DOCTOR WHEN . . .

- You suffer from noises in your ears that last for more than a few days.
- Your ear noises are accompanied by dizziness or pain.

FOOD THERAPY

"There's a major food connection here," says Paul Yanick, Ph.D., a research scientist in Milford, Pennsylvania. "Basically, a lack of magnesium might cause some people to suffer tinnitus." He recommends eating plenty of magnesium-rich foods, which may provide relief from tinnitus and help prevent new episodes. (For food sources of magnesium, see "Getting What You Need" on page 142.)

HERBAL THERAPY

If your doctor says that your tinnitus is the result of circulation problems, try ginkgo, which increases blood flow to the brain, says Varro E. Tyler, Ph.D., professor of pharmacognosy at Purdue University in West Lafayette, Indiana. Ginkgo capsules are sold in most health food stores. Check the label for dosage instructions—and to be sure that you're getting enough ginkgo to be effective, says Dr. Tyler. He recommends a dose of 120 milligrams daily of a concentrated, standardized ginkgo extract known as GBE (*Ginkgo biloba* extract). Ginkgo works slowly, and it may take weeks or months before you notice improvement, he adds.

HOMEOPATHY

In his book *The Family Guide to Homeopathy*, Andrew Lockie, M.D., suggests that taking one of the following 6C remedies three times daily for up to two weeks may help control tinnitus.

If you have a roaring sound in your ears accompanied by giddiness and deafness, try Salicylic acidum, says Dr. Lockie. If you have roaring with a tingling sensation and your ears feel clogged up, he recommends Carbonium sulphuratum. Kali iodatum is a good remedy for long-standing ringing in the ears with no other symptoms, he says.

All of these remedies are available in many health food stores. To purchase the remedies by mail, refer to the resource list on page 637.

REFLEXOLOGY

You may get some relief from tinnitus by working the ear, cervical spine and neck reflex points on your hands or feet, says St. Petersburg, Florida, reflexologist Dwight Byers, author of *Better Health with Foot Reflexology*. Byers also suggests working the points on the sides and bottoms of both big toes thoroughly, using whichever technique you find most comfortable.

To help you locate these points, consult the hand and foot reflex charts beginning on page 582. For instructions on how to work the points, see "Your Reflexology Session" on page 110.

RELAXATION AND MEDITATION

Relaxation and meditation techniques can help some people temporarily relieve tinnitus and are particularly effective if used as part of a comprehensive treatment program that includes medication, broad-band noise generators (commonly known as white noise machines), hearing aids and other therapies, says Pawel Jastreboff, Ph.D., professor of surgery and physiology at the University of Maryland School of Medicine and director of the University of Maryland Tinnitus and Hyperacusis Center, both in Baltimore. Dr. Jastreboff says stress makes it harder for a person who has tinnitus to ignore the annoying ringing in his ears. Relaxation counteracts that.

Pick one of the relaxation techniques described beginning on page 113 and practice it for at least 30 minutes a day for at least a week. Relaxation may not be helpful for everybody, so if at the end of the week the technique isn't working or your tinnitus seems worse, try another relaxation method or see your doctor, Dr. Jastreboff says.

SEE ALSO Hearing Problems

TOOTHACHE

Chew on this: That toe-curling, flesh-crawling, all-consuming pain caused by a toothache was probably instigated by something as simple as a tiny amount of bacteria penetrating the tooth's tissue and inflaming its pulp.

Actually, chewing on anything is probably the last thing you want to do when you have a toothache. Your first thought may be to berate yourself for not brushing and flossing better or to find a few choice words for a broken or loose filling. A cracked tooth or blow to the mouth can also trigger an inflammation. Toothache pain can be deep and throbbing and can cause extreme sensitivity. The natural remedies in this chapter—in conjunction with medical care and used with your dentist's approval—may help relieve the pain of a toothache, according to some health professionals.

SEE YOUR MEDICAL DOCTOR WHEN . . .

- You feel a sharp or recurring pain in one or more teeth.
- You have a tooth that had been hurting but that suddenly stops hurting.
- You feel tooth pain when eating or drinking something hot.

ACUPRESSURE

To ease the throbbing pain, press point LI 4 on the hand that's on the same side as your toothache, says Michael Reed Gach, Ph.D., director of the Acupressure Institute in Berkeley, California, and author of *Acupressure's Potent Points*. LI 4 is located in the webbing between your thumb and index finger, close to the bone at the base of the index finger. (For help in locating this point, refer to the illustration on page 565.) The point is on the large intestine meridian, which is a traditional acupressure pathway for relieving toothaches, according to Dr. Gach. He explains that the meridian flows from the hands and up the arms until it reaches the teeth and gums.

To press point LI 4, says Dr. Gach, hold it with your thumb on top of the webbing and your index finger underneath, then squeeze into the webbing, angling the pressure toward the bone that connects the index finger to the hand. He suggests holding the point for one minute as needed to relieve pain. He cautions that pressing this point can cause uterine contractions and is not recommended for pregnant women.

TOOTHACHE

FOOD THERAPY

"Take a couple of cloves from the spice rack and place them between the aching tooth and your cheek, much like you'd use chewing tobacco," says Richard D. Fischer, D.D.S., president of the International Academy of Oral Medicine and Toxicology and a dentist and homeopath in Annandale, Virginia. "This remedy has been known for centuries to relieve many kinds of toothaches." Dr. Fischer says to chew the cloves a little bit to release their juice, then leave them in place for a half-hour or so or until the pain subsides. He advises continuing the treatment until you can see a dentist.

HERBAL THERAPY

Try oil of clove to soothe the pain until you can get to the dentist, says Varro E. Tyler, Ph.D., professor of pharmacognosy at Purdue University in West Lafayette, Indiana. But don't use it full strength, he cautions: It's so strong that it can damage your tooth's nerve. Ask your pharmacist to recommend an over-the-counter preparation containing oil of clove (sometimes called eugenol), such as Orajel, and follow label directions for use, he says.

HOMEOPATHY

To relieve a throbbing toothache that develops suddenly, try a 30X dose of Belladonna every 30 to 60 minutes until the pain begins to diminish, says Richard D. Fischer, D.D.S., president of the International Academy of Oral Medicine and Toxicology and a dentist and homeopath in Annandale, Virginia. If cold weather or foods worsen your tooth pain and warmth and light pressure on the jaw make it feel better, he suggests a 30X dose of Magnesia phosphorica every 30 to 60 minutes as needed.

Belladonna and Magnesia phosphorica are available in many health food stores. To purchase the remedies by mail, refer to the resource list on page 637.

HYDROTHERAPY

For quick relief of a toothache, try a charcoal compress, says Agatha Thrash, M.D., a medical pathologist and co-founder and co-director of Uchee Pines Institute, a natural healing center in Seale, Alabama. Mix a heaping tablespoonful of activated charcoal powder (which is sold in most health food stores and some pharmacies) with enough water to make a paste, apply it to a strip of gauze and bite down on the gauze "so that the paste squishes around your aching tooth," says Dr. Thrash. "Your tooth should feel better in ten minutes."

TOOTHACHE

IMAGERY

Recall a time when you swam in ice-cold water or played in the snow. Imagine the sensations of that moment. Feel the chill of the water or snow penetrate your hands and feet so that they become almost numb. Now imagine that feeling of numbness surrounding your tooth, soothing it as if you were rubbing it with snow until all of the pain is gone, says Deena Margetis, a certified clinical hypnotherapist specializing in dental care in Annandale, Virginia. This imagery should last no longer than five minutes and can be repeated as often as needed, she adds.

REFLEXOLOGY

Work all of the points on the sides and bottoms of your toes, paying special attention to the middle of both big toes, says St. Petersburg, Florida, reflexologist Dwight Byers, author of *Better Health with Foot Reflexology*. To work these points, use whichever technique you find most comfortable.

To help you locate these points, consult the foot reflex chart on page 592. For instructions on how to work the points, see "Your Reflexology Session" on page 110.

RELAXATION AND MEDITATION

Focus on your pain and rate it from zero to ten, with ten being the worst pain you've ever experienced and zero being no pain. Now concentrate on places in your body that feel calm and are pain-free, such as your left foot or your right ear. Keep searching deeper into your body and mind for pain-free points. As you refocus your attention on the calm parts of yourself, the pain in your tooth will fade into the background, says Neil Fiore, Ph.D., a psychologist in Berkeley, California, and author of *The Road Back to Health: Coping with the Emotional Aspects of Cancer*. Use this technique whenever you have pain or worry about pain. If the pain increases, call your doctor.

VITAMIN AND MINERAL THERAPY

One way to soothe the pain of a toothache is to increase your intake of calcium and magnesium, says Richard D. Fischer, D.D.S., president of the International Academy of Oral Medicine and Toxicology and a dentist and homeopath in Annandale, Virginia. He recommends taking 500 milligrams of calcium and 200 to 300 milligrams of magnesium at the first sign of a toothache: "It's soothing to the nerves of your teeth."

TOOTH GRINDING

The stress of the daily grind can become a . . . well, a daily grind—the common habit of nighttime tooth gnashing or daytime jaw clenching known as bruxism.

Problem is, this mouth movement can wear down teeth—they literally grind down and may even become loose. Besides affecting looks, this can cause jaw pain, particularly when you wake up, and can make teeth more sensitive to hot and cold foods and drinks. If this grinding continues, you can dislocate your jaw or damage the jaw joint, causing headaches, neck and shoulder pain and ringing in your ears. The natural remedies in this chapter—in conjunction with medical care and used with the approval of your dentist—may help prevent or ease tooth grinding, according to some health professionals.

SEE YOUR MEDICAL DOCTOR WHEN . . .

- Your spouse says you grind or gnash your teeth while asleep.
- You notice that you're habitually gnashing your teeth or clenching your jaw muscle, as if chewing or biting something.
- You wake up with jaw pain, headaches or neck or shoulder pain.

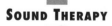

RELAXATION AND MEDITATION

Whenever you feel tension building in your jaw, do the progressive relaxation exercise described on page 122, suggests Deena Margetis, a certified clinical hypnotherapist in Annandale, Virginia, who specializes in dental care. When you've completed the exercise and your body feels relaxed, imagine all of the remaining tension draining out of your jaw, down your shoulder and arm and into your hand. Clench and unclench your fist until you feel the tension gently dissipate.

SOUND THERAPY

Try listening to music with a slow, relaxing beat just before going to bed, says Janalea Hoffman, R.M.T., a composer and music therapist based in Kansas City, Missouri. Many people find that the music calms them down and makes them less likely to grind their teeth while sleeping, according to Hoffman. Try playing the music for 20 to 30 minutes; it's okay to fall asleep while listening to it.

Make sure the music you listen to is 60 beats per minute or slower, Hoffman says. She recommends her tape *Musical Massage*; for other suggested pieces to relax by, see "Sailing Away to Key Largo" on page 129. Many of these pieces are available in music stores. For information on mail order, refer to the resource list on page 642.

VITAMIN AND MINERAL THERAPY

"Tooth grinding may be the result of a deficiency in calcium and magnesium," says Richard D. Fischer, D.D.S., a dentist and homeopath in Annandale, Virginia, and president of the International Academy of Oral Medicine and Toxicology. "Many people get relief by taking a 500-milligram supplement of calcium each day, along with 200 to 300 milligrams of magnesium. If the trouble continues, then increase the amounts to 1,000 milligrams of calcium and 400 to 600 milligrams of magnesium."

SEE ALSO Temporomandibular Joint Disorder

TYPE A PERSONALITY

If you're one of those hard-driving, time-pressured, workaholic type A personalities, chances are you wouldn't dream of taking the time to stop and smell the roses. Too bad, because research shows that if you don't, you might wind up pushing up daisies before your time.

What stresses your cardiovascular system—and puts you at increased risk of heart attack—are the anger, hostility, cynicism and extreme competitiveness that sometimes come with type A behavior. The natural remedies in this chapter, used with your doctor's approval, may help a type A personality relax, according to some health professionals.

SEE YOUR MEDICAL DOCTOR WHEN . . .

- Your type A behavior is starting to affect your health, causing headaches, body aches, racing heartbeat, high blood pressure or other symptoms.

AROMATHERAPY

Aromatherapy offers a number of ways for the type A personality to relax and unwind, says Los Angeles aromatic consultant John Steele. He recommends a combination of baths, massages and a diffuser (candle or electric), using a soothing oil such as lavender, ylang ylang, bergamot, melissa, jasmine, grapefruit, geranium, sandalwood, rose or neroli.

At the end of the day, draw yourself a hot bath scented with six to ten drops of essential oil, suggests Steele. He says to soak for 15 minutes, then massage your neck and shoulders with a blend of ten drops of essential oil per ½ ounce of carrier oil such as almond or sunflower (carrier oils are available in most health food stores). For deepest relaxation, he recommends using a diffuser or an aroma lamp to scent the room as you bathe.

For information on preparing and administering essential oils, including cautions about their use, see page 19. For information on purchasing essential oils, refer to the resource list on page 633.

FLOWER REMEDY/ESSENCE THERAPY

"The type A personality is very rigid and overreacts when things don't go according to plan," says Patricia Kaminski, co-director of the Flower Essence Society, a Nevada City, California, organization that studies and promotes the therapeutic use of flower remedies/essences. Such personalities can benefit from the Bach flower remedy Willow, according to Kaminski. "The willow is a strong, resilient tree that bends easily in the wind without breaking. This remedy encourages the same kind of flexibility in the person who takes it," she says. The Bach flower remedy Holly can be helpful for "emotional congestion," according to Kaminski. And the essence Scarlet Monkey Flower helps a person identify the sources of his anger and come to terms with it.

Flower remedies/essences are available in some health food stores and through mail order (refer to the resource list on page 635). For information on preparing and administering flower remedies/essences, see page 37.

IMAGERY

Picture walking along the bank of a river until you come to a bridge. Walk to the middle of the bridge and stare into the water. Pick out one drop of water in the river and imagine that it represents the current moment. Let that drop (or moment) expand until it is three feet wide. Then allow it to become as wide as the river.

Eventually, the drop should expand to the point that everything around you is in the current moment, says Dennis Gersten, M.D., a San Diego psychiatrist and publisher of *Atlantis*, a bi-monthly imagery newsletter. "Essentially, that imagery helps you live in the moment, which is difficult for type A's," he explains. He suggests doing this imagery for 10 to 20 minutes twice a day.

As an alternative, envision making a videotape of your fast and furious day. Now rewind the tape and play it in slow motion. Above this moving picture of your life, see the words "slow" and "easy" in pink, coral or salmon light, says Elizabeth Ann Barrett, R.N., Ph.D., professor and coordinator of the Center for Nursing Research at Hunter College of the City University of New York in New York City. She suggests doing this imagery once at the end of the day; it should take about ten minutes, she adds.

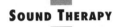

JUICE THERAPY

"Celery juice has a very soothing effect on the nervous system, so it's a wonderful tonic for the type A person," says Elaine Gillaspie, N.D., a naturopathic physician in Portland, Oregon. She recommends an eight-ounce blend of equal parts celery juice, carrot juice and water, taken at least once a day. "Celery juice also is a mild diuretic and may have a beneficial effect on high blood pressure," she notes.

For information on juicing techniques, see page 93.

SOUND THERAPY

Try spending 10 to 20 minutes each day listening to relaxing music, suggests Steven Halpern, Ph.D., composer, researcher and author of *Sound Health: The Music and Sounds That Make Us Whole.* To get started, turn on the music, then sit or lie comfortably, close your eyes and take a deep breath. Dr. Halpern suggests that you wear headphones to focus your full attention and to avoid distraction. He recommends, however, that you keep the speakers playing, so your body absorbs the sound energy. While the music plays, slow your breathing and let it become steady. Listen not just to the notes but to the silence between the notes. Dr. Halpern says this will keep you from analyzing the music, which will allow it to relax you.

Here are some suggested pieces of music: *Seapeace*, a New Age album by Georgia Kelly; *Spectrum Suite, Inner Peace* and *Comfort Zone*, all by Dr. Halpern; and any recording of Gregorian chants. For other selections, see "Sailing Away to Key Largo" on page 129.

Many of these pieces are available in music stores. For mail-order information, refer to the resource list on page 642.

VITAMIN AND MINERAL THERAPY

"If you're a type A, you can benefit from taking a magnesium supplement and an amino acid named GABA (gamma-aminobutyric acid), both of which can help mellow you out," says Julian Whitaker, M.D., founder and president of the Whitaker Wellness Center in Newport Beach, California. He recommends a daily 400-milligram supplement of magnesium. Follow the manufacturer's dosage suggestion for GABA, he adds. GABA is available in supplement form in most health food stores.

YOGA

Patience and relaxation are what you need, according to Alice Christensen, founder and executive director of the American Yoga Association. She says meditation (see page 153) for 20 to 30 minutes every day will help you find more of both. She also recommends the complete breath exercise (see page 152), which you can use several times per day—at work, on the commute, in bed or any other time you feel stressed or angry.

SEE ALSO Anger; Irritability

ULCERS

U lcers used to be painful little badges of honor. If you worked really hard, you got these little holes in your stomach or intestinal lining. That proved you were unrelenting and driven to succeed.

Not anymore. Researchers have discovered that stress and success aren't necessarily what causes ulcers. In many cases, the culprit is a bacterium called *Helicobacter pylori*, which anyone can get, regardless of occupation. Drinking coffee, taking too much aspirin, smoking and a bad diet can make things worse.

Ulcers form when the mucus lining of the stomach loses its ability to repel stomach acids. The acids, which digest food, begin to digest your stomach instead. This is a gastric ulcer. If the ulcer forms at the top of the small intestine, it's a duodenal ulcer. The natural remedies in this chapter—in conjunction with medical care and used with your doctor's approval—may help prevent or ease an ulcer, according to some health professionals.

SEE YOUR MEDICAL DOCTOR WHEN ...

- You feel burning, gnawing or aching just below your breastbone.
- You have pain that subsides after eating, then reappears two to three hours later.
- You don't feel pain but you spit up matter that looks like coffee grounds or have dark, tarry bowel movements.

AYURVEDA

Aloe vera gel is an excellent treatment for ulcers, says David Frawley, O.M.D., director of the American Institute of Vedic Studies in Santa Fe, New Mexico. He says to take one to two teaspoons three times daily, mixing it with enough honey or a nonacidic fruit juice to disguise the taste if you wish. "Aloe vera gel has a milder taste than the other bitter herbs, although it still doesn't taste very good," Dr. Frawley says. Aloe vera gel is safe to drink, he adds, but make sure you buy a product meant for internal use, not a gel that's for external use only. Ask your Ayurvedic practitioner or herbalist to recommend a brand that won't have a laxative side effect. It's available in most health food stores.

Ulcers are a symptom of excess pitta dosha, says Vasant Lad, B.A.M.S., M.A.Sc., director of the Ayurvedic Institute in Albuquerque, New Mexico. (For more information on the Ayurvedic doshas, see "All about Vata, Pitta and Kapha" on page 28.) For angry, hateful feelings accompanied by a burning sensation in the stomach, Dr. Lad recommends drinking a mixture of one cup of hot milk and one teaspoon of arrowroot powder (available in the baby food section of many supermarkets). Or you can make a tea by combining equal portions of cumin, coriander and fennel seeds and steeping roughly a teaspoon of this mixture in a cup of hot water for roughly ten minutes. Dr. Lad says to use this drink when your ulcer flares up or as a preventive measure whenever you're feeling angry.

FLOWER REMEDY/ESSENCE THERAPY

"I've seen many ulcer patients who don't let go of painful emotions, who hold their fears in their stomachs," says Susan Lange, O.M.D., of the Meridian Center for Personal and Environmental Health in Santa Monica, California. "The flower essence Dandelion helps them let go of that tension.

"Other people with ulcers can handle their own anxieties, but they absorb other people's problems like a sponge," she continues. "The California essence Pink Yarrow helps them distinguish between their own problems and someone else's."

Flower essences are available in some health food stores and through mail order (refer to the resource list on page 635). For information on preparing and administering flower essences, see page 37.

FOOD THERAPY

Eat more cabbage, says Allan Magaziner, D.O., a nutritional medicine specialist and head of the Magaziner Medical Center in Cherry Hill, New Jersey.

"Cabbage contains a lot of glutamine, an amino acid that has been shown to heal ulcers." His recommendation: Have at least one healthy serving of steamed cabbage each day for two weeks.

HYDROTHERAPY

For temporary relief of gastric ulcer pain, nothing beats activated charcoal, says Agatha Thrash, M.D., a medical pathologist and co-founder and co-director of Uchee Pines Institute, a natural healing center in Seale, Alabama. She suggests mixing two tablespoons of activated charcoal powder with a little water in the bottom of a tall glass (at least eight ounces). Continue stirring and adding water a little at a time until the glass is full, she says, then drink it with a straw. She says to follow the charcoal water with a glass of plain water. This treatment may be repeated hourly until pain subsides, she adds. Activated charcoal is available in most health food stores and some pharmacies.

REFLEXOLOGY

Work the solar plexus and stomach points on the bottoms of both feet, say Kevin and Barbara Kunz, reflexology researchers in Santa Fe, New Mexico, and authors of *Hand and Foot Reflexology*. They also suggest working the solar plexus, top of shoulder and stomach points on both hands.

To help you locate these points, consult the hand and foot reflex charts beginning on page 582. For instructions on how to work the points, see "Your Reflexology Session" on page 110.

RELAXATION AND MEDITATION

Daily thermal biofeedback increases blood flow in the digestive system, which helps heal and protect the lining of the stomach, says Steven Fahrion, Ph.D., director of research at the Life Sciences Institute of Mind-Body Health in Topeka, Kansas. To learn this simple ten-minute technique, see page 121.

SOUND THERAPY

If stress is contributing to your ulcer, relaxing music may help, says Janalea Hoffman, R.M.T., a composer and music therapist based in Kansas City, Missouri. She suggests listening to music with a slow, steady beat for about 30 minutes per day. Among the selections Hoffman recommends are her tapes *Deep Daydreams* and *Musical Massage*. For other relaxing selections, see "Sailing Away to Key Largo" on page 129. Many of these pieces are available in music stores. For mail-order information, refer to the resource list on page 642.

VITAMIN AND MINERAL THERAPY

Use the food sensitivity diet (see "Food Sensitivity: How to Discover the 'Healthy' Foods That Can Cause Disease" on page 52) to eliminate any foods that might have a role in causing the problem, says David Edelberg, M.D., an internist and medical director of the American Holistic Center/Chicago. He also suggests eliminating sugar, caffeine and alcohol from your diet and giving up smoking.

A person who has already developed an ulcer may want to use the following supplemental regimen to help control its symptoms, adds Dr. Edelberg: 10,000 international units of vitamin A twice a day; 50 milligrams of B-complex vitamins a day; 1,000 milligrams of vitamin C a day (use the buffered form); 400 international units of vitamin E a day; 500 milligrams of glutamine three times a day; one capsule of rice bran oil (gamma oryzanol) three times a day; two 380-milligram tablets of deglycyrrhizinated licorice four times a day—between meals and at bedtime—for one month; and 30 milligrams of zinc picolinate a day for one month. These dietary supplements, alone or in combination, are available in most health food stores, according to Dr. Edelberg.

URINARY TRACT INFECTIONS

A *Prevention* magazine survey found that urinary tract infections are the most common health problem among women; nearly half of those who responded to the questionnaire said they'd had at least one.

Infection occurs when a microorganism invades your bladder or your urethra, which carries urine from the bladder and out of the body. The result is burning or pain during urination, the urge to urinate frequently, lower back pain and sometimes blood in the urine. Though they're much more common in women, men can also develop urinary tract infections—especially those over age 50, who may have enlarged prostates.

Proper hygiene and drinking lots of fluids are both essential for preventing urinary tract infections. The natural remedies in this chapter—in conjunction with medical care and used with your doctor's approval—may help prevent urinary tract infections or speed their healing, according to some health professionals.

SEE YOUR MEDICAL DOCTOR WHEN . . .

- You notice blood in your urine.
- You have pain in your lower back or side.
- You have a fever, nausea or vomiting.

AROMATHERAPY

To speed the healing of a urinary tract infection, add 20 drops each of euca-lyptus and sandalwood essential oils to a hot bath, suggests Greenwich, Con-necticut, aromatherapist Judith Jackson, author of *Scentual Touch: A Personal Guide to Aromatherapy*. She says to soak in the tub for ten minutes. Juniper and thyme essential oils may be substituted for the eucalyptus and sandalwood if you prefer those scents, according to Jackson.

For information on preparing and administering essential oils, including cautions about their use, see page 19. For information on purchasing essential oils, refer to the resource list on page 633.

HERBAL THERAPY

Capsules of uva ursi, also called bearberry, may help treat urinary tract infec-tions, according to Varro E. Tyler, Ph.D., professor of pharmacognosy at Purdue University in West Lafayette, Indiana. These capsules are available in most health food stores, and Dr. Tyler says to follow the dosage recommenda-tions on the label. But there's a catch: In order for this remedy to work, ac-cording to Dr. Tyler, you must maintain alkaline urine by eating a diet rich in milk, vegetables, fruits and fruit juices. He also suggests taking two teaspoons of baking soda a day, a small dose with each of your meals. Do not use this remedy if you are watching your sodium intake, he adds.

HYDROTHERAPY

Water is the best way to treat any urinary tract infection, says Agatha Thrash, M.D., a medical pathologist and co-founder and co-director of Uchee Pines Institute, a natural healing center in Seale, Alabama. "People who get infec-tions usually don't drink enough water, so the urine sits in the bladder too long, and bacteria build up," says Dr. Thrash. She tells patients to drink "loads of water" at the first sign of an infection: 6 to 8 eight-ounce glasses a day for young, healthy people, 10 eight-ounce glasses for those over age 50 and 12 eight-ounce glasses for active people over 60, whose bodies need extra fluids, according to Dr. Thrash.

Along with drinking water, try contrast sitz baths to increase circulation in the pelvis, suggests Tori Hudson, N.D., a naturopathic physician and professor at the National College of Naturopathic Medicine in Portland, Oregon. Soak in a shallow hot bath for three to five minutes, then sit in a basin of cold water for 30 seconds. "Repeat this sequence three times, finishing with cold water," says Dr. Hudson. "And if you don't have two tubs, you can alternate hot and cold compresses to the pelvic area." You can use this treatment once or twice a day, she adds.

JUICE THERAPY

While drinking fluids is the best way to flush out the bacteria that cause urinary tract infections, some fluids are better than others, says Michael A. Klaper, M.D., a nutritional medicine specialist in Pompano Beach, Florida, and director of the Institute of Nutritional Education and Research, an organization based in Manhattan Beach, California, that teaches doctors about nutrition and its relationship to disease. He says that cranberry juice is probably the best, because it helps prevent bacteria from anchoring to bladder walls. "The key is to drink real cranberry juice, not those cranberry juice cocktails," he explains. "Those drinks are too sweet. It has to be really tart to work." If you can't find cranberry juice, look for cranberry juice concentrate that you can mix with water.

To stave off the problem, certified nutritionist Cherie Calbom, M.S., of Kirkland, Washington, co-author of *Juicing for Life*, suggests drinking 16 ounces of fresh cranberry juice per day. "Mix it with some fresh apple juice for the best taste," she suggests.

Like Dr. Klaper, she says to use fresh or frozen cranberries. "If you can't find them, use cranberry juice concentrate," she advises. "Mix ½ tablespoon of concentrate with a pint of fresh apple juice."

For information on juicing techniques, see page 93.

REFLEXOLOGY

Work the bladder and kidney points on the bottoms of your feet, say Kevin and Barbara Kunz, reflexology researchers in Santa Fe, New Mexico, and authors of *Hand and Foot Reflexology*. You can also use the corresponding golf ball technique (page 588) to work the kidney and adrenal gland points on both hands.

To help you locate these points, consult the hand and foot reflex charts beginning on page 582. For instructions on how to work the points, see "Your Reflexology Session" on page 110.

VAGINITIS

It doesn't take much to throw off the body's natural balance, especially in a sensitive area such as a woman's vagina. It can be irritated by any number of things, including infections, tampons, condoms, antibiotics, deodorant sprays, douches, sperm, even fluctuations in estrogen levels.

When that happens, the result is vaginitis, an inflammation of the vaginal area. The condition is marked by pain and itching and sometimes by unusual vaginal discharge.

Doctors often prescribe drugs to combat vaginitis. If you have medication, be sure to take it all, or the infection may quickly return. The natural remedies in this chapter—in conjunction with medical care and used with your doctor's approval—may help soothe the symptoms of vaginitis and speed healing, according to some health professionals.

SEE YOUR MEDICAL DOCTOR WHEN . . .

- You have deep pain in your pelvis or swollen glands in the groin area and are running a fever above 101°F.
- You have open sores in the vaginal area, whether they hurt or not.

FOOD THERAPY

While vaginitis can be caused by any number of culprits, it often results from an overgrowth of yeast and certain types of abnormal bacteria, says Elson Haas, M.D., director of the Preventive Medical Center of Marin in San Rafael, California, and author of *Staying Healthy with Nutrition*. According to Dr. Haas, yogurt containing live cultures has been proven to reduce the yeast and bacterial overgrowth. He advises eating one to two cups of yogurt a day for three or four days. Avoiding yeast products such as baked goods, alcohol and vinegar is also recommended, he says. For recurring yeast-related vaginitis, he suggests his three-week detoxification diet (see "Detoxing Your Ills" on page 48).

HERBAL THERAPY

Try a Saint-John's-wort or calendula salve to soothe the itching and irritation caused by vaginitis, says Barre, Vermont, herbalist Rosemary Gladstar, author of *Herbal Healing for Women* and other books about herbs. These products are sold in most health food stores, and Gladstar says to follow the application directions on the label.

HOMEOPATHY

For a burning, creamy yellow or green discharge that is worse in the evening and after eating and that may be accompanied by chills or irregular or no periods, try a 6X dose of Pulsatilla three times a day or a 30C dose once or twice a day until you begin to feel better, says Cynthia Mervis Watson, M.D., a family practice physician in Santa Monica, California, who specializes in homeopathy and herbal therapy. She says that a similar dose of Sepia will help if you have painful intercourse and an itchy yellow or green discharge.

To tame a burning vaginal discharge that causes skin rashes and that is worse from bathing, warmth or drinking alcohol, and if you are prone to getting skin rashes, Dr. Watson says to try a 6X dose of Sulphur three times a day or a 30C dose once or twice a day. If you have a swollen, burning, itchy vulva and a corrosive, acrid yellow discharge that is worse between periods, she suggests the same dosage of Kreosote.

A 6X dose of Graphites three times a day will help if you have a pale, thin, profuse, irritating white discharge that occurs in sporadic gushes and that may be worse in the morning or while walking, according to Dr. Watson. If you have a green, bloody discharge accompanied by a raw feeling that seems worse after urinating but better after washing with cool water, take a 6X dose of Mercurius three times a day or a 30C dose once or twice a day, she says.

All of these remedies are available in many health food stores. To purchase the remedies by mail, refer to the resource list on page 635.

HYDROTHERAPY

"Contrast sitz baths promote circulation and speed the body's natural healing process," says Tori Hudson, Ph.D., a naturopathic physician and professor at the National College of Naturopathic Medicine in Portland, Oregon. For instructions on setting up a contrast sitz bath, see "Hydrotherapy at Home" on page 78.

If you don't have two large basins, Dr. Hudson says to soak for three minutes in a hot, shallow bath, then stand up and hold a cold, wet towel between the legs and over the pelvis for 30 to 60 seconds. Repeat this cycle five times.

While douching with water, yogurt or apple cider vinegar is a common folk remedy for vaginitis, Dr. Hudson cautions against douching with anything if you have an infection. "Douching can actually force bacteria farther up into the vagina and can aggravate the condition," she says.

To prevent recurring vaginal infections, get into the habit of rinsing the perineal area (located between your anus and vaginal opening) after urinating or having a bowel movement, says Agatha Thrash, M.D., a medical pathologist and co-founder and co-director of Uchee Pines Institute, a natural healing center in Seale, Alabama. Keep a quart-size cup or jar near the toilet. For each rinse, add a tablespoon or two of apple cider vinegar to a quart of plain water. Slowly pour the mixture into the pubic hair while you're sitting on the toilet. "This protects the natural acid balance of the vaginal area, which is prone to yeast overgrowth if it becomes too alkaline," says Dr. Thrash.

SEE ALSO Yeast Infections

VARICOSE VEINS

Varicose veins—those squiggly, swollen knots of blue or red blood vessels—are ugly and often painful. They form when valves in the veins lose their elasticity and the walls of the veins weaken and develop balloonlike pockets. These pockets can trap blood and cause minor clots and inflammation. Varicose veins occur most often in the legs but can appear in your arms as well.

Since the tendency to develop them can be inherited, you may not be able to stop varicose veins altogether. But your attempts to avoid or remove them don't have to be in vain. The natural remedies in this chapter—in conjunction with medical care and used with your doctor's approval—may be helpful for those with varicose veins, according to some health professionals.

SEE YOUR MEDICAL DOCTOR WHEN . . .

- Your varicose veins become painful.
- You see red lumps in your veins that don't get smaller even when you raise your legs.
- You have varicose veins around your ankles that rupture and start to bleed.

AROMATHERAPY

Stimulate circulation in the legs with gentle massage, recommends aromatherapist Judith Jackson, author of *Scentual Touch: A Personal Guide to Aromatherapy.* She says to blend 12 drops each of cypress and geranium essential oils in four ounces of a carrier oil such as almond, soy or sunflower. (Carrier oils are available in most health food stores.) Then, she says, gently apply the mixture to the legs by stroking upward, in the direction of the heart. Don't massage directly on the veins, Jackson cautions; instead, massage the surrounding area and gently stroke the oil over the veins.

VARICOSE VEINS

For information on preparing and administering essential oils, including cautions about their use, see page 19. For information on purchasing essential oils, refer to the resource list on page 633.

FOOD THERAPY

"A high-fiber diet helps prevent straining of your stool, which can build up pressure and aggravate varicose veins," says Julian Whitaker, M.D., founder and president of the Whitaker Wellness Center in Newport Beach, California. He suggests trying to consume at least 30 grams of fiber a day. You can get this amount by building your meals around whole grains, legumes, fruits and vegetables, adding these foods to your diet as often as possible, he says.

Also, Dr. Whitaker says to eat plenty of blackberries and cherries, since they are rich in compounds that may prevent varicose veins or lessen the discomfort they cause.

HOMEOPATHY

At least four remedies can help control varicose veins, writes Andrew Lockie, M.D., in his book *The Family Guide to Homeopathy*. He suggests taking one of these 30C remedies every 12 hours for up to seven days.

For varicose veins that feel bruised and sore, try Hamamelis, according to Dr. Lockie. He recommends Pulsatilla if you feel chilly and if warmth and allowing your legs to hang down make your veins worse. Carbo vegetabilis is a good remedy for varicose veins that make the skin around them appear mottled and marbled, he says. If your legs look pale but redden easily and walking slowly relieves the weak, achy feeling, he says to try Ferrum metallicum.

All of these remedies are available in many health food stores. To purchase the remedies by mail, refer to the resource list on page 637.

HYDROTHERAPY

After eliminating contributing factors such as obesity, constipation and clothing that has tight waistbands, try alternating hot and cold baths to stimulate circulation in the legs, suggests Agatha Thrash, M.D., a medical pathologist and co-founder and co-director of Uchee Pines Institute, a natural healing center in Seale, Alabama. Use two buckets or plastic wastebaskets tall enough to submerge the legs up to the knees. Fill one container with enough comfortably hot water to cover the lower legs and the other container with the same amount of cold water. Soak your feet and legs in the hot water for about three minutes, then immerse them in the cold water for about 30 seconds. Repeat three times, finishing with the cold soak. You'll need to use this treatment once a day for at least one month to see results, according to Dr. Thrash. If you have diabetes, you should use warm (not hot) water, she adds.

JUICE THERAPY

Fresh fruit juices can be very helpful for those with varicose veins, says Cherie Calbom, M.S., a certified nutritionist in Kirkland, Washington, and co-author of *Juicing for Life*. Dark-colored berries such as cherries, blackberries and blueberries contain anthocyanins and proanthocyanidins, pigments that tone and strengthen the walls of the veins, Calbom explains. She adds that pineapples are rich in the enzyme bromelain, which helps prevent blood clots, an uncommon but serious complication of varicose veins.

"Juicing provides these nutrients in much higher concentrations than you can get by just eating the fruits," says Calbom. She suggests drinking eight ounces of fresh berry or pineapple juice, alone or diluted with another fruit juice, once or twice a day for maximum benefit.

For information on juicing techniques, see page 93.

MASSAGE

Never massage directly on varicose veins, warns Elaine Stillerman, L.M.T., a massage therapist in New York City. Still, a general leg massage can help reduce swelling in the veins, she says. Sit up comfortably on a sofa or bed, with your legs raised slightly on a pillow. Now use the effleurage stroke (page 570) to work up the entire leg from the ankle to the upper thigh. Again, remember not to touch the varicose veins. You can do this daily for about five minutes on each leg.

REFLEXOLOGY

Working your hands or feet may help with varicose veins, says Rebecca Dioda, a reflexologist with the Morris Institute of Natural Therapeutics, a holistic health education center in Denville, New Jersey. She recommends focusing on these reflex points: adrenal and parathyroid gland, digestive system (especially the liver), spine, heart and sciatic nerve.

To help you locate these points, consult the hand and foot reflex charts beginning on page 582. For instructions on how to work the points, see "Your Reflexology Session" on page 110.

YOGA

A special breathing exercise can help ease pain from varicose veins, according to Stephen A. Nezezon, M.D., yoga teacher and staff physician at the

Himalayan Institute of Yoga Science and Philosophy in Honesdale, Pennsylvania. His instructions: Start by lying on your back on the floor, arms at your sides, with your feet resting above you on a chair. Breathe deeply through your nose using the belly breath (see page 152). Dr. Nezezon says gravity helps pull blood from your legs. The deep breathing creates a pull in your chest cavity that also draws blood from the legs. Fresh blood then enters your legs, easing the pain. Do this exercise once a day for about ten minutes.

VISION PROBLEMS

The eye is one of nature's great feats of engineering, with millions of working parts that let you focus up close, far away and in between, all in spectacular color and three dimensions.

Of course, all of this complexity also means that things can sometimes get out of whack. There are nearsightedness, in which you have trouble focusing on distant objects, and farsightedness, where you can't see close-up things well. There are glaucoma, a buildup of fluid pressure that can damage your optic nerve, and cataracts, opaque lenses that fog your vision. Diabetes can cause detached retinas and other complications. And macular degeneration—the deterioration of the macula, the part of the eye that's responsible for distinguishing fine details—is the leading cause of blindness in people over age 50. Some of these problems require glasses, some may need surgery to fix, and some are irreversible. The natural remedies in this chapter—in conjunction with medical care and used with your doctor's approval—may help minimize vision problems, according to some health professionals.

SEE YOUR MEDICAL DOCTOR WHEN...

- Your vision is impaired, you have pain in your eye, you're light-sensitive, you have double vision or you have things floating through your field of vision.
- You have blurred vision and/or see rainbow halos around lights.
- You have something embedded in your eye.
- You have gotten hit in the eye.
- You have a dull ache around your eyes that persists for more than two days.
- You see flashes of light off and on for more than 20 minutes and you also feel faint.

FOOD THERAPY

Drink less coffee, says Jay Cohen, O.D., associate professor at the State University of New York College of Optometry in New York City. "One study about ten years ago looked at caffeine and the effect it has on the focusing system of the eye—and it's a negative effect." Other sources of caffeine to avoid, according to Dr. Cohen, include tea, chocolate and cola as well as many pain relievers.

He also advises eating an overall healthy diet that relies more on fresh fruits and vegetables than on refined sugars and high-cholesterol animal products. "My feeling is you should have the best possible diet for the best possible vision," says Dr. Cohen. Foods that are high in carotenes, such as broccoli, kale, cauliflower, peas, beets, green beans, brussels sprouts and cabbage, are especially good.

VITAMIN AND MINERAL THERAPY

A daily supplement that contains vitamin C, vitamin E and beta-carotene can help minimize vision problems associated with aging, such as farsightedness, says Jay Cohen, O.D., associate professor at the State University of New York College of Optometry in New York City. "Many studies show that people who take antioxidant vitamin supplements are at much lower risk of developing age-related changes in the eyes."

YOGA

You can strengthen eye muscles and improve vision with a series of simple yoga exercises, writes yoga teacher Rosalind Widdowson in her book *The Joy of Yoga*. She suggests doing the entire sequence of exercises described below once a day in the order listed.

She says that you can do all of these exercises sitting in a straight-back chair, with your feet resting comfortably on the floor.

Distancing. Put your left hand in your lap. Stretch your right arm straight out, at eye level, with your palm facing you. Make a gentle fist, then raise your index finger.

With both eyes, look down at your nose. Then switch your glance to your raised finger. Then look as far into the distance as you can. Switch back to your finger, then your nose. Do this five times. Repeat this exercise with your left arm extended and your right hand in your lap.

Widdowson says you should also do a set of these exercises first with one eye closed, then with the other closed.

Verticals/horizontals. Sit with both hands in your lap. Hold your head straight up, looking forward. With both eyes, look right, then straight ahead, then left and then straight again. Repeat five times.

After this, look up, then straight, then down and then straight again. Repeat five times.

Diagonals. Again, sit with both hands in your lap and your head held straight up. Start by looking up and right. Then in one smooth motion, move your glance diagonally until you're looking down and left. Return to looking up and right. Do this five times. Then switch, looking up and left, moving down and right and returning up and left. Repeat five times.

Circles. Sit with both hands in your lap and your head facing forward. Make a full circle with your eyes in a clockwise direction. Do this five times, then do five circles counterclockwise.

Expansion. Close your eyes tightly, then open them wide, looking at an object far off in the distance. Do this ten times.

SEE ALSO Cataracts; Eyestrain; Glaucoma; Night Blindness

WARTS

Give toads a break. You can't catch warts from them—not by petting them, holding them or even puckering up and kissing them. Actually, it's the guy next to you in the locker room or the child on the playground swing set who passes to you the virus that causes warts.

The virus enters the skin through a cut or scrape and sets up shop. One to eight months later, you get a wart. They are especially likely to grow on your fingers and hands but can also appear on your elbows, face and scalp. And you can make them spread by giving the virus a chance to invade surrounding areas through shaving, scratching or rubbing. Sometimes they go away on their own; sometimes they stick around for years. Even if a doctor removes a wart, the virus can remain in your skin and cause new warts to grow. The natural remedies in this chapter, used with your doctor's approval, may help prevent or treat warts, according to some health professionals.

SEE YOUR MEDICAL DOCTOR WHEN . . .

- You have a wart that grows in a place that prevents you from normal functioning, such as a fingertip.
- Your wart is painful, bleeds or changes shape or color.
- Your wart grows bigger than the eraser on a pencil.

FOOD THERAPY

Eat more foods rich in vitamin A and zinc, two nutrients important for healing and skin repair, says Allan Magaziner, D.O., a nutritional medicine specialist and head of the Magaziner Medical Center in Cherry Hill, New Jersey. (See "Getting What You Need" on page 142 for food sources of vitamin A and zinc.)

You may also get relief with this remedy recommended by Elson Haas, M.D., director of the Preventive Medical Center of Marin in San Rafael, California, and author of *Staying Healthy with Nutrition*. His instructions: In the morning, crush a vitamin A capsule, mix it with just enough water to make a paste and apply it directly to the wart. In the afternoon, apply a drop of castor oil; in the evening, apply a drop of lemon juice. This should help dissolve the wart.

HOMEOPATHY

If you have a large, painful wart near a fingernail or fingertip, try Causticum 6X, says Maesimund Panos, M.D., a homeopathic physician in Tipp City, Ohio, and co-author with Jane Heimlich of *Homeopathic Medicine at Home*. Dulcamara 6X will help destroy a wart that is hard, smooth and flattened, according to Dr. Panos. If your wart is painful, large and jagged, she suggests Nitric acid 6X. For a soft, fleshy wart that seems to be on a stalk, she says to try Thuja occidentalis 6X. Take any of these remedies three times a day until the wart disappears, she adds.

All of these remedies are available in many health food stores. To purchase the remedies by mail, refer to the resource list on page 637.

IMAGERY

Close your eyes, breathe out three times and imagine yourself at a cool, clear mountain stream, writes Gerald Epstein, M.D., a New York City psychiatrist, in his book *Healing Visualizations*. Picture the part of your body that has the wart. Remove the part, turn it inside out and wash it thoroughly in the stream. Envision all of the waste products as gray or black strands that are carried away in the swift current. Once the body part is clean, hang it out to dry in the sun. Imagine it healing from the inside, looking like all of the healthy cells around it. When it is dry, turn it right-side out, put it back on and notice that the wart has vanished. Open your eyes. Do this exercise three times a day, two to three minutes at a time, for 21 days.

WATER RETENTION

S ure, your body needs water to live. But there's no need to hoard it. You can do just fine without the swollen fingers, plumped-up legs and bloated belly that go along with a case of water retention.

Lots of things can cause your body to keep excess water, including too much salt in your diet, hormone changes, steroid medications, the menstrual cycle and even pregnancy. Most of the time, the condition is temporary and harmless, if somewhat uncomfortable. But if the swelling doesn't subside, or if you can leave an indentation in your skin by poking it with a finger, it could signal trouble with your liver, kidneys, heart or thyroid. The natural remedies in this chapter—in conjunction with medical care and used with your doctor's approval—may help ease water retention, according to some health professionals.

SEE YOUR MEDICAL DOCTOR WHEN . . .

- You have swelling in your abdomen or your extremities that lasts for more than a week and your skin "dents" when you poke it with a finger.
- You're pregnant and you notice sudden swelling, especially in your legs.

ACUPRESSURE

To improve the body's fluid balance, press the Sp 4 points, situated on the upper arch of each foot, one thumb-width from the ball of the foot, suggests Michael Reed Gach, Ph.D., director of the Acupressure Institute in Berkeley, California, and author of *Acupressure's Potent Points*. (For help in locating these points, refer to the illustration on page 566.) You can work both Sp 4 points simultaneously, says Dr. Gach, by placing the soles of your feet together, then pressing the point on your right foot with your right thumb and the point on your left foot with your left thumb. One minute of pressure on these points, three times daily, can help your body rid itself of excess fluids over the course of a couple of weeks, says Dr. Gach.

AROMATHERAPY

The essential oils geranium, cypress and juniper help alleviate water retention when added to your bath, according to Judith Jackson, an aromatherapist in Greenwich, Connecticut, and author of *Scentual Touch: A Personal Guide to Aromatherapy*. She suggests adding 20 drops each to a warm bath and soaking for ten minutes.

For information on preparing and administering essential oils, including cautions about their use, see page 19. For information on purchasing essential oils, refer to the resource list on page 633.

FOOD THERAPY

"Water retention often means that there's too much sodium in the diet," says Michael A. Klaper, M.D., a nutritional medicine specialist in Pompano Beach, Florida, and director of the Institute of Nutritional Education and Research, an organization based in Manhattan Beach, California, that teaches doctors about nutrition and its relationship to disease. His answer: Try to limit your sodium intake to 2,000 milligrams (less than one teaspoon) per day by eliminating condiments and other salt- and sodium-rich foods. He also suggests eating more foods high in potassium, which can offset sodium overload. (See "Getting What You Need" on page 142 for a list of potassium-rich foods.)

HERBAL THERAPY

Try a tea of dandelion greens and burdock root, says Barre, Vermont, herbalist Rosemary Gladstar, author of *Herbal Healing for Women* and other books about herbs. Dandelion greens are high in potassium and help create the proper water balance that the body needs, she explains, while burdock root is a mild, natural diuretic.

Here's Gladstar's recipe: Mix two parts dandelion greens, two parts burdock root and one part marshmallow root. (You can find these dried herbs in most health food stores or through mail order; for mail-order information, refer to the resource list on page 635.) Add three to four tablespoons of this herb mixture to a quart of cold water and bring to a low boil. Simmer for 15 minutes. Remove from the heat, strain to remove the dried herbs and cool. Gladstar says to drink three to four cups of this tea throughout the day.

JUICE THERAPY

The Diuretic Formula juice blend was developed by naturopathic physician Michael Murray, N.D., author of *The Complete Book of Juicing*, to ease water retention. His recipe: Juice a handful of dandelion greens, followed by two celery stalks and four carrots. He suggests drinking this blend twice a day, in conjunction with proper medical treatment.

For information on juicing techniques, see page 93.

WRINKLES

Remember when your mom used to say "Don't scrunch up your face, or it'll stay that way"? Well, she was right. Over the years, your skin develops a "memory" for your most common facial moves, including squinting, frowning and raising your eyebrows. The result, sorry to say, is wrinkles.

Other things cause wrinkles, too. Anything that robs your skin of moisture, such as too much scrubbing or the overuse of astringents, can lead to problems. But the worst offender is too much exposure to the ultraviolet rays of the sun. Experts recommend using a sunscreen with an SPF (sun protection factor) of 15 on your exposed skin every time you go outside. The natural remedies in this chapter, used with your doctor's approval, may help prevent or reverse wrinkling, according to some health professionals.

SEE YOUR MEDICAL DOCTOR WHEN . . .

- Your wrinkles are really bothering you and interfering with your feelings about your appearance.

ACUPRESSURE

To tone facial muscles, press both Facial Beauty points, St 3, which are situated at the bottom of each cheekbone, directly below the pupil, says Michael Reed Gach, Ph.D., director of the Acupressure Institute in Berkeley, California, and author of *Acupressure's Potent Points*. (For help in locating these points, refer to the illustration on page 564.) Dr. Gach recommends holding these points for one minute three times a day.

AROMATHERAPY

To minimize the appearance of wrinkles and help prevent new ones, Fair Oaks, California, aromatherapist Victoria Edwards suggests a skin-nourishing face oil that she says she discovered quite by accident. "I created it when my daughter had chickenpox to keep her skin from scarring, but I found out it is great for my skin as well," she explains.

To prepare, says Edwards, add one drop of rose and two drops of everlast (sometimes called immortelle or helichrysum) essential oils to one ounce of rose hip seed essential oil. She says to store the mixture in a dark glass bottle and apply it every morning, immediately after cleansing. This blend smells great and keeps skin hydrated, according to Edwards.

"It's a little expensive to prepare because of the rose oil," she admits. "But a six-month supply will cost under $100, less than what a lot of women pay at the cosmetic counter for products that don't do what they're supposed to."

For information on preparing and administering essential oils, including cautions about their use, see page 19. For information on purchasing essential oils, refer to the resource list on page 633.

MASSAGE

Two self-massage routines, done daily, can nourish and relax facial tissue and skin, says Monika Struna, author of *Self-Massage*. The first, called patting, is done while you stand with your feet about one foot apart. Lean forward slightly at the waist for balance. Then start patting your face as if you were gently slapping it with the bottom sides of your fingers. Your left hand should do the left side of your face, and your right hand should do the right side. Continue patting the cheeks and sides of your face for 15 to 20 seconds.

The second technique is called wrinkle release. Place the fingertips of your right hand on the right center of your forehead and the fingertips of your left hand on the left center of your forehead. Apply gentle to moderate pressure, so you can feel the layer of tissue beneath the outer skin. Then move your fingers back and forth as you would if you were washing your hair. Be careful not to move the fingers too far and stretch the skin. Do this for a few seconds, then move your fingers across the forehead to the sides of the face, down and back across the cheekbones. Continue moving your hands over your face, working your way down the left side with your left hand and the right side with your right hand. Struna says this will help relax and nourish the tissue under your skin, where wrinkles start. Continue for 30 to 60 seconds.

YEAST INFECTIONS

Most of the time, the fungus *Candida albicans* leads a quiet and harmless existence in a woman's vagina. But when something throws a woman's system out of balance, the fungus can grow rapidly and create an uncomfortable little problem—namely, a yeast infection.

The telltale signs of an infection are burning and itching in the vaginal area and a discharge that looks somewhat like cottage cheese. The most common trigger for a yeast infection is antibiotic medication, although the hormone shift during a woman's menstrual cycle can also lead to problems. Estimates show that nearly three in four American women will have a yeast infection sometime before menopause. The natural remedies in this chapter—in conjunction with medical care and used with your doctor's approval—may help prevent yeast infections or relieve their symptoms, according to some health professionals.

SEE YOUR MEDICAL DOCTOR WHEN...

- You notice itching or burning in the vaginal area.
- You see an unusual vaginal discharge.

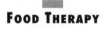

FOOD THERAPY

"Get off sugars and fermented foods," says Elson Haas, M.D., director of the Preventive Medical Center of Marin in San Rafael, California, and author of *Staying Healthy with Nutrition*. "These foods cause an overgrowth of yeast in the intestinal tract, which manifests itself into yeast infections." He recommends eliminating all refined sugars, breads and other baked goods, alcohol, caffeine and vinegar and going on his three-week detoxification diet (see "Detoxing Your Ills" on page 48).

Also, according to Dr. Haas, scientific research shows that some women find relief by eating yogurt containing acidophilus, which are friendly bacteria. "Adding yogurt to the diet helps when the yogurt contains acidophilus, which reduces yeast infections," adds Dr. Haas. He recommends one to two cups of acidophilus-containing yogurt every day for three or four days.

HYDROTHERAPY

To prevent recurring yeast infections, wash the area between the anus and the vagina every time you use the toilet, says Agatha Thrash, M.D., a medical pathologist and co-founder and co-director of Uchee Pines Institute, a natural healing center in Seale, Alabama. Keep a quart-size jar or bottle in the bathroom, fill it with plain water and rinse the genital and anal areas after urinating or having a bowel movement, while you're still sitting on the toilet. Pregnant women, those with diabetes and others prone to yeast infections should add two to three tablespoons of apple cider vinegar per quart of plain water. "This protects the natural acid balance of the vaginal area, which is prone to yeast overgrowth if it becomes too alkaline," says Dr. Thrash.

JUICE THERAPY

Women may be able to speed the healing of yeast infections and to prevent recurrences with daily doses of cranberry or blackberry juice, according to Elaine Gillaspie, N.D., a naturopathic physician in Portland, Oregon. If you can't find fresh or frozen berries, "be sure to use unsweetened cranberry concentrate, not bottled cranberry juice, since most brands are loaded with sugar or corn syrup, which encourages the buildup of yeast," she cautions. And because even fresh berry juices are rich in natural fruit sugars, she suggests diluting four ounces of juice with an equal amount of water to get an eight-ounce serving.

She also recommends juicing a clove of fresh garlic and adding it to your vegetable juices. "Nothing prevents yeast overgrowth as well as garlic does," says Dr. Gillaspie.

For information on juicing techniques, see page 93.

VITAMIN AND MINERAL THERAPY

Take more vitamin C, says Elson Haas, M.D., director of the Preventive Medical Center of Marin in San Rafael, California, and author of *Staying Healthy with Nutrition*. "Yeast grows better in an alkaline environment, and vitamin C is acidic, so it helps reduce the yeast." He recommends taking between 500 and 2,000 milligrams daily in supplement form.

SEE ALSO Vaginitis

ACUPRESSURE

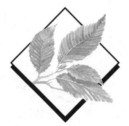

ILLUSTRATIONS

ACUPRESSURE POINTS—FRONT VIEW

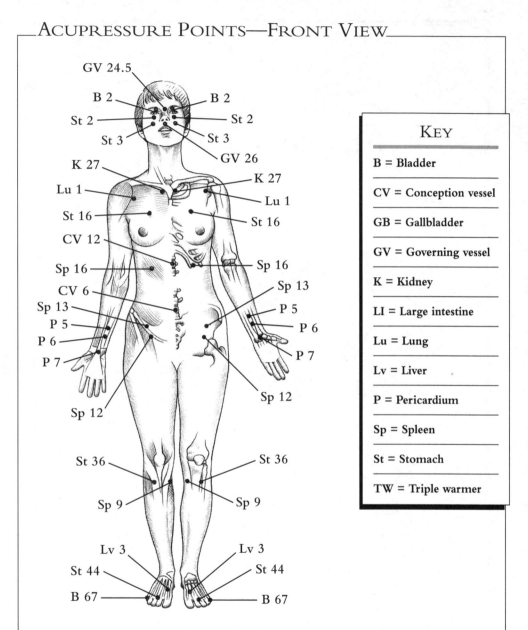

KEY

B = Bladder

CV = Conception vessel

GB = Gallbladder

GV = Governing vessel

K = Kidney

LI = Large intestine

Lu = Lung

Lv = Liver

P = Pericardium

Sp = Spleen

St = Stomach

TW = Triple warmer

This front view of the body shows self-care acupressure points on the meridians that correspond to the lungs, pericardium, bladder, stomach, liver, spleen and kidneys. It also shows points on the governing vessel, which is key to the central nervous system, and the conception vessel, which influences reproduction and digestion. Acupressurists contend that the meridians are invisible "wires" of energy, or chi, that run throughout the body.

ACUPRESSURE POINTS—BACK VIEW

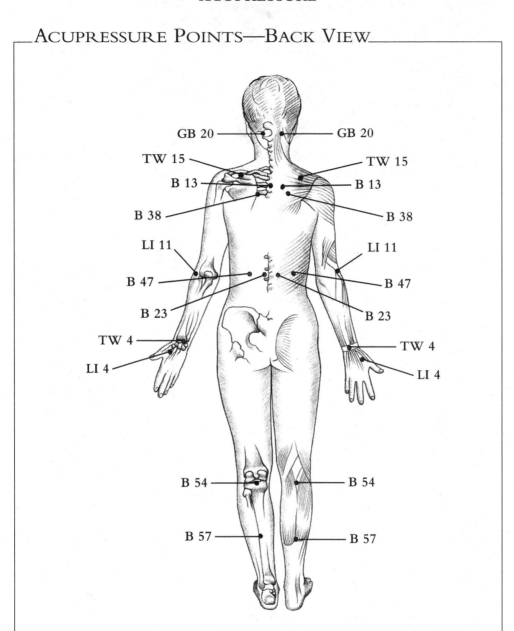

GB 20   GB 20

TW 15   TW 15

B 13   B 13

B 38   B 38

LI 11   LI 11

B 47   B 47

B 23   B 23

TW 4   TW 4

LI 4   LI 4

B 54   B 54

B 57   B 57

This back view of the body shows self-care accupressure points found along the large intestine, bladder, gallbladder and triple warmer meridians. Acupressurists believe that applying pressure at these points can help relieve pain and speed healing.

ACUPRESSURE POINTS—SIDE VIEW

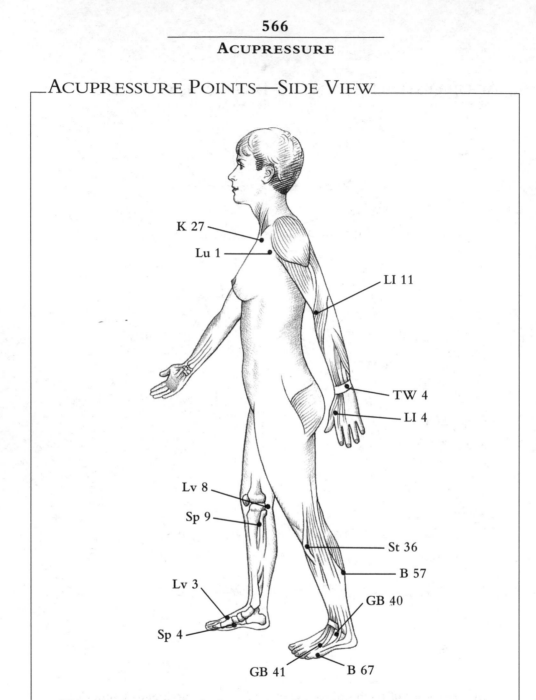

K 27

Lu 1

LI 11

TW 4

LI 4

Lv 8

Sp 9

St 36

B 57

Lv 3

GB 40

Sp 4

GB 41

B 67

   This side view of the body shows some of the self-care acupressure points found on the liver, large intestine, triple warmer, gallbladder, stomach, spleen, kidney, lung and bladder meridians. This location chart will help you find the pressure points that acupressurists say may ease pain and speed healing of specific medical problems.

ACUPRESSURE

ACUPRESSURE POINTS ON THE HEAD

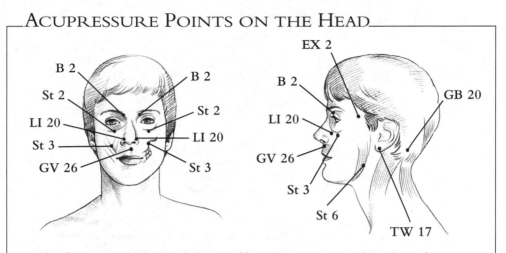

The front view of the head shows self-care acupressure points along the stomach, large intestine, bladder and governing vessel meridians. Acupressurists say that these particular pressure points may, among other things, help relieve headaches, sinus pain, acne and other skin problems and improve memory and concentration. The side view of the head reveals several self-care acupressure points associated with the bladder, large intestine, gallbladder, triple warmer, stomach and governing vessel meridians. EX 2, found near the temples, is an extra point not located directly on any meridian.

ACUPRESSURE ENERGY MERIDIANS—FRONT VIEW

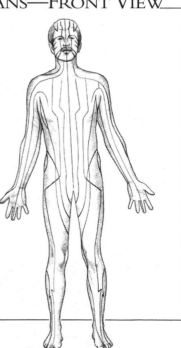

This illustration shows the six major meridians that flow up the front of the body. Each meridian is connected to a particular organ. The meridians shown here influence the lungs, heart, pericardium, liver, spleen and kidneys. Acupressurists say these meridians may also influence other parts of the body. Eye problems, for example, may be relieved by applying pressure on the liver meridian.

ACUPRESSURE ENERGY MERIDIANS—BACK VIEW

This illustration shows the six major meridians that flow down the back of the body. These meridians influence the small and large intestines, stomach, gallbladder, bladder and triple warmer, which helps control the transportation and distribution of fluids within the body, according to acupressure experts.

ACUPRESSURE ENERGY MERIDIANS—SIDE VIEW

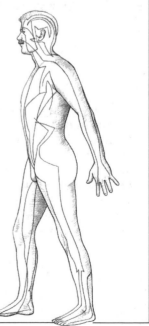

This is a side view of the major meridians of the body, including those that influence the kidneys, lungs, bladder, spleen and liver. Chinese medicine experts contend that these pathways are invisible "wires" of energy that need to be in balance in order to maintain health.

MASSAGE

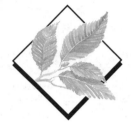

ILLUSTRATIONS

SWEDISH MASSAGE STROKES

EFFLEURAGE. Use your palms or fingertips to lightly stroke whatever part of the body you are massaging. Use long, gliding strokes and gentle pressure. Always stroke toward the heart. If you are using effleurage on the legs, for example, stroke upward from the ankles, as shown. On the arms, stroke from the wrist to the shoulder.

PETRISSAGE. Lightly grab the muscle you want to massage by placing your thumb on one side of it and your fingers on the other. Gently lift the muscle away from the bone and knead it by squeezing and rolling. Then let the muscle slip from your fingers. You can then pick it up with your other hand. Proceed up or down the muscle by moving your hand one to two inches after each stroke.

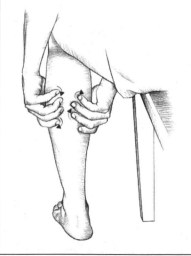

FRICTION. Use your fingertips and thumbs to make small, circular movements on the muscle you want to massage. Your fingertips don't slide over the skin; they are stationary and work through the skin to the muscle below. Vary the pressure, starting with light pressure and increasing it after a minute or two. For larger muscles such as the thigh or back, use your palm or the heel of your hand. Again, make the circular motion and vary the pressure.

TAPOTEMENT. Tap, chop or clap vigorously on the muscle you want to massage, using your fingertips, the sides of your hands, cupped palms or lightly closed fists. Use short, light, rapid strokes, as if you were tapping on a bongo drum. This should feel like quick rhythmic contact rather than a karate chop.

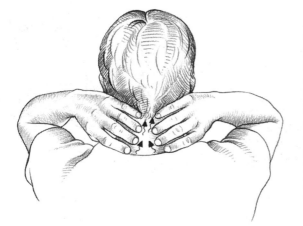

VIBRATION. Place one hand or both hands on the muscle you want to work, with your fingers spread. Then press down firmly and use your whole arm to transmit a trembling motion for several seconds. Move your hands continuously or lift them and move them a few inches. Repeat until the entire muscle has been covered. For a lighter version, use just your fingertips and press down more gently, as shown.

FOOT MASSAGE

1.

Place your left foot on the edge of a chair. Squeeze the foot lightly with both hands, moving your hands to cover the entire foot from the ankle to the toes. Pay special attention to any spots that feel stiff or sore; squeeze them for about ten seconds.

2.

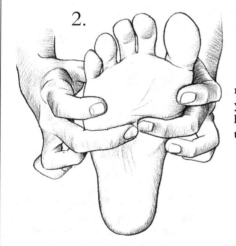

Apply a small amount of vegetable oil, massage oil or moisturizing lotion to your hands. Put the middle finger of each hand on the sole of your foot, just below the ball. Press for about ten seconds.

3.

With the oil still on your fingers, touch either side of your ankle with your fingertips. Make small, gentle circles around the ankle bone.

4.

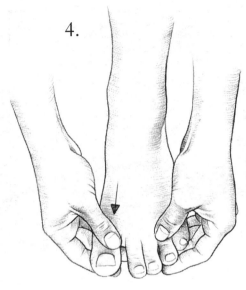

Hold your toes with your thumbs on top and fingers underneath. Slide your hands forward, pulling the toes gently away from the foot. Then roll each toe back and forth three times.

Sit down, placing your left foot over your right knee, with the sole facing you. Hold your ankle with your left hand. Use the fingertips on your right hand to make small circles all over the sole. Pay special attention to any areas that feel sore or painful.

Repeat the massage on your right foot.

5.

HEADACHE MASSAGE

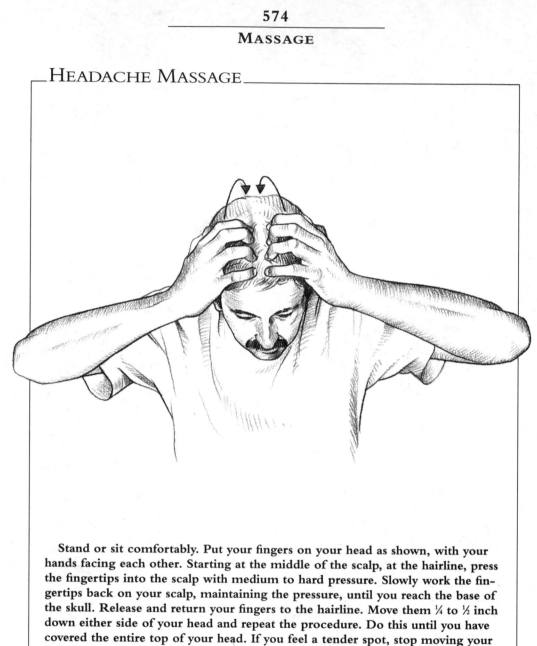

Stand or sit comfortably. Put your fingers on your head as shown, with your hands facing each other. Starting at the middle of the scalp, at the hairline, press the fingertips into the scalp with medium to hard pressure. Slowly work the fingertips back on your scalp, maintaining the pressure, until you reach the base of the skull. Release and return your fingers to the hairline. Move them ¼ to ½ inch down either side of your head and repeat the procedure. Do this until you have covered the entire top of your head. If you feel a tender spot, stop moving your fingertips and concentrate on that area for a few seconds longer. You can return to it another time, if it still hurts. Continue the massage for one to two minutes.

HELLERWORK

Before beginning this routine, stand with your feet shoulder-width apart. Slowly lift your shoulders as if shrugging, then roll them backward. Shrug again, then roll your shoulders forward. This helps loosen the shoulder joints in preparation for the massages below.

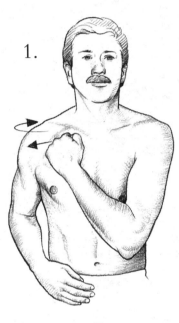

1.

Stand with your feet shoulder-width apart. Make a fist with your left hand, then position the fist just under the right collarbone as shown. (If you have trouble making a fist, you can use your fingertips instead.) Push the fist gently into the muscle. Then slide the fist slowly along the bottom of the collarbone toward the shoulder. As your fist moves, draw your right shoulder back slightly. Stop when your fist reaches the end of the shoulder joint. Repeat three times, moving your fist a little lower on your chest each time. Then repeat using the right fist on the left shoulder. This exercise, along with the next two, loosens muscles in the front of the chest and in the neck, allowing your shoulders to roll back.

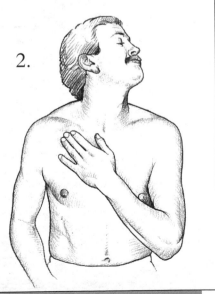

2.

Place the fingertips of your left hand under the right collarbone as shown. Pull down slightly. Now slowly tilt your head back. Jut your lower jaw forward and slowly turn your head to the left. Repeat. Shake your right arm to loosen it. Repeat this with the right fingertips under your left collarbone, slowly turning your head to the right.

(continued)

HELLERWORK—
CONTINUED

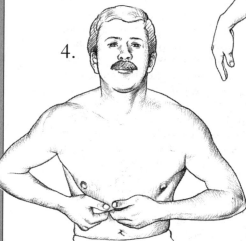

3.

With your left hand, lightly pinch the right pectoral muscle as shown. Lift the right arm straight out to the side, then overhead. Hold for several seconds, feeling the stretch across the top of the chest. Repeat, then shake the right arm to loosen it. Repeat using the right hand and left arm.

4.

Lean slightly forward at the waist. Reach under the bottom of your rib cage on the right side with the fingers of both hands. Take a deep breath as you straighten at the waist and pull up on your ribs. Hold for several seconds, release and repeat. Then repeat by pulling up on the bottom of the left ribs. This exercise expands the rib cage and increases breathing potential.

Make a fist with your right hand. Place the fist under the right ear as shown. Apply gentle pressure, then slowly turn your head to the left. Hold your fist steady, so it runs across the muscles of the neck as your head turns. Repeat three times, lowering the fist about one inch each time. Shake your arm and roll your shoulders when finished. Then repeat with the left fist under the left ear, turning the head to the right. This lengthens the neck and allows the shoulders to drop.

5.

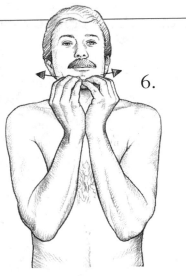

6.

Place your fingertips along the chin as shown. The little fingers from both hands should touch. Press firmly into your jawbone. Slowly move your hands apart, tracing the jawbone as you move toward the ears. Repeat. This reduces jowl size and jaw tension.

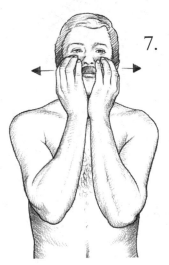

7.

Press your fingertips or the pads of your fingers firmly into the bottoms of your cheekbones. Your little fingers should be against the sides of your nose. Now slowly move your hands back toward the ears, tracing the ridge of bone as they go. Repeat. This lifts and lengthens the muscles and tissue around the cheekbones.

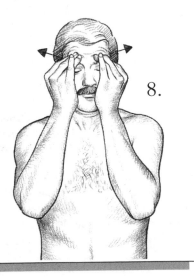

8.

Press your fingertips firmly into the bone just above the eyebrows. Lift the skin and muscle as you press into the bone. Now move your hands toward the edges of the face, keeping the pressure firm. Repeat. This reduces worry lines between your eyes.

LEG RUB FOR CONSTIPATION

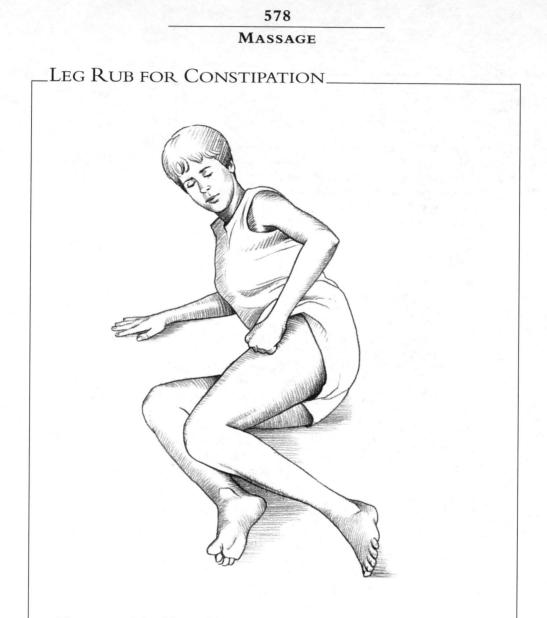

Lie on your right side on either the floor or a mat. Lift your shoulders and upper chest off the floor, supporting your upper body with the right elbow and forearm. Bend your knees slightly. Make a fist with your left hand and reach down to the outside of your left thigh. Place the fist just above the knee and draw it toward your hip. Apply even, firm pressure. When you reach the upper thigh, lift your fist and place it back down near the knee. Repeat for one to two minutes. When you finish with the left thigh, roll over and repeat on the right thigh. Use your right fist to apply the pressure.

TOWEL TRICK FOR HEADACHES

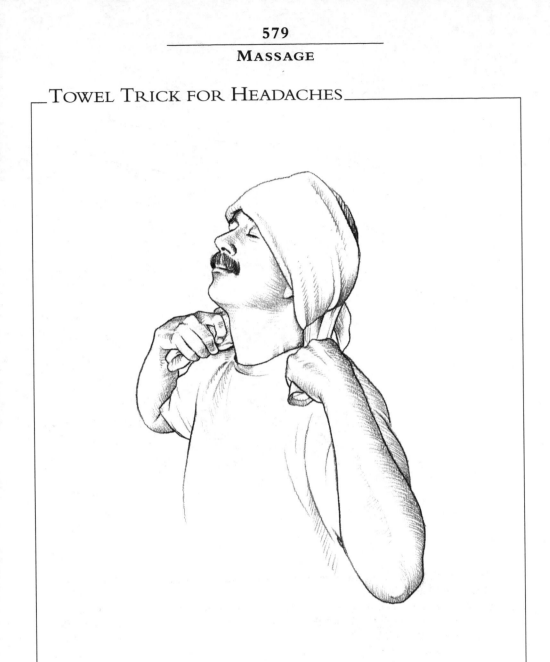

Fold a bath towel lengthwise into thirds. Sitting comfortably, lay the middle of the towel over your forehead and cross the ends behind your head, at the base of the skull. Pull the ends tightly so that you can feel pressure across your forehead. Breathing out as you count to five, tilt your head back. Keep the pressure constant. Hold it for 10 to 30 seconds. Repeat one or two times if needed.

TOWEL TRICKS FOR NECK PAIN

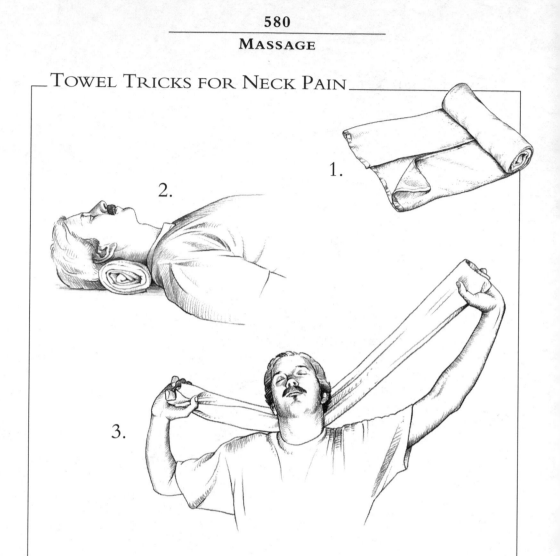

Fold a bath towel, bringing the sides to the middle until the edges touch (1). Roll the towel snugly.

Lie flat on your back on either the floor or a mat and place the towel under the curve of your neck (2). Hold this pose for 15 to 20 minutes. Once in a while you can move the roll higher or lower on your neck, experimenting to see what feels good. You should also do this massage by placing the towel under the small of your back and holding for 15 to 20 minutes. Again, you can move the towel up or down to see which placement feels best.

Then fold the bath towel into thirds lengthwise (3). Grab one end with your left hand and one end with your right hand. Place the middle of the towel behind your head, at the base of the skull. Let your head fall back, supported by the towel. Now pull the towel back and forth with your hands, allowing your head to be pulled with the towel. Breathe normally. You can continue doing this for up to five minutes.

REFLEXOLOGY

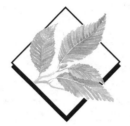

ILLUSTRATIONS

HAND POINTS AND TECHNIQUES

When a remedy calls for working a reflex point on your hand, look for the name of that point in the chart below. Next to the name you'll find one or more numbers. Look for the numbers in the illustrations beginning on page 585. These are the points you need to work. The chart also lists techniques that you can use to work the points. For instructions on the hand reflexology techniques, see the illustrations beginning on page 587.

For example, if a remedy calls for working the diaphragm point, first find the diaphragm in the chart. The number for the diaphragm point is 11. Go to the illustrations and find point 11. The chart also suggests using either the golf ball technique or the thumb walk. Try both and use the one that feels more comfortable.

Point Name	Point Numbers	Finger walk	Golf ball	Rotation on a point	Single finger grip	Thumb walk
				Techniques		
Adrenal gland	17		✓		✓	
Arm	5, 7		✓			✓
Bladder	22	✓	✓	✓	✓	✓
Brain	2		✓		✓	✓
Cervical spine	10, 32		✓			✓
Chest	8, 9, 35	✓	✓			✓
Colon	25, 26		✓			✓
Diaphragm	11		✓			✓
DIGESTIVE SYSTEM						
Colon	25, 26		✓			✓
Gallbladder	16		✓			✓
Liver	13		✓			✓
Pancreas	18		✓			✓
Small intestine	21		✓			✓
Stomach	14		✓			✓
Ear	4, 33	✓	✓		✓	✓
Esophagus	3, 32		✓		✓	✓
Eye	4, 33		✓		✓	✓
Face	2, 30		✓		✓	✓

(continued)

HAND POINTS AND TECHNIQUES—CONTINUED

Point Name	Point Numbers	Finger walk	Golf ball	Rotation on a point	Single finger grip	Thumb walk
Fallopian tube	39	✓		✓	✓	
Gallbladder	16		✓			✓
Head	1, 2, 30, 31		✓		✓	✓
Heart	9		✓			✓
Hip	37	✓		✓		
Ileocecal valve	24		✓		✓	✓
Intestine	21, 24, 25, 26		✓		✓	✓
Kidney	20		✓		✓	✓
Knee	37	✓		✓		
Leg	37	✓		✓		
Liver	13		✓			✓
Lung	9, 35	✓	✓			✓
LYMPHATIC SYSTEM						
Lymph drain	34, 39	✓			✓	✓
Spleen	15		✓			✓
Tonsil	3	✓			✓	✓
Lymph drain	34, 39	✓			✓	✓
Neck	3, 32	✓	✓		✓	✓
Ovary	27			✓	✓	✓
Pancreas	18		✓			✓
Parathyroid gland	3		✓		✓	✓
Pituitary gland	6		✓	✓	✓	✓
Prostate	28			✓	✓	✓
REPRODUCTIVE SYSTEM						
Fallopian tube	39	✓		✓	✓	
Ovary/testicle	27			✓	✓	✓
Uterus/prostate	28			✓	✓	✓

(continued)

HAND POINTS AND TECHNIQUES—CONTINUED

Point Name	Point Numbers	Techniques				
		Finger walk	Golf ball	Rotation on a point	Single finger grip	Thumb walk
Sciatic nerve	37			✓		
Shoulder	5, 7, 8		✓			✓
Sigmoid colon	26		✓			✓
Sinus	2, 3, 31, 32		✓			✓
Small intestine	21		✓			✓
Solar plexus	11		✓		✓	✓
Spine	10, 12, 19, 23, 29, 32	✓	✓	✓	✓	✓
Spleen	15		✓			✓
Stomach	14		✓			✓
Testicle	27			✓	✓	✓
Thoracic spine	12, 19		✓			✓
Throat	3	✓	✓		✓	✓
Thyroid gland	3, 32		✓	✓	✓	✓
Tonsil	3	✓			✓	✓
Top of shoulder	4, 33	✓	✓		✓	✓
Uterus	28			✓	✓	✓

REFLEX POINTS—LEFT PALM

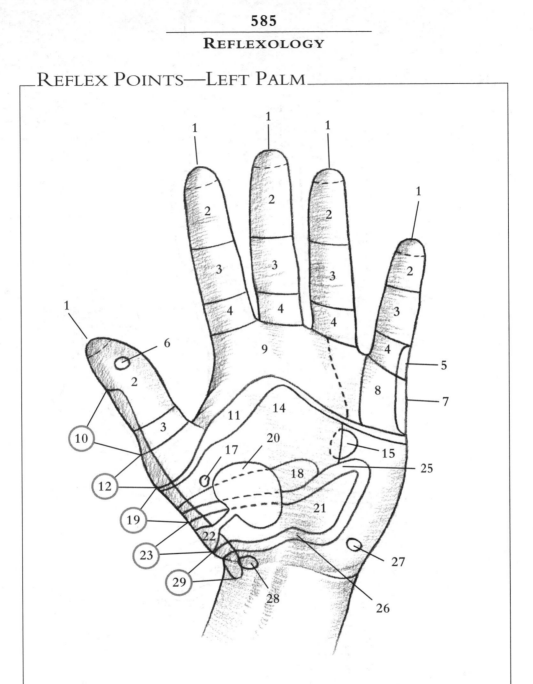

This illustration shows reflexology points located on the palm of the left hand. The numbers designating the points are also listed in the chart beginning on page 582, which shows which of the five techniques used in hand reflexology are best for applying pressure to each point. Experiment until you find the techniques that work best for you—the ones that apply the most pressure with the least effort.

REFLEX POINTS—RIGHT PALM

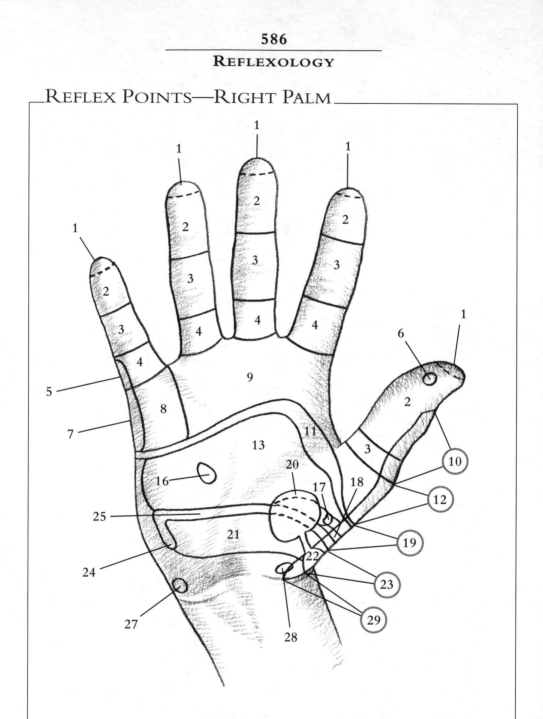

Use the illustration above to locate reflex points on the palm of your right hand. The numbers designating the points correspond to the numbers listed in the chart beginning on page 582. Refer to the chart to find out which of the five hand reflexology techniques you can use to work each point.

REFLEX POINTS—BACK OF HAND

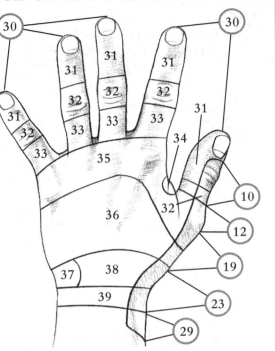

Hand reflexology isn't just for your palms. As shown here, there are many reflex points on the backs of your hands as well. The chart beginning on page 582 recommends the best techniques for applying pressure to each of these points. Always choose a technique that allows you to work a point well, but without a lot of effort.

FINGER WALK

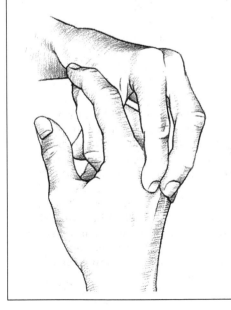

Use the edge of your index finger to "walk" on the hand, taking "bites" of the hand by bending the finger joint closest to the nail. Place your thumb on the other side of the hand you're working for extra leverage. Work each area at least four or five times before moving on to the next area. You should also work adjoining points before moving on.

GOLF BALL TECHNIQUES

When using these techniques, work each area at least four or five times before moving on to the next area. You should also work adjoining points before moving on.

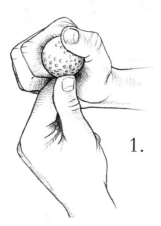

1.

To work the tips of your left fingers, hold the golf ball between the thumb and index finger of the right hand. Roll the ball gently from side to side over the tip of the left thumb. Repeat with each fingertip on the left hand, then switch the ball to the left hand and work the right fingertips.

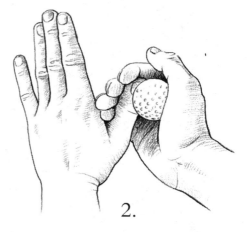

2.

To work the nails of the left hand, grasp the golf ball in the palm of your right hand. Trap your left thumb between the golf ball and your right hand and roll the ball gently over the nail on the left thumb. Repeat with each finger on the left hand, then switch hands and repeat.

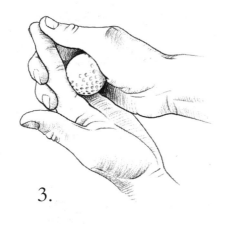

3.

To work the undersides of your left fingers, place a golf ball in your right palm. Wrap your right fingers behind the fingers you are working on and press comfortably with the golf ball. Start with the left index finger. Roll the ball slowly up and down the finger, keeping the ball tucked into your right palm. Repeat this with each finger on your left hand. Repeat on the fingers of your right hand, cupping the golf ball in your left palm.

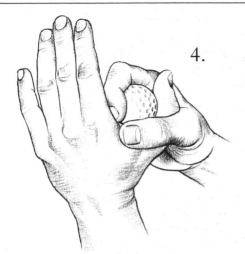

4.

To work the undersides of your thumbs, you'll need to switch your hand position a little. Start by cupping the golf ball with the index finger and middle finger of your right hand. Bend your other two fingers so that they're touching your right palm. Now place your left thumb on top of the golf ball and wrap your right thumb over the top of your left thumb. Roll the ball up and down the underside of the left thumb, applying pressure by squeezing with your right hand. Make sure you cover the entire area. Then switch the golf ball to your left hand and work on your right thumb.

You'll also need to work the area just below the base of the fingers on both hands. To do this for your left hand, first cup the golf ball in your right palm. Now place your right palm over your left palm so that the fingers on your right hand bend over the outside edge of your left index finger. Squeeze the ball against the upper left palm and roll it back and forth. Make sure you cover the entire area below all four fingers. Now switch hands and work the same reflex points on your right hand.

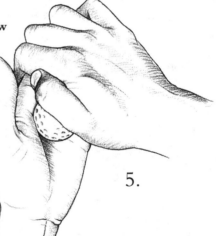

5.

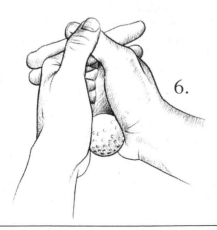

6.

To work the lower palms and heels of your hands, place the golf ball between your palms and interlace your fingers. Roll the ball between your hands, bending your wrists to move it around your palms. Vary the pressure by squeezing your hands closer together. Continue until you have worked the entire area.

ROTATION ON A POINT

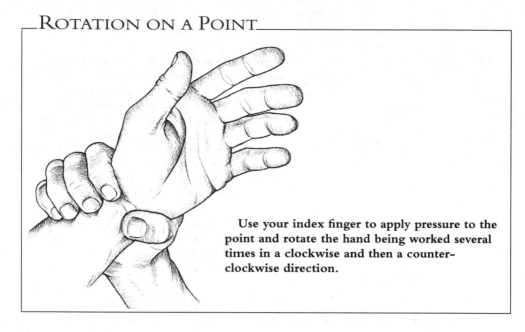

Use your index finger to apply pressure to the point and rotate the hand being worked several times in a clockwise and then a counter-clockwise direction.

SINGLE FINGER GRIP

This technique is used to apply pressure to a small area on the hand. To work your left hand, brace it against the palm of your right hand. Use the fingertip of your index or middle finger to locate and apply pressure to the reflex area. To work your right hand, reverse hand positions. With this technique, apply pressure, hold for a few seconds, then release. Work each area at least four or five times before moving on to the next area.

THUMB WALK

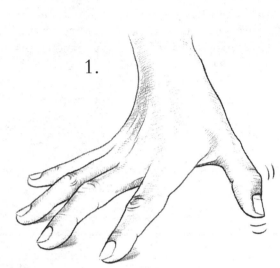

1.

The thumb walk is similar to the finger walk technique, except that you use the outside edge or tip of your thumb, slowly "walking" it along the area you want to work. Do this by bending only the joint that is closest to your thumbnail.

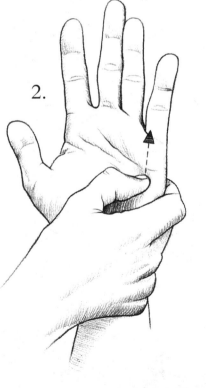

2.

Place your fingers on the back of the hand that you're working. The fingers should be directly underneath your thumb. This helps you apply more even pressure to the reflex areas. Now each time you bend and unbend the first joint of your thumb to move it forward, imagine that the thumb is taking tiny bites of the hand. Try to keep the pressure gentle but steady. Work each area at least four or five times before moving on to the next area. You should also work adjoining points before moving on.

FOOT POINTS AND TECHNIQUES

When a remedy calls for working a reflex point on your foot, look for the name of that point in the chart below. Next to the name you'll find one or more numbers. Look for the numbers in the illustrations beginning on page 596. These are the points you need to work. The chart also lists techniques that you can use to work the points. For instructions on the foot reflexology techniques, see the illustrations beginning on page 598.

For example, if a remedy calls for working the bladder point, first find the bladder in the chart. The number for the bladder point is 28. Go to the illustrations and find point 28. The chart also suggests using either rotation on a point or the thumb walk. Try both and use the technique that feels more comfortable.

Point Name	Point Numbers	Techniques			
		Finger walk	Hook and back up	Rotation on a point	Thumb walk
Adrenal gland	23			✓	✓
Arm	9	✓			✓
Ascending colon	33				✓
Bladder	28			✓	✓
Brain	1	✓			
Breast	49	✓			✓
Bronchial tube	12				✓
Cervical spine	8				✓
Chest	13, 49	✓			✓
Colon	33–38				✓
Diaphragm	17			✓	✓
DIGESTIVE SYSTEM					
Colon	33–38				✓
Duodenum	29				✓
Gallbladder	20			✓	
Liver	19				✓
Pancreas	24				✓
Small intestine	30				✓
Stomach	21				✓
Duodenum	29				✓

(continued)

FOOT POINTS AND TECHNIQUES—CONTINUED

Point Name	Point Numbers	Techniques			
		Finger walk	Hook and back up	Rotation on a point	Thumb walk
Ear	2, 3	✓			✓
Esophagus	15				✓
Eye	3	✓			✓
Fallopian tube	51	✓			
Gallbladder	20			✓	
Head	1–8	✓			✓
Heart	14				✓
Helper to eye	10			✓	✓
Helper to inner ear	47	✓			✓
Helper to thyroid	12				✓
Hip	58			✓	
Hip/sciatic nerve	59	✓			
Hypothalamus	5		✓		
Ileocecal valve	32		✓		
Intestine	29, 30, 32, 33, 35, 37, 38		✓		✓
Kidney	25			✓	✓
Knee	58			✓	
Leg	58			✓	
Liver	19				✓
Lower back	39, 40			✓	✓
Lower spine	39, 40			✓	✓
Lung	13				✓
Lymph drain for breast/chest	48	✓			
Lymph drain for groin	52	✓			
LYMPHATIC SYSTEM					
Lymph drain	48, 52	✓			
Spleen	22			✓	✓
Thymus	54				✓

(continued)

FOOT POINTS AND TECHNIQUES—CONTINUED

Point Name	Point Numbers	Techniques			
		Finger walk	Hook and back up	Rotation on a point	Thumb walk
LYMPHATIC SYSTEM—CONTINUED					
Tonsil	11, 45	✓			✓
Mammary gland	49	✓			
Neck	10, 11, 45	✓			✓
Nose	53	✓			
Ovary	60	✓			
Pancreas	24				✓
Parathyroid gland	11, 45				✓
Penis	55	✓			
Pituitary gland	6		✓		
Prostate	56	✓		✓	
Rectum	57	✓			
REPRODUCTIVE SYSTEM					
Fallopian tube	51	✓			
Mammary gland	49	✓			
Ovary/testicle	60	✓			
Seminal vesicle	51	✓			
Uterus/prostate	56	✓		✓	
Vagina/penis	55	✓			
Vas deferens	51	✓			
Sciatic nerve	42	✓			✓
Seminal vesicle	51	✓			
Shoulder	9	✓			✓

(continued)

FOOT POINTS AND TECHNIQUES—CONTINUED

Point Name	Point Numbers	Finger walk	Hook and back up	Rotation on a point	Thumb walk
Sigmoid colon	38		✓		✓
Small intestine	30				✓
Solar plexus	18				✓
Spine	8, 16, 39, 40, 41			✓	✓
Spleen	22			✓	✓
Stomach	21				✓
Tailbone	41				✓
Testicle	60	✓			
Thoracic spine	16			✓	✓
Throat	11, 45	✓			✓
Thymus	54				✓
Thyroid gland	11, 45	✓			✓
Tonsil	11, 45	✓			✓
Transverse colon	35				✓
Ureter	27				✓
URINARY TRACT					
Bladder	28			✓	✓
Kidney	25			✓	✓
Ureter	27				✓
Uterus	56	✓		✓	
Vagina	55	✓			
Vas deferens	51	✓			
Whole spine	8, 16, 39, 40, 41			✓	✓

REFLEX POINTS—SOLES OF FEET

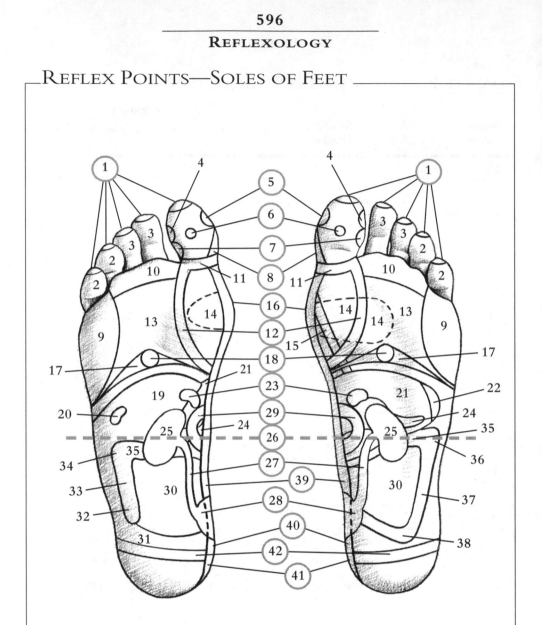

These illustrations show the reflexology points located on the soles of the feet. The numbers designating the points are also listed in the chart beginning on page 592, which shows which of the four techniques used in foot reflexology are best for applying pressure to each point. Experiment until you find the techniques that work best for you—the ones that apply the most pressure with the least effort.

REFLEX POINTS—TOP AND SIDE OF FOOT

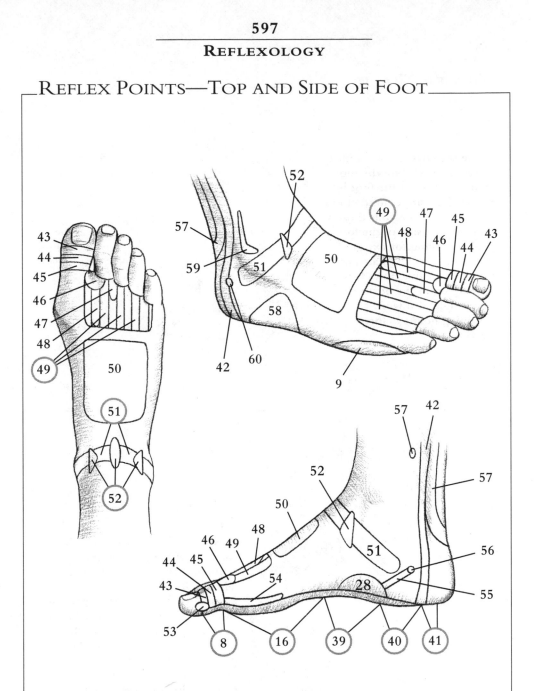

The tops and sides of the feet are also rich with reflex points, according to reflexology experts. Each of the points shown in these illustrations is also listed in the chart beginning on page 592. Use the chart to determine which foot reflexology techniques are best for applying pressure to a given point, then choose the technique that you can use comfortably while also giving the point a good "workout."

FINGER WALK

Use the edge of your index finger to "walk" on the foot, taking "bites" of the foot by bending the finger joint closest to the nail. Place your thumb on the other side of the foot you're working for extra leverage. Work each area at least four or five times before moving on to the next area. You should also work adjoining points before moving on.

HOOK AND BACK UP

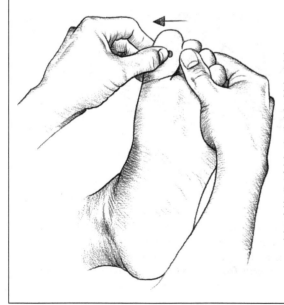

Use this technique to put pressure on a single reflex point on the foot. Place your thumb on the point and apply gentle pressure. Then pull the thumb back, keeping the pressure steady. Even though you're pulling slightly, the thumb should not slide off the point. Put your fingers behind your foot for leverage. Work each area at least four or five times before moving on to the next area. You should also work adjoining points before moving on.

ROTATION ON A POINT

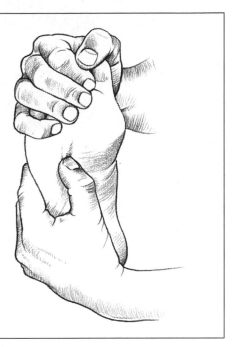

To work the foot, press the thumb lightly onto the reflex point and wrap the fingers around the foot for leverage. Then grasp the top of the foot with your other hand. Move the foot in a circular motion, pulling it down and putting gentle pressure on the thumb spot.

THUMB WALK

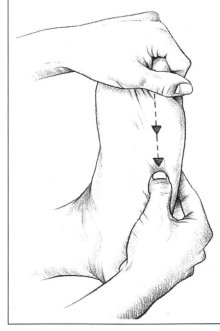

The thumb walk is similar to the finger walk technique, except that you use the outside edge or tip of your thumb, slowly "walking" it along the area you want to work. Do this by bending only the joint that is closest to your thumbnail.

Wrap your fingers around the foot that you're working so that they're directly underneath your thumb. This helps you apply more even pressure to the reflex areas. Now each time you bend and unbend the first joint of your thumb to move it forward, imagine that the thumb is taking tiny bites of the foot. Try to keep the pressure gentle but steady. Work each area at least four or five times before moving on to the next area. You should also work adjoining points before moving on.

RELAXATION AND MEDITATION

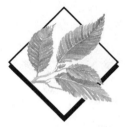

ILLUSTRATIONS

STRETCHED-BASED RELAXATION

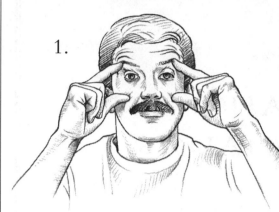

1.

Push up your eyebrows with your index fingers and push down on your cheeks with your thumbs. Hold this position for about ten seconds. Then release and let the muscles around your eyes relax.

After a minute of relaxing, let your head slowly drop toward your right shoulder for about ten seconds. Then slowly drop your head toward the left shoulder for another ten seconds. Be sure not to raise your chin, in order to prevent overextension of the head and neck muscles.

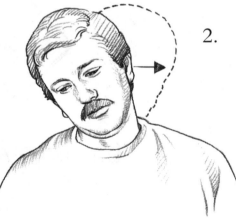

2.

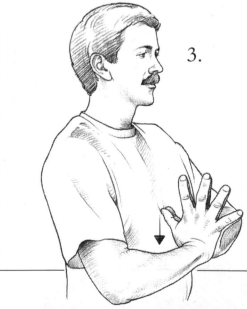

3.

Put your hands together as if you were praying. Then keeping your fingertips and palms together, spread your fingers as if you were creating a fan. Move your thumbs down along the midline of your body until you feel a light stretch in the lower arms. Hold this position for about ten seconds, then relax.

RELAXATION AND MEDITATION

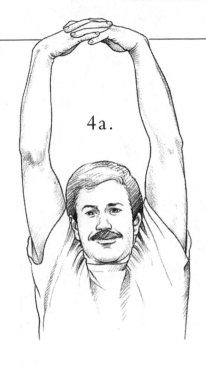

4a.

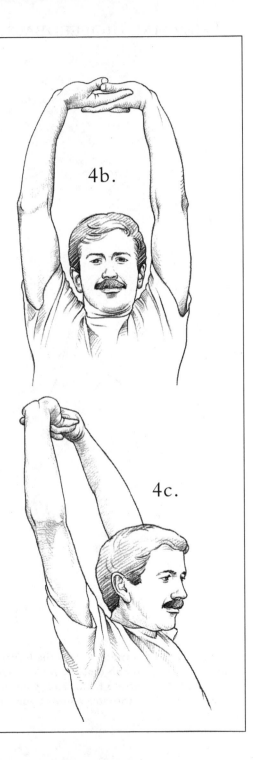

4b.

4c.

Interlock your fingers and raise your hands over your head as shown (4a). Straighten your elbows and rotate your palms outward (4b). Then let your arms move back over your head until you feel resistance (4c). Hold this position for about ten seconds, then quickly release and let your arms rest at your sides for one minute.

THERMAL BIOFEEDBACK

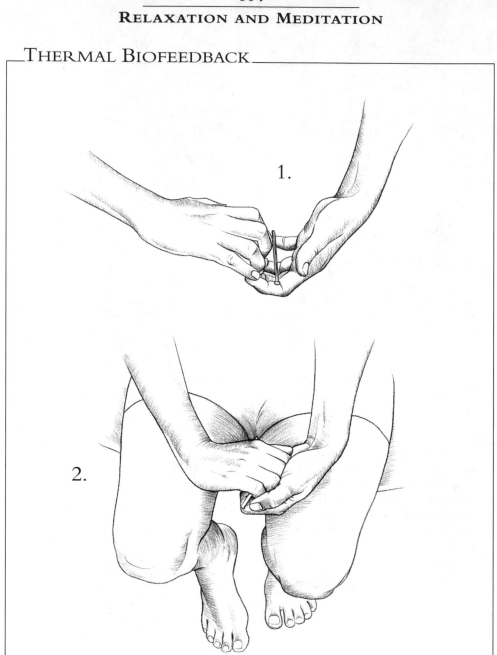

Place a thermometer across the fingers of one hand as shown (1). Touch your fingertips together so that the pinky finger of each hand is touching the index finger of the opposite hand. Roll your fingers together so that they form a ball around the thermometer and rest your hands comfortably in your lap (2).

YOGA

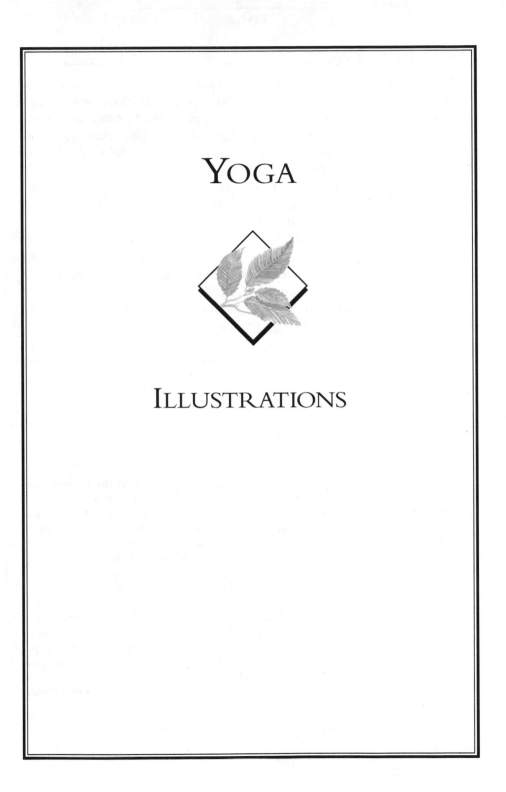

ILLUSTRATIONS

DAILY ROUTINE

The yoga exercises are shown in their ideal positions. Because levels of flexibility can vary greatly from person to person, if you're new to yoga, don't attempt or expect to do these positions perfectly. It is best to proceed at your own pace and comfort level. Consult your physician before attempting to do these exercises, especially if you have special medical needs or a chronic medical condition or if you are pregnant.

The first 16 poses should be part of your daily yoga routine, which should also include breathing exercises, relaxation and meditation. Pick three or four of these basic poses each day, alternating them from day to day to give your body a complete workout. Some of the basic poses have also been recommended for specific ailments. If you are suffering from a specific problem, make the recommended poses part of your daily yoga routine. For greater benefit, do them in the order listed.

The remaining poses, which are targeted to specific ailments, should be done in addition to your daily yoga routine.

MOUNTAIN POSE

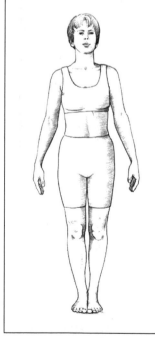

Stand with your feet close together; the inner bones of your ankles should touch, as should the edges of your big toes. Rock back on your heels and stretch the soles of your feet forward, then place your feet back down. Now raise your heels and stretch your soles back, then place your heels back on the floor.

Breathe normally. Stand with your knees locked gently. Tighten your thighs lightly and hold. Now tighten your buttocks and stomach muscles, keeping your back straight. Lift your rib cage by arching your back slightly, and pull your shoulders back. Relax your arms and let them hang normally at your sides. Keep your neck straight, and make sure your head is up and facing forward. Hold this position for 30 to 40 seconds, then relax. Repeat the pose one or two times.

YOGA

STANDING SUN POSE

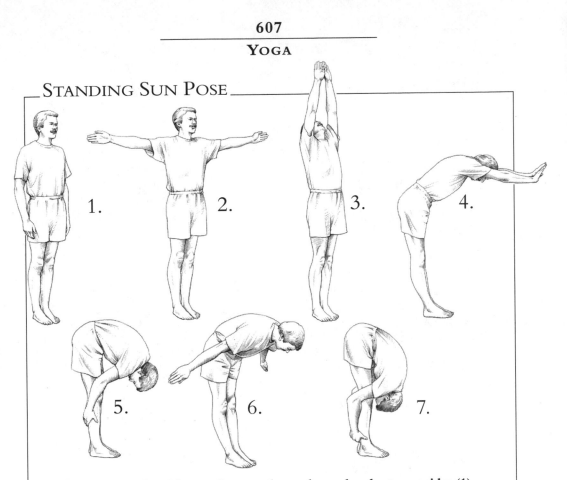

Stand up straight with your feet together and your hands at your sides (1). Exhale.

Inhale slowly as you raise your arms straight out from your sides (2). Continue lifting your arms until they are straight overhead (3). Look up and stretch gently.

Begin to exhale as you bend slowly from the hips (4). Continue to bend forward as you exhale completely. Grab the backs of your legs with your arms, elbows bent (5). Breathe evenly, letting your breath relax you into the pose. Inhale slowly, then exhale and let go of the muscle tension in your legs. Hold for several seconds.

Let go of your legs and inhale slowly. As you lift your body, bring your hands out at your sides and over your head (6). Exhale and lower your hands to your sides.

Repeat two times.

ADVANCED VERSION: As your muscles become more flexible, you may be able to draw your forehead forward toward your legs (7). Do not force yourself into this position. Instead, allow your body to relax and stretch downward as you exhale.

Repeat two times.

NOTE: If you have high blood pressure, consult your doctor before doing the standing sun pose.

TREE POSE

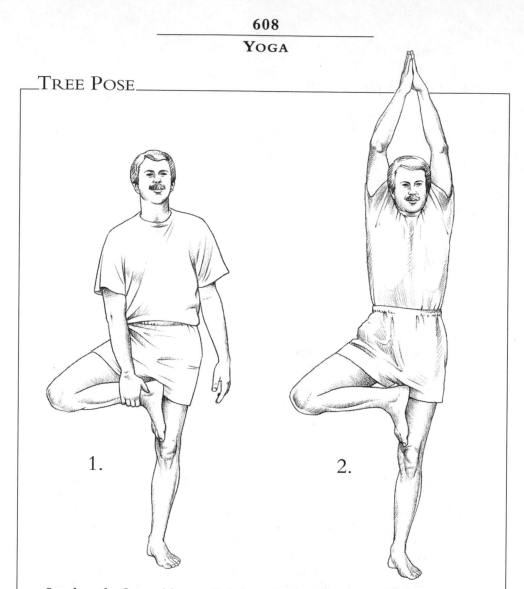

1.

2.

Stand on the floor with your feet close together. Bend your right leg and bring it slowly up your left leg, using your right hand for assistance (1). Use your left hand to hold on to a chair or wall for added balance. Put the sole of your right foot against the inside of your left leg, as high as you can reach comfortably.

When your balance is steady, raise both arms and place them together, palm to palm, high over your head (2). Focus on the wall in front of you to help with balance. Relax your stomach muscles and breathe normally. Hold this pose for 10 to 30 seconds, continuing to breathe normally. Relax and return to the standing position.

Repeat with your left leg.

NOTE: The elderly and people with advanced osteoporosis should not try this pose.

DANCER POSE

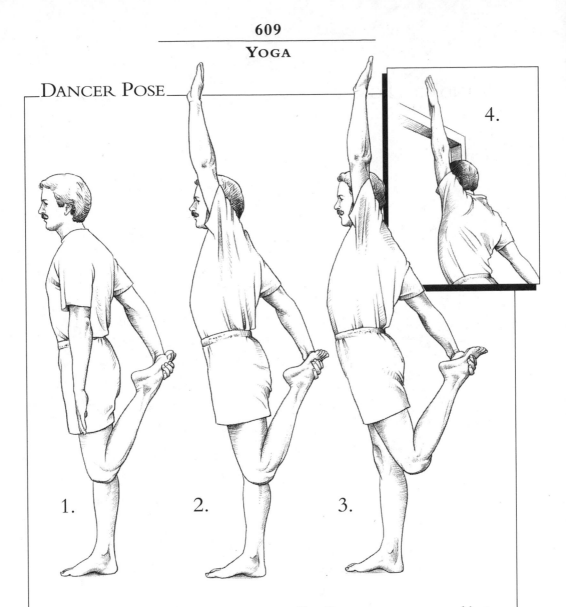

1. 2. 3. 4.

Stand up straight with your arms at your sides. Focus your eyes on an object across the room to help with balance. Bend your left knee and grab it behind your back with your right hand (1). Then lift your left arm, pointing your fingers at the ceiling (2).

Raise your left leg slowly back and away from your body (3). Keep your hand on your foot. When you reach a comfortable point, relax your abdominal muscles and breathe deeply from your stomach. Hold the pose for several seconds, then relax. Repeat with your right leg.

If you have trouble keeping your balance, stand in a doorway and place your hand flat over the door (4).

NOTE: People with lower back and disk problems should use caution with this pose. Get your doctor's approval first.

WINDMILL POSE

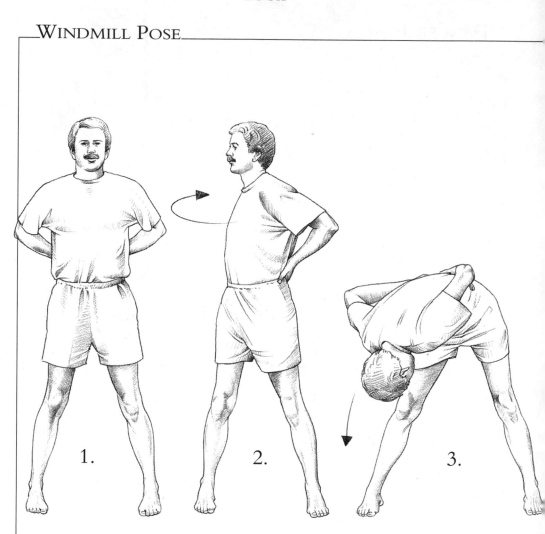

1. 2. 3.

Stand with your feet shoulder-width apart (1). Spread your fingers on both sides of your spine to support your lower back. Make sure your toes are pointed slightly inward. Begin to breathe in slowly.

As you continue to inhale, twist your torso slowly to the right (2). Your feet should remain in place.

Then begin to exhale. Bend forward at the waist, drawing your forehead as close to your right knee as possible (3). Without stopping, swing your head and

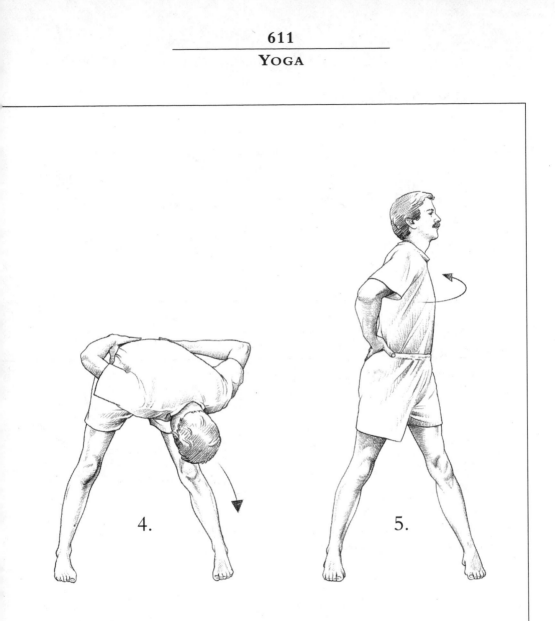

4.

5.

torso slowly toward your left knee (4). Make sure your hands remain on your back. You should finish exhaling when your head reaches your left knee.

Begin inhaling and lift your torso (5). As you straighten your body, keep it facing left. When you reach a full standing position, you should finish inhaling. Hold your breath and twist your body back to the right. Do three times in each direction.

NOTE: Use caution if you have lower back pain.

CORPSE POSE

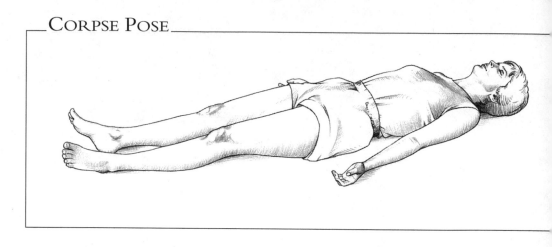

KNEE SQUEEZE

1.

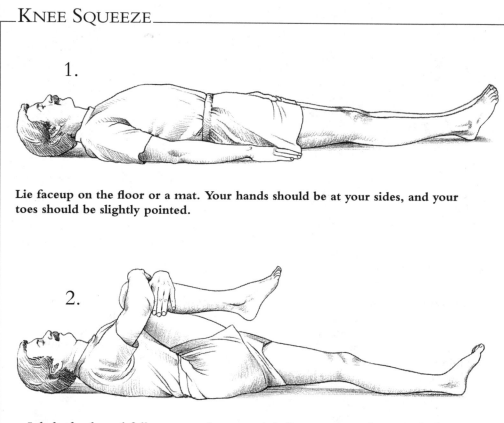

Lie faceup on the floor or a mat. Your hands should be at your sides, and your toes should be slightly pointed.

2.

Inhale slowly and fully as you raise your right knee to your chest. Grab the knee with both arms and hold it to your chest for a few seconds.

Lie on your back on either the floor or a mat. Your arms should be at your sides, with the palms of your hands facing up. Your legs should be straight, with your feet in a relaxed position. Relax all of your muscles, close your eyes and hold the pose for 30 seconds to several minutes, until your muscles completely relax. Breathe deeply and scan your body to feel any tension. If you feel tension, concentrate on the area and relax the muscles.

> NOTE: If you feel pain in your lower back, try bending your legs. Raise your knees and place your feet flat on the floor. Hold this position for 30 seconds to several minutes, following the instructions above.

3.

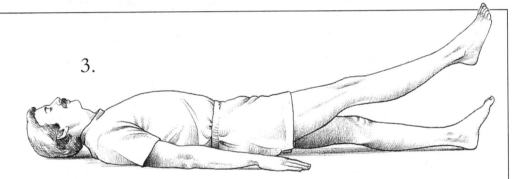

Then begin to exhale as you straighten your knee and lower it slowly to the floor. Repeat with the left leg. Do this a total of three times, alternating legs.

Next, breathe in completely, then lift both knees to your chest at the same time. Wrap your arms around both legs and hold for a few seconds, then breathe out and lower your legs.

4.

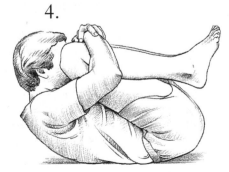

ADVANCED VERSION: After a few weeks, you can also raise your head and place your forehead between your knees as far as possible.

SPINE TWIST

1.

2.

3.

4.

Sit on the floor or a mat with your knees drawn close to your chest (1). Your hands should be on either side of your body, palms down.

Keeping your knees bent, lower your right leg and slide it under your left leg (2). Your right knee should be touching the floor, and your right heel should be tucked in front of your left buttock. Lift your left leg over your right knee and place your left foot on the outside of your right knee.

Lift your rib cage, straighten your spine and twist to the left (3). Place your left hand behind your right foot. Bring your right arm over your left leg and place your right hand in front of your right foot. Turn your shoulders and head so that they are facing left.

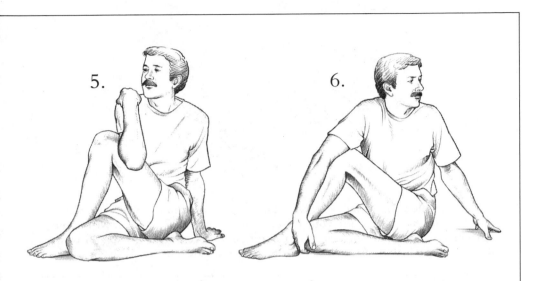

If you have difficulty bringing your right arm over your left leg, reach under your left leg and grab the back of your thigh (4). Then proceed to the last position in this sequence (7).

Bend your right arm, placing your right elbow on the outside of your left knee (5). Rock your left knee back and forth a few times with your right elbow. Then pull your left leg as far right as you can and straighten your right arm (6). Keep it on the outside of your left leg, and depending on your flexibility, grab your pants, right knee or left ankle with your right hand.

Place your left hand behind you as close to the base of your spine as possible (7). Be sure to keep your back straight. Breathe in deeply and look forward. As you start to exhale, gently twist your spine to the left, turning your head to the left and looking as far to the left as possible. Use your hands and arms only for balance; don't try to force your body farther by flexing your arm muscles. Hold this pose as you breathe gently for several seconds. Then unwind and repeat on the other side.

NOTE: Use extreme caution if you have problems with disks in your spine.

HEAD-TO-KNEE

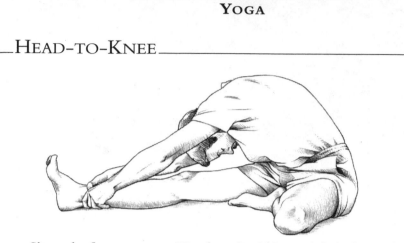

Sit on the floor or a mat. Your legs should be straight in front of you, with your feet together. Make sure your torso, neck and head are straight. Now bend your left knee and slide your left foot toward your crotch. Rest the sole of your left foot on the inside of your right thigh as high as possible.

SEATED SUN POSE

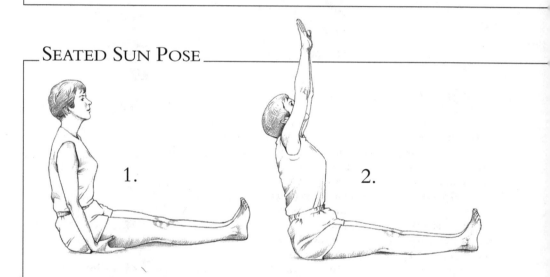

1.

2.

Sit on the floor or a mat with your legs straight in front of you, feet flexed and hands at your sides (1). Keep your back straight.

Exhale. Begin inhaling slowly, then lift your arms straight out to the sides and over your head (2). When your hands reach the top, hook your thumbs together and reach upward, looking up as you stretch.

Begin to exhale and bend forward slowly from your hips (3). Keep your arms parallel to your ears. Finish breathing out and grab your legs as far down as you can comfortably reach (4). Bend your elbows and use your arms to pull your torso toward your legs. If you can't bend your elbows, move your hands higher

Now take a deep breath as you lift your arms straight over your head. Stretch as high as possible and expand your chest. Begin to exhale and bend forward, with your back straight and your head between your arms. Bend forward as far as you can comfortably reach, keeping your head between your arms. Rest your hands on your right leg. Make sure to keep the back of your right knee touching the floor or mat. Relax. Hold the position for five to ten seconds, breathing normally.

If you want to stretch even more, stay in this position, take a deep breath and stretch forward from the base of your spine. As you exhale, try to bring your head farther down your right leg. When you reach as far as possible, breathe normally and relax. After five to ten seconds, begin to inhale and lift your head, neck and back. Keep your arms in line with your head as you straighten into the sitting position. Breathe out and slowly lower your arms. Repeat with the left leg, then do the complete sequence two more times.

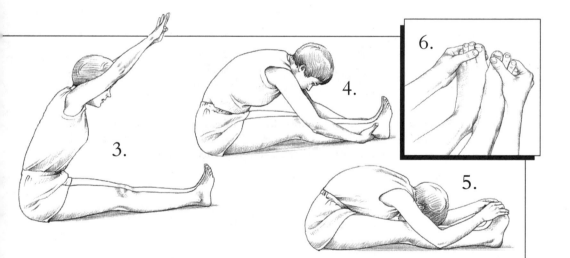

on your legs until you can. Hold this point for one or two seconds. If you are able to touch your toes with your elbows bent, grasp them for a second or two (5). Your thumbs should be on the tops of your big toes, with your index fingers on the bottoms (6).

Inhale slowly and begin to lift your chest back to the starting position. Your hands should be resting at your sides. Inhaling, lift your arms straight out and over your head again, hooking your thumbs together. Look up and stretch slowly. Begin to exhale and lower your arms. Repeat two more times.

BABY POSE

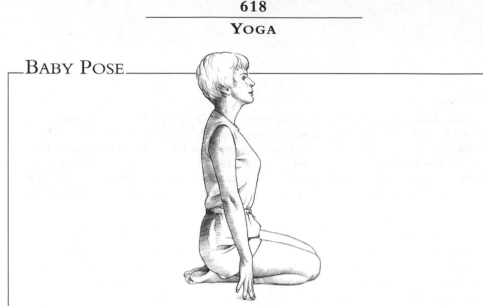

Sit on the floor with your knees bent and heels beneath your buttocks. Your arms should hang freely at your sides. The tops of your toes should be flat on the floor.

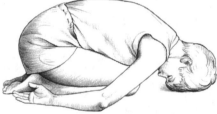

Lean forward slowly at the waist until the top of your forehead is touching the floor. Your arms should be resting on either side of your legs. Keep your neck straight and relaxed, and breathe normally. Hold for five minutes or less.

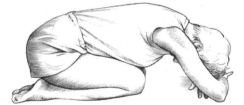

If this pose is uncomfortable, you can cross your arms and rest your forehead on your forearms. Again, be sure to keep your neck straight and relaxed.

If you have arthritis in your knees, you can do a variation of the baby pose while seated in a chair. Push your hips against the back of the chair and place your feet flat on the floor, slightly apart. Then lean forward at the waist, letting your head drop between your knees. Be sure to keep your neck straight and relaxed. Your arms should be hanging at your sides, with your hands near your ankles.

NOTE: Do not do this exercise if you have high blood pressure.

EASY BRIDGE POSE

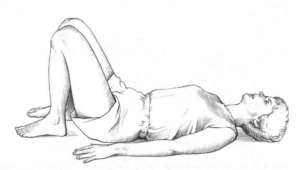

Lie on the floor or a mat. Your knees should be bent. Place your feet flat on the floor and as close to your buttocks as possible. Your hands should be at your sides, with palms down.

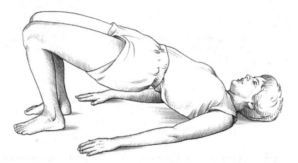

Breathe out slowly as you relax your head, neck and shoulders. As you start to breathe in, lift your hips off the floor slowly. Arch your back, with your shoulders and neck remaining on the floor. Hold this position for one or two breaths. Then slowly lower your hips to the floor as you exhale. Repeat two more times.

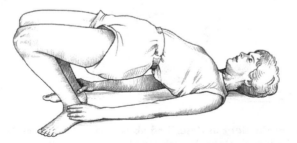

ADVANCED VERSION: Grab your ankles with your hands and proceed as described above.

NOTE: **Do not attempt this pose during the second half of pregnancy.**

HALF BOAT POSE

Lie flat on your stomach on either the floor or a mat. Your forehead should touch the floor, and your arms should be straight over your head with the palms also touching the floor. Your legs should remain together, with the muscles relaxed completely.

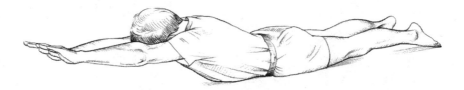

Take a deep breath as you slowly lift your arms, head and torso off the floor. Keep your head between your arms at all times. Breathe evenly. Hold for five seconds. Then breathe out, lower your arms, head and chest back to the floor, and relax. Repeat two more times.

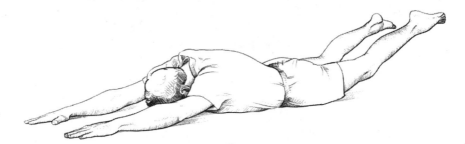

Stay facedown on the floor as described above. Move your feet 12 to 18 inches apart, keeping your legs straight. Breathe in slowly as you lift your legs and feet. Keep your upper body and arms relaxed. Breathe evenly and hold for five seconds. Then breathe out and slowly lower your legs back to the ground. Repeat two more times.

BOAT POSE

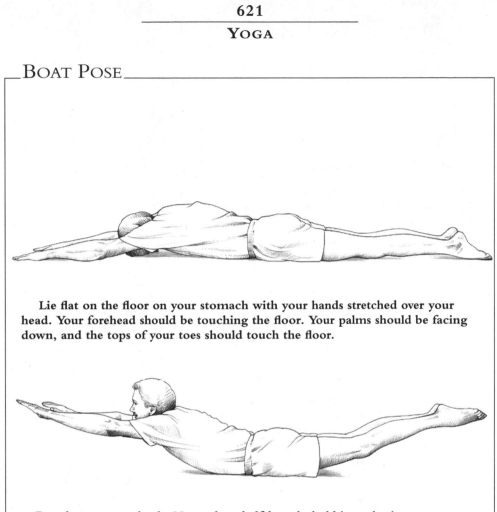

Lie flat on the floor on your stomach with your hands stretched over your head. Your forehead should be touching the floor. Your palms should be facing down, and the tops of your toes should touch the floor.

Breathe out completely. Now take a half-breath, hold it, and raise your arms and legs as high as you can. Lift your head and look up. Hold this pose for several seconds, then exhale and lower your limbs back to the resting position. Make sure you keep your arms straight, with no bend at the elbows or wrists. Your knees should also be straight, and your toes should be pointed. Repeat two more times.

NOTE: Before attempting the boat pose, use the half boat pose for at least one week.

COBRA POSE

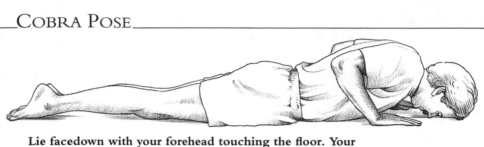

Lie facedown with your forehead touching the floor. Your toes should be pointed, with the tops of your toes touching the floor. Place your hands, palms down, on the floor next to your armpits.

Lift your head slowly off the floor as you begin to take a breath. Be sure to look straight up. Now lift your chest and stomach off the floor. Use the muscles of the back to lift, curling your spine as you rise. Don't push up with your arms, and make sure to keep your hipbone on the floor at all times. Your mouth should be closed, with your lower jaw jutting forward to stretch your throat muscles.

When your torso is off the floor, hold the pose for several seconds. Make sure your elbows remain bent at all times. Then begin to exhale and lower your body slowly to floor. The stomach should touch first, followed by the chest and forehead. Repeat two more times.

> NOTE: Women should avoid this pose during menstrual periods. Men and women should not attempt this pose if they have open wounds in the abdominal region or if they have undergone abdominal or pelvic surgery within the past several weeks.

LION POSE

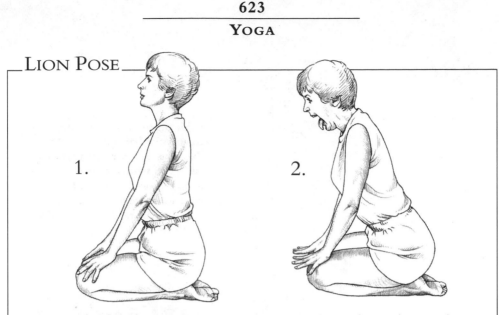

Sit on the floor or a mat with your knees bent and your feet under your buttocks (1). Keep your back straight and place your hands on your knees. Close your eyes and take a complete breath.

Open your eyes, lean forward slightly and exhale while making a growling sound (2). As you growl, open your mouth and stick out your tongue as far as possible. Spread your fingers wide. Repeat several times.

ALTERNATE NOSTRIL BREATH

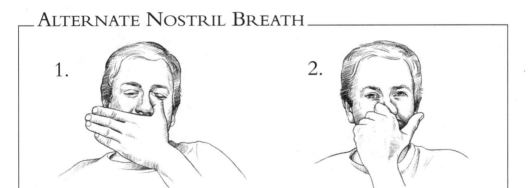

Sit in a comfortable position on the floor or in a chair. Press the thumb of your left hand against the left side of your nose, blocking the air passage (1). The other fingers on your left hand should reach straight across your face but should not touch the face. Breathe in slowly through your right nostril for a count of ten.

Let go with your thumb, but close the right nostril with the side of your index finger (2). Breathe out through the left nostril for a count of ten.

Repeat five times. Then switch hands and repeat five times, breathing in through the left nostril and out through the right nostril.

BUTTERFLY

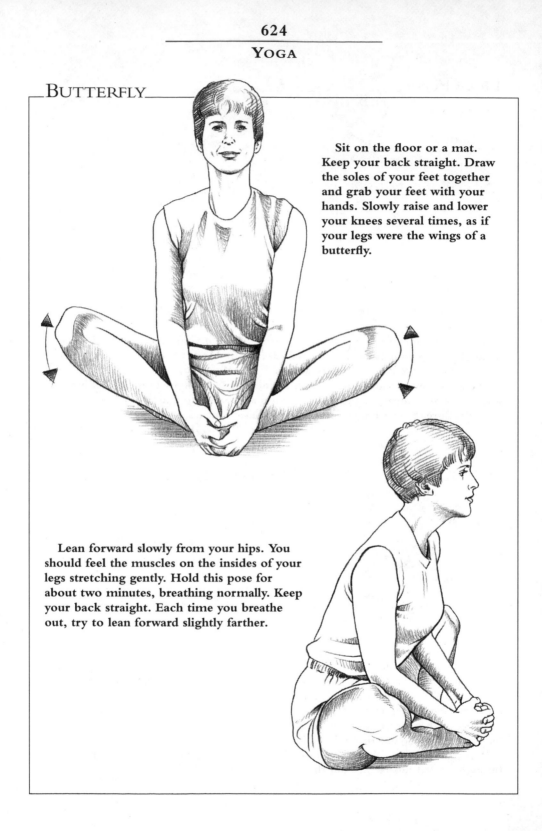

Sit on the floor or a mat. Keep your back straight. Draw the soles of your feet together and grab your feet with your hands. Slowly raise and lower your knees several times, as if your legs were the wings of a butterfly.

Lean forward slowly from your hips. You should feel the muscles on the insides of your legs stretching gently. Hold this pose for about two minutes, breathing normally. Keep your back straight. Each time you breathe out, try to lean forward slightly farther.

HAND EXERCISES FOR ARTHRITIS

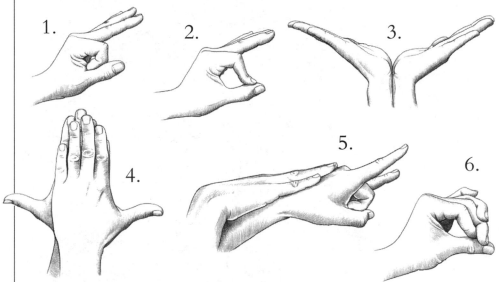

CURLING. Stretch your left arm straight in front of you. Keep your wrist straight and make the okay sign with your index finger curled onto the side of your thumb (1). The other fingers should be kept straight. Release the index finger and curl the middle finger, then the ring finger, then the pinky. Keep the other fingers straight at all times. Do six times with each hand.

CONTRACTING. Gently push together the tips of your thumb and index finger (2). Keep the other fingers straight. The first joint of your index finger should be bent slightly inward where it is pushed against the thumb. Repeat with your middle, ring and pinky fingers. Do six times with each hand.

FANNING. Press your palms together in front of your body at stomach level. Then open your fingertips and palms, bending back at the wrists (3). Then bringing your elbows together, move your wrists away from each other. Return to the original position. Do six times.

FISH. Place one palm on the back of your other hand (4). Your fingers should be straight, and your thumbs should stick out on either side. Rotate your thumbs in full circles six times. Then reverse direction and rotate six more times.

DEER. Hold your arms straight in front of you. Make a gentle fist with your left hand, then straighten the index and pinky fingers (5). Keep the thumb underneath, holding the other two fingers. Now put your right hand on the back of the left hand and gently "pet" the left hand. Do this six times, then switch hands and repeat six more times.

PEACOCK'S TAIL. Hold your left hand straight in front of you. Push together the tips of your thumb and index finger (6). Then wrap your middle finger over your index finger, using your right hand for assistance. Follow by wrapping your ring finger over your middle finger and your pinky over your ring finger. Unfold the fingers and relax. Do this six times, then switch hands and repeat six more times.

LEG UP, LEG OUT

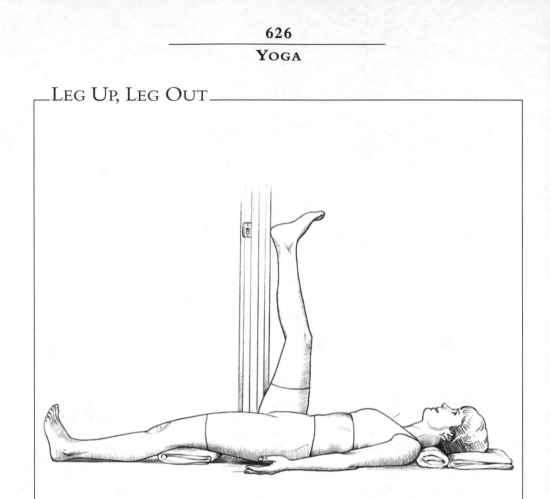

To do this exercise, find a place where you can stretch one leg up a wall and the other straight on the floor, such as a doorway. Sit with your right side close to the wall or doorway. Then supporting your trunk with your arms, lie down and extend your right leg up the wall or the inside of the doorway. Once you're in this position, cushion your neck with a rolled-up towel and your head with a folded towel. Keep your left leg bent, with the foot on the floor. Let your arms rest easily at your sides.

Adjust the position of your buttocks so that your right leg can be fully straightened and your sacrum (the triangular-shaped bone just above your tailbone) can rest solidly on the floor. If you can't completely straighten your right leg, move your buttocks away from the wall or doorway until you can straighten your leg while maintaining a comfortable hamstring stretch.

Once the buttocks are positioned, slowly stretch out your left leg. If your lower back hurts when your left leg is outstretched on the floor, place a rolled blanket behind your knee so that your lower back is comfortable. Hold this position for 30 to 60 seconds, then repeat with your left leg raised. Continue to alternate legs until you have done the exercise three or four times with each leg. Do two or three sets of this exercise once or twice a day.

NECK ROLL

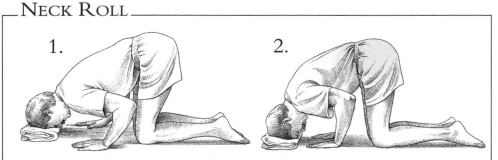

1.   2.

Kneel on the floor or a mat (1). Place your forehead on the floor or on a folded towel if the floor is uncomfortable and position your hands underneath your shoulders.

Breathe out slowly as you roll your head forward gently (2). Do not push too far; you should feel a pleasant stretch in the back of your neck. Return to the starting position, then repeat slowly 20 times.

NOTE: Do not attempt this pose if you have pain in your neck or other neck problems.

PIRIFORMIS STRETCH

To stretch out a tight piriformis muscle, sit on the edge of a blanket folded four to six inches high, with your knees bent and your feet flat on the floor in front of you. Take your left foot under your right knee and place it on the floor next to the outside of your right buttock. Place your right foot on the floor next to the outside of your left thigh. Feel your weight resting equally on both sitting bones. From this base, allow your spine to lengthen upward as you gently lift your breast-bone.

Stabilize your trunk by holding your right knee with both hands. If your right foot won't reach the floor, or if the stretch in your right buttock is too intense, place your right foot next to or in front of your right knee instead.

If the stretch is still too intense or you feel radiating pain down your leg, raise the height of the padding to decrease the intensity of the stretch. If you don't feel any stretch in your right buttock, gently pull your right knee across your body toward the left side of your chest.

Stay in the pose for 20 seconds to several minutes. Then repeat with your left leg bent. Do two to four sets once or twice a day. As your piriformis muscles stretch out over a period of months, gradually decrease the height of your blanket until you can sit on the floor.

YAWNING

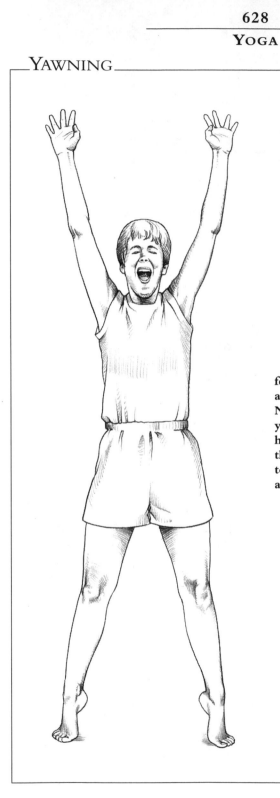

Stand up straight with your feet about shoulder-width apart and your hands at your sides. Now stand on your toes and lift your arms straight over your head. Force yourself to yawn three times, then lower your heels to the floor and slowly drop your arms. Repeat six times.

PART III

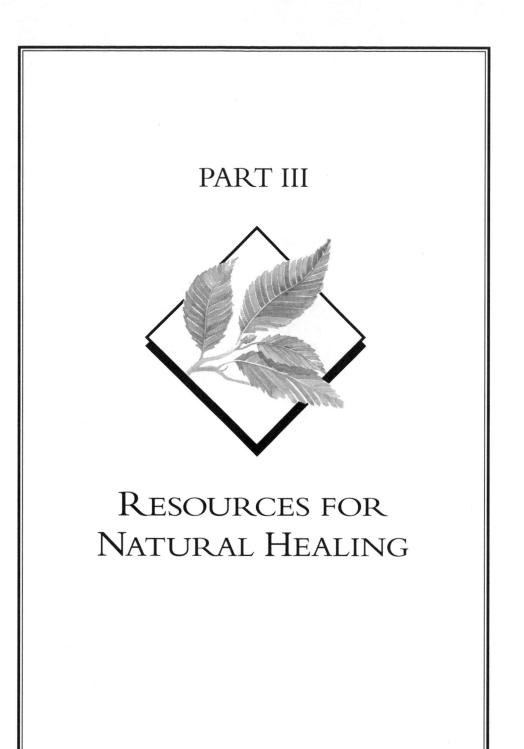

Resources for
Natural Healing

RESOURCES

If you're interested in more information on any of the alternative healing methods discussed in this book, the list below should help you. You'll find organizations that can provide you with self-help material or refer you to a qualified alternative practitioner in your area, along with suppliers of herbs, essential oils and other remedies recommended in Part II and books, audio- and videotapes for your reference.

ACUPRESSURE

ORGANIZATIONS

Acupressure Institute
1533 Shattuck Ave.
Berkeley, CA 94709
Offers *The Hands-On Health Care Catalog*, featuring charts, books and videotapes.

American Oriental Bodywork Therapy Association
6801 Jericho Tpk.
Syosset, NY 11791
Publishes a national directory of licensed practitioners and instructors that is available for a fee.

G-Jo Institute
P.O. Box 848060
Hollywood, FL 33084
An educational organization emphasizing natural health that provides publications and home study courses on acupressure and other self-help topics.

Jin Shin Do Foundation for Bodymind Acupressure
366 California Ave., Suite 16
Palo Alto, CA 94306
Offers classes, books, charts and tapes.

Jin Shin Jyutsu, Inc.
8719 E. San Alberto Dr.
Scottsdale, AZ 85258
Provides training, books and materials as well as practioner referrals.

BOOKS

Beinfield, Harriet. *Between Heaven and Earth: A Guide to Chinese Medicine.* New York: Ballantine Books, 1992.

Gach, Michael Reed. *Acupressure's Potent Points: A Guide to Self-Care for Common Ailments.* New York: Bantam Books, 1990.

Gach, Michael Reed. *Acu-Yoga: Self-Help Techniques to Relieve Tension.* Briarcliff Manor, N.Y.: Japan Publications, 1981.

Gach, Michael Reed. *Arthritis Relief at Your Fingertips: Your Guide to Erasing Aches and Pains without Drugs.* New York: Warner Books, 1990.

Lundberg, Paul. *The Book of Shiatsu.* St. Louis: Fireside Books, 1992.

Masunga, Shizuto, and Wataru Ohashi. *Zen Shiatsu: How to Harmonize Yin and Yang for Better Health.* Briarcliff Manor, N.Y.: Japan Publications, 1977.

Reid, Daniel. *The Complete Book of Chinese Health and Healing.* Boston: Shambhala, 1994.

Wagner, Lindsay, and Robert M. Klein. *Lindsay Wagner's New Beauty: The Acupressure Facelift.* New York: Prentice Hall, 1987.

Yamamoto, Shizuko. *Barefoot Shiatsu: Whole-Body Approach to Health.* Briarcliff Manor, N.Y.: Japan Publications, 1979.

Yamamoto, Shizuko. *The Shiatsu Handbook.* Eureka, Calif.: Turning Point Publications, 1986.

ALTERNATIVE MEDICINE

ORGANIZATIONS

American Association of Naturopathic Physicians
2366 Eastlake Ave. E., Suite 322
Seattle, WA 98102
For a fee, offers a national referral directory, which lists all U.S. members of the association, and an information brochure.

American Holistic Health Association
Suzan Walter, President
P.O. Box 17400
Anaheim, CA 92817-7400
Grassroots movement promoting a holistic approach to wellness. Offers booklets, a newsletter and networking lists of self-help resources. Open to all.

American Holistic Medical Association
4101 Lake Boone Trail, Suite 201
Raleigh, NC 27606
Publishes a national referral directory of M.D.'s and D.O.'s who practice holistic medicine, including information about their schooling and philosophy of practice. The directory is available by mail order for a fee.

Bastyr University
144 NE 54th St.
Seattle, WA 98105
Offers a four-year program leading to a doctor of naturopathic medicine degree. Master of science degree in acupunture and certification in midwifery also available. Write for a catalog.

National College of Naturopathic Medicine
11231 SE Market St.
Portland, OR 97216
Offers a four-year graduate program to prepare students for licensure and the general practice of naturopathic medicine. Post-doctoral programs are being developed in naturopathic obstetrics, homeopathy and classical Chinese medicine.

BOOKS

Burton Goldberg Group. *Alternative Medicine: The Definitive Guide.* Puyallup, Wash.: Future Medicine Publishing, 1993.

RESOURCES

AROMATHERAPY

ORGANIZATIONS

Aromatherapy Seminars
1830 S. Robertson Blvd., #203
Los Angeles, CA 90035
1-800-677-2368
Conducts introductory seminars and aromatherapy training courses at a number of locations across the country.

National Association for Holistic Aromatherapy
P.O. Box 17622
Boulder, CO 80308-7622
1-800-566-6735
Provides a newsletter, a correspondence course, books and directories of aromatherapy schools and practitioners.

SOURCES FOR ESSENTIAL OILS

Herba-Aromatica
c/o Galina Lisin
25063 Oakridge Ct.
Hayward, CA 94541
Lisin, an aromatic consultant, has an in-house laboratory where she formulates her own oils.

Jeanne Rose Aromatherapy
219 Carl St.
San Francisco, CA 94117
Provides study courses and aromatherapy first-aid kits, a line of exotic essential oils, books on herbs and aromatherapy and various lectures and seminars.

Leydet Aromatics, Inc.
P.O. Box 2354
Fair Oaks, CA 95628
Essential oils and other aromatherapy supplies.

Origins
767 5th Ave.
New York, NY 10153
1-800-ORIGINS (for location of nearest store)
1-800-723-7310 (to order)
A cosmetics company that uses aromatherapy oils in some of its products.

Phybiosis
Suite JR
P.O. Box 992
Bowie, MD 20718
Essential oils, aromatic diffusers of various styles and prices and body care products.

BOOKS

Ackerman, Diane. *A Natural History of the Senses.* Avenel, N.J.: Random House Value Publishing, 1993.

Blevi, Viktor, and Gretchen Sween. *Aromatherapy.* New York: Avon Books, 1993.

Jackson, Judith. *Scentual Touch: A Personal Guide to Aromatherapy.* (out of print; check your library)

Rose, Jeanne. *Aromatherapy: Applications and Inhalations.* Berkeley, Calif.: North Atlantic Books, 1992.

Sadler, Julie. *Aromatherapy.* New York: Sterling Publishing, 1994.

Tisserand, Robert B. *The Art of Aromatherapy: The Beautifying and Healing Properties of the Essential Oils of Flowers and Herbs.* Rochester, Vt.: Destiny Books, 1987.

AYURVEDA

ORGANIZATIONS

American Institute of Vedic Studies
1701 Santa Fe River Rd.
Santa Fe, NM 87501
Provides certification courses and publications on Ayurveda. Not a treatment center.

Ayurvedic Institute
P.O. Box 23445
Albuquerque, NM 87192-1445
Herbs, oils and remedies formulated by Vasant Lad, B.A.M.S., M.A.Sc., director of the institute.

The Maharishi International University
1000 N. 4th St.
D. B. 1155
Fairfield, IA 52557
Four-year undergraduate program; Ayurvedic clinic on campus. Also offers books, videotapes, audiotapes and Maharishi Ayurveda products, including herbal formulas, hair and skin care products and foods. Write for a catalog.

SOURCES FOR AYURVEDIC HERBS

Bazaar of India Imports
1810 University Ave.
Berkeley, CA 94703
Herbs, oils, soaps, books, incense.

Planetary Formulas
P.O. Box 533
Soquel, CA 95073
Write for a catalog of Ayurvedic and Chinese herbs.

Quantum Publications, Inc.
P.O. Box 598
South Lancaster, MA 01561
1-800-858-1808
Catalog of *Ageless Body, Timeless Mind* products, a line of herbal formulas from author Deepak Chopra, M.D.

BOOKS

Chopra, Deepak. *Ageless Body, Timeless Mind: The Quantum Alternative to Growing Old.* New York: Crown Publishing Group, 1993.

Chopra, Deepak. *Creating Health: How to Wake Up the Body's Intelligence.* Boston: Houghton Mifflin, 1987.

Chopra, Deepak. *Perfect Health: The Complete Health Mind-Body Guide.* New York: Harmony Books, 1990.

Chopra, Deepak. *Quantum Healing: Exploring the Frontiers of Body, Mind, Medicine.* New York: Bantam Books, 1990.

Frawley, David. *Ayurvedic Healing: A Comprehensive Guide.* Sandy, Utah: Passage Press, 1989.

Lad, Vasant. *Ayurveda, The Science of Self-Healing: A Practical Guide.* Twin Lakes, Wis.: Lotus Press, 1984.

Lonsdorf, Nancy, Veronica Butler and Melanie Brown. *A Woman's Best Medicine: Health, Happiness and Long Life through Ayurveda.* New York: The Putnam Publishing Group, 1995.

Svoboda, Robert E. *Prakruti: Your Ayurvedic Constitution.* Albuquerque, N.M.: Geocom, 1989.

FLOWER REMEDY/ ESSENCE THERAPY

SOURCES FOR FLOWER REMEDIES/ESSENCES

Capitol Drugs, Inc.
4454 Van Nuys Blvd.
Sherman Oaks, CA 91403
1-800-858-8833
Bach flower remedies, homeopathic remedies, herbs, nutritional supplements, kits, educational services.

Flower Essence Services
P.O. Box 1769
Nevada City, CA 95959
1-800-548-0075
English and California flower essences, books on flower essence therapy.

The Flower Essence Society
Patricia Kaminski, Co-director
P.O. Box 459
Nevada City, CA 95959
1-800-548-0075
An organization that studies and promotes the therapeutic use of flower remedies/essences.

Nelson Bach USA, Ltd.
Wilmington Technology Park
100 Research Drive
Wilmington, MA 01887
1-800-319-9151
Manufactures and distributes the 38 Bach flower essences as well as Rescue Remedy, a blend of five essences used for emergency stress relief.

BOOKS

Kaminski, Patricia, and Richard Katz. *Flower Essence Repertory.* Nevada City: Calif.: Flower Essence Society, 1992.

Kaslof, Leslie J. *The Traditional Flower Remedies of Dr. Edward Bach: A Self-Help Guide.* New Canaan, Conn.: Keats Publishing, 1993.

Vlamis, Gregory. *Bach Flower Remedies to the Rescue.* Rochester, Vt.: Inner Traditions, 1990.

FOOD THERAPY

BOOKS

Barnard, Neal. *Food for Life: How the New Four Food Groups Can Save Your Life.* New York: Crown Publishing, 1994.

Haas, Elson. *Staying Healthy with Nutrition: The Complete Guide to Diet and Nutritional Medicine.* Berkeley, Calif.: Celestial Arts, 1991.

Mindell, Earl. *Earl Mindell's Food as Medicine.* New York: Simon & Schuster, 1994.

Ornish, Dean. *Dr. Dean Ornish's Program for Reversing Heart Disease.* New York: Random House, 1990.

HERBAL THERAPY

ORGANIZATIONS

American Botanical Council
P.O. Box 201660
Austin, TX 78720
Publishes the journal *Herbalgram*, available for a fee. Write for a catalog.

The American Herbalists Guild
P.O. Box 1683
Soquel, CA 95073
Directory of herbal education.

Herb Research Foundation
1007 Pearl St., #200 F
Boulder, CO 80302
General information on herbs.

SOURCES FOR HERBAL REMEDIES

Capitol Drugs, Inc.
4454 Van Nuys Blvd.
Sherman Oaks, CA 91403
1-800-858-8833
Herbs, homeopathic remedies, nutritional supplements, kits, educational services, Bach flower remedies.

Capitol Drugs, Inc.
8578 Santa Monica Blvd.
West Hollywood, CA 90069
1-800-858-8833
Herbs, homeopathic remedies, supplements, books.

Gaia Herbs
12 Lancaster County Rd.
Harvard, MA 01451
Almost 300 herbal extracts, salves, oils and alcohol-free products.

Herb Pharm
P.O. Box 116
Williams, OR 97544
Tinctures.

Herb Products Co.
11012 Magnolia Blvd.
P.O. Box 898
North Hollywood, CA 91603-0898
Herb products and essential oils.

Simplers Botanical Co.
Box 39
Forestville, CA 95436
Herbal extracts and formulas, aromatherapy oils, skin care products and books.

BOOKS

Foster, Steven. *Herbal Renaissance: Growing, Using and Understanding Herbs in the Modern World*. Layton, Utah: Smith, Gibbs, Publisher, 1993.

Gladstar, Rosemary. *Herbal Healing for Women*. New York: Simon & Schuster, 1993.

Green, James. *The Male Herbal*. Freedom, Calif.: Crossing Press, 1991.

Hoffman, David. *The New Holistic Herbal*. Rockport, Mass.: Element Books, 1991.

Moore, Michael. *Medicinal Plants of the Mountain West*. Santa Fe, N.M.: Museum of New Mexico Press, 1979.

Rose, Jeanne. *Jeanne Rose's Modern Herbal*. New York: Perigee Books, Berkley Publishing Group, 1987.

Tyler, Varro E. *Herbs of Choice: The Therapeutic Use of Phytochemicals*. Binghamton, N.Y.: Haworth Press, 1994.

Weiss, Rudolf Fritz. *Herbal Medicine*. Portland, Ore.: Beaconsfield Publishing, 1985.

RESOURCES

HOMEOPATHY

ORGANIZATIONS

International Foundation for Homeopathy
2366 Eastlake Ave. E, Suite 325
Seattle, WA 98102
General information, training, referrals.

National Center for Homeopathy
801 N. Fairfax St., Suite 306
Alexandria, VA 22314
Offers an information packet that includes a directory of practitioners and resources in the United States and Canada. Also publishes newsletters and sponsors classes and conferences for members.

National College of Naturopathic Medicine
11231 SE Market St.
Portland, OR 97216
A national center for homeopathic education.

New England School of Homeopathy
356 Middle St.
Amherst, MA 01002
1-800-637-4440
Courses, seminars, journals.

SOURCES FOR HOMEOPATHIC REMEDIES

Annandale Apothecary
3299 Woodburn Rd.
Annandale, VA 22003
Homeopathic remedies, nutritional products, books.

Bierer's Pharmacy
146 S. Main St.
Lexington, VA 24450
1-800-552-6779
Homeopathic remedies, mail-order service.

Biological Homeopathic Industries
11600 Cochiti SE
Albuquerque, NM 87123
1-800-621-7644
Combination homeopathic remedies, therapeutic information.

Boericke & Tafel
2381 Circadian Way
Santa Rosa, CA 95407
1-800-876-9505, ext. 100
Homeopathic remedies.

Boiron, The World Leader in Homeopathy (East Coast)
6 Campus Blvd., Bldg. A
Newtown Square, PA 19073
1-800-BOIRON-1
Homeopathic remedies, kits, books, educational materials.

Boiron, The World Leader in Homeopathy (West Coast)
98C W. Cochran St.
Simi Valley, CA 93065
1-800-BLU-TUBE
Homeopathic remedies, kits, books.

Budget Pharmacy
3001 NW 7th St.
Miami, FL 33125
1-800-221-9772
Homeopathic remedies, books, tapes.

Capitol Drugs, Inc.
4454 Van Nuys Blvd.
Sherman Oaks, CA 91403
1-800-858-8833
Homeopathic remedies, herbs,
nutritional supplements, kits, educational services, Bach flower
remedies.

Capitol Drugs, Inc.
8578 Santa Monica Blvd.
West Hollywood, CA 90069
1-800-858-8833
Homeopathic remedies, herbs,
supplements, books.

Dolisos America, Inc.
3014 Rigel Ave.
Las Vegas, NV 89102
1-800-365-4767
Homeopathic remedies.

**Fairfax Medical Center
Pharmacy**
10721 Main St.
Fairfax, VA 22030
1-800-723-7455
Homeopathic remedies.

Five Elements Center
115 Rte. 46, Bldg. D, Suite 29
Mountain Lakes, NJ 07046
1-800-248-0884
Homeopathic remedies, educational
materials.

**Homeopathic Educational
Services**
2124 Kittredge Street, #N
Berkeley, CA 94704
1-800-359-9051
Homeopathic remedies, books, tapes,
software.

Homeopathic Informational Resources, Ltd.
Oneida River Park Dr.
Clay, NY 13041
1-800-289-4447
Homeopathic remedies, books,
videotapes, software, audiotapes.

Longevity Pure Medicine
9595 Wilshire Blvd., #502
Beverly Hills, CA 90212
Homeopathic products.

**Luyties Pharmacal Company/Nu
Age Laboratories/Formur
Publishers/Walker Pharmacal**
4200 Laclede Ave.
St. Louis, MO 63108
1-800-325-8080
Homeopathic remedies, kits, books.

The Medicine Shoppe
6307 York Rd.
Baltimore, MD 21212-2699
Homeopathic remedies, kits, books.

Newton Laboratories, Inc.
612 Upland Trail
Conyers, GA 30207
1-800-448-7256
Homeopathic remedies, educational
materials.

Northeast Homeopathic (a division of Acton Pharmacy)
563 Massachusetts Ave.
Acton, MA 01720
1-800-552-4956
Homeopathic remedies.

Powell Pharmacy, Inc.
11085 Little Patuxent Pkwy.
Columbia, MD 21044
Homeopathic remedies, vitamins.

RESOURCES

Standard Homeopathic
210 W. 131st St.
Box 61067
Los Angeles, CA 90061
1-800-624-9659
Homeopathic remedies, books.

Washington Homeopathic Products, Inc.
4914 Del Ray Ave.
Bethesda, MD 20814
1-800-336-1695
Maker of homeopathic remedies.

BOOKS

Lockie, Andrew. *The Family Guide to Homeopathy: Symptoms and Natural Solutions.* New York: Simon & Schuster, 1993.

Lockie, Andrew, and Nicola Geddes. *The Women's Guide to Homeopathy.* New York: St. Martin's Press, 1994.

Panos, Maesimund, and Jane Heimlich. *Homeopathic Medicine at Home.* Los Angeles: Jeremy P. Tarcher, 1981.

Reichenberg-Ullman, Judyth. *The Patient's Guide to Homeopathic Medicine.* Edmonds, Wash.: Picnic Point Press, 1994.

Ullman, Dana. *Discovering Homeopathy: Your Introduction to the Science and Art of Homeopathic Medicine.* Berkeley, Calif.: North Atlantic Books, 1991.

Ullman, Dana. *Homeopathic Medicine for Children and Infants.* Los Angeles: Jeremy P. Tarcher, 1992.

VIDEOTAPES

Video Remedies, Inc.
P.O. Box 290866
Davie, FL 33329-0866
1-800-733-4874
Homeopathic first-aid videotapes.

HYDROTHERAPY

ORGANIZATIONS

Desert Springs Therapy Center
66705 E. Sixth St.
Desert Hot Springs, CA 92240
Provides patients with short- or long-term hydrotherapy treatments for various illnesses and conditions.

Uchee Pines Institute
Agatha Thrash, M.D., Co-director
30 Uchee Pines Rd., Suite 75
Seale, AL 36975
Publishes a newsletter and provides information on various types of natural therapy, including hydrotherapy, exercise, herbs and nutrition. A quarterly health journal is available for a fee.

BOOKS

Dail, Clarence, and Charles Thomas. *Hydrotherapy: Simple Treatments for Common Ailments.* Brushton, N.Y.: TEACH Services, 1989.

Thrash, Agatha, and Calvin Thrash. *Home Remedies: Hydrotherapy, Massage, Charcoal and Other Simple Treatments.* Seale, Ala.: New Lifestyle Publishing, 1981.

IMAGERY

ORGANIZATIONS

The Academy for Guided Imagery
P.O. Box 2070
Mill Valley, CA 94942
1-800-726-2070
Offers books and audiotapes of imagery exercises as well as a directory of imagery practitioners.

BOOKS

Achterberg, Jeanne, Barbara Dossey and Leslie Kolkmeier. *Rituals of Healing: Using Imagery for Health and Wellness.* New York: Bantam Books, 1994.

Epstein, Gerald. *Healing Visualizations: Creating Health with Imagery.* New York: Bantam Books, 1989.

Rossman, Martin L. *Healing Yourself: A Step-by-Step Program for Better Health through Imagery.* New York: Pocket Books, 1994.

Sheikh, Anees, ed. *Eastern and Western Approaches to Healing: Ancient Wisdom and Modern Knowledge.* New York: John Wiley & Sons, 1989.

NEWSLETTERS

Atlantis, The Imagery Newsletter
4016 Third Ave.
San Diego, CA 92103
Practical, how-to-do-it imagery techniques.

JUICE THERAPY

ORGANIZATIONS

American Association of Naturopathic Physicians
2366 Eastlake Ave., Suite 322
Seattle, WA 98102
Publishes a referral directory and an information brochure, both available for a fee. The directory contains the names of all member physicians in the United States; the brochure explains naturopathic medicine and lists naturopathic colleges in the United States.

MANUFACTURERS OF JUICERS

Omega Products, Inc.
6291 Lyters Ln.
P.O. Box 4523
Harrisburg, PA 17111
Omega juicer.

Plastaket Manufacturing Co., Inc.
62220 E. Hwy. 12 (Victor Rd.)
Lodi, CA 95240
Champion juicer.

Vita-Mix Corp.
Dept. PRO 193
8615 Usher Road
Cleveland, OH 44138
1-800-VITAMIX
Vita-Mix juicer.

BOOKS

Blauer, Stephen. *The Juicing Book: A Complete Guide to the Juicing of Fruits and Vegetables for Maximum Health and Vitality.* Wayne, N.J.: Avery Publishing, 1989.

Calbom, Cherie, and Maureen B. Keane. *Juicing for Life: A Guide to the Health Benefits of Fresh Fruit and Vegetable Juicing.* Wayne, N.J.: Avery Publishing, 1992.

Murray, Michael T. *The Complete Book of Juicing: Your Delicious Guide to Healthful Living.* Rocklin, Calif,: Prima Publishing, 1992.

MASSAGE

ORGANIZATIONS

American Massage Therapy Association
820 Davis St., Suite 100
Evanston, IL 60201-4444
847-864-0123
Offers referrals to qualified therapists.

Associated Bodywork and Massage Professionals
28677 Buffalo Park Rd.
Evergreen, CO 80439-7347
1-800-8-MASSAGE, ext. 0 (referrals)
1-800-458-2267 (subscriptions)
Offers referrals to qualified therapists. Also publishes *Massage & Bodywork* magazine, available by calling the 800 number listed above.

BOOKS

Lawrence, D. Baloti, and Lewis Harrison. *Massageworks: A Practical Encyclopedia of Massage Techniques.* (out of print; check your library)

Stillerman, Elaine. *Mother Massage: A Handbook for Relieving the Discomforts of Pregnancy.* New York: Delta, 1992.

Struna, Monika. *Self-Massage: Touch Techniques to Relax, Soothe and Stimulate Your Body.* (out of print; check your library)

West, Ouida. *The Magic of Massage: A New and Holistic Approach.* Mamaroneck, N.Y.: Hastings House, 1990.

REFLEXOLOGY

ORGANIZATIONS

International Institute of Reflexology
P.O. Box 12642
St. Petersburg, FL 33733-2642
Offers referrals to reflexologists trained by the institute, seminars, books and reflexology charts.

Laura Norman and Associates, Reflexology Center
41 Park Ave., Suite 8A
New York, NY 10016
1-800-FEET FIRST
Call for private appointments (in Manhattan). Also offers training classes (beginner through certification), books, audiotapes, videotapes and aromatherapy foot care products.

Reflexology Research
P.O. Box 35820
Albuquerque, NM 87176
1-800-713-6711
Call to order books and charts as well as for general information about reflexology. Also offers private reflexology sessions (in Santa Fe, New Mexico) and training and certification classes.

RESOURCES

BOOKS

Byers, Dwight. *Better Health with Foot Reflexology*. St. Petersburg, Fla.: Ingham Publishing, 1987.

Kunz, Kevin, and Barbara Kunz. *Hand and Foot Reflexology: A Self-Help Guide*. St. Louis: Fireside Books, 1992.

Norman, Laura. *Feet First: A Guide to Foot Reflexology*. St. Louis: Fireside Books, 1988.

RELAXATION AND MEDITATION

ORGANIZATIONS

Association for Transpersonal Psychology
P.O. Box 3049
Stanford, CA 94305
Newsletters, professional journals, conferences, directories and other services.

Institute of Noetic Sciences
P.O. Box 909
Sausalito, CA 94966
Quarterly review and bulletin, resource guide for books and audiotapes, conferences.

Mind/Body Health Sciences, Inc.
393 Dixon Rd.
Boulder, CO 80302
Newsletter/catalog of books and audiotapes on meditation.

BOOKS

Borysenko, Joan. *Minding the Body, Mending the Mind*. New York: Simon & Schuster, 1988.

Davis, Martha, Elizabeth Robbins Eshelman and Matthew McKay. *The Relaxation and Stress Reduction Workbook*, 4th ed. Oakland, Calif: New Harbinger Publications, 1995.

Eliot, Robert S. *From Stress to Strength: How to Lighten Your Load and Save Your Life*. New York: Bantam Books, 1994.

Fiore, Neil A. *The Road Back to Health: Coping with the Emotional Side of Cancer*. Berkeley, Calif.: Celestial Arts, 1991.

LeShan, Lawrence. *Meditating to Attain a Healthy Body Weight*. New York: Doubleday and Company, 1994.

Shaffer, Martin. *Life after Stress*. New York: Plenum Press, 1982.

SOUND THERAPY

ORGANIZATIONS

American Assocation for Music Therapy, Inc.
P.O. Box 80012
Valley Forge, PA 19484
Write for general information on music therapy and membership, a listing of publications and subscriptions to newsletters.

National Association for Music Therapy
8455 Colesville Rd., Suite 930
Silver Spring, MD 20910
Offers referrals to qualified music therapists and general information on music therapy.

Sound Listening and Learning Center

2701 East Camelback, Suite 205
Phoenix, AZ 85016
Provides individual and group programs for children and adults as well as workshops focusing on the power of sound and personal growth. Free brochure and catalog available.

SOURCES FOR AUDIOTAPES

Inner Peace Music

c/o Steven Halpern, Ph.D.
P.O. Box 2644
San Anselmo, CA 94979
1-800-909-0707
Music for relaxation, health and well-being.

Institute for Music, Health and Education

Don G. Campbell, Founder
P.O. Box 4179
Boulder, CO 80306
1-800-490-4968
General information, correspondence courses in music and sound healing and a catalog of books and audiotapes.

Rhythmic Medicine

c/o Janalea Hoffman, R.M.T.
P.O. Box 6431
Shawnee Mission, KS 66206
1-800-487-8120
Cassettes, CDs and a book on therapeutic music.

BOOKS

Bassano, Mary. *Healing with Music and Color: A Beginner's Guide.* York Beach, Maine: Samuel Weiser, 1992.

Campbell, Don G. *Music: Physician for Times to Come.* Wheaton, Ill.: Quest, 1991.

Campbell, Don G. *Music and Miracles.* Wheaton, Ill.: Quest, 1992.

Campbell, Don G. *The Roar of Silence: Healing Powers of Breath, Tone and Music.* Wheaton, Ill.: Quest, 1989.

Halpern, Steven. *Sound Health: The Music and Sounds That Make Us Whole.* (out of print; check your library)

Scarantino, Barbara Anne. *Music Power: Creative Living through the Joys of Music.* (out of print; check your library)

VITAMIN AND MINERAL THERAPY

ORGANIZATIONS

American College for Advancement in Medicine

P.O. Box 3427
Laguna Hills, CA 92654
Offers listing of all association physicians nationwide, books and other literature.

SOURCES OF VITAMIN AND MINERAL SUPPLEMENTS

Capitol Drugs, Inc.

4454 Van Nuys Blvd.
Sherman Oaks, CA 91403
1-800-858-8833
Nutritional supplements, homeopathic remedies, herbs, kits, educational services, Bach flower remedies.

RESOURCES

Capitol Drugs, Inc.
8578 Santa Monica Blvd.
West Hollywood, CA 90069
1-800-858-8833
Supplements, homeopathic remedies, herbs, books.

Powell Pharmacy, Inc.
11085 Little Patuxent Pkwy.
Columbia, MD 21044
Vitamins, homeopathic remedies.

BOOKS

Gerson, Richard F. *The Right Vitamins.* (out of print; check your library)

YOGA

ORGANIZATIONS

American Yoga Association
513 S. Orange Ave.
Sarasota, FL 34236
1-800-226-5859
Call for guidelines on how to find a qualifed yoga instructor, general information about yoga and a listing of books, audiotapes and videotapes.

Himalayan International Institute of Yoga Science and Philosophy
R.R. 1, Box 400
Honesdale, PA 18431
1-800-822-4547
Call for a guide to programs and a catalog of products and publications.

International Association of Yoga Therapists
109 Hillside Ave.
Mill Valley, CA 94941
Send a self-addressed, stamped envelope for referrals to teachers in your area.

Rocky Mountain Institute of Yoga and Ayurveda
P.O. Box 1091
Boulder, CO 80306
Write for information about courses and seminars and for appointments at the institute with yoga therapists.

BOOKS

Christiansen, Alice. *The American Yoga Association Beginner's Manual.* St. Louis: Fireside Books, 1987.

Monro, Robin, R. Nagarantha and H. R. Nagendra. *Yoga for Common Ailments.* St. Louis: Fireside Books, 1990.

Samskrti and Veda. *Hatha Yoga Manual I,* 2nd ed. Honesdale, Pa.: Himalayan Publishers, 1985.

Schatz, Mary Pullig. *Back Care Basics: A Doctor's Gentle Yoga Program for Back and Neck Pain Relief.* Berkeley, Calif.: Rodmell Press, 1992.

Widdowson, Rosalind. *The Joy of Yoga.* (out of print; check your library)

NEWSLETTERS

Yoga for Today
Rudra Press
Box 13390
Portland, OR 97213-0390
1-800-876-7798
Send a legal-size self-addressed, stamped envelope for a free copy.

VIDEOTAPES

Collage Video Specialties, Inc.
5390 Main St., Dept. 1
Minneapolis, MN 55421
1-800-433-6769

COMMON DEGREES IN ALTERNATIVE MEDICINE

You're familiar with an M.D.—but what about an M.Ac. or a D.Hom.? These are just two of the many degrees that are granted by a wide variety of the boards, schools and associations of alternative medicine. The list below gives you many of the alternative degrees that are currently available and should help you tell whether an alternative practitioner is well-trained or not.

A.P. (Acupuncture Physician)
Signifies state certification in Florida. The state now grants the title certified acupuncturist.

B.A.M.S. (Bachelor of Ayurvedic Medicine and Surgery)
Indian college degree equivalent to an M.D. but in Ayurvedic medicine; requires four years of graduate studies. There are no state-recognized certification exams or titles in the United States. Most Ayurvedic practitioners have either an N.D. or an M.D. degree and practice under that title.

C.A. (Certified Acupuncturist)
Signifies board certification in acupuncture and licensure to practice granted by the state medical board.

C.A.M.T. (Certified Acupressure Massage Therapist)
Qualifications depend on the school from which the degree is received. No state or federal regulation.

C.A.T. (Certified Acupressure Therapist)
One thousand hours of training are required to become an acupressure therapist. An additional 150 hours of training at a fully approved school are needed for certification.

C.M.T. (Certified Music Therapist)
The American Association for Music Therapy (AAMT) grants this designation to graduates of music therapy programs at AAMT-approved schools who complete clinical internships of 900 hours.

D.Ac. (Diplomate of Acupuncture)
Indicates that the acupuncturist has passed an exam given by the National Commission for the Certification of Acupuncturists.

COMMON DEGREES IN ALTERNATIVE MEDICINE

D.H.A.N.P. (Diplomate of Homeopathic Academy of Naturopathic Physicians)
N.D.'s who pass the certification exam given by the Homeopathic Academy of Naturopathic Physicians may use these initials to indicate that they are also homeopaths. A minimum of one year in practice is required before one may sit for the D.H.A.N.P. exam.

D.Hom. (Diplomate of Homeopathic Medicine)
This degree, along with an M.D., used to be granted by Hahnemann Medical College (now Hahnemann University School of Medicine) in Philadelphia, the last medical school to offer training in homeopathy. It has not been granted since the late 1940s.

D.Ht. (Diplomate of Homeotherapeutics)
This designation is awarded to M.D.'s and D.O.'s after they pass an exam consisting of a presentation of ten cases treated with homeopathic medicine with three years of follow-up, a written exam, an oral exam and a casetaking supervised by a panel of doctors.

D.O.M. (Doctor of Oriental Medicine)
Synonymous with O.M.D. Both abbreviations are used.

L.Ac. (Licensed Acupuncturist)
Indicates a state license or a diploma from a European school. Synonymous with C.A.

L.M. (Licensed Midwife)
Indicates state licensing; requirements vary greatly between states.

L.M.T. (Licensed Massage Therapist)
The national certification exam is given by the National Certification Board of Therapeutic Massage and Body Work, which is accredited by the National Commission for Certifying Agencies. Most states require a minimum of 500 hours of in-class training.

M.Ac. (Master of Acupuncture)
Graduate of an M.Ac. education program. This usually requires two years of study plus a year of supervised practice.

M.A.Sc. (Master of Ayurvedic Science)
Indian college degree that requires three years of post-graduate studies, including an internship of two years. This is in addition to the four years of graduate work necessary to earn a B.A.M.S.

Ms.T., M.T. (Massage Therapist)
A generic term that doesn't necessarily entail certification or licensure.

Common Degrees in Alternative Medicine

N.D. (Doctor of Naturopathy)

N.D. licensure laws require a resident pre-med course of at least four years and 4,000 hours of study at a college recognized by the state examining board. N.D.'s are considered the general practitioners of the natural healing world.

O.M.D. (Oriental Medical Doctor)

This title generally indicates some additional training beyond state licensure to practice acupuncture. It also is sometimes taken by Chinese M.D.'s who are licensed medical doctors in China but not in the United States and by U.S. practitioners who complete O.M.D. degree programs at foreign schools. If you are considering treatment from someone who calls himself an O.M.D., note if he also uses the initials C.A., L.Ac., Lic.Ac. or R.Ac., all of which usually indicate state licensure or qualification.

R.Ac. (Registered Acupuncturist)

State registration; in Vermont, registration does not include a review of qualifications.

R.M.T. (Registered Music Therapist)

Requirements for this title, granted by the National Association for Music Therapy (NAMT), include a four-year degree in music therapy from an NAMT-approved school and a six-month, full-time supervised clinical internship (1,040 hours total). Use of this designation does not indicate state licensure.

CREDITS

"What's Your Dosha?" on page 33 is reprinted by permission of the Putnam Publishing Group from *A Woman's Best Medicine* by Melanie Brown, Ph.D., Veronica Butler, M.D., and Nancy Lonsdorf, M.D. Copyright © 1993 by Melanie Brown, Ph.D., Veronica Butler, M.D., and Nancy Lonsdorf, M.D.

The illustrations on pages 585, 586 and 587 are from the book *Hand and Foot Reflexology* by Kevin and Barbara Kunz. Copyright © 1984. Used by permission of the publisher, Prentice Hall/A Division of Simon & Schuster.

The illustrations on pages 596 and 597 are adapted from *Feet First: A Guide to Foot Reflexology.* Copyright © 1988 by Laura Norman. Illustrations copyright © 1988 by Laura Norman and Ivey Barry. Reprinted by permission of Simon & Schuster, Inc.

The captions to the illustrations for stretching relaxation on pages 602 and 603 are adapted from *Stretch Relaxation: A Training Manual* by Charles Carlson, Ph.D., and Frank Collins. Copyright © 1986 by Charles Carlson, Ph.D., and Frank Collins. Reprinted by permission.

The captions to the illustrations for leg up, leg out on page 626 and the piriformis stretch on page 627 are adapted from *Back Care Basics: A Doctor's Gentle Yoga Program for Back and Neck Pain Relief* by Mary Pullig Schatz, M.D. Copyright © 1992 Mary Pullig Schatz, M.D. Reprinted with permission of Rodmell Press, 2550 Shattuck Avenue, #18, Berkeley, CA 94704.

The imagery remedies for specified conditions are adapted from *Healing Visualizations* by Gerald Epstein. Copyright © 1989 by Gerald Epstein. Used by permission of Bantam Books, a division of Bantam Doubleday Dell Publishing Group, Inc.

INDEX

Note: Underscored page references indicate boxed text and tables.
Boldface references indicate illustrations.

A

Abdomen, pain in, 514–16
Abrasions, skin, 260–61
Acetylsalicylic acid, in aspirin, 56
Acidification of blood, as cause of hot flashes, 421
Acidophilus, as treatment for
cold sores, 247
hair loss, 334
Acidum hydrofluoricum, as treatment for sweating, 530
Acne, 23, 161–65
Aconite
first-aid uses of, 71
as treatment for
headache, 341
panic attacks, 454
Activated charcoal, as treatment for
diarrhea, 277
digestive problems, 77, 80
flatulence, 306
heartburn, 347
indigestion, 377
nausea and vomiting, 440
poisoning, food, 315
sore throat, 510
stomachache, 516
ulcers, 544
Acupressure. *See also* Acupressure points; Meridians (channels of energy)
acupuncture vs., 11
Chinese medicine and, 13
goal of, 11

healing effect of touch and, 18
history of, 11
professionals, selecting, 12
techniques, 11, 15–16
as treatment for
acne, 161
allergies, 166
ankle, swollen, 13
anxiety, 178
arthritis, 182–83
asthma, 188–89
backache, 195
breastfeeding problems, 207
chronic fatigue syndrome, 236
chronic illness, 16
colds, 240–41
constipation, 252
cough, 257
depression, 265
dermatitis and eczema, 270
dizziness, 280
emotional problems, 13–14
eyestrain, 293
foot pain, 317–18
hangover, 335
headache, 338–39
heartburn, 345–46
hiccups, 358–59
impotence, 369
insomnia, 386
joint pain, 402
leg cramps, 410

memory problems, 414
menstrual problems, 423
migraine headache, 426
motion sickness, 432
muscle cramps and pain, 435
nausea and vomiting, 438
neck pain, 441–42
pain, 11, 13
premenstrual syndrome, 471–72
repetitive strain injury, 486–87
sinus problems, 501
sprains, 512
stomachache, 514–15
stress, 11
temporomandibular joint disorder, 531–32
toothache, 535
water retention, 557
wrinkles, 559
types of, 12
workout, 17, 18
Acupressure points
back view, **565**
in Chinese medicine, 14–15
front view, **564**
on head, **567**
meridians and, 14–15
in pairs, 16
side view, **566**
Acupuncture, 11
Acu-yoga, 12
Additives, food, health problems from, 45, 310

649

INDEX

INDEX

INDEX

INDEX

INDEX